Surgical Pathology of Hepatobiliary Tumors

Wen-Ming Cong
Editor

Surgical Pathology of Hepatobiliary Tumors

PEOPLE'S MEDICAL PUBLISHING HOUSE

Springer

Editor
Wen-Ming Cong
Department of Pathology
Eastern Hepatobiliary Surgery Hospital
Second Military Medical University
Shanghai, China

The print edition is not for sale in China Mainland. Customers from China Mainland please order the print book from: People's Medical Publishing House.

ISBN 978-981-10-3535-7   ISBN 978-981-10-3536-4 (eBook)
DOI 10.1007/978-981-10-3536-4

Library of Congress Control Number: 2017932888

Printed on acid-free paper

This Springer imprint is published by Springer Nature
The registered company is Springer Nature Singapore Pte Ltd.
The registered company address is: 152 Beach Road, #21-01/04 Gateway East, Singapore 189721, Singapore

Foreword

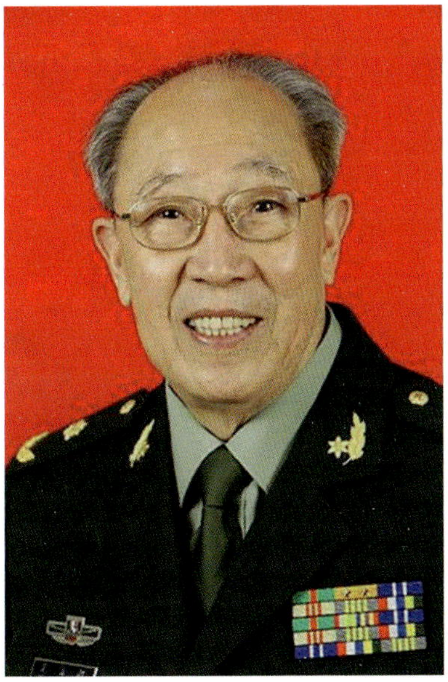

China has a high incidence of hepatobiliary tumors at present and even in the forthcoming decades. With rapid development in the field of hepatic surgery, pathology should play a more supportive role in the improvement of clinical diagnosis and treatments. In order to greatly improve the long-term therapeutic effects of hepatocellular carcinoma (HCC), researchers and clinicians are making huge efforts of developing standardized individual clinic mode to diagnose and treat hepatic tumors, which would lead to more emphasis on the research and understanding of the pathobiological features of HCC. Now there is an increasing realization that exploration of clinic mode to treat HCC in the perspective of biological characterization is an optimal way to greatly improve the efficacy of early diagnosis and treatment, and the instructive function of HCC diagnosis and treatment standards on individualized treatment is limiting without the involvement of the pathobiological characterization of HCC.

This book *Surgical Pathology of Hepatobiliary Tumors*, based on the former edition published 15 years ago, was reedited by a group of experts with Professor Wen-Ming Cong as the editor in chief, who is the director of the Department of Pathology of Eastern Hepatobiliary Surgery Hospital (EHBH). In this book our experience in the pathological diagnosis of hepatobiliary tumors of more than 40,000 cases over 30 years in EHBH is summed up, and a new histological classification of hepatobiliary tumors termed as "Three Types and Six Subtypes" is advanced. Aiming to reveal the recent developments of surgical pathology of hepatobiliary in the perspective of pathobiology of tumors, this book contains descriptions of more than 100 tumors of the liver and intrahepatic bile duct, with updated information in picture-illustrated composing style and broad clinical practicability and guidance. It is the most systemic and thorough reference book on pathological diagnosis of hepatobiliary tumors and will be greatly useful for clinicians, pathologists, and researchers of medical basis or other disciplines.

I wish to see close cooperation between liver cancer surgeons and the pathologists, innovative researches focusing on key clinical concerns and demands, and active exploration of new mode and methods of pathological diagnosis, further developing technology architecture of diagnostic pathology which is scientific, objective, and standardized, playing a more supportive basis role in improving clinical long-term curative effect of HCC. This book *Surgical Pathology of Hepatobiliary Tumors* is a beneficial exploration on the above facets and deserves my sincere congratulations on its publication. I should be very glad to recommend this book to my peers.

Academician of Chinese Academy of Sciences
President of Eastern Hepatobiliary Surgery Hospital
Second Military Medical University
200438, Shanghai, China

Meng-Chao Wu

Preface

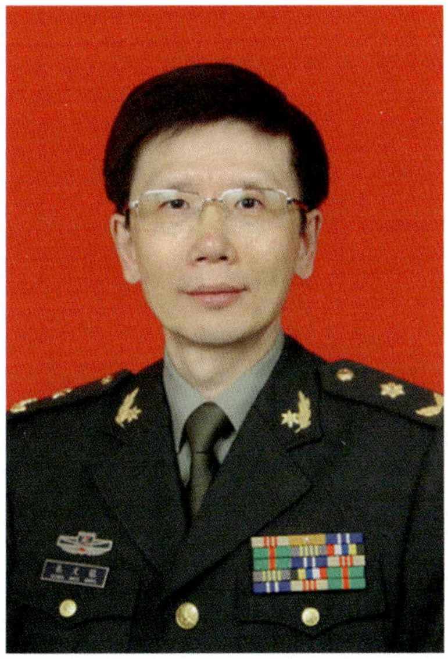

It has been 15 years since I drew the outline of the former edition of *Diagnostic Surgical Pathology of Hepatobiliary Tumors* when I was a visiting scholar of the Department of Pathology at the University of Pittsburgh Medical Center (UPMC) in 1999. As the first Chinese book on pathological diagnosis of hepatobiliary tumors, it has gained much attention and recognition and become one of the frequently used reference books due to its useful guide for improving the pathological diagnosis of hepatobiliary tumors. However, during the past 15 years, integration and mutual promotion of the molecular biology and molecular pathology of liver cancer have been witnessed, and new concepts such as heterogenicity, pathobiological features, molecular classification, and individualized treatment have emerged and been accepted as the basic guidance in modern clinical therapeutics of liver cancer. Furthermore, Chinese scholars have made innovative achievements in molecular pathology and histopathological diagnosis of liver cancer. With much experience in clinical pathological diagnosis and with new hepatic lesions, understanding, and concepts and methods put forward, we are ready to rewrite this book. Receiving much encouragement and support from my teacher, Professor Meng-Chao Wu, a world-famous Chinese hepatobiliary surgery scientist and surgeon, being considered as the "father of Chinese hepatobiliary surgery," we finished the recompiling of the book after one year's intense work and present it to everyone here.

The disciplines we stick to throughout our writing is emphasizing the integration of basic research, pathological diagnosis, and clinical practice, introducing recent developments and scientific achievements, focusing on the philosophy and mode of diagnosing liver cancer pathobiologically, and illustrating the theories, concepts, pathological features, and diagnostic techniques, in the aim of providing the readers with a reference book which helps improve the pathological theories and diagnosis of liver cancer. Therefore, we put emphasis on the new concepts and knowledge in surgical pathology of hepatobiliary tumors. Based on our new histological classification of hepatobiliary tumors termed as "Three Types and Six Subtypes," we described the histological classification of more than 100 entities of the liver and intrahepatic bile ducts in detail with a selection of over 600 pictures to illustrate the pathological features and biological behavior of these tumors. We have omitted the chapter "Pathological Diagnosis of Liver Transplantation," the contents of which were demonstrated in our published book *Clinical Pathology of Liver Transplantation* in 2011. To elucidate the pathological features of hepatic tumors in children systematically, we added the chapter "Hepatic Tumors in Children." It should be explained that tumors of the same type will be referred to in different parts of the book to maintain its integrity, because they can be seen in both adults and children. Besides, some tumors of the liver can also be seen in intrahepatic and extrahepatic bile ducts and gallbladder. A glossary of terms is included for the reader's convenience. In particular, Professor Thung SN, who was the director of the Department of Pathology of Mount Sinai School of Medicine in New York, USA, was invited to write the chapter "Biopsy and Pathologic Diagnosis of Hepatic Tumor." I hope this will be helpful for the improvement of the level of hepatic pathological diagnosis on small biopsy tissue samples.

I am particularly grateful to my supervisor, Professor Meng-Chao Wu, an Academician of the Chinese Academy of Sciences, for his precious advice on the compiling and his kindness to write the preface. Academician Meng-Chao Wu has been so kind and attentive to me and offering careful guidance on my learning, working, and research for the past several decades for which I've been grateful and respectful. Academician Meng-Chao Wu is a pioneer and chief founder of Chinese hepatic surgery and has devoted much attention to the development of our Department of Pathology. The establishment of the new Department of Pathology in the An-Ting new district of EHBH was brought into a new era under his support. Academician Meng-Chao Wu pointed out in the preface that "the instructive function of HCC diagnosis and treatment standards on individualized treatment is limiting without the involvement of the pathobiological characterization of HCC," which makes us be more aware of the heavy responsibilities and glorious mission of pathologists, as tissue samples are the most important and direct carrier of biological features of liver cancer.

I would particularly thank the world-renowned expert in liver cancer and Academician of the Chinese Academy of Engineering, Professor Zhao-You Tang, who was invited to make a brilliant exposition on the fundamental roles of pathobiological characteristics in improving the level of diagnosis and treatment of hepatocellular carcinoma. Academician Tang begins his article with "pathology is a prerequisite for a cancer surgeon to make decisions, I am grateful for the contributions made by pathologists," which allows us to deeply feel his profound understanding and ardent love of the subject of pathology. I am extremely honored that Academician Tang has been the Chairman of the dissertation committee for my both master's and doctor's degree theses, and I always have a deep respect for the care and guidance from him.

I would particularly thank the world-famous expert in liver cancer, Academician of the Chinese Academy of Engineering, Professor Hong-Yang Wang, who was invited to make a profound analysis and prediction on the development trend of the research on molecular biology of hepatocellular carcinoma. Academician Wang brilliantly pointed out that liver cancer molecular typing and individual treatment are the only way to overcome the liver cancer. Academician Wang led an Innovative Research Groups of the National Natural Science Foundation of China on liver cancer and significantly promotes the academic research level of hepatocellular carcinoma of China, and our pathology team also got a lot of concern and guidance from Academician Wang.

I would like to thank Professor Thung SN from the Department of Pathology of Mount Sinai School of Medicine in New York, USA, Professor Yuan Ji from the Department of Pathology of Shanghai Zhongshan Hospital, and Professor Xiang-Ru Wu from the Department of Pathology of Shanghai Xinhua Hospital, who are successful experts in hepatopathological study, and their preciseness and elaboration in writing represent the basic discipline of the book to explore the new diagnostic mode of pathobiological characteristics of liver cancer.

And I would also like to thank Hui Dong, Xin-Yuan Lu, You-Wen Qian, Qian Zhao, Yu-Yao Zhu, Long-Hai Feng, Sheng Xia, Guang-Zhi Jin, Zhi-hong Xian, and Hua Yu et al. who are all my colleagues for their hard work in data collection and sorting and technical support for the compiling of the book. Their meticulous statistical work on the archival data from the Department of Pathology over 30 years provides the readers with representative data of the Chinese population. Among them, Hui Dong, PhD; You-Wen Qian, PhD; and Yu-Yao Zhu, MS undertook the serious work on formatting the final manuscript, picture editing, and text proofreading.

In the light of pathological diversity of hepatobiliary tumors, there is controversy about some concepts and understanding, and studies on liver cancer cover a wide research area with rapid developments of clinical diagnosis and treatment, which altogether bring a great challenge to the writing of the book. Despite our efforts to perfect the book, there may still be some omissions and inadequacies. We would appreciate it very much if readers will kindly point out our errors for future revision of this book.

Department of Pathology
Eastern Hepatobiliary Surgery Hospital
Second Military Medical University
200438, Shanghai, China

Wen-Ming Cong

Contents

Editors and Contributors

Academic Consultant

Meng-Chao Wu Academician of Chinese Academy of Sciences, Eastern Hepatobiliary Surgery Hospital, Second Military Medical University, Shanghai, China

Editor

Wen-Ming Cong Department of Pathology, Eastern Hepatobiliary Surgery Hospital, Second Military Medical University, Shanghai, China

Special Guest Authors

Zhao-You Tang Academician of Chinese Academy of Sciences, Liver Cancer Institute, Zhongshan Hospital, Fudan University, Shanghai, China

Swan N. Thung Professor & Director of Division of Hepatopathology, Department of Pathology, The Mount Sinai Medical Center, New York, USA

Hong-Yang Wang Academician of Chinese Academy of Sciences, International Cooperation Laboratory on Signal Transduction, Eastern Hepatobiliary Surgery Hospital, Second Military Medical University, Shanghai, China

Contributors

Hui Dong Department of Pathology, Eastern Hepatobiliary Surgery Hospital, Second Military Medical University, Shanghai, China

Long-Hai Feng Department of Pathology, Eastern Hepatobiliary Surgery Hospital, Second Military Medical University, Shanghai, China

Yuan Ji Zhong-shan Hospital, Fudan University, Shanghai, China

Guang-Zhi Jin Department of Pathology, Eastern Hepatobiliary Surgery Hospital, Second Military Medical University, Shanghai, China

Xin-Yuan Lu Department of Pathology, Eastern Hepatobiliary Surgery Hospital, Second Military Medical University, Shanghai, China

You-Wen Qian Department of Pathology, Eastern Hepatobiliary Surgery Hospital, Second Military Medical University, Shanghai, China

Xia Sheng Department of Pathology, Eastern Hepatobiliary Surgery Hospital, Second Military Medical University, Shanghai, China

Stephen C. Ward Department of Hepatic Pathology, Mount Sinai School of Medicine, New York, USA

Xiang-Ru Wu Xin Hua Hospital, Shanghai Jiao Tong University School of Medicine, Shanghai, China

Qian Zhao Department of Pathology, Eastern Hepatobiliary Surgery Hospital, Second Military Medical University, Shanghai, China

Yu-Yao Zhu Department of Pathology, Eastern Hepatobiliary Surgery Hospital, Second Military Medical University, Shanghai, China

Zhen Zhu Department of Pathology, Eastern Hepatobiliary Surgery Hospital, Second Military Medical University, Shanghai, China

Academic Secretary

Hui Dong Department of Pathology, Eastern Hepatobiliary Surgery Hospital, Second Military Medical University, Shanghai, China

1 My View on the Biological Features and Surgical Treatment of Liver Cancer

Zhao-You Tang

Pathology is the prerequisite for oncology surgeons to make decisions. I can only feel grateful for the contribution made by my fellow pathologists. Having the honor to write a passage for the introduction to this monograph, I am even more overwhelmed. After all, I'm only a clinician, not a basic research fellow. Fortunately there are the two words "my view" in my title. Therefore this passage will just be my personal opinions from the clinical perspective for the reference of those engaged in the same pursuit.

In 2012 the article "Two Hundred Years of Cancer Research" [1] by DeVita and Rosenberg was published on *The New England Journal of Medicine*, in which the "cellular origin of cancer" put forward by Virchow in 1863 has laid the "pathological foundation" for modern oncology and become the gold standard for cancer diagnosis and the basis for treatment decisions, and Watson et al. discovered the double helix structure of DNA in 1953, EGF and its EDFR in 1979, p53 anti-oncogene in 1981, etc., all these initiating the research of molecular biology and suggesting that the context of cancer research has been gradually transformed from "pathology" to "pathology-biology." The establishment of the "pathological foundation" of cancer has focused the attention of the great cancer-fighting army on one thing, i.e., employing all available means to eliminate pathologically confirmed tumors, which leads to the development of tumor-eliminating treatments such as surgery, radiotherapy, chemotherapy, interventional therapy (e.g., TACE), and local treatment, hence the substantial progress of curative effect in cancer treatment.

As an oncology surgeon, I've realized the distinct differences of liver cancer from the pathological and biological perspectives. For example, in terms of diagnosis, the former focuses on appearance and answers questions of whether it is cancer or what cancer it is, while the latter focuses on biological features, i.e., how is its degree of malignancy. In terms of treatment, the former is about eliminating tumor, while the latter is aimed at decreasing the potentiality of cancer invasion and metastasis and improving the body's cancer-fighting ability. In terms of means of application, the former has surgery, radiotherapy, chemotherapy, local treatment, interventional therapy, the latest VEGF-targeted molecular targeted curative agent, etc., while the latter emphasizes biological treatment like differentiation inducing therapy and immunotherapy. In terms of prognostic indicator, the former values biological features of morphologic correlation like degree of differentiation, while the latter values biological features of molecular correlation like prognostic molecular predictor. In terms of efficacy evaluation, the former values the effective rate for tumor (complete remission, partial remission, etc.), while the latter values overall survival rate and quality of life.

Now that there is still a long way to go before cancer is conquered, this transformation of context gives us new ideas from the clinical perspective. It is expected that in the future trend of cancer treatment, tumor elimination will still be the most important goal of treatment. Nevertheless, besides the elimination of primary tumor, another important goal will be the modification of residual tumor to decrease its degree of malignancy and the modification of body to increase its cancer-fighting ability. In this way, "transforming the bad" or "surviving with tumor" becomes another "end point" of treatment.

1.1 Surgical Treatment in the Pathological Context

Surgical treatment plays a decisive role in improving the curative effect of liver cancer in the twentieth century. In the 1950s, the regular hepatectomy of liver cancer for the first time improved the curative effect for liver cancer substantially. Started in the 1960s and confirmed in the 1990s, the

Z.-Y. Tang (✉)
Academician of Chinese Academy of Sciences, Liver Cancer Institute, Zhongshan Hospital, Fudan University, Shanghai, China
e-mail: zytang88@163.com

W.-M. Cong (ed.), *Surgical Pathology of Hepatobiliary Tumors*, DOI 10.1007/978-981-10-3536-4_1

liver cancer treatment method liver transplantation made part of unresectable relatively small liver cancer treatable, thus extending the benefits to more liver cancer patients. In the 1970s, alpha fetoprotein was used for screening, and the curative effect of resection was doubled through early detection, early diagnosis, and early treatment, especially the local resection of small liver cancer (≤5 cm). In the 1980s, thanks to combined therapy such as surgical hepatic artery ligation, intubation infusion chemotherapy, and radiotherapy, resection after downstaging (reduction) made radical cure possible for a small number of patients with unresectable liver cancer. The rise of local treatment like TACE and radiofrequency ablation has obviously extended the benefits to more patients, among which some were cured after resection of reduced tumor. All of these efforts are aimed at "tumor elimination." During the past half century, the survival rate of inpatients at the Liver Cancer Research Institute of Zhongshan Hospital, Fudan University (hereinafter referred to as this Institute) has indeed experienced improvement every 10 years, which is attributable to surgical treatment, especially the resection of small liver cancer.

In the "pathological context," efforts during the past half century are mainly aimed toward "eliminating tumors as many as possible," which include:

1. Surgery-related: researches on improving resection rate, decreasing operative mortality rate, resection of tumor along its edges, operation method in strict accordance with intrahepatic anatomy, reducing tumor spread during operation, etc.
2. Liver transplantation to treat liver cancer, which is also mainly for the purpose of eliminating tumor even more completely
3. Preoperative and postoperative treatment-related: researches on how to further eliminate residual cancer, such as postoperative radiotherapy, chemotherapy, application of TACE, and application of molecular targeted curative agent sorafenib

However, even though all these efforts have improved curative effect to a certain extent, none of them can solve the problem completely, the greatest bottleneck being postoperative cancer metastasis and recurrence.

Apparently, the metastasis of cancer originates from the cancer cells left behind. And there are two possibilities for the recurrence of cancer: metastatic tumor and another primary tumor, the latter of which falls into the category of cancer prevention. Therefore, the main barrier to improving the curative effect of surgical treatment for liver cancer is cancer metastasis. The most obvious evidence is that in about 40 years, despite the growth of cases of small liver cancer resection at this Institute by hundreds of times, the five-year survival rate is still wandering below 60%.

1.2 Biological Hallmarks of Cancer

The "biological hallmarks of cancer" is a very comprehensive issue, and it would be quite difficult to summarize in one passage. In 2011 the article "Hallmarks of Cancer: The Next Generation" by Hanahan was published in *Cell*, which may provide a brief summary of the biological hallmarks of cancer [2]. Including a few upcoming hallmarks, ten hallmarks are listed: (1) sustaining proliferative signaling, (2) evading growth suppressors, (3) resisting cell death, (4) enabling replicative immortality, (5) inducing angiogenesis, (6) activating invasion and metastasis, (7) reprogramming of energy metabolism, (8) avoiding immune destruction, (9) tumor promoting inflammation, and (10) genome instability and mutation. Among which, based on my understanding, the former six hallmarks are related to cancer cells, while the latter four involve the whole body, e.g., metabolic regulation, immune function, inflammation-triggered cancer, genetic mutation, and instability. Therefore, cancer originates from cells. However, instead of simple cytopathic effect, this process involves the whole body which is under the influence of external environment and hereditation.

From the clinical perspective, I believe "activating invasion and metastasis" is of the uttermost importance among the abovementioned ten hallmarks of cancer. This is the major biological feature that makes cancer different from benign tumor. Without the potentiality for invasion and metastasis, cancer will become benign tumor, while most of the other hallmarks serve the feature of "invasion and metastasis."

Since the understanding of the biological hallmarks of cancer invasion and metastasis has been updated significantly in recent years, proper adjustment should be made in the surgical treatment of liver cancer. (1) It was once believed that the enhancement of the potentiality for cancer metastasis is the result of clone screening during cancer progression. Now it is believed that cancer metastasis is a systemic issue; apart from targeting at metastasis, cancer treatment should also attach importance to systemic intervention, which may change the potentiality for cancer metastasis. As mentioned above, four out of the ten cancer hallmarks of the next generation are related to systemic regulation. It is also pointed out in literature that general conditions and intrahepatic tumor control are risk factors of extrahepatic metastasis [3], which also signifies that the prevention of cancer metastasis requires systemic intervention. (2) It was understood that cancer metastasis is a phenomenon of advanced-stage cancer.

Now it is understood that cancer metastasis doesn't manifest advanced stage of cancer, and prevention should start early. In our cooperation with the Americans, the comparison of small and big liver cancer reveals only seven genetic differences, while 153 genetic differences are discovered in the comparison of liver cancer with and without metastasis, suggesting that the genetic change of cancer metastasis occurs during the stage of primary tumor, and even small liver cancer can have strong metastatic potential [4]. This also explains why sometimes the recurrence and metastasis of small liver cancer happens very fast after resection and suggests the importance of early intervention. (3) It was once believed that metastasis is possible for all cancer cells. Now it's believed that it's just the cancer stem cells. For example, the EpCAM-positive liver cancer cells are stem-like cells; therefore, cancer stem cells are an important target of the anti-metastasis research [5]. I discovered that treatment with oxaliplatin in nude mouse model for human liver cancer can upregulate stem cell markers (e.g., EpCAM and CD90), while the "Song You Yin" containing five kinds of traditional Chinese medicine can downregulate those markers, reduce metastasis, and prolong survival time [6]. (4) It was once believed that cancer metastasis is in the nature of cancer cells, while now it is believed that immune inflammatory microenvironment is a key factor for cancer metastasis. During our collaboration with the Americans, it was discovered that 17 genes related to immunity and inflammation (not related to cancer metastasis) in the microenvironment around cancer can predict metastasis [7]. In 1889, Paget put forward the "seed and soil" theory of cancer metastasis, emphasizing that seed needs the right soil for growth. However, the discovery in the twenty-first century suggests that the performance of seed can also be influenced by different soils. Existing literature shows that the interaction between cancer stem cells and the microenvironment results in metastasis [8]. This Institute also finds that "Song You Yin" can improve microenvironment and inhibit cancer metastasis through downregulating the cytokines secreted by activated hepatic stellate cells [9]. Thus, a new field of intervention was discovered in anti-metastasis research. (5) It was usually believed that cancer cells could only become more malignant. Now it has been noticed that the potentiality for cancer metastasis can be bidirectional, i.e., it can either become worse or better. Therefore, "transforming the bad" is an important direction of research. It has always been believed that the metastasis potential of cancer gets increasingly enhanced during its development through clone screening, and the latest research also suggests that various cancer-killing therapies promote metastasis of residual cancer. However, differentiation inducing therapy and some Chinese medicine treatment can reduce the potential for metastasis.

All of these new ideas suggest the anti-metastasis research should not only be targeted at cancer cells, especially cancer stem cells, but also microenvironment, which is under the regulation of the whole body. Therefore, besides tumor elimination therapy, researchers should also focus on differentiation inducer, anti-inflammatory agent, immunotherapeutic agent, matrix metalloproteinase, fat metabolism, and other measures of systemic intervention. For instance, for cancer stem cells, the guiding principle of elimination and modification at the same time from the biological property point of view is more comprehensive than simple elimination advocated in the past. Above is the common problem of cancer metastasis. Despite the "individuality" of the biological hallmarks of liver cancer, their "commonness" is the most important. Therefore, the above analysis and statement is also suitable for liver cancer.

1.3 Outlook for Surgical Treatment in the Context of Pathology-Biology

For the past century, we have made every attempt to eliminate liver cancer once it's been confirmed by pathology. Since the 1990s, the development of molecular biology and systems biology has made us realize that similar to other cancers, liver cancer is not only local lesion but also systemic lesion. In addition to tumor elimination, goals of the clinical treatment of liver cancer should also include modification of tumor and body in the hope of transforming the bad residual cancer or reducing its invasion and metastasis potential and increasing the body's cancer-fighting ability so as to achieve "surviving with cancer." Since it's been proven that even the most radical surgical resection cannot ensure, there are no circulating tumor cells (CTC) left behind. Furthermore, as to the various existing therapies, we should not only recognize their efficacy and side reaction but also notice the "opposite effect" [10] and take countermeasures. This is a shortcut to improving the efficacy of tumor elimination therapy. I believe the conceptual change will broaden the perspective of liver cancer surgery research significantly.

It is expected that in the twenty-first century to improve the efficacy of liver cancer surgery, the goal will be changed from simple elimination of tumor to modification of tumor and body on the basis of elimination of as many tumors as possible. There are multiple ways to improve the efficacy of liver cancer surgery, some of which can promote efficacy significantly, such as early diagnosis and treatment, while others are less impressive, such as researches on distal and proximal resection in liver cancer surgery, surgical indications and complications, etc. Some can improve efficacy substantially, like the research on new therapy; and some improve efficacy in treating certain subgroups of liver cancer, such as the research on indications for some therapy. Later I'll talk about methods that may greatly improve the efficacy of liver cancer surgery. The following divisions are only for the purpose of emphasizing analysis from different perspectives. As a matter of fact, they are interrelated and inseparable.

1.3.1 Early Diagnosis and Treatment Is Still Important but Limited

It's been over 40 years since the research on small liver cancer started since the 1970s, but the UICC still puts forward the slogan that "early discovery can save life." This is because the 10-year survival rate of patients who have received small liver cancer resection is twice as high as that of patients of large liver cancer resection, and there is a negative correlation between the size of liver cancer and the post-resection survival rate. As mentioned earlier, the improvement of prognosis of liver cancer inpatients at this Institute is also attributable to the increase of the percentage of small liver cancer resection. The prognosis of liver cancer is improving in the USA, which can also be attributed to early diagnosis and treatment [11], and the same is true for the increase of liver cancer survival rate in Italy in the past 20 years [12]. The rise of local treatment (such as radiofrequency ablation, which is in fact an extension of surgical resection) and liver transplant in recent years has extended the benefits to more patients of small liver cancer.

Even though there is still more to be researched about early diagnosis and treatment (e.g., genome and proteome technologies can help in the early diagnosis of over half AFP negative liver cancer), the efficacy of various early treatment methods is reaching the limit: as has been noted, the 5-year survival rate of small liver cancer resection hasn't improved in 40 years; and according to the statistics of 1305 cases, the 5-year survival rate after radiofrequency ablation is merely 59.7%, even for small liver cancer of only 2.2 cm in diameter [13]. This suggests that the bottleneck is still liver metastasis and recurrence after treatment.

Therefore, research on the prevention of metastasis and recurrence of small liver cancer after early diagnosis and treatment will be the key to further improvement of the efficacy of early diagnosis and treatment, which first of all requires predictors of metastasis of small liver cancer after treatment. Even though this Institute has done some research on this [14], more exploration is still needed for it to enter clinical routine.

The past decades have proved that continuing to adopt the method of elimination after surgical resection can keep improving efficacy, but it can't solve the problem completely. Therefore, we must search for a way out from wider perspectives. I believe the way out is to consider this problem from the perspective of pathology-biology instead of just pathology, i.e., change the strategy of simple elimination to both elimination and modification. For metastasis and recurrence of existing cancer focus, it has already been proven that treatments like resection, radiofrequency ablation, and TACE can improve efficacy. However, for a few residual cancers escaping treatment, the strategy of continued elimination has little effect. There is a lot more to be explored from the biological perspective, such as systemic intervention of nerve, immunity, endocrine secretion, metabolism, anti-inflammation, etc. For instance, this Institute found during experimental research that the combined use of interferon-a and "Song You Yin" after palliative resection of liver cancer can inhibit the enhancement of the metastasis potential of residual cancer induced by palliative resection, thus prolonging survival time [15].

1.3.2 The Combined Treatment Model Will Be Changed

Cancer is a complex disease triggered by multiple factors, involved by various genes, and formed in different stages. It is both a local lesion and a systemic lesion. Therefore, combined treatment is the long-term strategic direction. The functions of combined treatment in surgical treatment are: first, making those with no indications of surgical resection resectable, and second, further improving the efficacy of surgical treatment. The invasion and metastasis potential of cancer is changeable (either for worse or for better); if it can be changed for the better, then surviving with tumor will become a goal. In general, combined surgical treatment can be divided into two categories:

First is the "tumor elimination + tumor elimination" model: the combined and sequential application of surgical treatment and other tumor elimination methods (radiofrequency ablation, intervention, radiotherapy, and chemotherapy) is a strategy based on the pathological context. Atypical example of combined treatment of such model is "resection after downstaging (regression)," which results in failure to improve prognosis of liver cancer resection. I have been engaged in such researches since the late twentieth century [16]. Now the latest literature still has reports such as that gemcitabine + oxaliplatin makes some advanced liver cancer patients treatable [17]. There is still a lot of room for the development of this combined treatment model, e.g., experimental research discovers that the molecular targeted curative agent sorafenib can reduce metastasis and recurrence after liver cancer surgery [18].

Second is the "tumor elimination + tumor/body modification" model: the combined and sequential application of tumor elimination therapy (including surgical treatment) and methods to modify tumor and body reflects the measures taken in the context of pathology-biology. (1) In the case of surgical treatment + biotherapeutic agent, since as early as 2000, this Institute has already discovered that interferon-a can reduce recurrence by inhibiting angiogenesis in experimental research [19] and confirmed its clinical value in clinical randomized controlled trial [20]. (2) In surgical treatment + anti-inflammatory treatment, surgical treatment may cause inflammation and hypoxia, which reinforce each other [21]; like this, some anti-inflammatory agents have already become potential auxiliary anticancer agent [22]. It has already been reported that taking aspirin can lower liver cancer incidence rate among patients of chronic liver diseases [23]. (3) In surgical treatment + antiviral (HBV/HCV) treatment, as reported in literatures, long-acting interferon + ribavirin can reduce postoperative recurrence of C hepatitis-related liver cancer [24]. (4) In surgical treatment +differentiation inducing therapy, arsenic trioxide treatment is effective for a certain type of leukemia, and the working mechanism is to make leukemic cells better differentiated [25]. This Institute also discovered that arsenic trioxide can induce the differentiation of $CD133^+$liver cancer cells, reducing the recurrence of liver cancer after resection in tumor-bearing mice and prolonging survival time. (5) In surgical treatment + traditional Chinese medicine, experimental research by our Institute found out that tanshinone IIA, the extract from salvia miltiorrhiza, can inhibit metastasis after palliative resection of liver cancer and prolong the survival time of tumor-bearing mice. One of its mechanisms of action is normalization of tumor blood vessel endothelium, improving tumor hypoxia through the regulation of HIF-1α, inhibiting the EMT of liver cancer cells, and inhibiting the metastasis of liver cancer [26]. (6) And in surgical treatment + other non-elimination tumor treatments, in the early years, hepatic artery ligation wasn't one of the surgical treatment methods that can resect liver cancer, similar to the principle of TACE in recent years. Our experimental research finds out that even though simple artery ligation inhibits tumor, it promotes the spread of cancer and does not prolong animals' survival time. In comparison, combining the use of P13K inhibitor LY294002 can inhibit the EMT caused by hypoxia, thus improving efficacy [27]. This Institute has further confirmed that the mechanism of promoting metastasis of residual cancer by hypoxia is the activation of β-catenin [28]. As to the combination of surgical treatment and systemic intervention, it will be talked about later.

1.3.3 The Residual Cancer Metastasis-Promoting Effect of Tumor Elimination Therapy Will Be Brought to Attention

As the major means of cancer treatment, tumor elimination therapy, including surgical treatment, has been applied for over a century and definite efficacy has been achieved, but the total prognosis of the entire group of liver cancer patients is still not satisfactory. In the past more emphasis was laid on the side effects of tumor elimination therapy and less on its "counteraction," which is mainly promoting the metastasis of residual cancer. Reports on this have been on the increase, and researches have been carried out in this Institute for many years. The research on the mechanism of this "counteraction" and its intervention will help to further improve the efficacy of tumor elimination therapy.

In recent years, this Institute has established nude mice and cell model of human liver cancer with high metastasis potential [29, 30], and experimental research based on the application of this model suggests palliative resection, radiotherapy, chemotherapy, hepatic artery ligation, and the latest molecular targeted therapy featuring anti-VEGF can all promote the residual cancer's metastasis potential. Its mechanism is to induce EMT through hypoxia, inflammation, immune suppression, etc., accompanied by a series of genetic changes. According to my discovery, palliative resection can promote the metastasis of residual cancer, partly through upregulating VEGF andMMP2/TIMP2 [15]; radiotherapy promotes late metastasis of residual cancer mainly through the EMT induced by TMPRSS4 [31]; the metastasis-promoting effect of hepatic artery ligation and hypoxia mainly induces intratumoral hypoxia and EMT [27], while the activation of β-catenin by hypoxia is an important mechanism of the metastasis-promoting effect [28]; and oxaliplatin chemotherapy induces EMT, accompanied by downregulating E-cadherin and promoting pulmonary metastasis [32]. The residual cancer metastasis-promoting effect of sorafenib this Institute discovered is related to downregulating HTATIP2 through JAK-STAT3 signaling pathways [33], inhibiting natural killer cells [34], and inhibiting the interleukin-12b from host [35]. In recent years, an increasing number of literatures have reported about the cancer-promoting effect of tumor elimination therapy, e.g., radiotherapy causes the death of cancer cells, and strong growth stimulating signals are generated through the apoptosis mechanism to promote the proliferation of residual cancer [36]; anti-angiogenesis therapy improves the invasion of residual cancer [37]. Therefore when other tumor elimination methods are applied in combined surgical treatment, intervention to the metastasis-promoting effect of tumor elimination therapy should be considered as a whole.

This Institute has found quite a few clinically used irrelevant drugs with certain effects of intervening in the "counteraction" of tumor elimination therapy: (1) Cytokine, such as interferon-a, can prolong the survival time after palliative resection [15]. (2) Anti-inflammatory agent like zoledronic acid can improve the efficacy of sorafenib through eliminating tumor-related macrophage (anti-inflammation) [38]. (3) Traditional Chinese medicine also has certain effect in intervening with the "counteraction." This Institute found the small complex prescription "Song You Yin" of five kinds of traditional Chinese medicine can prolong nude mice's survival time through inducing apoptosis and downregulating MMP2 and VEGF [39]; this Institute also found that after oxaliplatin (chemotherapy) treatment, the metastasis potential of residual cancer is enhanced, and this enhancement can be inhibited by Song You Yin [32]; another discovery is that Song You Yin can reinforce the effect of interferon and inhibit the enhancement of metastasis potential after palliative resection [15]. What's noticeable is that tanshinone IIA, one ingredient of Song You Yin, can prolong the survival time after palliative resection through vascular normalization [26]. (4) This Institute also discovered that tyroserleutide, a tripeptide, could inhibit the metastasis-promoting effect of radiotherapy [40]. All of these provide potential clinical methods for further improvement of the efficacy of tumor elimination therapy.

1.3.4 Cancer Metastasis and Recurrence Will Focus on Systemic Intervention

The ultimate bottleneck of all surgical treatments, including liver transplant for liver cancer, is still the recurrence and metastasis of cancer. The invasion and metastasis potential of cancer result from the interaction of external environment (including treatment measures), body, microenvironment, and cancer cells. For this reason, in the intervention with metastasis, we should attach importance to the weak links, including microenvironment and systemic intervention, and the microenvironment is usually under systemic regulation. Of cause, we should also give full play to existing therapies in the prevention and treatment of liver cancer metastasis. As a matter of fact, previously tumor elimination therapy has been adopted continuously, such as re-resection of recurrence and metastasis, local treatment, TACE, radiotherapy, chemotherapy, and VEGF-targeted molecular targeted treatment. Even though it also improved efficacy, the problem has never been solved completely. In this section, we will focus on the discussion of systemic intervention, which is based on the biological hallmarks of cancer.

Modern oncology is based on pathology; once confirmed with cancer through microscopy, people would try to eliminate it by every possible means. With the development of molecular biology, our horizon is elevated from cellular level to molecular level, which on one hand makes tumor elimination therapy more precise and on the other hand consequently ignores systemic action. The scientific development in recent years gradually brings our attention to the importance of systemic intervention for cancer.

1. Nervous system: as reported in literature, the invasion and metastasis of tumor cells is led by neurotransmitters, and tumor cells express multiple neurotransmitters, thus supporting the theory that psychosocial factors are related to tumor progression [41]; some believe the function of nervous system in the onset of cancer is transmitting the information of cancer cells to the brain through body fluids and nerve pathways so that the brain can regulate the growth of tumor through the neuroendocrine-immune system [42]. Therefore, intervention through the nervous system is worth considering.
2. Immune system: it has been found out that immunity not only protects the host but also promotes tumor growth [43], thus cooling the immunization therapy. Another problem of immunization therapy is that the tumor antigenicity is too weak to induce enough immune reaction. In recent years, it has been discovered that the relevant antigen-4 (CTLA-4) and antibody of anti-cytotoxic T lymphocyte can reinforce the antitumor effect significantly. This immunization therapy targets at the immunocyte to improve its anticancer immune reaction and avoids the problem of tumor antigen [44]. Even though the new immunity drug Yervoy (ipilimumab) can markedly prolong the survival time of advanced melanoma patients, it is only effective to 20–30% of patients and often accompanied by severe or even fatal autoimmune response. Besides, it was also discovered that the molecular targeted curative agent imatinib achieves anticancer effect through immunostimulation and that long-acting interleukin-10 can promote tumor immunity and be used in treatment. All this information suggests that the new immunotherapeutic agent deserves our attention.
3. Endocrine system: the close relationship between the endocrine system and cancer has already been noticed in early years; in recent years, besides estrogen and androgen, attention has been paid to thyroid hormone, progesterone [45], etc.
4. Metabolic intervention: this has become a hot field in recent year; ATP consumption promotes cancer metabolism [46]; the metabolism of tumor cells is related to lipoclasis; adipocyte can promote cancer metastasis and provide energy for the rapid growth of tumor [47]. The proliferation of liver cancer is mainly related to glycometabolism but not angiogenesis; and long-acting arginine can stabilize conditions of advanced liver cancer.

What's worth mentioning is that an article in 2012 claims elevated level of whole-body PTEN (tumor-suppressor gene) can lead to relatively normal metabolic state, increase in energy consumption, and decrease in fat accumulation and help to prevent cells from cancerization [48]. Some even believe that cancer is metabolic disintegration [49]. All of this suggests the importance of metabolic intervention. Most of the abovementioned anti-inflammatory agent and traditional Chinese medicine are also systemic intervention in nature. The greatly emphasized idea of "change of lifestyle" in recent years, especially moderate exercises, is also put forward from the perspective of systemic intervention.

It is not expected that systemic intervention alone can eliminate an existing tumor, which still requires tumor elimination therapy such as surgery. However, to neglect the limited residual cancer after tumor elimination therapy may lead to death as a result of cancer metastasis and recurrence. The modification of residual cancer and transformation of body are exactly what's needed to control residual cancer.

1.3.5 Personalized Treatment Will Be Divided into Holistic and Molecular Levels

Different liver cancer patients have commonness as well as individuality. This is because the etiological factors, genetic background, general conditions, etc. of different patients are not identical, and its influence leads to different biological phenotypes of cancer, which are expressed as molecular signatures that are not entirely the same. Considering the development of molecular biology, in 2009, Hayden published an article in *Nature*, expressing that "personalized cancer therapy gets closer." Nevertheless, the implementation of personalized therapy has prerequisites:

1. We need to figure out the biological features of different individuals before shooting at the target—we should research on prognostic markers and establish molecular classification of cancer. For instance, during our collaboration with the Americans, it was discovered that interferon is better suited for those with low expression of miR-26a and not suitable for those with high expression [50]—this provides basis for personalized interferon therapy for liver cancer patients.
2. We need to search for the key relevant molecules from cancer cells, microenvironment, and body, which is a quite complex thing itself. Quite a few related molecules have been discovered by now, but arrangement and screening are needed before they can be transformed for clinical use.
3. Then design molecular targeted curative agent. Currently most molecular targeted curative agents are targeted at single molecular, but the trend will be multiple targets. More importance has been attached to glycoconjugate again in recent years, which suggests the horizon must be broadened in the search of target molecule.

Above is the personalized therapy at the molecular level. Actually the concept of personalized therapy has already existed in traditional Chinese medicine, i.e., "treatment based on differentiation," which refers to personalized treatment with a holistic view. I believe this is also necessary for personalized therapy; this and molecular-level personalized treatment are mutually dependent and complementary. Nevertheless, to achieve molecular-level personalized therapy with a holistic view will be quite difficult indeed.

1.3.6 The Biological Hallmarks of Liver Cancer Will Be the Key to Success of Surgical Treatment

At the beginning of the twenty-first century, biology will be the key factor influencing the development of liver cancer surgery. Tumor elimination through surgery and other cancer-killing methods will still be the main and basic method, but modification of residual cancer and body is the key to further improvement of efficacy. The comprehensive treatment under the guidance of new concept will play an important role. All in all, according to the new concept of cancer metastasis, we should attach great importance to the application of the "modification" strategy, which includes modification of the residual cancer to transform the bad and modification of the body to increase its cancer-fighting ability. In order to achieve this goal, systemic intervention will be the key point.

References

1. DeVita VT, Rosenberg SA. Two hundred years of cancer research. N Engl J Med. 2012;366:2207–14.
2. Hanahan D, Weinberg RA. Hallmarks of cancer: the next generation. Cell. 2011;144:646–74.
3. Uchino K, Tateishi R, Shiina S, et al. Hepatocellular carcinoma with extrahepatic metastasis: clinical features and prognostic factors. Cancer. 2011;117:4475–83.
4. Ye QH, Qin LX, Forgues M, et al. Predicting hepatitis B virus-positive metastatic hepatocellular carcinoma using gene expression profiling and supervised machine learning. Nat Med. 2003;9:416–23.
5. Yamashita T, Ji J, Budhu A, et al. EpCAM-positive hepatocellular carcinoma cells are tumor-initiating cells with stem/progenitor cell features. Gastroenterology. 2009;136:1012–24.
6. Jia QA, Ren ZG, Bu Y, et al. Herbal compound "Songyou Yin" renders hepatocellular carcinoma sensitive to oxaliplatin through inhibition of stemness. Evid Based Complem Altern Med. 2012;2012:908601.
7. Budhu A, Forgues M, Ye QH, et al. Prediction of venous metastases, recurrence, and prognosis in hepatocellular carcinoma based on a unique immune response signature of the liver microenvironment. Cancer Cell. 2006;10:1–13.

8. Malanchi I, Santamaria-Martínez A, Susanto E, et al. Interactions between cancer stem cells and their niche govern metastatic colonization. Nature. 2011;481:85–9.
9. Jia QA, Wang ZM, Ren ZG, et al. Herbal compound "Songyou Yin" attenuates hepatoma cell invasiveness and metastasis through downregulation of cytokines secreted by activated hepatic stellate cells. BMC Complem Altern Med. 2013;13:89.
10. Yamauchi K, Yang M, Hayashi K, et al. Induction of metastasis by cyclophosphamide pretreatment of host mice: an opposite effect of chemotherapy. Cancer Res. 2008;15(68):516–20.
11. Altekruse SF, McGlynn KA, Dickie LA, et al. Hepatocellular carcinoma confirmation, treatment, and survival in surveillance, epidemiology, and end results registries, 1992–2008. Hepatology. 2012;55:476–82.
12. Santi V, Buccione D, Di Micoli A, et al. The changing scenario of hepatocellular carcinoma over the last two decades in Italy. J Hepatol. 2012;56:397–405.
13. Kim YS, Lim HK, Rhim H, et al. Ten-year outcomes of percutaneous radiofrequency ablation as first-line therapy of early hepatocellular carcinoma: analysis of prognostic factors. J Hepatol. 2013;58:89–97.
14. Pang JZ, Qin LX, Ren N, et al. Loss of heterozygosity at D8S298 is a predictor for long-term survival of patients with Tumor-Node-Metastasis Stage I of hepatocellular carcinoma. Clin Cancer Res. 2007;13:7363–9.
15. Huang XY, Huang ZL, Wang L, et al. Herbal compound "Songyou Yin" reinforced the ability of interferon-alfa to inhibit the enhanced metastatic potential induced by palliative resection of hepatocellular carcinoma in nude mice. BMC Cancer. 2010;10:580–9.
16. Tang ZY, Yu YQ, Zhou XD, et al. Cytoreduction and sequential resection: a hope for unresectable primary liver cancer. J Surg Oncol. 1991;47:27–31.
17. Zaanan A, Williet N, Hebbar M, et al. Gemcitabine plus oxaliplatin in advanced hepatocellular carcinoma: a large multicenter AGEO study. J Hepatol. 2013;58:81–8.
18. Feng YX, Wang T, Deng YZ, et al. Sorafenib suppresses postsurgical recurrence and metastasis of hepatocellular carcinoma in an orthotopic mouse model. Hepatology. 2011;53:483–92.
19. Wang L, Tang ZY, Qin LX, et al. High-dose and long-term therapy with interferon-alfa inhibits tumor growth and recurrence in nude mice bearing human hepatocellular carcinoma xenografts with high metastatic potential. Hepatology. 2000;32:43–8.
20. Sun HC, Tang ZY, Wang L, et al. Postoperative interferon alpha treatment postponed recurrence and improved overall survival in patients after curative resection of HBV-related hepatocellular carcinoma: a randomized clinical trial. J Cancer Res Clin Oncol. 2006;132:458–65.
21. Eltzschig HK, Carmeliet P. Hypoxia and inflammation. N Engl J Med. 2011;364:656–65.
22. Dinarello CA. Anti-inflammatory agents: present and future. Cell. 2010;140:935–50.
23. Sahasrabuddhe VV, Gunja MZ, Graubard BI, et al. Nonsteriodal anti-inflammatory drug use, chronic liver disease, and hepatocellular carcinoma. J Natl Cancer Inst. 2012;104:1808–14.
24. Hsu, et al. Postoperative peg-interferon plus ribavirin associated with reduced recurrence of hepatitis C virus-related hepatocellular carcinoma. Hepatology. 2013;58:150–7.
25. Zhang XW, Yan XJ, Zhou ZR, et al. Arsenic trioxide controls the fate of the PML-RARa oncoprotein by directly binding PML. Science. 2010;328:240–3.
26. Wang WQ, Liu L, Sun HC, et al. Tanshinone IIA inhibits metastasis after palliative resection of hepatocellular carcinoma and prolongs survival in part via vascular normalization. J Hematol Oncol. 2012;5:69–79.
27. Liu L, Ren ZG, Shen Y, et al. Influence of hepatic artery occlusion on tumor growth and metastatic potential in a human orthotopic hepatoma nude mouse model: relevance of epithelial-mesenchymal transition. Cancer Sci. 2010;101:120–8.
28. Liu L, Zhu XD, Wang WQ, et al. Activation of beta-catenin by hypoxia in hepatocellular carcinoma contributes to enhanced metastatic potential and poor prognosis. Clin Cancer Res. 2010;16:2740–50.
29. Sun FX, Tang ZY, Liu KD, et al. Establishment of a metastatic model of human hepatocellular carcinoma in nude mice via orthotopic implantation of histologically intact tissues. Int J Cancer. 1996;66:239–43.
30. Tian J, Tang ZY, Ye SL, et al. New human hepatocellular carcinoma (HCC) cell line with highly metastatic potential (MHCC97) and its expression of the factors associated with metastasis. Br J Cancer. 1999;81:814–21.
31. Li T, Zeng ZC, Wang L, et al. Radiation enhances long-term metastasis potential of residual hepatocellular carcinoma in nude mice through TMPRSS4-induced epithelial–mesenchymal transition. Cancer Gene Ther. 2011;18:617–26.
32. Xiong W, Ren ZG, Qiu SJ, et al. Residual hepatocellular carcinoma after oxaliplatin treatment has increased metastatic potential in a nude mouse model and is attenuated by Songyou Yin. BMC Cancer. 2010;10:219–30.
33. Zhang W, Sun HC, Wang WQ, et al. Sorafenib down-regulates expression of HTATIP2 to promote invasiveness and metastasis of orthotopic hepatocellular carcinoma tumors in mice. Gastroenterology. 2012;143:1641–9.
34. Zhang QB, Sun HC, Zhang KZ, et al. Suppression of natural killer cells by sorafenib contributes to prometastatic effects in hepatocellular carcinoma. PLoS One. 2013;8:e55945.
35. Zhu XD, Sun HC, Xu HX, et al. Antiangiogenic therapy promoted metastasis of hepatocellular carcinoma by suppressing host-derived interleukin-12b in mouse models. Angiogenesis. 2013;16:809–20.
36. Huang Q, Li F, Liu X, et al. Caspase 3-mediated stimulation of tumor cell repopulation during cancer radiotherapy. Nat Med. 2011;17:860–6.
37. Casanovas O. Cancer: limitation of therapies exposed. Nature. 2012;484:44–6.
38. Zhang W, Zhu XD, Sun HC, et al. Depletion of tumor-associated macrophages enhances the effect of sorafenib in metastatic liver cancer models by antimetastatic and antiangiogenic effects. Clin Cancer Res. 2010;16:3420–30.
39. Huang XY, Wang L, Huang ZL, et al. Herbal extract "Songyou Yin" inhibits tumor growth and prolongs survival in nude mice bearing human hepatocellular carcinoma xenograft with high metastatic potential. J Cancer Res Clin Oncol. 2009;135:1245–55.
40. Jia JB, Wang WQ, Sun HC, et al. A novel tripeptide, tyroserleutide, inhibits irradiation-induced invasiveness and metastasis of hepatocellular carcinoma in nude mice. Investig New Drugs. 2010;29:861–72.
41. Entschladen F, Drell 4th TL, Lang K, et al. Tumour-cell migration, invasion, and metastasis: navigation by neurotransmitters. Lancet Oncol. 2004;5:254–8.
42. Ondicova K, Mravec B. Role of nervous system in cancer aetiopathogenesis. Lancet Oncol. 2010;11:596–601.
43. Schreiber RD, Old LJ, Smyth MJ, et al. Cancer immunoediting: integrating immunity's roles in cancer suppression and promotion. Science. 2011;331:1565–70.
44. Weiner LM, Murray JC, Shuptrine CW. Antibody-based immunotherapy of cancer. Cell. 2012;148:1081–4.
45. Joshi PA, Jackson HW, Beristain AG, et al. Progesterone induces adult mammary stem cell expansion. Nature. 2010;465:803–7.
46. Israelsen WJ, Vander Heiden MG. ATP consumption promotes cancer metabolism. Cell. 2010;143:669–71.

47. Nieman KM, Kenny HA, Penicka CV, et al. Adipocytes promote ovarian cancer metastasis and provide energy for rapid tumor growth. Nat Med. 2011;17:1498–503.
48. Garcia-Cao I, Song MS, Hobbs RM, et al. Systemic elevation of PTEN induces a tumor-suppressive metabolic state. Cell. 2012;149:49–62.
49. Krall AS, Christofk HR. Cancer: a metabolic metamorphosis. Nature. 2013;496:38–40.
50. Ji JF, Shi J, Budhu A, et al. MicroRNA expression, survival, and response to interferon in liver cancer. N Engl J Med. 2009;361:1437–47.

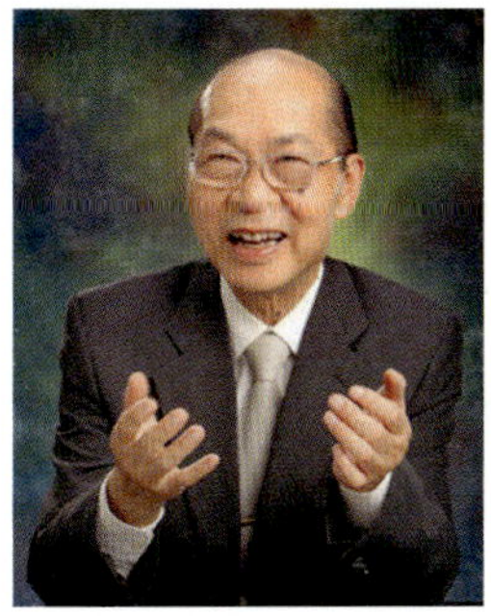

Zhao-You Tang is an Academician of Chinese Academy of Sciences, Department of Liver Surgery, Liver Cancer Institute, Zhongshan Hospital, Fudan University, Shanghai, China.

2 Thinking on Innovative Research of Liver Cancer and Clinical Transformation

Hong-Yang Wang

In recent years, the global economy and society have been developing in fluctuations and oscillations. Despite the significant progress achieved in medicine, science, and technology, the ongoing globalization and urbanization are challenging the nation's ability to protect public health. The threat to human health posed by complex diseases such as malignant tumor, diabetes, hypertension, and coronary heart disease has not been weakened with the socioeconomic development; on the contrary, it even showed an increasing trend. As far as cancer is concerned, February 4 is the World Cancer Day. On February 3, 2014, the World Cancer Report was published by the International Agency for Research on Cancer (IARC), the official cancer organization under WHO. The report pointed out that cancer is one of the main causes for death globally, causing 8.2 million deaths in 2012. Throughout the world, cancers with the highest fatality rate include lung cancer (1.5 million), liver cancer (745,000), gastric cancer (723,000), colorectal cancer (694,000), etc. The report predicted that in the future 20 years, the annual number of new cancer cases in the world would increase to 22 million; meanwhile, the annual number of cancer deaths will increase from 8.2 million to 13 million [1]. The situation for global cancer prevention and control is very severe.

Even though the cancer incidence rate in China is not the highest, because of its tremendous population base, in 2012, 3.07 million cancer cases were newly diagnosed in China, accounting for 21.8% of the world's total, and 2.2 million people died from cancer, accounting for 26.9% of the total number of cancer deaths worldwide. As far as liver cancer is concerned, over 50% of the world's newly diagnosed liver cancer cases are in China, whose liver cancer deaths account for about 51% of the world's total. The reason is that China is one of the regions of high viral hepatitis B prevalence. Over a hundred million hepatitis B virus carriers are important susceptible populations, and over 85% of liver cancer patients in China have evidence of hepatitis B viral infection.

Usually the incidence of liver cancer is accompanied by the typical "hepatitis-liver cirrhosis-liver cancer" process, but the pathogenesis from hepatitis to liver cancer is yet to be clarified. At present, screening and follow-up for high-risk populations is one of the important strategies for liver cancer control. In reality, China is lacking in convenient and effective means of liver cancer warning and surveillance for susceptible populations and does not have a scientific and reasonable molecular typing system. In the clinical diagnosis and treatment of liver cancer, difficult problems exist, such as nonspecific treatment method, high recurrence and metastasis rate, lack of basis for personalized treatment, few innovative efficient drugs, etc. Many hepatitis patients would turn pale at the mentioning of liver cancer because of the all-time high fatality rate of liver cancer, and the difficulty to cure hepatitis and treat liver cancer is also consuming an excessive amount of the already insufficient health resources.

The completion of the Human Genome Project and the progress of integrative biology and systems biology made it possible for early tumor prevention and early intervention of higher efficiency. With the development of medicine, a "4P" medical model has been proposed, i.e., preventive, predictive, personalized, and participatory. This model has initiated a new approach of medical research on tumor transformation. Once the breakthrough happens, it may bring about revolutionary changes to tumor prevention and control. Translational medicine is dedicated to filling the gap between basic experimental R&D and clinical application and shortening the time needed for a new diagnosis and treatment method to go from the laboratory to clinical stage. As a "B2B (bench to bedside)" continuous research and application development process, transitional medicine is now more commonly used in researches on malignant tumor including liver cancer. The key links of transitional medicine research are identification of biomarkers (the new parameter for the diagnosis and surveillance of tumor genesis and progression)

H.-Y. Wang (✉)
Academician of Chinese Academy of Sciences, International Cooperation Laboratory on Signal Transduction, Eastern Hepatobiliary Surgery Hospital, Second Military Medical University, Shanghai, China
e-mail: hywangk@vip.sina.com

W.-M. Cong (ed.), *Surgical Pathology of Hepatobiliary Tumors*, DOI 10.1007/978-981-10-3536-4_2

through screening and R&D of new diagnosis technology, new treatment strategy, and new method. In recent years, China has gradually increased its investment in liver cancer research; initiated a batch of national scientific research programs, targeted at the key scientific problems of liver cancer; gathered teams with advantages in liver cancer research; established a technological innovation system combining production, study, research, and application; tackled key problems through collaboration; promoted the basic and clinical research on liver cancer; obtained a batch of important molecular markers through screening; actively explored new strategies of biotherapy for liver cancer; and implemented standardized combined therapy with enthusiasm and achieved initial success. Once the new products, new technologies, and new plans resulting from relevant researches are approved, they will be put into clinical use and application in high-risk areas. These practices will become valuable exploration of the innovative liver cancer research and clinical translation. Apparently, China is welcoming new leaps forward facing the challenges of liver cancer prevention and treatment.

2.1 Early Warning and Early Diagnosis Are the Breakthrough Points for Innovative Research on Liver Cancer

Based on the change of medical model and research idea, right now throughout the world, the key point for liver cancer prevention and control is screening for new markers, accelerating the transformation into clinical application, and improving the ability of risk prediction and early diagnosis of liver cancer. At present, the early diagnosis rate of liver cancer is extremely low in China, which greatly impacted the effect of liver cancer treatment. Considering China's huge population base of chronic hepatitis B virus carriers and chronic hepatitis B patients, a systemic analysis targeted at these high-risk groups and liver cancer patients can help to achieve breakthrough in the prevention and early diagnosis and treatment of liver cancer and improve the level of liver cancer prevention and control faster.

A hot area of liver cancer research is screening for liver cancer-related markers or determining spectral pattern with various high-throughput "omics" technologies. Through large-scale screening for warning and diagnosis markers, China's liver cancer researchers have already found out a batch of markers with proprietary intellectual property right and good prospect in clinical application, especially the important serological warning, early diagnosis, and pathological diagnostic markers such as MXR7 (GPC3), DKK1, and miRNA. Through multicenter and large-sample clinical cases, it has been confirmed that the combined use of these molecular markers and AFP can improve the accuracy rate of liver cancer diagnosis significantly [2]. Recently, many technical plans of hepatoma-specific early diagnostic reagent with proprietary intellectual property rights have been formed, some of which have been used in industrialization R&D through collaboration with enterprises, and will be applied and popularized in China's hepatopathy diagnosis and treatment units and high-risk areas after obtaining CFDA approval. They will play a key role in increasing the early diagnosis rate of liver cancer, improving the treatment effect, and lowering the fatality rate.

2.2 Research on Molecular Regulation Network Will Provide New Drug Target for Biotherapy of Liver Cancer

The genesis and progression of liver cancer result from the combination of genetic and environmental factors. It is a multilevel multistage dynamic development process, and the recurrence and metastasis caused by invasive growth is also a process of the steric effect of liver cancer cells and microenvironment, which involves the complex regulation network [3]. At present, we still lack specific prevention and treatment measures, the crucial reasons being the pathogenesis of highly heterogeneous liver cancer is not clarified and the panoramic analysis of the dynamic regulation mechanism of liver cancer is not completed.

The systematic understanding of the genesis and progression of liver cancer and the network regulation mechanism of inflammation-cancer transformation is of vital importance to obtaining specific drug target and also an important scientific problem in the research on liver cancer prevention and treatment, especially the research on the systematic regulation of signal transduction network of liver cancer cells and microenvironment and the research on interaction of host nervous system, hormone endocrine system, immune system, etc. and their role in the genesis and progression of liver cancer; they update and enrich concepts about the prevention, diagnosis, and treatment of liver cancer; provide new targets applicable to the research and development of new drugs for liver cancer; and ultimately realize effective and specific multi-target therapy.

2.3 Metabolic Abnormality Is Closely Linked with the Genesis and Progression of Liver Cancer

During the genesis and progression of malignant tumor, cellular metabolic features have experienced fundamental changes, promoting the malignant proliferation of tumor cells. The relationship between metabolic abnormality and tumor has never been neglected since the 1920s when Otto Warburg first reported about the Warburg effect, i.e., under well-oxygenated conditions, the glycolysis of tumor cells will also be greatly reinforced. In recent years, the content of the Warburg effect has been further expended: the metabolic features of tumor cells are significantly different from those of normal tissues in terms of nucleic acid, protein, enzymatic system, and glycometabolism [4]. Research shows that many metabolic pathways such as fatty acid, glutamine, serine, and choline metabolism have changed in tumor cells, all of which are collectively referred to as metabolic reprogramming [5].

The liver is the main metabolic organ of the human body with extensive participation in metabolic processes such as the absorption, synthesis, decomposition, storage, and transport of substances like sugar, protein, lipoid, and vitamins. If liver cells become cancerous, the original powerful metabolic capability of liver cells may very likely be "kidnapped" to create conditions for tumor growth. Evidence-based medical researches indicate a close relationship between metabolic diseases such as obesity, diabetes, and cardiovascular diseases and the genesis and progression of malignant tumors including liver cancer. The latest research shows that DMBG, the drug originally used for diabetes treatment, can reduce the risk of liver cancer and improve the prognosis of liver cancer patients [6].

Research on the interaction between the metabolic reprogramming of liver cancer cells and the body's metabolic state and further clarification of the internal regulation network of metabolic phenotypes of liver cancer through interdisciplinary collaboration of cancer systems biology, metabonomics, bioinformatics, molecular imaging, epidemiology, etc. can not only help to understand the pathogenesis of liver cancer but also target at critical node points of the energy metabolism of liver cancer, interfere with cellular metabolic abnormality, and provide new ideas and strategies for the diagnosis, prevention, and treatment of liver cancer [7].

2.4 Liver Cancer Stem Cells Promote the Genesis and Progression and Recurrence and Metastasis of Liver Cancer

Recent researches indicate that tumor does not consist of homogeneous tumor cells. A small part of cells are equipped with the ability of self-renewal and continuous proliferation to form new tumor colony, and these tumor cells are referred to as cancer stem cell (CSC) or tumor-initiating cell (TIC) [8]. The traditional method of chemotherapy can inhibit the growth of tumor, but may lead to the accumulation of cancer stem cells, the existence of which may be the reason for tumor recurrence and metastasis and tolerance to chemotherapy [9, 10]. In-depth research on the signal regulation network of cancer stem cells in search for suitable therapeutic target is an international frontier scientific issue of liver cancer research. Clinical trials targeted at cancer stem cell therapy for rectal cancer and breast cancer have already begun in foreign countries, and the research results are worth expecting.

As far as liver cancer is concerned, the inflammatory microenvironment caused by chronic liver diseases like chronic viral hepatitis, alcoholic liver disease, and nonalcoholic fatty liver promotes the activation and proliferation of liver stem cells, and during this process, malignant transformation of stem cells may occur. Plenty of evidence suggests that cancer stem cells play an important role in the progression of liver cancer—they participate in the genesis, recurrence and metastasis, and resistance to radiotherapy/chemotherapy. Some molecular markers with close relationship to phenotypes such as invasive growth of liver cancer stem cells and tolerance to chemotherapy (e.g., CD133, CD24, CD44, CD90, EpCAM, and OV6) have also been discovered one after another [11–13]. GWAS analysis and in-depth mechanism research based on high-throughput technology indicate some signaling pathways that have played an important role in the development and regeneration of liver (such as Wnt/β-catenin, TGF-β, and IL-6/STAT3) give rise to abnormal activation due to reasons like mutation and participate in the regulation of the proliferation and activation of liver cancer stem cells [14–16]. Recently, Chinese scholars have obtained monoclonal antibody of subunit α2δ1m that identifies voltage-dependent calcium channel through the method of whole cell immunity, which can decrease the content of cancer stem cells in hepatic cellular cancer, and its combined use with Doxorubicin inhibits the tumor growth in liver cancer tumor-bearing animal model significantly [17]. This research discovered and proved a new functional marker and therapeutic target of cancer stem cells of hepatic cellular cancer and made positive attempt at intervention strategy.

The research on cancer stem cells deepens our understanding of the biological hallmarks of liver cancer stem cells. However, like other cancer stem cells, the research on liver cancer stem cells still need to clarify a lot of question, e.g., whether the stem cell niches participating in the self-renewal regulation of liver cancer stem cells also exist in liver [18]; what is the percentage of liver cancer stem cells in liver cancer cells; and what method can accurately recognize and separate liver cancer stem cells, etc. We believe that the clarification of these problems and technological breakthroughs can open up new possibilities for the early diagnosis, prevention, and treatment of liver cancer.

2.5 Molecular Typing and Personalized Therapy Are the Only Ways to Cure Liver Cancer

Since December 1971, when the American president Nixon signed the National Cancer Act and thereby began over 40 years of war on cancer, the world's total expenditure on cancer research has exceeded 200 billion USD, and over 1 million articles have been published. Even though the situation for prevention and control is still serious, cancer research is not entirely fruitless. The rise of personalized therapy for cancer in the past few years is one of the important breakthroughs. The promotion of molecular typing for breast cancer, lung cancer, and leukemia and the corresponding personalized therapies have improved efficacy markedly. Screening for specific groups of patients based on molecular markers and application of compound or antibody that blocks relevant signaling pathways to inhibit the growth of malignant tumor have become new ideas for tumor prevention and control.

At present, radical treatment (hepatectomy, liver transplantation, local ablation) is the major means for liver cancer patients to achieve long-term survival [19]. Nevertheless, postoperative recurrence and metastasis and lack of effective chemotherapy drugs are important issues constraining the further improvement of efficacy for liver cancer, and neither secondary surgical resection nor liver transplantation can effectively improve the prognosis of live cancer. Research results suggest that liver cancer is highly heterogeneous, i.e., there are many different genotypes of liver cancer, their genesis and progression are related to multiple pathway abnormalities, and relatively great differences exist among different patients, which explains the difficulty of the R&D of molecular-targeted drugs targeted at liver cancer. Therefore, the screening for molecular diagnostic markers of liver cancer, molecular typing, and development of personalized targeted drugs are vital issues of the innovative research on liver cancer. The development of translational medicine bridges the gap between basic research and clinical practice. On one hand, the liver cancer regulation network node molecules and markers discovered in basic research can be tested in clinical observation; on the other hand, the problems discovered clinically can be answered through basic research, so as to better understand the biological hallmarks of different types of liver cancer and guide its prevention and treatment. New ideas of molecular typing of liver cancer have been put forward by domestic and international scholars during the preliminary exploration of molecular typing and personalized treatment of liver cancer, but most of these typing methods are still going through preclinical research, yet to be confirmed by large sample clinically, and not mature enough for actual application [20–22].

Sorafenib is an oral multitarget tyrosinase inhibitor. SHARP and ORIENTAL clinical researches confirmed that sorafenib is comparatively efficient and safe for advanced hepatic cellular cancer. This initiated a new era of targeted drug treatment of liver cancer, and sorafenib quickly became the standard treatment drug for advanced liver cancer [23]. Nevertheless, in clinical practices, it can be observed that the efficacy of sorafenib for certain patients is not obvious, and some patients of short survival time cannot wait long enough to see its efficacy after receiving sorafenib for treatment [24]. Such phenomenon has triggered thoughts about personalized application of sorafenib to treat liver cancer. As a matter of fact, earlier some scholars have already conducted exploratory research on the application of molecular makers to choose target population suitable for sorafenib treatment. However, since no ideal biomarkers have been found, the pathogenesis of liver cancer is complex, and patients usually have underlying diseases such as hepatitis and hepatic cirrhosis, so far no ideal biomarkers can guide the choice of patients for the clinical use of sorafenib. The SHARP research and subsequent work made a preliminary assessment of biomarkers of predictive significance to sorafenib treatment for cancer, and results indicate relevance between molecular markers such as AFP, c-Kit, IGF-2, and HGF and whether patient can benefit from sorafenib treatment, but further confirmation is still needed.

Personalized therapy on the basis of molecular typing is the developing trend of future liver cancer treatment. Searching from better indicators on the molecular level, further improving the plan and choosing groups for treatment, and conducting personalized treatment under the guidance of molecular markers will provide new opportunities for the targeted treatment of liver cancer.

2.6 Prospect

In the past, due to the immaturity of the research system of translational medicine, laboratory research and clinical research usually go their separate ways. It would take decades before the new tumor markers and therapeutic targets discovered in a lab can be put into clinical application after verification, and the problems and difficulties encountered in clinical work could not be explained and solved efficiently in time. Besides, subject to flaws like long cycle and low throughput, traditional research technologies suggest very limited information for tumor. Over a relatively long period of time, the innovative research of liver cancer couldn't be advanced rapidly, only very few diagnosis markers were used for routine clinical practice, and treatment measures lacked personality [25]. However, with the appeal of scientists and national attention to liver cancer prevention and treatment in recent years, a batch of major plans of scientific research has been implemented; the National Liver Cancer Science Center is about to be completed and put into use, and the innovative research of liver cancer faces unprecedented new opportunities. Meanwhile, the development of systems biology theory and technologies deepens out understanding of the biological hallmarks of liver cancer with the discovery of many biomarkers of vital importance to the diagnosis or treatment of liver cancer. The collaboration between basic research labs and clinical diagnosis and treatment units is becoming closer each day; translational research on liver cancer is moving forward quickly, and the cycle from innovative laboratory discovery to clinical application is being shortened continuously. New strategies of early warning, early diagnosis, molecular typing, and targeted intervention will initiate the stage of prevention and clinical personalized treatment as soon as possible, bringing hopes of finally conquering liver cancer—the major threat to people's health for many years!

References

1. Ferlay J, Soerjomataram I, Ervik M. GLOBOCAN 2012 v1. 0, Cancer Incidence and Mortality Worldwide: IARC CancerBase No. 11. Lyon: International Agency for Research on Cancer 2013; 2014.
2. Shen Q, Fan J, Yang XR, et al. Serum DKK1 as a protein biomarker for the diagnosis of hepatocellular carcinoma: a large-scale, multicentre study. Lancet Oncol. 2012;13(8):817–26.
3. Aravalli RN, Steer CJ, Cressman EN. Molecular mechanisms of hepatocellular carcinoma. Hepatology. 2008;48(6):2047–63.
4. Warburg O, Wind F, Negelein E. The Metabolism of Tumors in the Body. J Gen Physiol. 1927;8(6):519–30.
5. Ward PS, Thompson CB. Metabolic reprogramming: a cancer hallmark even warburg did not anticipate. Cancer Cell. 2012;21(3):297–308.
6. Zheng L, Yang W, Wu F, et al. Prognostic significance of AMPK activation and therapeutic effects of metformin in hepatocellular carcinoma. Clin Cancer Res. 2013;19(19):5372–80.
7. Chen HP, Shieh JJ, Chang CC, et al. Metformin decreases hepatocellular carcinoma risk in a dose-dependent manner: population-based and in vitro studies. Gut. 2013;62(4):606–15.
8. Driessens G, Beck B, Caauwe A, et al. Defining the mode of tumour growth by clonal analysis. Nature. 2012;488(7412):527–30.
9. Jordan CT, Guzman ML, Noble M. Cancer stem cells. N Engl J Med. 2006;355(12):1253–61.
10. Schepers AG, Snippert HJ, Stange DE, et al. Lineage tracing reveals Lgr5+ stem cell activity in mouse intestinal adenomas. Science. 2012;337(6095):730–5.
11. Ma S, Chan KW, Hu L, et al. Identification and characterization of tumorigenic liver cancer stem/progenitor cells. Gastroenterology. 2007;132(7):2542–56.
12. Sell S, Leffert HL. Liver cancer stem cells. J Clin Oncol. 2008;26(17):2800–5.
13. Yamashita T, Wang XW. Cancer stem cells in the development of liver cancer. J Clin Invest. 2013;123(5):1911–8.
14. Yang ZF, Ho DW, Ng MN, et al. Significance of CD90+ cancer stem cells in human liver cancer. Cancer Cell. 2008;13(2):153–66.
15. Lee TK, Castilho A, Cheung VC, et al. CD24(+) liver tumor-initiating cells drive self-renewal and tumor initiation through STAT3-mediated NANOG regulation. Cell Stem Cell. 2011;9(1):50–63.
16. Yang W, Wang C, Lin Y, et al. OV6(+) tumor-initiating cells contribute to tumor progression and invasion in human hepatocellular carcinoma. J Hepatol. 2012;57(3):613–20.
17. Zhao W, Wang L, Han H, et al. 1B50-1, a mAb raised against recurrent tumor cells, targets liver tumor-initiating cells by binding to the calcium channel alpha2delta1 subunit. Cancer Cell. 2013;23(4):541–56.
18. Wagers AJ. The stem cell niche in regenerative medicine. Cell Stem Cell. 2012;10(4):362–9.
19. Bruix J, Sherman M. Management of hepatocellular carcinoma: an update. Hepatology. 2011;53(3):1020–2.
20. Avila MA, Berasain C, Sangro B, et al. New therapies for hepatocellular carcinoma. Oncogene. 2006;25(27):3866–84.
21. Villanueva A, Toffanin S, Llovet JM. Linking molecular classification of hepatocellular carcinoma and personalized medicine: preliminary steps. Curr Opin Oncol. 2008;20(4):444–53.
22. Ji J, Shi J, Budhu A, et al. MicroRNA expression, survival, and response to interferon in liver cancer. N Engl J Med. 2009;361(15):1437–47.
23. Llovet JM, Ricci S, Mazzaferro V, et al. Sorafenib in advanced hepatocellular carcinoma. N Engl J Med. 2008;359(4):378–90.
24. Cheng AL, Kang YK, Chen Z, et al. Efficacy and safety of sorafenib in patients in the Asia-Pacific region with advanced hepatocellular carcinoma: a phase III randomised, double-blind, placebo-controlled trial. Lancet Oncol. 2009;10(1):25–34.
25. Llovet JM, Pena CE, Lathia CD, et al. Plasma biomarkers as predictors of outcome in patients with advanced hepatocellular carcinoma. Clin Cancer Res. 2012;18(8):2290–300.

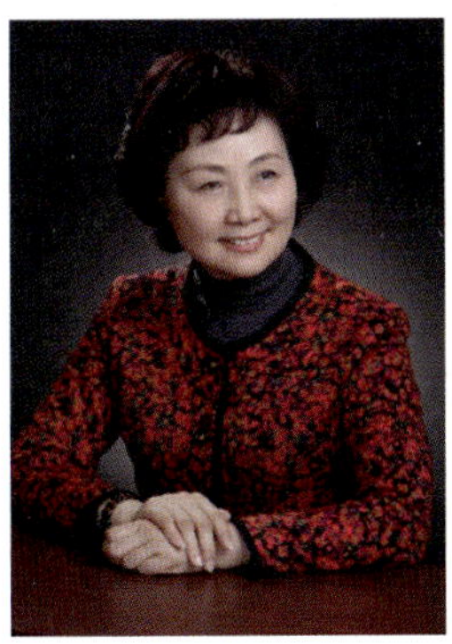

Hong-Yang Wang is an Academician of Chinese Academy of Sciences, International Cooperation Laboratory on Signal Transduction, Eastern Hepatobiliary Surgery Hospital, Second Military Medical University, National Center for Liver Cancer, Shanghai, China.

Researches on Surgical Pathology of Hepatobiliary Tumors in EHBH

3

Wen-Ming Cong

I would have introduced some influential historic events in the development of hepatic surgical pathology on the basis of review of literature at the beginning of the article as usual. However, it would be very difficult for me to carry it out mainly due to my limited knowledge and information. Thus, based on our previous studies and books and articles written by many experts from different viewpoints on the history and future of hepatic surgical pathology, I endeavored to narrow down the coverage to make it a brief retrospection of our over 30 years' experience in China's only specialized hospital of hepatobiliary surgery and introduce several celebrated foreign experts on hepatic pathology, who have helped and supported us with important impact on our work. This is a retrospection as well as expression of inspiration and gratefulness, for we have progressed and improved greatly through learning from predecessors' great books and articles and their precious advice.

3.1 American Hepatopathologist Professor Hugh A. Edmondson

Professor Edmondson was a former director of the Department of Pathology, School of Medicine, University of Southern California, who advanced the well-known and widely adopted Edmondson-Steiner Grading of hepatocellular carcinoma (HCC) with four grades in 1954. He also suggested that the higher grade the HCC is, the more likely it will metastasize. Furthermore, the terms such as fibrolamellar carcinoma of the liver, focal nodular hyperplasia of the liver, adenomatous hyperplasia of the liver, and mesenchymal hamartoma of the liver were also firstly named by Professor Edmondson.

Early in 1979 when the Center for China PLA hepatobiliary surgery, Changhai Hospital, the Second Military Medical University (SMMU), was established, Professor Meng-Chao Wu, as the Director of the Center, set up the lab of hepatobiliary surgery to train postgraduates on related fields of expertise. And I began my study on pathology of hepatic tumors for Master's and Doctor's degrees under the supervision of Professor Meng-Chao Wu in 1984 and 1987, respectively. Professor Wu then became an Academician of Chinese Academy of Sciences with much reputation, as he internationally pioneered in the research of pathobiological features of small hepatocellular carcinoma (SHCC), etc. At that time I was supervised to study the pathobioloical characterization of SHCC. But at that time, there were few books on the liver pathology in the SMMU's library then except a book named by *Tumors of the Liver and Intrahepatic Bile Ducts: Atlas of Tumor Pathology* [1], which was the most authoritative monograph on the topic of pathology of hepatic tumors, edited by Professor Edmondson and colleagues and published by American Force Institute of Pathology (AFIP) in 1958. This atlas of pathology illustrates around thirty kinds of liver tumors from three aspects, namely, benign liver tumors, malignant liver tumors, and tumor-like lesions with a few of black-and-white photographs, and is like an illuminative tutor to guide our pathological practice and is greatly beneficial. I admire Professor Edmondson a lot for his classic naming and profound understanding of various liver tumors as early as in the 1950s.

Thanks to the increasingly rapid development of hepatic surgery in our hospital, it has become our unique advantage to accumulate experience in pathological diagnosis of liver diseases. We have firstly reported several diseases within or without the coverage of Professor Edmondson's books, such as the pathological characterizations of special lesions of focal nodular hyperplasia of the liver [2], focal fatty change of the liver [3], hepatic angiomyolipoma [4], adenomatous hyperplasia of the liver [5], hepatic primary chondrosarcoma [6], multiple primary malignant tumors of the liver [7], etc. Since 1988, we published a series of papers on the pathobiological features of SHCC and proposed a new concept that an HCC of nearly 3 cm in diameter may reach an important

W.-M. Cong (✉)
Department of Pathology, Eastern Hepatobiliary Surgery Hospital, Second Military Medical University, Shanghai, China
e-mail: wmcong@smmu.edu.cn

W.-M. Cong (ed.), *Surgical Pathology of Hepatobiliary Tumors*, DOI 10.1007/978-981-10-3536-4_3

turning point for the critical transformation, changing from relatively benign behavior to a more aggressive progression, and the 3 cm cutoff seems to be the best definition for SHCC [8–14]. In 1997, we reported the results of clinical pathological characteristics of 3160 cases of hepatobiliary tumors excised surgically [15]. We edited and published Chinese first monograph *Surgical Pathological Diagnosis of Hepatobiliary Tumors in 2002* [16]. Since the previous histological classification of hepatic and intrahepatic bile duct tumors, proposed by the World Health Organization (WHO) with about thirty histological types, could not meet the clinical need of pathodiagnosis and treatment, we suggested a new histological classification of hepatobiliary tumors with over 100 kinds of lesions into three types (tumorlike lesions, benign tumors, malignant tumors) and six subtypes (hepatocyte, cholangiocyte, muscular or fibrous or adipose, vascular and lymphatic, neuroendocrine, and miscellaneous tumors) based on the review of the current literature and our experience in pathodiagnosis of hepatobiliary tumors in over 40,000 cases within over 30 years and have a relatively comprehensive understanding of the constructive characteristics of different hepatobiliary tumors (Tables 3.1, 3.2, and 3.3) [17, 18].

Under the leadership of Academician Meng-Chao Wu, we have made great progresses in the exploration of pathological diagnosis and molecular pathology of hepatobiliary tumors, resulting in the development from pathological group in the lab of hepatobiliary surgery to the Department of Pathology in a Grade A Tertiary Specialized Hospital of hepatobiliary surgery. The number of cases diagnosed in our Department of Pathology per year has gradually risen from less than one hundred, to several thousand, and to approximate ten thousand. Up to now, our Department has successfully applied and finished ten projects supported by the National Natural Science Foundation of China and several projects supported by the Army and Shanghai Municipal Foundations, including the training plan for 100 outstanding cross-century academic leaders of Shanghai health system and the fund for military outstanding young- and middle-aged experts of medical and health. We achieved the "Silver Star in Science and Technology" from PLA General Logistics Department, National Science and Technology Progress Award (third class), Medical Science and Technology Progress Award of PLA (second class, twice), Medical Achieve Awards of PLA (first class), Chinese Medical Science and Technology Awards (second class), Shanghai Science and Technology Awards (first class) and Shanghai Medical Science and Technology Awards (first class), and so forth. And we are also honored to have become one of the principal members of the Innovative Research Team Integrating Clinical and Basic Research of Liver

Table 3.1 Histological types of tumorlike lesions of hepatic and intrahepatic bile ducts

Hepatocellular tumorlike lesions	**Miscellaneous tumorlike lesions**
Focal nodular hyperplasia	Mesenchymal hamartoma
Nodular regenerative hyperplasia	Inflammatory pseudotumor
Partial nodular transformation	Inflammatory myofibroblastic tumor
Precancerous lesions	Pseudolymphoma
Compensatory hyperplasia	Pseudolipoma
Focal fatty change	Solitary necrotic nodules
Accessory lobe	Peliosis hepatis
Bile duct tumorlike lesions	Sarcoidosis
Biliary hamartoma	Nodular extramedullary hematopoiesis
Simple hepatic cysts	Cystic echinococcosis
Polycystic liver diseases	Liver abscess
Caroli disease	Malacoplakia
Congenital choledochal cyst	Ectopic tissues
Congenital hepatic fibrosis	Larva migrans
Ciliated hepatic foregut cyst	Hepatic infarction
Epidermoid cyst	
Endometrial cyst	
Peribiliary cysts	
Cyst of the accessory liver	
Alimentary duplication cyst	
Biloma	
Mesothelial cyst	

Table 3.2 Histological types of benign tumors of hepatic and intrahepatic bile ducts

Hepatocellular tumors	**Neurological and endocrinic tumors**
Hepatocellular adenoma	Neurilemmoma
Hepatic adenomatosis	Neurofibroma
Bile duct tumors	Plexiform neurofibroma
Bile duct adenoma	Neurofibromatosis
Biliary cystadenoma	Paraganglioma
Intraductal papillary neoplasms of the bile ducts	Adrenal rest tumor
Biliary adenofibroma	Pancreatic rest tumor
Vascular and lymphatic tumors	Gastrinoma
Cavernous hemangioma	Vasoactive intestinal peptide tumor
Hemangioblastoma	Somatostatinoma
Infantile hemangioendothelioma	**Miscellaneous benign tumors**
Lymphangioma	Teratoma
Lymphangiomatosis	Mesothelioma
Muscular, fibrous, and adipose tumors	Myxoma
Leiomyoma	Chondroma
Solitary fibrous tumor	Langerhans cell histiocytosis
Angioleiomyolipoma	Spongiotic pericytoma
Lipoma	
Myelolipoma	

Table 3.3 Histological types of malignant of hepatic and intrahepatic bile ducts

Hepatocellular tumors	**Neurological and endocrine tumors**
Hepatocellular carcinoma	Neuroendocrine neoplasms
Fibrolamellar hepatocellular carcinoma	Malignant peripheral nerve sheath tumor
Combined hepatocellular-cholangiocarcinoma	**Miscellaneous malignant tumors**
Dual-phenotype hepatocellular carcinoma	Carcinosarcoma
Hepatoblastoma	Yolk sac tumor
Bile duct tumors	Chorioepithelioma
Intrahepatic cholangiocarcinoma	Malignant teratoma
Bile duct cystadenocarcinoma	Malignant rhabdoid tumor
Mucin-producing intrahepatic cholangiocarcinoma	Gastrointestinal stromal tumors
Special types of intrahepatic cholangiocarcinoma	Malignant melanoma
Vascular and lymphatic tumors	Malignant mesothelioma
Angiosarcoma	Synovial sarcoma
Malignant hemangiopericytoma	Osteoclast-like giant cell tumors
Epithelioid haemangioendothelioma	Desmoplastic small round cell tumor
Kaposi sarcoma	Histocytic sarcoma
Lymphoma	
Follicular dendritic cell tumor	
Extramedullary plasmacytoma	
Muscular, fibrous, and adipose tumors	
Leiomyosarcoma	
Rhabdomyosarcoma	
Fibrosarcoma	
Liposarcoma	
Malignant fibrous histiocytoma	
Undifferentiated(embryonal) sarcoma	
Myofibroblastic sarcoma	
Osteosarcoma	
Chondrosarcoma	

Cancers of The Second Military Medical University, the National Science and Technology Progress Award of China in 2012, which was led by Academician Meng-Chao Wu and Academician Hong-Yang Wang in EHBH.

3.2 British Hepatopathologist Professor Anthony PP

Professor Anthony worked in the Department of Pathology of Royal Devon and Exeter Hospital, University of Exeter, and he took part in constructing WHO Histological Classification of Hepatic and Intrahepatic Bile Duct Tumors in 2002. Professor Anthony firstly suggested the concept of liver cell dysplasia (LCD) in 1973 [19] and defined it as the result of chronic integration of HBV in hepatic cells which is a premalignant lesion, and the patients with liver cirrhosis complicated by LCD are at significantly higher risks to develop HCC and should be followed up with serum AFP testing. The above important concepts are still very classic even today and remain to be the research focus. At the beginning of our research in pathology of hepatic carcinoma, we were faced with the question of how to observe and understand LCD; related articles written by Professor Anthony became our key reference and guidance, based on which we reported the findings that DNA ploidy and nuclear atypia index in LCD were between normal and hepatic cells and HCC cells in 1988 [20, 21], demonstrating abnormal proliferating cell populations at different stages of premalignant progression, consistent with the basic features of premalignant lesions. Later, we reported in situ hybridization and immunohistochemistry of HBV, AFP mRNA and P21, DNA content and nuclear atypia via image dissector in premalignant condition of liver cancer in the first National Youth Academic Conference held by Chinese Pathological Society, Chinese Medical Association in Xiamen City in November, 1991, and won the Outstanding Research Paper Awards. Thereafter, we kept on conducting the research in genomic instability and proteomic screening of diagnostic markers related to premalignant lesions, such as dysplastic nodules [22] and hepatocellular adenoma [23].

When we were planning to compile Surgical Diagnostic Pathology of Hepatobiliary Tumors, I wrote to Professor Anthony to consult him about premalignant lesions of liver cancers and invited him to participate in writing the book on December 2, 2001. Though he wrote back to say that he was not able to write related articles because he had already retired despite his identity as an emeritus professor and honorary advisor in pathology on December 19 of the same year, he showed great encouragement and provided a list of reference books to us. He believed the book would be very outstanding in the field due to its wide-range coverage and adequate pathological materials with proper utilization. Much to my surprise, he mentioned that he had paid an academic visit in Shanghai in 1983 when I just graduated and started to work in the SMMU, and I felt very pity that I hadn't attend his lecture.

3.3 American Hepatopathologist Professor Anthony J. Demetris

Professor Demetris is the Director of the Division of Liver Transplantation Pathology of the University of Pittsburgh Medical Center (UPMC), Pennsylvania, USA, and the Director of Liver Steering Committee of International Banff Working Group on organ transplantation pathology. Professor

Demetris took the lead in developing the well-adopted International Criteria for liver transplantation pathology including acute rejection activity index (RAI) [24], and he received the honorable title of Starzl Professor of Transplant Pathology, belonging to the working group led by Professor Thomas E. Starzl who successfully performed the world's first liver transplantation. The first liver transplantation in our hospital was performed by Academician Meng-Chao Wu working group in 1978, and we reported the first pathological diagnosis of liver biopsy in 3 patients with posttransplantation complications in the Conference of diagnostic pathology of PLA in 1996. With more experience accumulated in liver transplantation pathodiagnosis, we realized much difference of theory and practice between liver transplantation pathodiagnosis and general surgical pathodiagnosis, and it was difficult for us to ensure the accuracy of each pathodiagnosis via liver biopsy due to the inadequate knowledge and training of liver transplantation pathodiagnosis. Hence, as a visiting scholar, I went to the Division of Liver Transplantation Pathology of Starzl Transplantation Institute in UPMC in 1999, which is one of the largest centers of organ transplantation in America. Pathodiagnosis of organ transplantations, mainly including the liver, kidney, heart, lung, small intestine, etc., was performed, and abundant data on transplantation pathology could be obtained in UPMC. Thanks to Professor Demetris's meticulous and thoughtful arrangement for my study there, I learned a lot from Professor Demetris and other pathological experts, receiving much advice and guidance in transplantation pathology.

During my study in the department of pathology, UPMC, I also learned how to investigate tumor genomic instability from Professor Sydney D Finkelstein's group. In his lab, radioisotope labeling DNA sequencing was used to screen tumor suppressor genes and loss of heterozygosity (LOH) profiles of microsatellites to investigate the biological features of tumors. Their researching idea and method meet the working characteristics and practical demand of molecular diagnostic pathology as well in our department. Professor Finkelstein has original insights into molecular pathology and was very supportive of my interest in the study of LOH features of tumor suppressor genes and microsatellites of HCC and intrahepatic cholangiocarcinoma (ICC). He helped me with the designing and conducting of the research, and I got abundant experimental data with an original article published with the direction of Professor Finkelstein [25]. Meanwhile, I took advantage of the rich collection of literature and the convenience of online search in the library of UPMC and completed the synopsis of the book *Surgical Diagnostic Pathology of Hepatobiliary Tumors*, fulfilling the preliminary work to compile the book before my return to homeland in 2000.

With the strong support of experts in the field of pathology, such as Professor Nai-Xin Zhang, who was then the Director of the Chinese Society of Pathology (CSP), I undertook the group leader of the National Pathology Cooperation Group of Hepatobiliary Tumors and Liver Transplantation in October, 2002. In the meantime, the book of Diagnostic Surgical Pathology of Hepatobiliary Tumors was finally published, in which we added the chapter of Pathodiagnosis of Liver Transplantation for the first time in China [10]. In 2005, our Pathology Cooperation Group took the lead in reporting the results of a multicenter pathology study of 665 cases with 1123 liver biopsies after liver transplantation [26], which was referred to as one of the most influential papers in the related field by BioMedLib of Biomedical Library, University of Minnesota. From 2007 to 2009, our Pathology Cooperation Group took the lead in organizing pathological experts to constitute Guidelines I and II for pathological diagnosis and grading of common diseases after liver transplantation [27, 28], had held several national conferences on liver transplantation pathology, and published a series of papers on the pathodiagnosis of special complications post-liver transplantation, such as a special subtype of acute rejection named as central perivenulitis and small-for-size syndrome [29–31], and we have also made reports of pathology of liver transplantation in several Chinese academic conference on Organ Transplantation. In 2010, we completed the research of pathodiagnosis via liver biopsy of 1147 cases of liver transplantation and won the second prize of Medical Achievements of PLA. And we edited the first domestic monograph of *Clinical Pathology of Liver Transplantation* in 2011 [32]. Right now, the *Practice guidelines for the pathological diagnosis of liver transplantation* (V2016) has been published.

Besides, our Department was equipped with an automatic DNA sequencer under the support of Academician Meng-Chao Wu in 2002, and we also applied the new detection items for genomic instability and study strategy based on paraffin section cutting learned from UPMC to analyze single nucleotide polymorphism (SNP) of HCC, genomic instability of hepatocellular adenoma, and clonal origin model of recurrent hepatocellular carcinoma (RHCC), which have become an important molecular pathological technique platform in our Department.

3.4 American Hepatopathologist Professor Kamal G. Ishak

Professor Ishak was the Director of the Department of Hepatic and Gastrointestinal Pathology in AFIP of American. He was the first person to suggest that hepatoblastoma was independent of HCC in 1967, reported hepatic angioleiomyolipoma in 1976, reported undifferentiated sarcoma of the liver in 1978, reported hepatic epithelioid hemangioendothelioma in 1984, and advanced the famous Ishak Index which is widely used to assess the degree of histological activity in chronic hepatitis in 1995. He has given lectures on hepatic pathology in American-Canadian annual meetings of pathology for 30 years and is one of the editors in chief of *Tumors of the Liver and Intrahepatic Bile Ducts*. Atlas of tumors pathology (2001 Edition) took part in constructing WHO Histological Classification of Hepatic and Intrahepatic Bile Duct Tumors (2000 Edition). During my study in UPMC, I had a chance to meet him. He showed great interest in the medical scale, academic research, hepatic surgery quantity, and the number of pathological specimens in our hospital and gladly accepted my invitation to visit our Department.

From October 27 to October 28 in 2002, the press conference of Surgical Diagnostic Pathology of Hepatobiliary Tumors and a national seminar of pathology of hepatobiliary tumors were held in Shanghai Medical College of Fudan University and Eastern Hepatobiliary Surgery Hospital, the Second Military Medical University, separately. The conference and seminar were mainly organized by the well-known pathologist Professor Shi-Neng Zhu, former vice president of Shanghai Medical University, and coeditors in chief of Diagnostic Surgical Pathology of Hepatobiliary Tumors. Professor Ishak gave the invited lecture of Malignant Hepatic tumors and attended the foundation ceremony of National Pathology Cooperation Group for Hepatobiliary Tumors and Liver Transplantation of Chinese Pathological Society held in the Department of Pathology, Eastern Hepatobiliary Surgery Hospital, the Second Military Medical University along with other pathologists including Professor Nai-Xin Zhang, the director of division of Pathology, Chinese Medical Association, and Professor De-Wen Wang, the director of Malitary Professional Pathology Committee. Professor Ishak kindly presented me with two books written by him and his colleagues and kindly gave his invaluable advice and suggestions on pathology of hepatic tumors to us [33].

Professor Ishak is expert at investigating new lesions and making new viewpoints based on observation under light microscope in a scientific attitude, which inspired us a lot. Academician Zhao-You Tang suggested that it is difficult to greatly improve the efficacy of early diagnosis and treatment of liver cancers without the researches from biological aspects, and we should conform to the pathological and biological researching trend to further tackle the task of curing liver cancers [34]. Academician Meng-Chao Wu also suggested that the instructive function of HCC diagnosis and treatment standards on individualized treatment is limiting without the involvement of the biological characterization of HCC, on which the research should be reinforced to foster the concept transformation of treatment [35]. They all illustrated clearly the researching trend to molecular diagnosis, molecular classification, and molecular target identification in pathology of liver cancers. Therefore, we began to put emphasis on new pathological diagnosis of HCC and new molecular pathodiagnostic method to improve the diagnostic effectiveness with the support of Academician Meng-Chao Wu [36–40]. And the criterion of tumor diameter less than 3 cm as the standard volume of pathological SHCC was adopted in diagnosis, management, and treatment of HCC (V2011) proposed by Ministry of Health of the People's Republic of China [41], which was the result of comparison between animal and human HCC models and could reflect the benign-to-malignant biological transformation and long-term prognosis. In addition, we demonstrated the characteristics of HCC immunohistochemical diagnostic profile [42], screening new biomarkers for tumor diagnosis [43, 44], genetic polymorphisms in genetic susceptibility of HCC [45], finding a new subtype of dual phenotype HCC (DPHCC), which is characterized by expressing both HCC and ICC biomarkers and highly aggressive [46], and we have carried on a series of investigations on the clonal origination and molecular detection of recurrent hepatocellular carcinoma (RHCC) [10, 47, 48] and put forward six molecular subtypes of RHCC clonal origins [49]. These findings may provide reference for RHCC individualized therapeutic strategy clinically.

Our multidisciplinary research conducted by our Department of pathology with other clinic departments and laboratories, supported by Academician Meng-Chao Wu, won the First Prize of Military Medical Achievements in 2014. In 2015, with the support of the seven Chinese Societies, we have presided over the "Practice guidelines for the pathological diagnosis of primary liver cancer: 2015 update" [50]. Right now, we are taking the lead to develop the *Diagnostic Criteria for Primary Liver Cancer of China*, which is organized by the National Health and Family Planning Commission.

3.5 American Hepatopathologist Professor Swan Nio Thung

Professor Thung is the Director of the Department of Pathology of Mount Sinai Medical Center and has published many influential papers with Professor Josep M Llovet, who is in charge of the projects on liver cancers in Mount Sinai Medical Center and is one of the major founders of Barcelona Classification of Liver Cancers (BCLC). At the Fifth Annual conference of international Academy of Pathology in Hong Kong, I made a report of clinicopathologic features of 3160 cases of primary hepatic tumors in November, 1996. As an important component of this conference, an international seminar on hepatic pathology was held by International Liver Pathology Study Group, consisting of 15 world famous pathologists including Professor Thung. This group holds a symposium in different cities around the world annually. And I'd like to quote the words written in her thesis "The magnificence of liver biology and pathology is best revealed through the window of the microscope," which was introduced in the foreword of the proceedings by the president of this seminar, and it's the very moment that we began to pay attention to the work of Professor Thung.

For above reasons, I invited Professor Thung to give us a lecture on"Special acute rejection: pathological diagnosis and differentiation," at the Second Symposium of National Pathodiagnosis on Liver transplantation held in Eastern Hepatobiliary Surgery Hospital, the Second Military Medical University, in June, 2009. The lecture evoked great repercussions, and there was a heated discussion on the pathological sections of American and Chinese liver transplantation cases. Thus, we decided to invite her to be a visiting professor of the Second Military Medical University with the strong support from the hospital and the university. Professor Thung showed much responsibility and concern and helped us a lot, including the revision of a paper reporting a rare RHCC patient, who received three surgeries and was diagnosed as HCC, sarcocarcinoma combining cholangiocarcinoma and fibrosarcoma, and recurrent fibrosarcoma of the liver, separately [7]. As Professor Thung published a representative research paper *The Microvasscular Invasion (MVI) of HCC* [51], in April 2015, I invited him to come to Shanghai to give us a brilliant academic report about MVI in the conference on "Practice guidelines for the pathological diagnosis of primary liver cancer: 2015 update" of China, which is organized by Chinese Society of Liver Cancer and China Anti-Cancer Association. Considering the difficulty in the pathodiagnosis of small specimen biopsy via liver tumor puncture, we invited Professor Thung to write the chapter of biopsy and pathologic diagnosis of hepatic tumor. We believe it will be beneficial for our readers.

3.6 Conclusions

In conclusion, there are many famous hepatic pathologists and experts, who give us great support and invaluable help, though we cannot list them all in this chapter. And I would like to say that we are doing what we should do to get a better understanding of the development of hepatosurgical pathology both at home and abroad. We have the deep realization of the shortcomings compared to other departments of pathology, and we know there is still a long way to go to reach the goals to standardize pathodiagnosis in the hepatic tumors, systematize molecular pathodiagnosis, and promote scientific pathobiological diagnosis. We should make more efforts to finally bring about effective therapies of liver cancers. My tutor, Academician Meng-Chao Wu once said, "The solitary goal of my life is to treat liver cancers, and it is the only mission for me to overcome the difficulties in treating liver cancers." We should keep on working and progressing with the inspiration of him.

It's such coincidence that the publication date of this book is just around the 94th birthday of my teacher, Academician Meng-Chao Wu, and the opening date of An-Ting New District of Eastern Hepatobiliary Surgery Hospital, the Second Military Medical University. And we would like to dedicate this book to them.

References

1. Edmondson HA. Tumors of the liver and intrahepatic bile ducts, Atlas of tumors pathology. Washington DC: Armed Forces Institinte of Pathology; 1958.
2. Cong WM, Wu MC, Chen H, et al. Two cases of focal nodular hyperplasia of the liver. J Clinic Hepatol. 1991;7(2):112–2.
3. Cong WM, Wu MC. Four cases of focal hepatic steatosis. Acad J Sec Mil Med Univ. 1992;13(1):93–4.
4. Cong WM, Wu MC, Chen H. Hepatic angiomyolipoma: one case report. Chin J Surg. 1992;30(10):618–8.
5. Cong WM, Wu MC, Chen H. Three cases of hepatic adenomatous hyperplasia. Chin Med J. 1993;73(4):212–2.
6. Zhu Z, Guo J, Dong H. Primary chondrosarcoma of the liver: a case report and review of the literature. J Med Coll PLA. 2011;26(3):128–33.
7. Zhao Q, Su CQ, Dong H, et al. Hepatocellular carcinoma and hepatic adenocarcinosarcoma in a patient with hepatitis B virus-related cirrhosis. Semin Liver Dis. 2010;30(1):107–12.
8. Cong WM, Wu MC. Significance of clinicopathology in quantitative measurement of DNA content in hepatocellular carcinoma. J Med Coll PLA. 1988;3(2):153–6.
9. Cong WM, Wu MC. The biopathologic characteristics of DNA content of hepatocellular carcinomas. Cancer. 1990;66(3):498–501.
10. Cong WM, Wu MC, Zhang XZ. Characteristic changes of DNA stemlines during hepatocarcinogenesis in rats. Chin Med J. 1992;105(7):535–8.
11. Cong WM, Wu MC, Chen H. Clinicopathological characteristics of small hepatocellular carcinoma (An analysis of 93 Cases). Chin J Oncol. 1993;15(5):372–4.
12. Cong WM, Wu MC. Progress and prospect on the clinicopathological study of small hepatocellular carcinoma. Chin J Hepatobiliary Surg. 2011;17(5):353–6.
13. Lu XY, Xi T, Lau WY, et al. Pathobiological features of small hepatocellular carcinoma: correlation between tumor size and biological behavior. J Cancer Res Clin Oncol. 2011;137(4):567–75.
14. Cong WM, Wu MC. Small hepatocellular carcinoma - current and future approaches. Hepatol Int. 2013;7(3):805–12.
15. Cong WM, Wu MC, Wang Y, et al. Primary liver tumors in China: a clinicopathological study of 3, 160 cases. Oncol Rep. 1997;4(3):649–52.
16. Cong WM. A color atlas of pathology of hepatobiliary tumors. Shanghai: Shanghai Scientific and Technological Education Publishing House; 2002.
17. Cong WM, Dong H, Tan L, Sun XX, Wu MC. Surgicopathological classification of hepatic space-occupying lesions: a single-center experience with literature review. World J Gastroenterol. 2011;17(19):2372–8.
18. Cong WM. Surgical pathology of hepatobiliary surgery tumors: People's Medical Publishing House; 2015.
19. Anthony PP, Vogel CL, Barker LF. Liver cell dysplasia: a premalignant condition. J Clin Pathol. 1973;26(3):217–23.
20. Cong WM, Wu MC, Zhang XZ. Quantitative studies on DNA content and morphologic features of liver cell dysplasia. Chin J Cancer. 1988;7(3):177–9

21. Cong WM, Wu MC, Zhang XZ. Quantitative studies on the DNA content and morphological features of liver cell dysplasia. Chin J Cancer Res. 1989;1(3):21–3.
22. Dong H, Cong WM, Xian ZH, et al. Using loss of heterozygosity of microsatellites to distinguish high-grade dysplastic nodule from early minute hepatocellular carcinoma. Exp Mol Pathol. 2011;91(2):578–83.
23. Liu HP, Zhao Q, Jin GZ, et al. Unique genetic alterations and clinicopathological features of hepatocellular adenoma in Chinese population. Pathol Res Pract. 2015;211(12):918–24.
24. Demetris A, Adams D, Bellamy C, et al. Update of the international banff schema for liver allograft rejection: working recommendations for the histopathologic staging and reporting of chronic rejection. An International Panel Hepatology. 2000;31(3):792–9.
25. Cong WM, Bakker A, Swalsky PA, et al. Multiple genetic alterations involved in the tumorigenesis of human cholangiocarcinoma: a molecular genetic and clinicopathological study. J Cancer Res Clin Oncol. 2001;127(3):187–92.
26. Cong WM, Zhang SY, Wang ZL, et al. Pathological diagnosis of 1123 liver biopsies from 665 liver transplantations. Chin J Pathol. 2005;34(11):716–9.
27. Chinese Pathological Group of Hepatobiliary Tumor and Liver Transplantation. Guidelines of pathology diagnosis and classification of common lesions after liver transplantation (I). Chin J Organ Transplant. 2008;29(1):49–51.
28. Chinese Pathological Group of Hepatobiliary Tumor and Liver Transplantation. Guidelines of pathology diagnosis and classification of common lesions after liver transplantation(II). Chin J Organ Transplant. 2009;30(10):626–8.
29. Cong WM, Lu XY, Dong H, et al. Clinicopathological classifications and significance of acute rejection after liver transplantation:an analysis on 1 120 liver biopsies. Chin J Clin Exp Pathol. 2011;27(2):117–20.
30. Cong WM, Dong H. Histological observation of small-for-size syndrome after liver transplantation: a cas report. Chin J Organ Transplant. 2010;31(10):635–6.
31. Cong WM, Wang ZL. Review and reflection of the development of liver transplantation pathology in China. Organ transplant. 2011;2(3):121–4.
32. Cong WM. Clinical pathology of liver transplantation. Beijing: Military Medical Science Press; 2011.
33. Ishak KG, Goodman ZD, Stocker JT. Tumors of the liver and intrahepatic bile ducts, Atlas of tumor pathology. Washington DC: Armed Forces Institinte of Pathology; 2001.
34. Tang ZY. Looking for the treatment trends of liver cancer from a biological standpoint. Chin J Hepatobiliary Surg. 2009;15(6):401–2.
35. Wu MC. Progress in the diagnosis and treatment of primary liver cancer. CAMS. 2008;30(4):363–5.
36. Cong WM, Wu MC. More emphasis on pathobiological features of hepatic tumors. Chin J Surg. 2010;48(15):1121–4.
37. Cong WM, Wu MC. Surgical pathological features of tumors of the liver and intrahepatic bile ducts. Chin J Hepatobiliary Surg. 2008;14(5):358–60.
38. Cong WM, Wu MC. Review and outlook on hepatic surgicopathology in China. Chin J Hepatol. 2013;21(2):90–2.
39. Cong WM. Thinking about the establishing a pathobiological diagnostic mode for hepatobiliary tumors. Chin J Clin Exp Pathol. 2013;29(1):3–5.
40. Cong WM, Wu MC. New ideas for the molecular pathological diagnosis of hepatocellular carcinoma and new strategies for the clinic treatment. Chin Med J. 2014;94(20):1521–3.
41. Ministry of Health of the People's Republic of China. Practice guideline for diagnosis and treatment of primary liver cancer (V2011). J Clin Hepatol. 2011;27(11):1141–59.
42. Dong H, Cong WL, Zhu ZZ, et al. Immunohistochemical diagnosis on hepatocellular carcinoma and intrahepatic cholangiocarcinoma. Chin J Oncol. 2008;30(9):702–5.
43. Jin GZ, Li Y, Cong WM, et al. iTRAQ-2DLC-ESI-MS/MS based identification of a new set of immunohistochemical biomarkers for classification of dysplastic nodules and small hepatocellular carcinoma. J Proteome Res. 2011;10(8):3418–28.
44. Jin GZ, Yu WL, Dong H, et al. SUOX is a promising diagnostic and prognostic biomarker for hepatocellular carcinoma. J Hepatol. 2013;59(3):510–7.
45. Zhu ZZ, Cong WM, Liu SF, et al. A p53 polymorphism modifies the risk of hepatocellular carcinoma among non-carriers but not carriers of chronic hepatitis B virus infection. Cancer Lett. 2005;229(1):77–83.
46. Lu XY, Xi T, Lau WY, et al. Hepatocellular carcinoma expressing cholangiocyte phenotype is a novel subtype with highly aggressive behavior. Ann Surg Oncol. 2011;18(8):2210–7.
47. Cong WM, Wu MC, Chen H, et al. Studies on the clinical significance of the clonal origins of recurrent hepatocellular carcinoma. Chin Med Sci J. 1992;7(2):101–4.
48. Zhu YY, Gu YJ, Lu XY, et al. Clone analysis of two cases of postoperative late recurrence of hepatocellular carcinoma. Chin J Oncol. 2014;36(6):450–2.
49. Wang B, Xia CY, Lau WY, et al. Determination of clonal origin of recurrent hepatocellular carcinoma for personalized therapy and outcomes evaluation: a new strategy for hepatic surgery. J Am Coll Surg. 2013;217(6):1054–62.
50. Chinese Society of Liver Cancer. Chinese Society of Hepatology, Chinese Society of Pathology, et al. Practice guidelines for the pathological diagnosis of primary liver. Cancer: update. World J Gastroenterol. 2016;22(42):9279–87.
51. Roayaie S, Blume IN, Thung SN, et al. A system of classifying microvascular invasion to predict outcome after resection in patients with hepatocellular carcinoma. Gastroenterology. 2009;137(3):850–5.

4 Clonal Origins of Postoperative Recurrent Hepatocellular Carcinoma

Wen-Ming Cong

In the traditional view, recurrent hepatocellular carcinoma (RHCC) is a sign of tumor metastasis and late stage of development, and it has lost the chance of radical cure [1]. But with the deepening understanding of the theory of clonal origin in HCC, more and more evidence showed that there are two major patterns for clonal origin of RHCC, namely, monoclonal or monocenter origin and polyclonal or multicenter origin [2–4]. However, these two patterns are difficult to determine accurately based on clinical manifestations and histomorphological observations. Therefore, to carry out study of RHCC clonal origin model, looking for molecular markers of tumor clone detection, and establishing the corresponding molecular pathological examination method, is not only an important basic theoretical problem but also a practical guidance for the clinical understanding of clonal origin patterns of RHCC, scientifically formulating individualized strategy to prevent and treat RHCC and improving therapeutic effectiveness and long-term survival rate of RHCC [5].

4.1 Occurrence of Recurrent Hepatocellular Carcinoma

It has been estimated that the global annual number of new cases and deaths of primary hepatocellular carcinoma (primary hepatocellular carcinoma, PHCC) were both more than 600,000 in the world, of which more than 50% occurred in China [6]. As the number of cases of surgical resection of PHCC increases, the incidence of RHCC has risen accordingly. According to different authors' reports, the 5-year cumulative recurrence rates after excision of PHCC can reach 60–100%, with liver recurrent tumors accounted for 80–95% [7]. The number of RHCC surgeries in our department was 830 cases during a period of 26 years from 1985 to 2011 and has been increasing significantly in the last 5 years, including cases with multiple recurrences and surgeries, according to incomplete statistics (Fig. 4.1). Therefore, the study on the histogenesis and pathogenesis of RHCC is of practical significance to formulate clinical individualized therapeutic strategy for RHCC.

W.-M. Cong (✉)
Department of Pathology, Eastern Hepatobiliary Surgery Hospital, Second Military Medical University, Shanghai, China
e-mail: wmcong@smmu.edu.cn

4.2 Clonal Origin of Recurrent Hepatocellular Carcinoma

4.2.1 Monoclonal and Polyclonal Origin

The origin of RHCC has long been a major concern and discussion subject since at least 20 years ago [2]. Two major origin patterns of RHCC are concerned. One is intrahepatic metastasis (IM) origin, derived from intrahepatic micrometastases which cannot be recognized with the naked eyes and excised entirely during surgery due to the microvascular invasion (MVI) [8–10], and the residual cancer cells will proliferate post-surgery of PHCC. Obviously, IM pattern has the same clonal origin with the primary tumor and is also termed as monoclonal or single center origin. The other is multicentric occurrence (MO) origin, derived from cancer-adjacent hepatocytes, or de novo tumor clone, which undergo long-term genomic variation leading to carcinogenesis, due to persistent HBV/HCV infection in the patients of chronic hepatitis or liver cirrhosis [11–13].

4.2.1.1 IM-RHCC

Monoclonal origin hypothesis of tumor was proposed in the 1970s that tumors are derived from accumulation of mutation and clonal proliferation of single cells in the tumor cell population. RHCC is traditionally considered as monoclonal in origin, arising from intrahepatic metastasis or recurrence of the residual cancer cells post PHCC surgery, which prompted the initiation of clinical course into the late stage of invasion and metastasis.

W.-M. Cong (ed.), *Surgical Pathology of Hepatobiliary Tumors*, DOI 10.1007/978-981-10-3536-4_4

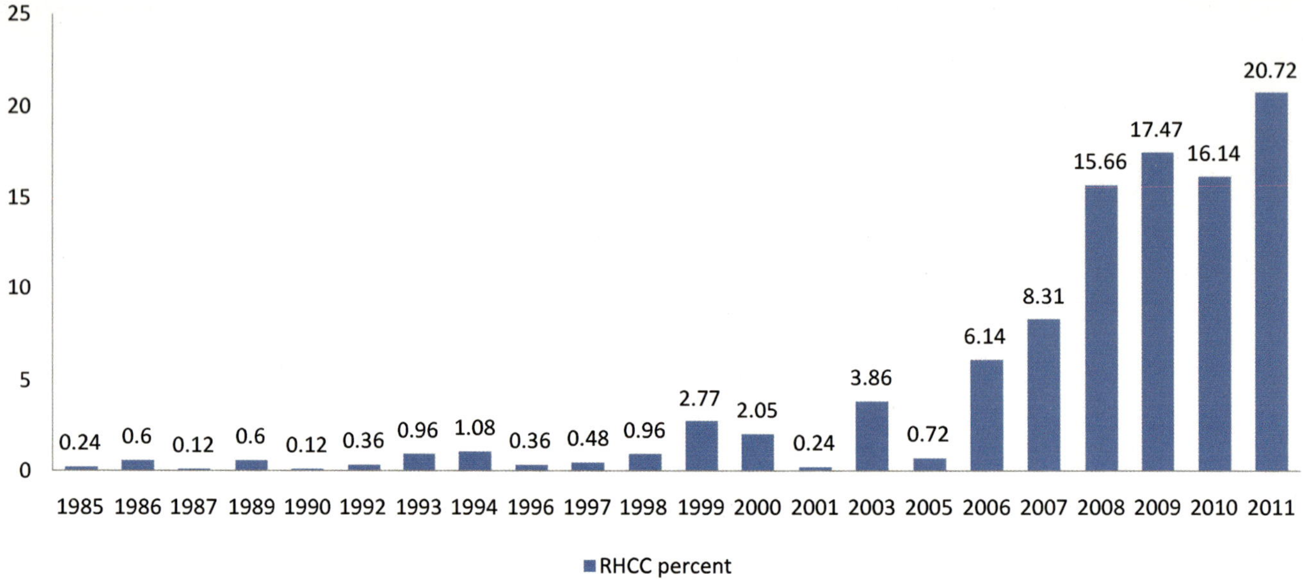

Fig. 4.1 Surgical resection of RHCC in Eastern Hepatobiliary Surgery Hospital

As we know, an adult liver contains about 500 thousand–1 million hepatic lobules, mainly composed of liver cell plates and hepatic sinusoid, and each lobule is surrounded by 3–4 portal areas, containing vasculature of interlobular artery, interlobular vein, and interlobular bile ducts, which facilitates the MVI and intrahepatic metastasis of HCC and is the histological basis for IM-RHCC. The reported incidence of MVI in PHCC is 15% to more than 60% [8–10], and the larger the tumor is, the higher risk of MVI is, which is the reason that more than 80% of the RHCC are mainly within the liver. According to our statistics of a group of HCC cases, the MVI rate in small HCC (≤3 cm in diameter) was 6.9%, among which even a microcarcinoma (0.6 cm in diameter) has also been observed with MVI [14]. Moreover, MVI has been recognized as one of the most important pathological indicators of both postoperative recurrence and metastasis risk and clinical prognosis after surgery [15].

4.2.1.2 MO-RHCC

The monoclonal theory of tumor proposed in 1976, that monoclonal proliferation is one of the main features of the tumor, laid an important theoretical foundation for the differentiation of tumor lesions and proliferative lesions, supported by most researchers considering multiple nodules, recurrent lesions, satellite lesions, and extrahepatic metastasis as monoclonal in origin. Until the late 1980s, with the development of molecular biological techniques which promoted the research of clonal origin of HCC, MO-RHCC was then discovered.

More attention has been paid to the mechanism of polyclonal origin of RHCC since the late 1990s. One of the reasons is the fact that more than 80% of PHCC patients in China have HBV-related chronic hepatitis or liver cirrhosis. HBV-DNA integrate into the genome of the host liver cell randomly, and precancerous lesions such as atypical hyperplasia and dysplastic nodules distribute throughout the liver with heterochronous carcinogenesis and multicenter origins. These contribute to the pathological basis of MO-RHCC. According to current RHCC molecular detection, the proportion of MO-RHCC is about 15–30%.

The interval between PHCC excision and RHCC occurrence is variable from less than 1 year to more than 10 years, making it difficult to preserve paired fresh tissue specimens for a long period to detect molecular clones. Supported by the National Natural Science Foundation of China, the author explored the microsatellite LOH pattern difference detection and determined the six molecular clone types or origin patterns of RHCC, via screening loss of heterozygosity (LOH) of high-frequency microsatellite DNA: type I, single nodular polyclonal RHCC via de novo tumor clone; type II, single nodular monoclonal RHCC via intrahepatic metastasis of PHCC; type III, single nodular monoclonal RHCC with its intrahepatic metastasis nodules; type IV, polyclonal and multinodular MO-RHCC; type V, single nodular polyclonal RHCC with its intrahepatic metastasis nodules; and type VI, combined polyclonal MO-RHCC and metastatic nodules from PHCC [16].

Differences of the above six types reflect the different mechanisms and pathways of RHCC providing a reference for clinical treatment of RHCC patients individually based on the clonal characteristics of HCC. As reported in the current literature, MO-RHCC and IM-RHCC constituted 15–30% and 70–85% of total RHCC, respectively, and the patients' average survival times post-surgery were

130 months and 80 months ($P < 0.05$), respectively, suggesting the better curative effect of reoperation for MO-RHCC [17].

4.2.2 Multifocal Growth and Multicentric Origin

Field cancerization theory was proposed by Slaughter in 1953 and remains to constitute the theoretical basis of pathogenesis of epithelial tumor. He hypothesized that one or multiple precancerous epithelial cells underwent sequential tumor genetic or epigenetic transformation to form primary field tumor (PFT) due to the impact of carcinogenic factors, whose persistent existence would facilitate the same genetic mutation and the formation of second field tumor (SFT) derived from the precancerous epithelial cells around the PFT [18, 19]. Theoretically, the molecular range of precancerous lesions is larger than the actual range of solid tumors. And dynamic multistage evolution and clonal selection of precancerous lesions in the region would lead to multifocal tumors with or without heterochrony. Different from tumors with multicentric origins, if PFT, SFT, and local recurrence (LR) of PFT share the same molecular variation or genetic alterations, they are determined as the same or monoclonal origin. However, if a tumor derives from another region, it's determined as a second primary tumor (SPT) and is a multicentric origin tumor. Thus, not all multifocal or recurrent tumors are multicentric origin tumors arising from de novo tumor clone, and it is apparently difficult to differentiate the clonal origins of PET, SFT, LR, and SPT clinically or histologically despite their different pathogenesis.

Slaughter's field cancerization hypothesis has already been confirmed in a variety of common epithelial tumors and is a practical reference for the investigation of clonal origin of RHCC. Studies have shown the significant difference among genetic methylation frequencies of HCC tissues, surgical margin, chronic hepatitis, and liver cirrhosis, suggesting the regional canceration in the liver, which reveals the variation and complexity of pathogenesis and origins of RHCC. Previous discussions of RHCC diagnosis, prevention, and treatment are more related to IM-RHCC, while we now should take the prevention and treatment of MO-RHCC into account, including the determination of molecules of PHCC, the prevention and repairing of genetic mutations and the progression of precancerous lesions in HBV/HCV infection areas, and early identification of precancerous cells with normal morphology and highly malignant tendency in the field. So, local canceration hypothesis is of practical significance to guide surgical resection, prevention, diagnosis, and treatment of PHCC. It can be deduced from the hypothesis that hepatic cells around HCC(T) have already had the genetic mutations to varying degrees and are in different stages of canceration in the patients with HBV/HCV infection, while their morphology remains basically normal. And these precancerous cells will continue the process of carcinogenesis to form LR or SPT after the so-called radical excision. Therefore, only when the PFT and all the cells with cancerous genetic mutations and biochemical alterations are excised will it be possible to completely prevent the recurrence of all forms of monoclonal tumor relapses or new tumor rerecurrences theoretically (Fig. 4.2).

Moreover, the clonal origin of liver tumors may involve malignant transformation and clonal selection within different tissues in terms of hepatic progenitor cells (HPCs). As mentioned above, determination of the clonal nature of tumors should be based on molecular pathology due to the complex and diverse clone types of RHCC. Microsatellite loss of heterozygosity (LOH) was applied for clone identification to diagnose the first case of multi-origin primary malignant tumors of the liver, which received the first HCC resection and later resection of intrahepatic cholangiocarcinoma and fibrosarcoma [20]. To improve molecular pathodiagnosis in the deparment of pathology, great importance should be attached to set up tumor molecular cloning detection methods [21].

4.3 Clinical Features of Recurrent Hepatocellular Carcinoma

4.3.1 Pathological Diagnostic Criteria

Shimada et al. described the characteristics of multiple nodular intrahepatic metastasis (IM) of HCC grossly and microscopically including ① obvious derivation from portal vein tumor thrombus, ② multiple satellite nodules around the primary tumor, and ③ histological similarities between solitary tumors adjacent to the primary tumor [22]. As to RHCC, IM can be diagnosed if the recurrent tumor has a moderate to low degree of differentiation and a similar or lower grade to the original tumor. Besides, the Liver Cancer Study Group of Japan put forward the histological diagnostic criteria of MO including [23] ① moderately to poorly differentiated primary tumor and highly differentiated recurrent tumor, ② highly differentiated PHCC and RHCC, ③ RHCC with precancerous lesions or highly differentiated HCC surrounding poorly differentiated HCC or nodule-in-nodule appearance, and ④ RHCC with higher differentiation than that of PHCC. And the diagnostic criterion for IM is RHCC with poorer differentiation than that of PHCC. However, these histological criteria can't be applied to diagnose most RHCC, due to the extremely small proportion of highly differentiated HCC and high-grade dysplastic nodules (HGDN) in clinical practice. Moreover, the determination of differentiation degree and precancerous lesions is not completely object, easily affected

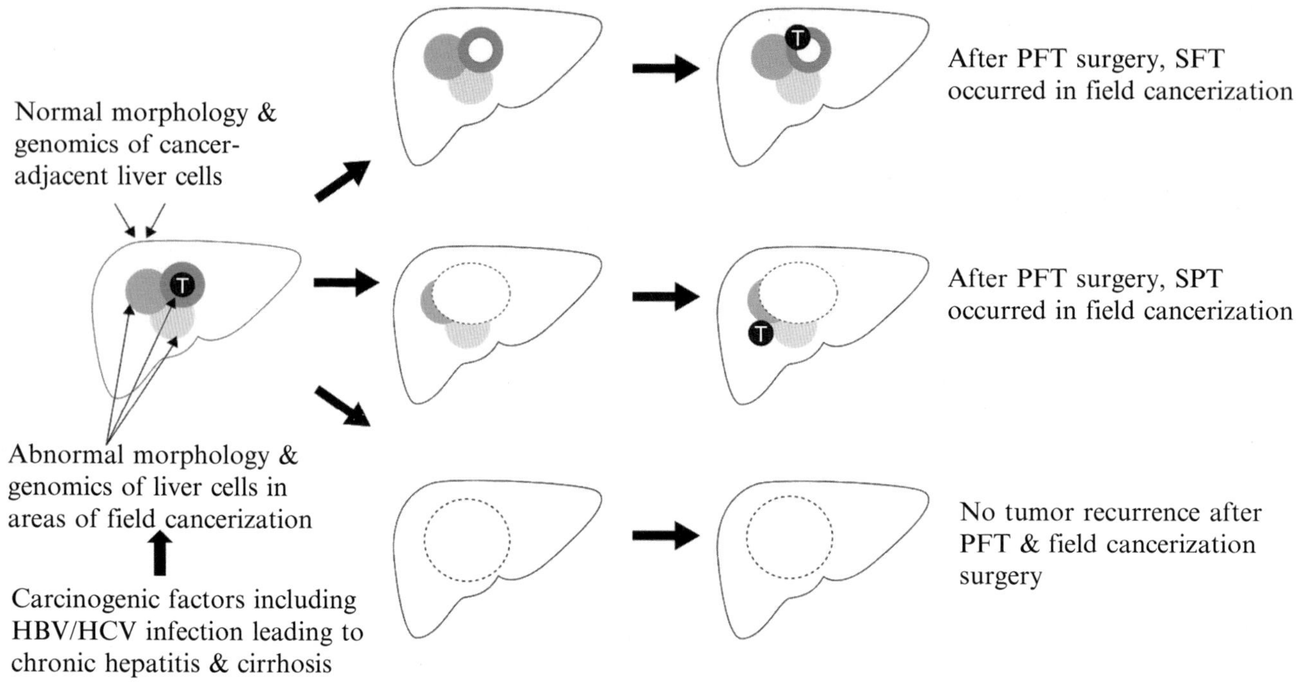

Fig. 4.2 Schematic diagram of the relationship between HCC and regional carcinogenesis and treatment mode

by subjective factors such as the working experience of the pathologists. Thus it is inaccurate to determine the clonal origin of RHCC simply based on the morphohistology of the tumors.

4.3.2 Clinical Diagnostic Criteria

Differentiation between recurrence of a residual lesion and a de novo tumor post-surgery is a key to develop therapeutic strategy and predict clinical prognosis scientifically. However, due to the inaccuracy of determining the clonal origin of a RHCC according to clinical manifestations, doctor's experience plays a major role. Currently, single center recurrence (IM-RHCC) refers to recurrence within 2 years post-surgery (short-term recurrence), and multicentric recurrence (MO-RHCC) refers to recurrence more than 2 years after tumor excision (long-term recurrence). Li et al. [24] detected the pattern of P53 mutation via PCR-SSCP and divided 12 cases into two groups, single center recurrence (6.5 ± 3.25 months) and multicenter recurrence (33.8 ± 17.8 months). They concluded that recurrence within 2 years post-surgery derived from single center or multicenters, while recurrence more than 2 years after surgery mainly derived from multicenters and thus was secondly primary carcinoma. However, our previous researches on molecular clone detection showed there was overlap of recurrence interval between IM-RHCC and MO-RHCC. For instance, in a molecular clone detection, monoclonal origin or recurrence of residual lesions was found in a RHCC 8 years post-surgery [4]. The author also reported a patient who occurred hepatic and colon metastasis from breast cancer 13 years after the surgery of breast cancer, and the patient received a second surgery for the metastatic tumors [25], indicating that residual cancer cells could stay silent or in a tumor-dormant state in vivo for a long time and proliferate again due to certain microenvironment changes even to metastasize.

The difference of serum AFP levels between PHCC and paired RHCC patients was also found to be associated with the difference of clonal origins. The recurrence intervals in group A (significantly different serum AFP levels between PHCC and RHCC patients) and group B (similar serum AFP levels between PHCC and RHCC patients) were 34.1 ± 3.8 months and 24.6 ± 2.7 months, respectively ($P < 0.05$), and recurrence intervals in group A type II and group B type II (recurrent tumors of different liver lobes) were 39.4 ± 5.9 months and 21.3 ± 4.1 months ($P < 0.05$), suggesting RHCC in group A has the features of MO-RHCC, such as the relatively longer growth periods of neoplasms in multistage growth pattern, and the difference of serum AFP levels may also reflect differences in tumor cell clone characteristics. Huang et al. [26] divided 82 RHCC into IM type and MO type post-surgery according to histological criteria; the recurrence intervals were 10.78 ± 7.9 months and 47 ± 31.69 months ($P < 0.001$), suggesting a possible relationship between recurrence intervals and tumor clonal origins. In principle, IM-RHCC-derived residual tumor post the first HCC excision is usually complicated with MVI or satellite foci formation, and this should primarily consider multi-modality therapy including interventional therapy (such as radiofrequency ablation, hepatic artery embolization chemotherapy, and biological therapy), while MO-RHCC is a de novo tumor in nature and is more suitable to be excised or treated by liver transplantation, the same effect of which can be acquired with the first surgery of PHCC. On this basis, the author proposed the relevance between clonal origin types and individualized treatment modes of RHCC (Fig. 4.3).

Yasui et al. [11] demonstrated a comparative study between 18 cases of MO-HCC and 64 cases of multinodular IM-HCC post surgery, and the results showed that 3-year survival rates and 3-year disease-free survival rates in MO-HCC group were 39% and 70%, respectively, which were significantly higher than those in IM group. However, total post-surgery survival rates in the two groups showed no significant difference despite patients of MO group were in the later AJCC stages at the time of surgery. Arii et al. [27] reported the survival rates of reoperation at 1 year and 3 years in HCC patients with intrahepatic recurrence were 100% and 80% in MO group and 91.7% and 38.1% in IM group, respectively, suggesting a better prognosis of surgical treatment in patients with MO-RHCC. Poon et al. [12] reported 246 cases of HCC post radical resection including 80 cases of early recurrence (≤1 year) and 46 cases of late recurrence (>1 year), among which 9 cases were diagnosed as IM receiving re-excision in early recurrence group and 6 cases were diagnosed as MO receiving re-excision in late recurrence group. The median survival time in the late recurrence group was significantly longer than that in early recurrence group (29.6 months vs. 15.8 months, $P = 0.005$). Huang et al. [26] divided the 82 postoperative cases of RHCC into IM group (54.9%) and MO group (45.1%) histologically, and the results showed significantly lower postoperative recurrence rate, higher postoperative overall survival, and recurrence-free survival rate in MO-RHCC group compared with IM-RHCC ($P < 0.001$). Matsuda et al. [13] reported 29 cases of RHCC with 31 excisions, divided into MO group (18 cases), IM group (4 cases), and undefined group (4 cases) histologically, and the 1-, 3-, and 5-year survival rates of patients were 100%, 69.7%, and 58.1% in MO group and 57.1%, 14.3%, and 14.3% in IM group ($P = 0.0016$).

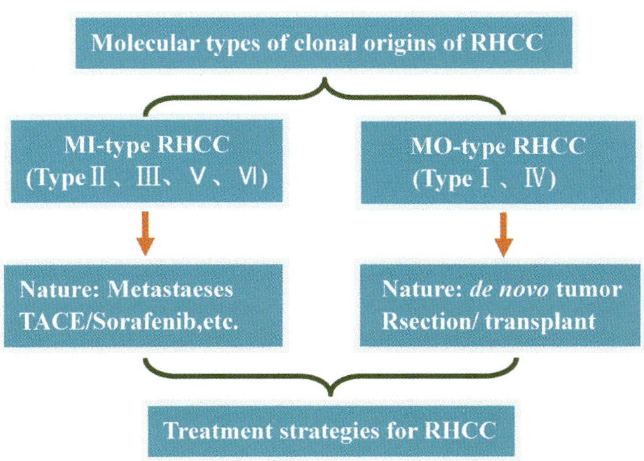

Fig. 4.3 Schematic diagram of clone classifications and individual diagnosis and treatment pattern of RHCC

As to liver transplantation for HCC patients, the core indicators in widely adopted criteria including Milan criteria, Pittsburgh criteria, and UCSF criteria are the diameter of the tumor, tumor thrombus in main vessels, and number of tumor nodules. It has begun to attract attention on the impact of clonal origin of multinodular HCC on long-term survival in liver transplantation patients. Finkelstein et al. [29] reported better postoperative survival in liver transplantation patients of multinodular MO-HCC compared with that of IM-HCC group, indicating the objective reference of molecular diagnosis in TNM staging, liver transplantation recipient screening, and prognosis assessment. Gehrau et al. [29] present a HCC diagnosis flow chart, and they proposed that patients with multiple HCC (>2 nodules) combined with molecular detection as MO type can be delivered in the assessment for liver transplantation, and for patients of IM type, TACE and targeted drug therapy with sorafenib would be the better choice.

4.4 Molecular Pathodiagnosis of HCC Clonal Origin

The existence of MO-RHCC and IM-RHCC has been confirmed by using molecular biological techniques, including DNA ploidy analysis, p53 gene mutation analysis, HBV-DNA integration analysis, X-chromosome inactivation pattern (XCIP) detection, comparative genomic hybridization (CGH) analysis, DNA methylation profile analysis, microsatellite LOH, chromosomal LOH, microRNA (miRNA) profile analysis, etc. [30–32]. Cheung et al. [33] studied 22 HCC nodules in six patients using cDNA microarrays containing 23,000 genes and found clonal relevance among HCC nodules via integrated analysis of 90 metastasis-related genes' differential expression, p53 gene mutation pattern and protein expression, HBV integration pattern, and comparative genomic hybridization of genes, but which is limited in clinical application because of its complicated process, heavy workload and high cost, and so forth. Microsatellite DNA is a good marker for overall stability of cellular genome and can facilitate PCR analysis with denser loci and more accurate location. Hence, analysis of chromosome with multiple high-frequency LOHs and a panel of microsatellite loci is beneficial to improve the accuracy in diagnosing the clonal origin of RHCC. Ng et al. [34]

compared microsatellite LOH, p53 mutation type, and HBV-DNA integration mode in terms of their properties in differentiating the clonal origin of multinodular HCC and concluded that microsatellite LOH is most widely used, suitable for samples with small DNA content, such as samples obtained via fine needle aspiration biopsy or liver biopsy and formalin-fixed paraffin-embedded (FFPE) tissue.

However, different detection methods and diagnostic criteria will cause significant difference in the proportions of molecular clonal patterns of RHCC. Ng et al. [34] reported 11 cases of nodular HCC with 25 nodules, among which MO-HCC and IM-HCC accounted for 36% and 64%, respectively. Morimoto et al. [35] reported 19 cases of RHCC with 52.6% MO-RHCC, 26.3% IM-RHCC, and 21.1% undefined cases. In another report conducted by Huang et al. [26], 54.9% IM-RHCC and 45.1% MO-RHCC were defined in 82 postoperative cases according to histological criteria.

It is worth noting that whole-genome microarray has been used to predict the prognosis and risks of intrahepatic recurrence and metastasis via screening of differentially expressed gene profile in RHCC after liver transplantation [28, 29]. And it can also be used to determine the clonal pattern, as shown in the report of miRNA expression profiles of ten cases of RHCC that expressions of miR-602, miR-451, miR-144, and miR-486-5p were significantly upregulated (>2.0 times) and expressions of miR-55 lb., mir-96, and miR-502-3p were significantly downregulated (<0.5 times) in early RHCC within 1 year after surgery, probably related to early recurrence of RHCC [36].

Tao et al. [37] analyzed the genomic variations of tumor tissues in six different regions (T1–T6) of the primary tumor (R0) excised in a RHCC and two recurrent tumors (R1, R2) using the methods of next-generation sequencing (NGS) of exon capture and whole-genome sequencing and detected 214 point mutations, including 205 point mutations (95%) detected in all three tumors, 24 mutations associated with amino acid changes, and 22 major domain insertions and deletions/copy number variations (>1 MB). They demonstrated the R0 tumor cell populations with these somatic mutations consist of four lineages (π0–π3) and are highly clonal, among which π0 cells contain all background mutations but without obvious proliferation. In addition, three protein-encoding mutations (CCNG1, P62, and an insertion and deletion/fusion gene, such as APC) were found to be the promoter mutation, and each lineage may hold only one lineage-specific protein-encoding mutation that initiates the proliferation and metastasis of R2 and R3 tumor cell populations. Furthermore, Alsinet et al. [38] suggested that a small amount of highly invasive and proliferative cells with the new mutation in the primary tumor cell population could form a new tumor nodule and continue to form new tumor nodules through similar clonal selection and proliferation. These results and analysis enrich our understanding in clonal heterogeneity of HCC, clonal selection mechanism during HCC development, and diversity and complexity of RHCC. Therefore, it is necessary to apply new technologies and new theories to the systemic investigation of the pathogenesis and diagnosis and treatment strategies of RHCC.

4.5 Prospection

The application of molecular cloning technique provides guidance for individualized clinical diagnosis and treatment of multiple and recurrent tumors. For instance, traditional classification according to the diameter and recurrent interval divides recurrent head and neck squamous cell carcinomas into LR and SPT, while they are classified into three types, LR, SFT, and SPT, using molecular biological detection methods. As to therapeutic strategy, radiotherapy or re-excision applies to postoperative minimal residual cancer which is highly risky to develop LR, regular diagnostic biopsy or chemotherapy applies to precancerous cells intra- or peri-surgical region which indicate high risk of developing SFT, and routine follow-ups apply to those without precancerous cells and the risk of developing SFT is low [37]. It is worthy of reference to integrate molecular diagnosis and therapeutic strategy in the study of RHCC.

At present, only a few researches on molecular cloning diagnosis of HCC have been reported abroad which focus more on the clonal analysis of multinodular HCC [14], and the results are similar with ours that interventional therapy is a preference for multinodular IM-HCC, while reoperation is suitable for multinodular MO-HCC. However, there are at least six subclonal patterns in multinodular HCC and therefore should be treated with comprehensible strategy according to the clinical pathological features of individuals.

In summary, with the rapid development of molecular tumor surgery, investigation on integrated treatment mode based on molecular clonal diagnosis and clinical individualized treatment of RHCC and multinodular HCC is promising in surgical diagnosis and treatment strategy of HCC. Further researches on molecular hepatopathology should be focused on the establishment of accurate identification and detection methods for tumor clonal origin and molecular boundary, predicting the risk of tumor recurrence, formulating the classifications and treatment pathways of RHCC according to molecular clonal evidence [17].

References

1. Tang ZY. Another discussion on the study of relapse and metastasis after adical surgery of liver cancer. Chin J Hepatobiliary Surg. 2001;7(11):643–5.

2. Cong WM, Wu MC, Chen H, et al. Studies on the clinical significance of the clonal origins of recurrent hepatocellular carcinoma. Chin Med Sci J. 1992;7(2):101–4.
3. Cong WM. Pathobiological characteristics of recurrent hepatocellular carcinoma. Chin J Prac Surg. 1995;15(5):269–71.
4. Zhu YY, Gu YJ, Lu XY, et al. Clone analysis of two cases of postoperative late recurrence of hepatocellular carcinoma. Chin J Oncol. 2014;36(6):450–2.
5. Cong WM. The pathological mechanisms of recurrence and metastasis of hepatocellular carcinoma and the evaluation strategies. Chin J Hepatol. 2016;24(5):324–6.
6. Gospodarowicz MK, Cazap E, Jadad AR. Cancer in the world: a call for international collaboration. Salud Publica Mex. 2009;51(Suppl 2):s305–8.
7. Nagano Y, Shimada H, Ueda M, et al. Efficacy of repeat hepatic resection for recurrent hepatocellular carcinomas. ANZ J Surg. 2009;79(10):729–33.
8. Eguchi S, Takatsuki M, Hidaka M, et al. Predictor for histological microvascular invasion of hepatocellular carcinoma: a lesson from 229 consecutive cases of curative liver resection. World J Surg. 2010;34(5):1034–8.
9. Sumie S, Kuromatsu R, Okuda K, et al. Microvascular invasion in patients with hepatocellular carcinoma and its predictable clinicopathological factors. Ann Surg Oncol. 2008;15(5):1375–82.
10. Roayaie S, Blume IN, Thung SN, et al. A system of classifying microvascular invasion to predict outcome after resection in patients with hepatocellular carcinoma. Gastroenterology. 2009;137(3):850–5.
11. Yasui M, Harada A, Nonami T, et al. Potentially multicentric hepatocellular carcinoma: clinicopathologic characteristics and postoperative prognosis. World J Surg. 1997;21(8):860–4.
12. Poon RT, Fan ST, Ng IO, et al. Different risk factors and prognosis for early and late intrahepatic recurrence after resection of hepatocellular carcinoma. Cancer. 2000;89(3):500–7.
13. Matsuda M, Fujii H, Kono H, et al. Surgical treatment of recurrent hepatocellular carcinoma based on the mode of recurrence: repeat hepatic resection or ablation are good choices for patients with recurrent multicentric cancer. J Hepatobiliary Pancreat Surg. 2001;8(4):353–9.
14. Lu XY, Xi T, Lau WY, et al. Pathobiological features of small hepatocellular carcinoma: correlation between tumor size and biological behavior. J Cancer Res Clin Oncol. 2011;137(4):567–75.
15. Chinese Society of Liver Cancer, Chinese Society of Hepatology, Chinese Society of Pathology, et al. Practice guidelines for the pathological diagnosis of primary liver cancer: 2015 update. World J Gastroenterol. 2016;22(42):9279–87.
16. Wang B, Xia CY, Lau WY, et al. Determination of clonal origin of recurrent hepatocellular carcinoma for personalized therapy and outcomes evaluation: a new strategy for hepatic surgery. J Am Coll Surg. 2013;217(6):1054–62.
17. Cong WM, Wu MC. New insights into molecular diagnostic pathology of primary liver cancer: advances and challenges. Cancer Lett. 2015;368(1):14–9.
18. Leemans CR, Braakhuis BJ, Brakenhoff RH. The molecular biology of head and neck cancer. Nat Rev Cancer. 2011;11(1):9–22.
19. Braakhuis BJ, Brakenhoff RH, Leemans CR. Second field tumors: a new opportunity for cancer prevention? Oncologist. 2005;10(7):493–500.
20. Zhao Q, Su CQ, Dong H, et al. Hepatocellular carcinoma and hepatic adenocarcinosarcoma in a patient with hepatitis B virus-related cirrhosis. Semin Liver Dis. 2010;30(1):107–12.
21. Cong WM, Dong H, Wang B, et al. Discussion on the clinical and pathological characteristics of recurrent liver cancer. Chin J Prac Surg. 2009;29(1):71–3.
22. Shimada K, Sakamoto Y, Esaki M, et al. Analysis of prognostic factors affecting survival after initial recurrence and treatment efficacy for recurrence in patients undergoing potentially curative hepatectomy for hepatocellular carcinoma. Ann Surg Oncol. 2007;14(8):2337–47.
23. Liver Cancer Study Group of Japan. The general rules for the clinical and pathological study of primary liver cancer. Jpn J Surg. 1989;19(1):98–129.
24. Li LQ, Peng T. Clonal origin of recurrent hepatocellular carcinoma and its relationship with time of recurrence. Chin J Hepatobiliary Surg. 1999;5(1):11–3.
25. Cong WM, Zhao X. A case of surgical resection of the liver and colon metastases after a mastectomy for breast cancer 13 years later. Chin J Prac Surg. 1999;19(6):335–5.
26. Huang ZY, Liang BY, Xiong M, et al. Long-term outcomes of repeat hepatic resection in patients with recurrent hepatocellular carcinoma and analysis of recurrent types and their prognosis: a single-center experience in China. Ann Surg Oncol. 2012;19(8):2515–25.
27. Arii S, Yamaoka Y, Futagawa S, et al. Results of surgical and nonsurgical treatment for small-sized hepatocellular carcinomas: a retrospective and nationwide survey in Japan. The Liver Cancer Study Group of Japan. Hepatology. 2000;32(6):1224–9.
28. Finkelstein SD, Marsh W, Demetris AJ, et al. Microdissection-based allelotyping discriminates de novo tumor from intrahepatic spread in hepatocellular carcinoma. Hepatology. 2003;37(4):871–9.
29. Gehrau R, Mas V, Archer KJ, et al. Molecular classification and clonal differentiation of hepatocellular carcinoma: the step forward for patient selection for liver transplantation. Expert Rev Gastroenterol Hepatol. 2011;5(4):539–52.
30. Das T, Diamond DL, Yeh M, et al. Molecular signatures of recurrent hepatocellular carcinoma secondary to hepatitis C virus following liver transplantation. J Transplant. 2013;2013:878297.
31. Mas VR, Fisher RA, Archer KJ, et al. Genes associated with progression and recurrence of hepatocellular carcinoma in hepatitis C patients waiting and undergoing liver transplantation: preliminary results. Transplantation. 2007;83(7):973–81.
32. Lou C, Du Z, Yang B, et al. Aberrant DNA methylation profile of hepatocellular carcinoma and surgically resected margin. Cancer Sci. 2009;100(6):996–1004.
33. Cheung ST, Chen X, Guan XY, et al. Identify metastasis-associated genes in hepatocellular carcinoma through clonality delineation for multinodular tumor. Cancer Res. 2002;62(16):4711–21.
34. Ng IO, Guan XY, Poon RT, et al. Determination of the molecular relationship between multiple tumour nodules in hepatocellular carcinoma differentiates multicentric origin from intrahepatic metastasis. J Pathol. 2003;199(3):345–53.
35. Morimoto O, Nagano H, Sakon M, et al. Diagnosis of intrahepatic metastasis and multicentric carcinogenesis by microsatellite loss of heterozygosity in patients with multiple and recurrent hepatocellular carcinomas. J Hepatol. 2003;39(2):215–21.
36. Barry CT, D'souza M, Mccall M, et al. Micro RNA expression profiles as adjunctive data to assess the risk of hepatocellular carcinoma recurrence after liver transplantation. Am J Transplant. 2012;12(2):428–37.
37. Tao Y, Ruan J, Yeh SH, et al. Rapid growth of a hepatocellular carcinoma and the driving mutations revealed by cell-population genetic analysis of whole-genome data. Proc Natl Acad Sci U S A. 2011;108(29):12042–7.
38. Alsinet C, Villanueva A, Llovet JM. Cell population genetics and deep sequencing: a novel approach for drivers discovery in hepatocellular carcinoma. J Hepatol. 2012;56(5):1198–200.

Tumor-Like Lesions of the Liver and Intrahepatic Bile Duct

5

Wen-Ming Cong, Yuan Ji, Xin-Yuan Lu, Long-Hai Feng, and Guang-Zhi Jin

5.1 Hepatocellular Tumor-Like Lesions

5.1.1 Focal Nodular Hyperplasia

Yuan Ji
Zhong-shan Hospital, Fudan University,
Shanghai, China

5.1.1.1 Pathogenesis and Mechanism

Focal nodular hyperplasia (FNH) was first reported by Edmondson in 1958, and the first case of FNH in China was reported in 1991 [1, 2]. FNH is a common benign tumor-like lesion with incidence rates of 0.6~3% in populations [3] and accounts for 8% among primary liver tumor [4] ranking the second common tumor or tumor-like lesion after liver hemangioma. Clonal feature detection of FNH showed that 50–100% of the liver cells were polyclonal and characteristic genetic mutations have not been found in FNH while vessel maturation-related gene (ANGPT1 and ANGPT2) changes were found in FNH. Compared with normal liver tissue, liver cirrhosis, and other hepatic tumors, the levels of ANGPT1 and ANGPT2 in FNH increased indicating vessel changes play a role in the formation of FNH, while others demonstrated the activation of β-catenin pathway without mutation of β-catenin [5].

5.1.1.2 Clinical Features

WHO proposed that 80–90% FNH cases occurred in women aged 30–40 years old, three quarters of the patients had a history of oral contraceptive in 2010. In China, FNH was reported to occur in patients aged 30–40 years with the ratio of male to female 1.8:1 to 1.6:1. Most of the patients had no history of oral contraceptive [6, 7], no clinical symptoms, and the disease was accidentally discovered in physical examination. A few cases had abdominal pain or other symptoms due to compression of the large masses on the surrounding organs, and they had no history of chronic hepatitis and liver cirrhosis with normal serum AFP, CEA, and CA19-9.

Imaging is an important method for the diagnosis of FNH. The sensitivity and specificity of FNH detection in regular contrast-enhanced CT examination and MRI are 75% and 92% and 70% and 98% [8], respectively. The images in ultrasound type B show that FNH has a variety of performances with clear boundaries, and the echoes can be stronger, equal, or weaker compared with the echoes of the normal liver tissue, with linear star-shaped echoes in the center of the image. In color Doppler examination, obvious blood flow can be observed inside the lesions indicating rich vasculature with trophic arteries in the center and star-shaped radiation branches. In CT inspection, FNH usually presents equal or low density in common scan, rapid enhancement in arterial phase, equal or low density in portal venous phase, and relatively high density in cases with a central scar. As to MRI examination, FNH presents equal signals in T1 phase, slightly higher or equal signals in T2 phase, and high signals for scars.

5.1.1.3 Gross Features

FNH is usually a solitary nodular gray-yellow mass similar to the color of the surrounding liver tissue, with a clear boundary and a medium texture, the size of which varies in the range of several millimeters to centimeters in diameter (Fig. 5.1a, b). Forty percent of the lesions present a fibrous scar in the center (Fig. 5.1a). A few cases have multiple FNH with smaller lesions, and central scars and nodular shape are not obvious (Fig. 5.1c), and the surrounding liver tissue is soft, delicate, and gray-red.

Y. Ji
Zhong-shan Hospital, Fudan University, Shanghai, China

W.-M. Cong (✉) • X.-Y. Lu • L.-H. Feng • G.-Z. Jin
Department of Pathology, Eastern Hepatobiliary Surgery Hospital, Second Military Medical University, Shanghai, China
e-mail: wmcong@smmu.edu.cn

W.-M. Cong (ed.), *Surgical Pathology of Hepatobiliary Tumors*, DOI 10.1007/978-981-10-3536-4_5

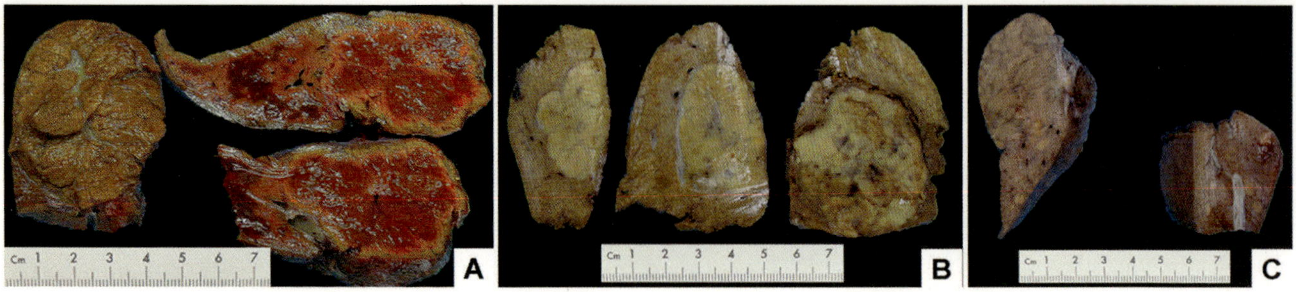

Fig. 5.1 Focal nodular hyperplasia. (**a**) Mass magin is clear and the fibrous scar can be seen in the center of the lesion; (**b**) The color of the mass is similar with the surrounding livers, nodular appearance; (**c**) multi-mininodular lesions with unconspicuous scar or nodular appearance

5.1.1.4 Microscopic Features

There is clear boundary between the tumor and surrounding liver tissue, with disappearance of the normal structure of hepatic lobules in the tumor lesions. FNH can be classified into classical FNH and nonclassical FNH according to microscopic features.

Classic FNH, accounted for more than 90% in FNH [7], consists of proliferated liver cells, bile duct, fibrous tissue, and vascular malformation, with varying amounts of inflammatory cells (Fig. 5.2) and a nodular performance (Fig. 5.2a). In the center of the lesions are scars formed by fibrous hyperplasia and vascular malformation. The vascular malformation has abnormal vascular intimal thickening due to fibrosis, uneven vessel wall thickness, and poor internal elastic membrane formation (Fig. 5.2b). The central scar tissue protrudes fibers to segment the entire lesion in nodular appearance, and it is very difficult to distinguish the obvious heperplasia of the fibers from liver cirrhosis (Fig. 5.2a, b), which is the reason for the previous term of "focal hepatic cirrhosis" for FNH. The liver cells in the lesion are similar to normal hepatic cells without atypia in funicular arrangement within two layers. Hyperplasia of small bile ducts is arranged in clusters in the boundary of fibrous tissue and liver cells, some of which are in poor tubular formation (Fig. 5.2c). And varying amounts of lymphocytes infiltrated the interstitial fibrous tissue. A proportion of liver cells in the lesion have changes such as fatty degeneration, and extramedullary hematopoiesis occurs in some interstitial tissues, and FNH complicated by metastasis adenocarcinoma has also been reported (Fig. 5.2d) [7]. The surrounding liver tissue of FNH is non-cirrhotic, though some may have fatty degeneration or be accompanied by HCC or cholangiocarcinoma.

Nonclassical FNH is rare and considered to be variants of FNH. Previous classification of nonclassical FNH includes telangiectatic FNH, mixed hyperplastic and adenomatous FNH, and atypical FNH. Telangiectatic FNH has been reported to be monoclonal and is similar to hepatocellular adenoma in molecular variation, with significantly different clinical manifestation from classic FNH, such as frequent rupture and bleeding. Thus, it has been classified as a special subtype of hepatocellular adenoma [9]. Few reports of other two subtypes are found in the literature, and there are no widely adopted diagnostic criteria for them.

Multiple FNH has a low incidence and was reported to be complicated by hemangioma or congenital absence of the portal vein [10, 11]. The number of lesions can be more than 20, and it has postoperative recurrence risk.

5.1.1.5 Immunohistochemistry

Catenin pathway activation leads to higher expression of downstream glutamine synthetase (GS) in FNH. The most important immunohistochemical markers are GS, CD34, CK7, and Ki-67 (Fig. 5.3). GS is expressed in hepatic cells around hepatic veins in a map-like distribution, and CD34 is mostly expressed in liver sinusoids diffusedly with focal distribution in some cases, while CK7 can be used to detect and outline the proliferated small bile ducts and Ki-67 suggests low proliferation index of FNH, mostly <1%. Other markers expressed in HCC are not detected in FNH, such as glypican-3, HSP70, and AFP.

5.1.1.6 Differential Diagnosis

FNH should be differentiated from hepatocellular adenoma and HCC. Hepatocellular adenoma is a hepatocellular clonal proliferated lesion without bile duct and occurs mainly in young adults aged 30–40 years old with no history of hepatitis or liver cirrhosis, which is easily differentiated from FNH. However, in inflammatory hepatocellular adenoma with reaction of bile duct, GS is a helpful indicator for differentiation according to its map-like pattern in FNH, diffused distribution in hepatocellular adenoma with β-catenin mutation, and negative result in other types of hepatocellular adenoma. HCC occurs mainly in older men with the history of chronic hepatitis and liver cirrhosis, containing atypical tumor cells with increased cell karyoplasmic ratio, thickened liver plates often more than three layers, and positive results of immunohistochemistry detection including alpha-fetoprotein (AFP), glypian-3 staining, and HSP70.

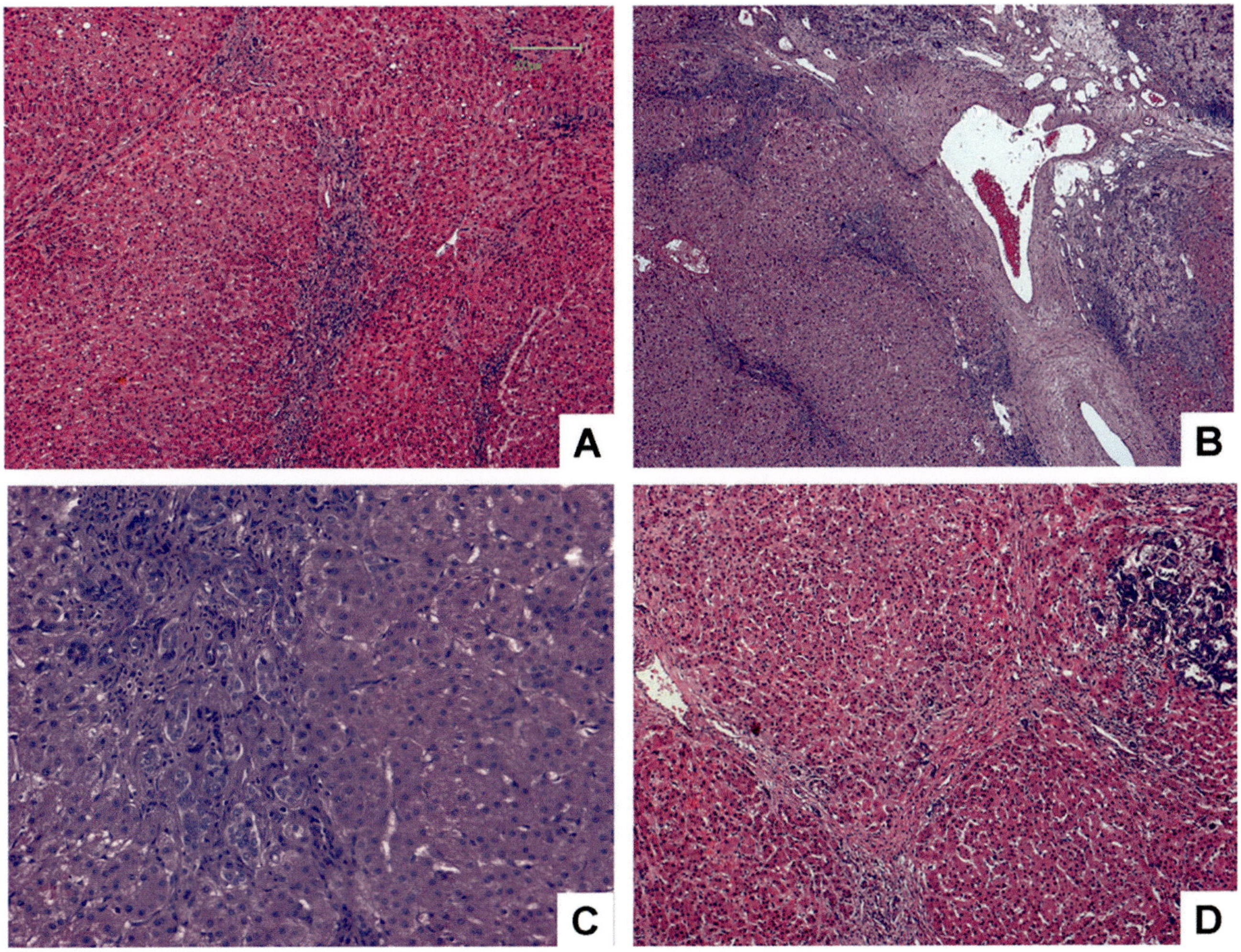

Fig. 5.2 FNH. (**a**) Hyperplasia fibrous segment the entire lesion in nodular appearance; (**b**) the center of the lesions is scars formed by hyperplasia fibrous and vascular malformation; (**c**) hyperplasia of small bile ducts, and inflammatory cells infiltrated; (**d**) FNH combined with adenocarcinoma metastatic

5.1.1.7 Treatment and Prognosis

In a follow-up study of 30 patients with 34 FNH lesions by ultrasound examination every 3–6 months over an average period of 42 months, the results showed that the lesions remained stable in 24 cases (70.6%), deteriorated in 1 case (2.9%), and improved or disappeared in 9 cases (26.5%). In the six patients with disappeared lesions, older age and longer period were independent factors, and their average period for the disappearance of lesions was 59 ± 30 months [12]. FNH presents no malignant transformation but may occasionally rupture and bleed [13]. For asymptomatic small lesions, regular follow-up is recommended, and surgical treatment should be applied to those with large tumor masses, significant symptoms, undefined diagnosis, or rapid tumor growth during clinical observation [6].

5.1.2 Nodular Regenerative Hyperplasia

Wen-Ming Cong and Xin-Yuan Lu
Department of Pathology, Eastern Hepatobiliary Surgery Hospital, Second Military Medical University, Shanghai, China

5.1.2.1 Pathogenesis and Mechanism

Nodular regenerative hyperplasia (NRH) was first described as a "miliary liver adenomatosis" by Ranstrom in 1953 and named as NRH by Steiner in 1959. The mechanism involves hepatic portal vein blood flow disorder caused by various factors, such as portal vein tumor thrombus derived from primary or metastatic hepatic tumors, hematopathy, blood disease, the toxicity of chemotherapy drugs (including

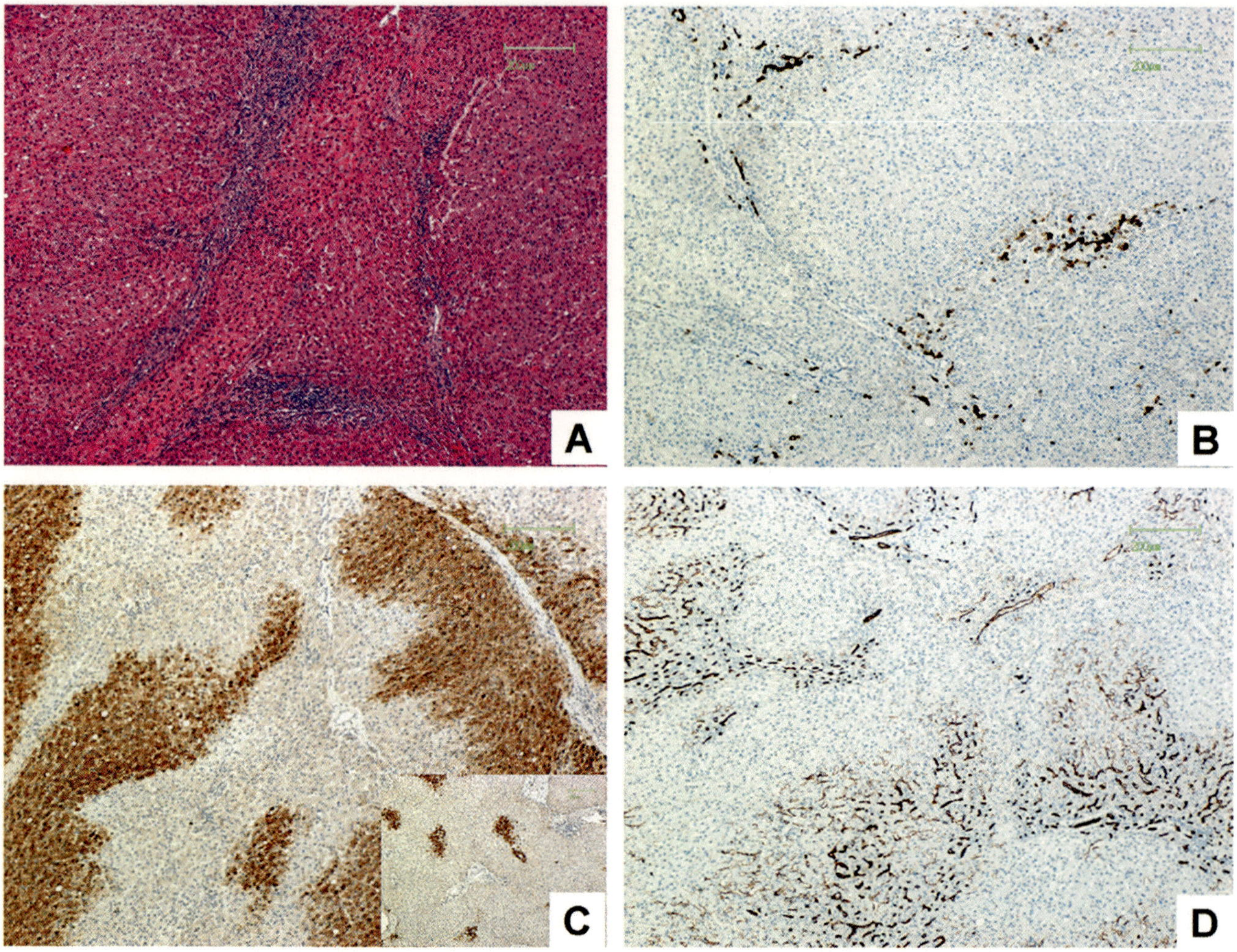

Fig. 5.3 Classic FNH. (**a**) The liver tissue was segment into nodules by fibrous, small bile hyperplasia ducts and inflammatory cells infiltrated in fibrous scar; (**b**) CK7 staining showed hyperplasia of small bile ducts in the boundary of fibrous tissue and liver cells; (**c**) GS staining showed positive cells distributed like a map, while the positive cells in the normal liver tissue were located in the periphery of the small hepatic vein showed as the *right-down* figure; (**d**) CD34 staining showed rich blood sinus distributed in focal or diffused

thiopurine drugs, anti-retroviral drugs [14, 15]), connective tissue disease, primary biliary cirrhosis (PBC), primary sclerosing cholangitis (PSC), hepatopulmonary syndrome (HPS) after liver transplantation, Budd-Chiari syndrome, immunological diseases (Felty syndrome, rheumatoid arthritis, splenomegaly, and leukopenia), myeloproliferative disease, tuberculosis, lymphoma, macroglobulinemia, polycythemia, renal transplantation, and HIV infection [16]. The common characteristics of the above diseases are endothelial inflammation and microvascular thrombosis inside the portal vein, resulting in deposition of red blood cells in Disse spaces of liver sinusoids and small branches of portal vein, causing obstruction or reduction in number, leading to sinusoidal obstructive syndrome (SOS), noncirrhotic intrahepatic portal hypertension (NCIPH), and further ischemic atrophy of the involved liver parenchyma and secondary reactive hyperplasia related to increasing blood flow of other small branches of portal vein, thus forming diffuse nodular hyperplasia without fibrous septa [17].

5.1.2.2 Clinical Features

NRH is the second most common cause of non-cirrhotic portal hypertension, with hepatosplenomegaly, portal hypertension, and other complications, such as esophageal varices and ascites, in half or more patients. NRH occurs mostly in adults. Jinjing Liu et al. reported 22 cases of NRH with an average age of 43 years old (22–70 years old) [18]. In the Department of Pathology, Eastern Hepatobiliary Surgery Hospital, Second Military Medical University, eight cases of NRH have been diagnosed since 1982, with male to female ratio of 7:1, aged 29–55 years old with an average of 44 years old. Lin Fang et al. reported a male patient of 34 years old who was admitted because of 1 year's fatigue and abdominal distension in 2011 [19]. And the color Doppler ultrasound suggested liver cirrhosis, splenomegaly, and portal hypertension, and liver MRI demonstrated multiple small nodules in the liver, compression and attenuation of the hepatic vein, and enlargement of the spleen and splenic vein. Liver puncture biopsy showed complete structure of liver tissue, crowded liver plates, nodular hyperplasia of liver cells with no fibrous enclosure, and atrophy of surrounding liver cells due to compression. Albuquerque [20] reported a case of familial NRH in 2013 in which the mother and daughter both had NRH with non-cirrhotic portal hypertension and similar complications including variceal hemorrhage and hepatopulmonary syndrome.

5.1.2.3 Gross Features

Lesions are diffuse nodules in the liver with a granular envelope, similar to small cirrhotic nodules, with brown or yellowish brown section lighter than the color of the surrounding normal liver tissue. The common size of the lesions is within 5 mm in diameter, usually 1–3 mm; thus, they were called micronodular transformation (Fig. 5.4). In a few cases, the nodular size reaches 5 cm due to nodular fusion.

5.1.2.4 Microscopic Features

Liver lobules with NRH nodular hyperplasia contain diffused nodules instead of normal tissue with disorderly structure and similar size compared to normal tissue. The proliferated liver cells show no atypia and are arranged into 1–2 layers of liver plates which go in various directions and interleaved with each other instead of converging into central vein. Hepatocellular boundary is observed between the nodules with no fibrous septa (Fig. 5.5), and reticular staining shows inter-nodular atrophy of the liver tissue and collapse of reticular scaffold. Usually, NRH nodules distribute around portal vein branches, especially in the portal area. In almost all cases, small branches of portal vein less than 0.05 cm in diameter contain general stenosis and occlusive lesions which are rarely observed in punctured tissues. Hepatic cells are enlarged or weakly dyed with loose and translucent cytoplasm, due to varying amounts of intracellular glycogen and fatty vacuoles, and internodular hepatic cells show atrophy with decreased volumes and red-dyed cytoplasm due to compression, thus forming the specific structure of bright region and dark region. Lysozyme staining shows the endothelial cells in the hepatic sinusoids and Kupffer cells inside the nodules. Besides, each NRH nodule often involves only one portal area and is also known as single acinar regenerative nodules.

Based on the above, the diagnostic criteria of NRH include: ① diffused hepatocellular hyperplasia nodules in the whole liver, ② intranodular hyperplasia and atrophy of liver cells, ③ no fibrous envelope around the regenerative nodule, and ④ no or rare inflammation in the portal area.

5.1.2.5 Differential Diagnosis

NRH are similar to small nodular cirrhosis both clinically and in gross appearance. In NRH, the nodules are soft, and the internodular boundary is unclear with gradual transition between intra- and extra-nodular liver cells. Non-internodular fibrous septa are the main histological feature to differentiate NRH from cirrhosis regenerative nodules. Masson trichrome staining shows no fibrous envelope around the nodules. NRH should also be differentiated from hepatic focal nodular hyperplasia, hepatocellular adenoma, congenital hepatic fibrosis (CHF), and HCC (Table 5.1). Liver puncture biopsy

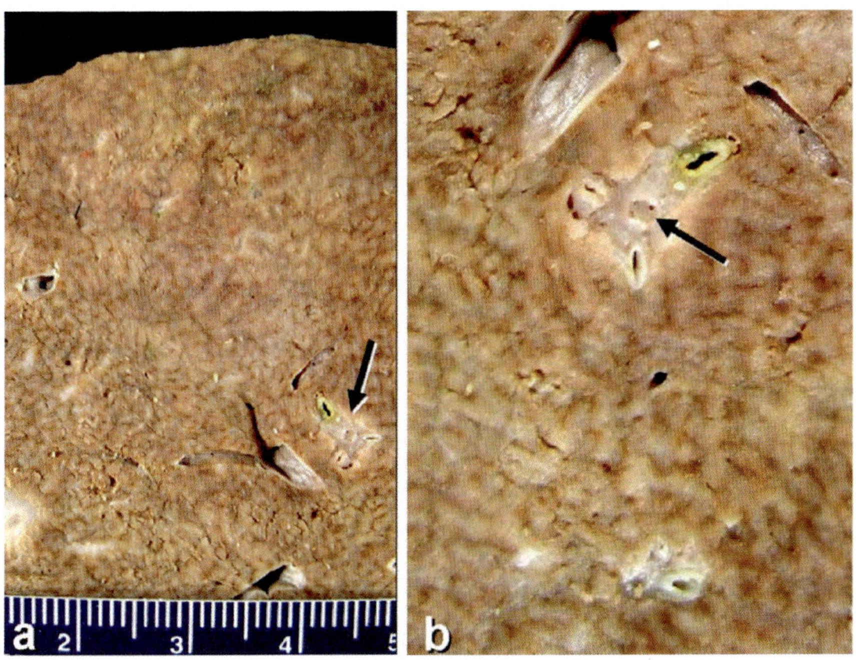

Fig. 5.4 Nodular regenerative hyperplasia. Small nodules ≤ 3 cm in diameter, the portal vein tumor thrombus in the liver metastasis of breast cancer is indicated by the arrow (Cite from Turk AT)

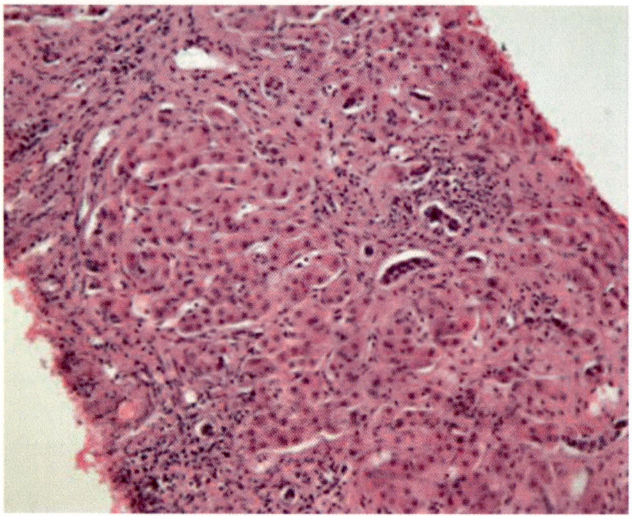

Fig. 5.5 Liver biopsy tissue showed hepatocellular hyperplasia nodules

Table 5.1 Differential diagnosis of common nodular regenerative hyperplasias

Diseases	Pathological features
Nodular regenerative hyperplasia	Multiple lesions in the liver, consistent in size, without internodular fibrous septa, with stenosis, occlusion, or malformation/ deviation of branches of the portal vein
Regenerative nodules in hepatic cirrhosis	A single lesion or multiple lesions with obvious inflammation and necrosis, various sizes, surrounded by inflammatory fibrous tissue
Focal nodular hyperplasia	A single nodule with stellate scar in the center consisting of multi-branched fibrous tissue which is rich in thick-walled vessels, and the vessel wall contains fibromuscular hyperplasia and concentric or eccentric stenosis in the vessels.
Hepatocellular adenoma	A single tumor or a few large tumor nodules, without portal area involvement

can be used to diagnose but with much difficulty, and an open wedge liver biopsy is alternative when necessary [21].

5.1.2.6 Treatment and Prognosis

NRH is a benign lesion and should receive symptomatic treatment due to the increase in the size and number of lesions, and the major complications are portal hypertension and late-term liver failure. The prognosis of NRH is generally good if the portal hypertension is well treated. Radomski et al. (2000) reported four cases of liver transplantation in NRH patients, who survived with normal hepatic function during the 2–4 years' follow-up. Alhosh et al. [22] reported a case of a 3-year-old boy who was diagnosed as NRH and received the first liver transplantation, and he received a second liver transplantation 2 years later due to hepatopulmonary syndrome with good recovery, normal hepatic function, improved hepatopulmonary syndrome, and normal oxygen saturation both at rest and in activity [22]. There is no evidence of canceration of NRH; however, Sood et al. [21] reported HCC in a 44-year-old woman with Turner syndrome, and the relevance of HCC and Tuner syndrome should be further investigated [23].

5.1.3 Partial Nodular Transformation

5.1.3.1 Pathogenesis and Mechanism

Partial nodular transformation (PNT) was first named by Sherlock and colleagues in 1966, though similar lesions were first reported early in 1090. PNT is an independent lesion, and more than ten cases have been reported, while some people regard it as a variant of NRH. PNT is characterized by large nonfibrous hyperplastic nodules formed by hepatocellular in nonfibrous or non-cirrhotic liver, which is also called non-cirrhotic nodule, primarily distributed along larger intrahepatic portal vein branches or portal tracts in periportal area. The pathogenesis of PNT is considered to be obstruction of the vessels in the hepatic hilar region or major branches of intrahepatic portal veins or hepatic veins, such as thrombosis in Felty syndrome (characterized by rheumatoid arthritis, with splenomegaly and reduction of white blood cells), which facilitates the communication of the obstructed vessels with the main portal veins in the portal area, resulting in regional hypoperfusion leading to atrophy of the liver parenchyma, and portal hyperperfusion to form fusion of multiple nodules. Hoso et al. (1996) reported a case of multiple PNT surrounding the intrahepatic tumor thrombus in the main portal vein, and the largest nodule was 8 cm in diameter without a fibrous envelope. PNT caused by secondary thrombosis were also reported in literature, due to occlusion of portal venous branches and portal cirrhosis in patients with idiopathic portal hypertension (IPH). Wanless et al. (1985) reported one case of a 29-year-old male with patent ductus venous, 15 mm in length and 15 mm in diameter. In this case, a portion of the portal venous blood was directly drained into the inferior vena cava via the umbilical vein, and several fistulae communicated the patent ductus venous with left hepatic vein and inferior vena cava, leading to dysplasia of intrahepatic portal venous vasculature and hyperplasia of partial liver parenchyma, which contributed to the formation of two 4 cm-in-diameter PNT nodules.

5.1.3.2 Clinical Features

Patients' clinical manifestation is characterized by presinusoidal portal hypertension.

5.1.3.3 Gross Features

PNT appears to be multiple nodules in varying sizes, with diameter of 0.3–4 cm, and is also called macronodular transformation.

5.1.3.4 Microscopic Features

The hyperplastic nodules distribute surrounding main branches of portal veins with blood or tumor thrombus in them. The nodules consist of proliferated liver cells and show the arrangement of 2–3 layers of liver plates via reticular fiber staining, with visible capillary bile duct and bile thrombi. Internodular region is composed of atrophic liver cells, without the formation of fibrous septum in Masson staining. Though PNT and NRH are similar histologically, PNT nodules tend to form larger nodules which are often several centimeters in diameter and are located mainly in the hepatic hilar region or along main branches of portal vein, while NRH are distributed diffusedly.

Supplementary: Idiopathic Portal Hypertension

Idiopathic portal hypertension (IPH) is classified as a benign nodular hepatocellular lesion, as well as NRH and FNH, and is related to liver hemodynamic disorder, characterized by increased flow resistance of presinusoidal portal veins and portal hypertension. IPH commonly appears in diffused lesions, due to chronic ischemia leading to hepatic parenchymal atrophy and nodular regeneration. However, nodular hyperplasia has been discovered in many cases. In addition, IPH, also known as non-cirrhotic portal fibrosis (NCPF) [24], shows undefined boundary without fibrous septa under the microscope. The portal fibrous tissue and bile ducts proliferate and stretch out into the hepatic parenchyma, with mild edema and infiltration of lymphocytes, and there is no interface inflammation or necrosis of hepatocytes. And the liver tissue is surrounded by incomplete fibrous envelope forming nodules with occlusion in small branches of portal veins and cirrhosis of central vein. IPH-related hepatic nodular lesions are benign disease with rare report of canceration.

5.1.4 Precancerous Lesions

Wen-Ming Cong, Long-Hai Feng, and Guang-Zhi Jin
Department of Pathology, Eastern Hepatobiliary Surgery Hospital, Second Military Medical University,
Shanghai, China

Among precancerous lesions, dysplastic foci (DF) and dysplastic nodule are of the most importance [25].

5.1.4.1 Dysplastic Foci

Pathogenesis and Mechanism

Dysplastic foci (DF), first proposed in the international consensus of terminology of hepatic nodular lesions by International Working Group (IWP) of World Gastroenterology Organisation in 1995, were defined as small liver cell dysplasia (LCD) with a diameter <1 mm which cannot be identified by radiological imaging or with the naked eye [26, 27]. DF are often multiple lesions in patients with chronic hepatitis, especially those with liver cirrhosis. LCD was described by British pathologist Anthony in 1973 for the first time, and he suggested that LCD was a precancerous lesion of HCC. Later Japanese researchers, Watanabe et al., classified LCD into two major types, small-cell dysplasia and large-cell dysplasia, in 1983, which are now known as small cell change and large cell change, in which DF is consisted mainly of small cell change or large cell change.

Microscopic Features

1. Small cell change. Small liver cells with decrease in size and increase in nucleocytoplasmic ratio, and the cytoplasm is basophilic. The nucleus is mildly pleomorphic and atypical, darker in color and crowded-like. In some LCD, multinuclei is the major characteristic. The proliferative activity of small cell change is higher than that of the surrounding liver tissue, similar to the performance of early HCC (Fig. 5.6a). The risk of canceration of small cell change-dominated DF with rapid proliferation is generally considered higher [28].
2. Large cell type. Hepatocytes in this type increase in size in proportion to their nuclei, resulting in normal nucleocytoplasmic ratio, with normal cellular density and cytoplasmic staining, while nuclear envelopes thicken and shrink, and atypia of hepatocytes with pleomorphic and dark-stained nuclei is commonly observed (Fig. 5.6b). Large cell change was previously considered as the feature of LCD by Anthony; however, whether LCD is a precancerous lesion is still in discussion, and WHO classification has not defined the property of LCD. Based on the literature, LCD with a history of HBV-/HCV-related liver cirrhosis is an important precancerous lesion supported by most researched. Since 1988, we have reported the results that the DNA ploidy and quantitative features of nuclear morphology are between that of normal liver cells and HCC cells, in consistent with the basic feature of precancerous lesion, suggesting LCD is atypia of cell population in various precancerous stages [29, 30].

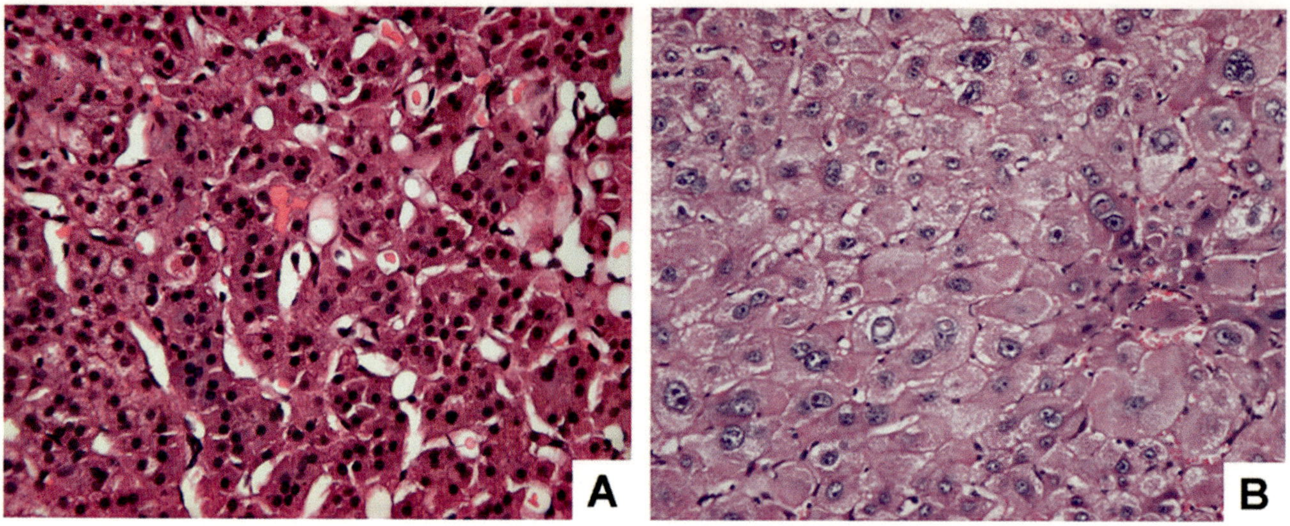

Fig. 5.6 Liver cell dysplasia. (**a**) Small cell change: hepatocyte was decreased in cytoplasm and size, increased in nucleocytoplasmic ratio, and occasional nuclear division; (**b**) large cell change: hepatocyte was increased in size and their nuclei, nucleocytoplasmic ratio was almost normal, and multinucleate hepatocyte was observed

Clinicopathological Significance

The occurrence of DF and LCD is relevant to the risk of HCC. Studies have shown that the incidences of LCD in the tissue of simple liver cirrhosis and pericarcinomatous hepatic cirrhosis were 6.9% and 64.5%, respectively, and the risk ratio of HCC in non-liver cirrhosis male patients with or without LCD was 13:1. The average age of liver cirrhosis patients without LCD was younger by 4–10 years than that of patients with LCD, while the average age of liver cirrhosis patients was younger by 3–6 years than patients with HCC, based on which we deduce that it would take 7–16 years for the development of liver cirrhosis to LCD to HCC. Thus, if crowded or clustered LCD is found in the pericarcinomatous liver cirrhosis tissue, it is necessary to pay more attention to them and follow up for a longer time. And it has been calculated that the risk of HCC derived from small cell change and large cell change (odds ratio, OR) was 6.33 and 3.88, respectively, suggesting that small cell change is more likely to cancerate.

5.1.4.2 Dysplastic Nodule

Pathogenesis and Mechanism

Dysplastic nodule (DN) is a nodular lesion, different from the surrounding liver tissue in morphology such as size, color, texture, section, etc., and was previously named adenomatous hyperplasia. It primarily occurs in patients with HBV-/HCV-related chronic hepatitis or liver cirrhosis, as well as chronic hepatic injuries, such as chronic alcoholic liver cirrhosis. DN is classified into low-grade dysplastic nodule (LGDN) and high-grade dysplastic nodule (HGDN) according to the degree of atypia of hepatocytes inside the lesion, and the common characteristic is the clonal proliferation of cell populations, including accumulation of intracellular iron and copper, fatty, and hyaline degeneration of hepatocytes, and eosinophilic degeneration, all of which do not exist in the surrounding liver tissue.

Clinical Features

Up to now, a total of 135 cases of DN have been diagnosed in the Department of Pathology, Eastern Hepatobiliary Surgery Hospital, Second Military Medical University, since 2005, with 57 cases of simple DN and 57.8% cases complicated by other diseases such as HCC, intrahepatic cholangiocarcinoma, hepatocellular adenoma, and cavernous hemangioma. Among them, more patients are male with a male to female ratio of 5.83:1, and the onset age ranged 27–75 years with an average of 54.6 years, and 95.7% of the patients had a history of viral hepatitis or cirrhosis, and three patients had chronic schistosomiasis liver disease. Most patients had no obvious clinical manifestation and were found to have liver lesions on examination. The main clinical manifestations include upper abdominal discomfort, abdominal pain, and other nonspecific digestive system symptoms. Some of the patients have portal hypertension due to liver cirrhosis or corresponding clinical symptoms and signs when complicated by HCC. In our hospital, serum AFP in LGDN and HGDN patients ranged 0–1210 U/L and 1.5–355.9 U/L, respectively. Ultrasound B examination often presents an inhomogenously hypoechoic area. CT images demonstrate hypodense area with irregular arterial enhancement and slightly lower density than the surrounding normal liver tissue in the portal and late phases of enhanced CT scanning. MRI shows hypointensity, isointensity, or hyperintensity on

T1WI and hyperintensity on T2WI, and enhanced MRI demonstrates the similar change as CT images that irregular enhancement of the lesion is observable with decreased signals in venous phase and balance phase.

Gross Features

DN occurs more in the right lobe of the liver, with a single lesion or multiple lesions, or even more than ten nodules in some cases, among which the degrees of atrophy may be different and some nodules may have cancerated. The average diameters of LGDN and HGDN lesions are 1.85 (0.5–4.1) cm and 2.56 (0.6–5.2) cm. DN is gray-white, obviously different from the color of the surrounding liver tissue. The cut surface shows lesion bulge out of the surrounding liver parenchyma, gray-yellow or gray-white in color, with a small amount of hemorrhage and necrosis, with a complete thin envelope or an ill-defined boundary (Fig. 5.7).

Microscopic Features

The histological criteria of DN were proposed by International Consensus Group for Hepatocellular Neoplasia (ICGHN) in 2009 [31].

1. LGDN. The nodules have an ill-defined boundary, and there is a fibrous septum to separate it from the surrounding liver cirrhosis which is a pseudoenvelope. Large cell change is visible in some lesions while small cell change is rare. The cells increase in density with uniform arrangement. Despite the existence of large cell change, there is no atypia or pseudoglandular tubes, with insignificant broadening of hepatic trabecula, mild capillarization in hepatic sinusoid, and few isolated arteries without concomitant bile duct (Fig. 5.8). LGDN has a blood supply of portal vein and is difficult to distinguish it from large regenerative nodules (LRN) morphologically, and ICGHN has grouped LRN into LGDN [25].

2. HGDN. The nodules in HGDN have a well- or ill-defined boundary and have no fibrous envelope, with mild atypia in cell morphology and structure and cannot be diagnosed as HCC. The cell density increases (two times the surrounding liver tissue), and the liver cells are arranged in irregular trabecula, with pseudoglandular tubes, with significant broadening of hepatic trabecula (Fig. 5.9). Small cell change is more commonly seen, with hyaline degeneration or fatty degeneration of liver cells. Different from HCC, there are a few portal structures in HGDN, with increased isolated arteries without concomitant bile duct (Fig. 5.10). And reticular structure disappears with ductular reaction visible suggesting the lesions may be nonmalignant with no stromal invation (nodular lesions with ill-defined boundary present invasion of the portal area and fibrous septa). In addition, we've found that HGDN has loss of heterozygosity (LOH) and instability of multiple genomic microsatellites which need further investigation for application in diagnosis and differential diagnosis [32]. Thus, present criteria on the differential diagnosis of HGDN and well-differentiated sHCC need further improving via active practice to achieve a broader consensus [33–35].

3. Nodule in nodule. Well-differentiated carcinomous micronodules can be identified via imaging or by the naked eye, with stromal invasion, which indicates invasion of carcinomous cells into the intranodular portal area and fibrous septa, in DN, especially HGDN. The nodules

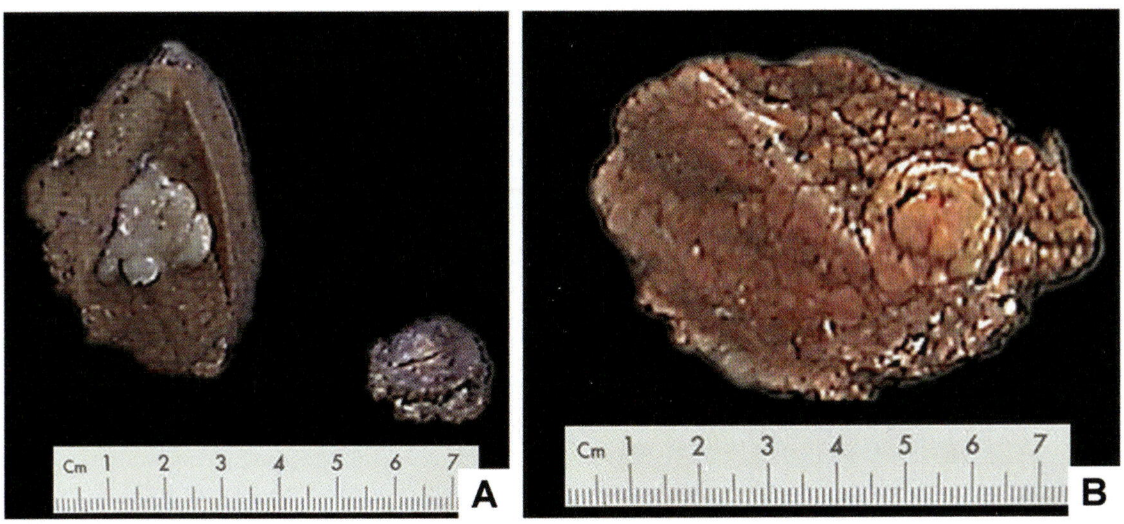

Fig. 5.7 Dysplastic nodule. (**a**) Small hepatocellular carcinoma in liver specimen, small nodule at right was LGDN resected simultaneously; (**b**) HGDN, the nodule had a roughly clear boundary, and no fibrous envelope

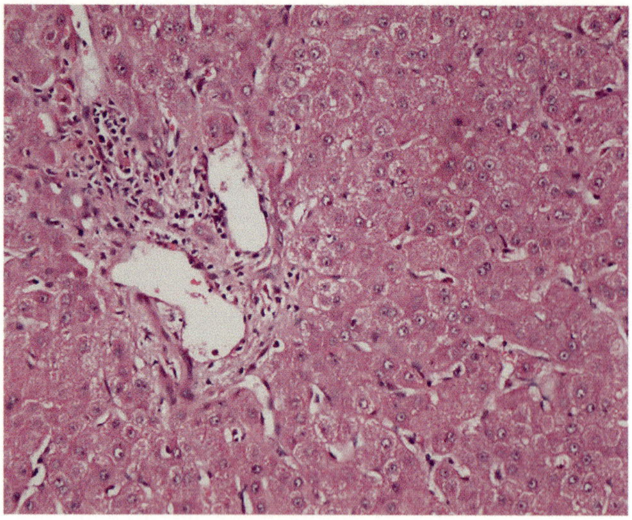

Fig. 5.8 LGDN portal structure was basically integral

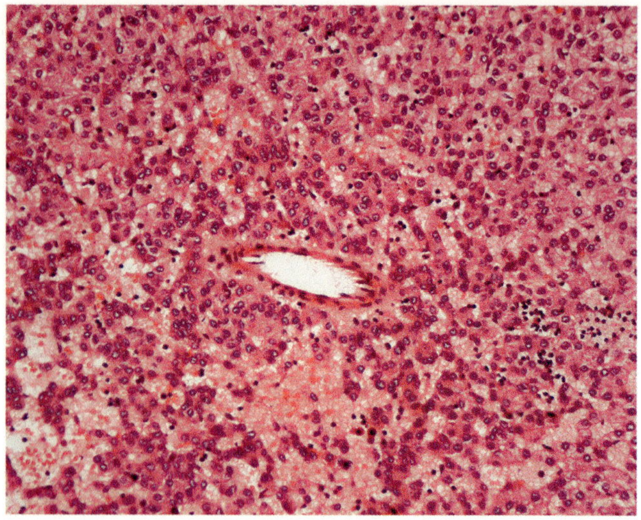

Fig. 5.10 Isolated arteries without concomitant bile duct

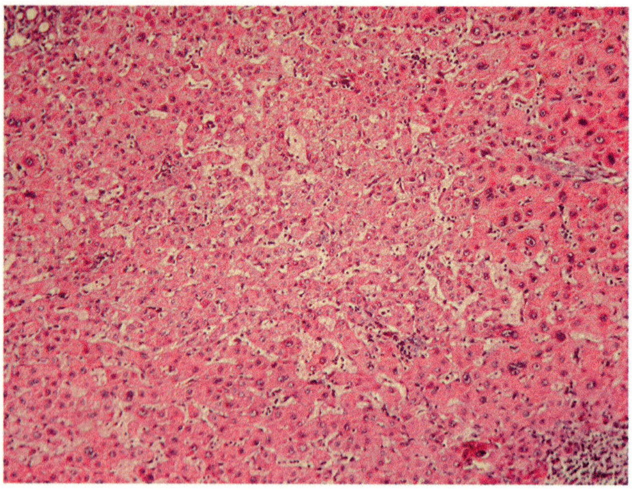

Fig. 5.9 HGDN trabecula was broadened in the central region of the lesion; atypical hyperplasia was obvious in the peripheral region

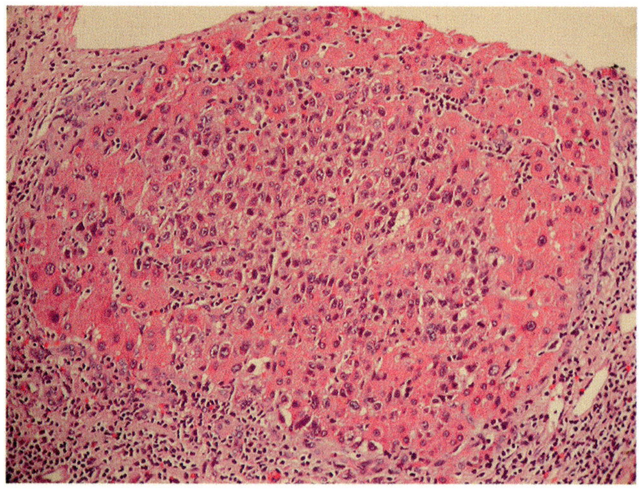

Fig. 5.11 HGDN, nodule in nodule of cancerization in the center of HGDN, expansive growth and transition with peripheral hepatic cell plate

grow aggressively and gradually replace the surrounding liver tissue with atypia (Fig. 5.11). We have diagnosed 30 cases of single HGDN in the Department of Pathology, Eastern Hepatobiliary Surgery Hospital, Second Military Medical University, since 2005, 13 cases (43.3%) of which presented nodule in nodule [36].

Immunohistochemistry

CK7 and CK19 are important markers to define ductular reaction and invasion. Nodules in HGDN present bile duct stain in the portal area, with increased Ki-67 index, and CD34 staining reveals the level of capillarization in hepatic sinusoid, which is related to the degree of carcinomous differentiation [37]. And DN with positive GPC-3, especially HGDN with positive GPC-3, is a late phase of precancerous lesions [38]. Kim Kwang Shik et al. screened a group of differentially expressed protein in DN and HCC tissues using proteomic methods, and the results showed that the expression levels of ACY1 and SUOX decrease in LGDN, HGDN, and WD-SHCC successively, contrary to the expression situation of protein P62. And the combination of SUOX, CD34, and AKR1B10 tests is beneficial in the differential diagnosis of DNA and WD-SHCC [39].

Differential Diagnosis

1. Focal nodular hyperplasia. The proliferated hepatocytes are well differentiated, cluster to form nodules, almost without a background of chronic hepatitis or liver cirrhosis. A typical fibrous scar is helpful in the diagnosis. And in nontypical scar cases, microvessels distributed along

the fibrous scar in CD34 immunohistochemistry are an evidence for diagnosis.
2. Hepatocellular adenoma. Hyaline degeneration and fatty degeneration may be observed in liver cells, sometimes with mild atypical hyperplasia and pseudoglandular tube. And diffuse, dialated, and thin-walled small vessels and vascular purpura-like changes are evidences for diagnosis.
3. Well-differentiated sHCC. Cell density increases and intertrabecular space widens, with expansive growth and invasion of the stroma or adjacent liver tissue. CD34 staining shows significant increase of microvessel density.

Treatment and Prognosis

Cancerous property of DN is the most important feature for clinical pathology. Reports showed the risk ratio for canceration of HGDN, LGDN, and LRN is 16.8, 2.96, and 1, respectively. Surgical treatment, including radiofrequency ablation and surgical resection, is the preferred choice for HGDN with radical effects in precancerous lesions. Given the high risk of HGDN canceration, the postoperative patients in early or start-up phase of HCC should be closely followed up [40]. Tommaso et al. [25] proposed the risk assessment of developing HCC in DN patients (Table 5.2).

Table 5.2 Risk assessment of developing HCC in DN patients

Major indicators	Risk
Diameter	
<1 cm	Low
>1.5 cm	High
Nodular image in arterial phase	
Low to moderate vasculature	Low
Rich vasculature	High
Enhanced MRI	
Moderate or high density	Low
Low density	High
Follow-up imaging	
Stable nodules	Low
Enlargement of nodules	High
With enhancement in arterial phase	Low
Without enhancement in arterial phase	High
Complication of HCC	
With	Low
Without	High
Pathological feature	
LGDN	Low
HGDN	High

5.1.5 Compensatory or Segmental Hyperplasia

The causes of compensatory or segmental hyperplasia of liver (CLH) include occlusion of portal vein or hepatic vein (Budd-Chiari syndrome), primary sclerosing cholangitis (PSC), stenosis or obstruction of the major bile duct (Allagille syndrome), and so forth, all of which lead to atrophy of involved liver parenchyma and partial or complete compensatory hyperplasia of other hepatic lobes, especially the caudate lobe, due to the its independent drainage in Budd-Chiari syndrome, while other lobes' drainage is dependent on the hepatic vein. Imaging shows that CLH was a nodular lesion of several centimeters in diameter close to the liver capsule. Histologically, compensatory or segmental hyperplasia of the liver tissue remains the portal area and central vein, with normal hepatocytes and atrophic liver cells in the surrounding regions. It should be differentiated from hepatocellular adenoma and well-differentiated HCC.

5.1.6 Focal Fatty Change

5.1.6.1 Etiology and Mechanism

Focal fatty change (FFC), first reported by Simon in 1934 as focal fatty infiltration, is a benign tumor-like lesion without any invasive property. According to radiological performance, non-diffuse hepatic adipose infiltrations are classified into four types: focal, multifocal, hepatolobular or hepatic segmental, and liver focal fatty sparing. The causes of FFC have not been well defined, and reports abroad suggested that FFC may be related to alcoholic liver disease, steroids, diabetes, and abnormal increase of portal venous supply induced by various factors. We have reported several cases with the history of hepatitis B in some FFC patients, indicating the involvement of hepatitis in the pathogenesis of FFC.

5.1.6.2 Clinical Features

FFC is often discovered in adults. A total of 42 cases have been diagnosed in the Department of Pathology, Eastern Hepatobiliary Surgery Hospital, Second Military Medical University, with a male to female ratio of 1.1:1 and an average age of 48.7 years old (range 26–85 years old). The patients had no obvious symptoms, presented strong echoes in ultrasound B examination. In CT scanning, focal low-density areas with clear or undefined boundaries are detected, with relatively decreased enhancement compared to the nor-

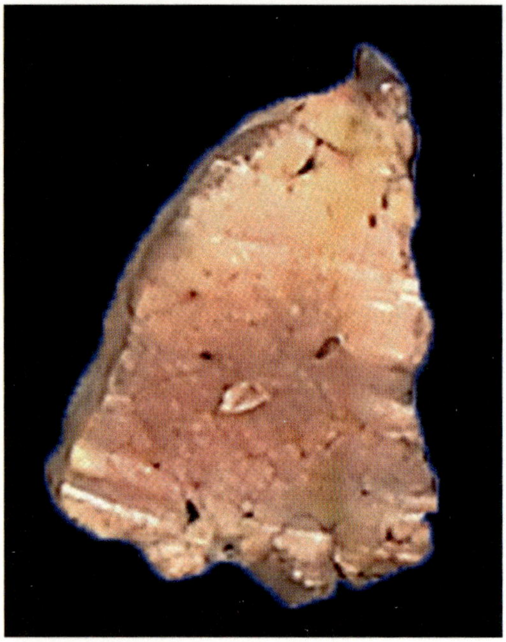

Fig. 5.12 Focal fatty change in the lesion area is located in the *upper part* of the specimen, *light yellow*, without coating

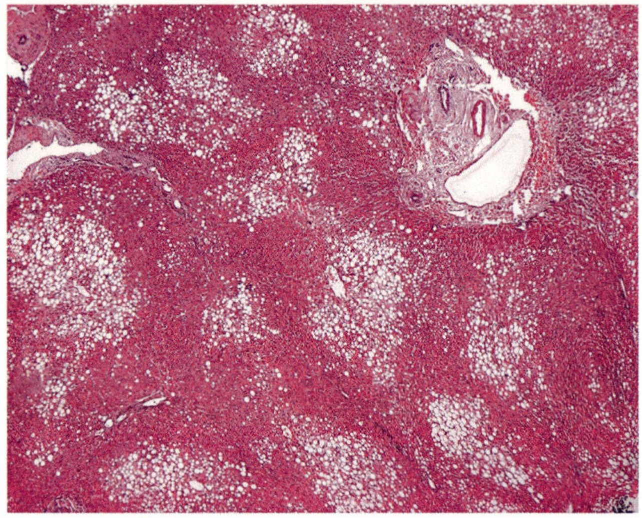

Fig. 5.13 Focal fatty change. Focal hepatic steatosis in the lesion area, distribution along the central vein

mal liver tissue; thus, it is difficult to differentiate it from HCC, especially multifocal FFC which is like metastasis. In MRI T1 phase, FFC shows regional high signal with relatively weak enhancement; however, it is difficult to differentiate it from HCC in cases of heterogeneous fatty livers whose MRI is extremely similar to that of HCC. When clinical symptoms are inconsistent with imaging findings or there is contradictory diagnostic evidence, cautious decisions on therapeutic strategy should be made. And a liver puncture biopsy is the best choice to diagnose undefined lesions [41, 42].

5.1.6.3 Gross Features

The lesions may be solitary or multiple, nodular in some cases, or appear in combination with other hepatic diseases such as liver cirrhosis and mostly seen in the right lobe of the liver, colored light yellow or dark red, 3–5 cm in diameter or larger than 10 cm in diameter in some cases, as tender as the liver but with no capsule, and one can distinguish it from the liver due to the difference in color and luster between them (Fig. 5.12). Although the imaging study suggests intrahepatic nodules, they can rarely be identified by the naked eye; thus, a guidance of ultrasound B should be introduced to detect the lesions.

5.1.6.4 Microscopic Features

The liver cells of fatty change in the lesion is focal or in the form of small patches, with macrovesicular lipid droplets in most of the cells. Lesions are located around the central vein or form fusion lesions, with no atypia of liver cells. Mallory bodies can be observed in the cytoplasm of hepatic cells in patients of alcoholic hepatic disease with no reconstruction of hepatic lobules, and portal area is visible with expansion and congestion of portal venous branches (Fig. 5.13). The degree of fatty change in the surrounding areas shows a gradient decrease, and liver cirrhosis occurs in patients with severe or long-term disease.

5.1.6.5 Differential Diagnosis

The clinical pathological significance of FFC lies in the differential diagnosis from tumors. Liver puncture biopsy results show a transition region between FFC and normal liver tissue, which is beneficial for diagnosis. In severe FFC, it should be differentiated from lipoma and well-differentiated liposarcoma. Lipoma has the same immunohistochemistry profile of liver cells and should be identified from lipid-rich well-differentiated HCC; well-differentiated liposarcoma has significant atypia, and lipid-rich angioleiomyolipoma contains a small amount of epithelioid cells surrounding adipocytes, which is positive in immunohistochemical HMB45 staining, and proliferation of small vessels different from the central vein. The key point to different FFC from hepatic adipose infiltration is the distribution of fatty change, as the former is characterized by fatty change surrounding the central vein and macrovesicular lipid droplets in most of the cells, and the latter diffuse or focal fatty change.

5.1.6.6 Treatment and Prognosis

FFC is a benign disease and should receive symptomatic treatment instead of any special treatment.

5.1.7 Accessory Lobe

Wen-Ming Cong and Xin-Yuan Lu
Department of Pathology, Eastern Hepatobiliary Surgery Hospital, Second Military Medical University, Shanghai, China

Accessory lobe is a type of congenital liver anatomic variations, consisting of normal liver tissue, with an incidence rate of 0.44%, and is often discovered in open or laparoscopic surgeries or autopsy, either connected to liver tissue or located in areas, such as the posterior or superior surface of the right lobe of the liver, gallbladder bed [43], or even thoracic cavity in the form of herniation in some reports [44]. Accessory lobe contains independent systems of the hepatic artery, portal vein, bile duct, and hepatic vein and can be classified into four types, according to the direction of bile drainage and the condition of Glisson's capsule: type I, drainage to intrahepatic bile duct of the normal liver; type II, drainage to the extrahepatic bile duct; and type III, drainage to the extrahepatic bile duct and shares hepatic envelope with the normal liver. Ruiz Hierro et al. [45] reported the resection of type I accessory lobe in the abdominal cavity in a 13-year-old child, which was 10 cm × 7 cm × 10 cm in size with focal nodular hyperplasia [45].

5.2 Bile Duct Tumor-Like Lesions

5.2.1 Biliary Hamartoma

Wen-Ming Cong
Department of Pathology, Eastern Hepatobiliary Surgery Hospital, Second Military Medical University, Shanghai, China

5.2.1.1 Pathogenesis and Mechanism

Biliary hamartoma (BH) was first reported by von Meyenburg in 1918 and is a combination of various components; thus, it is called von Meyenburg complex (VMC). It is also known as biliary microhamartoma (BMH) or multiple biliary hamartomas, due to the small and multiple lesions. BH is a rare focal developmental disease of the bile duct, accounting for 0.6–5.6% of autopsy cases and 0.6% of regular liver puncture biopsy cases. The pathogenesis of BH may involve the developmental malformation or abnormal reconstruction of bile duct plates (the precursor of the normal bile ducts) in embryo phase. In terms of embryology, intrahepatic bile duct plats derive from hepatic portal area to terminal development and reconstruction and are bilayer cylindrical in the embryo liver. The fetus bile duct plates in postnatal livers are known as bile duct malformation or hepatobiliary fibrous polycystic disease. The malformation is located in the primary branches of intrahepatic bile duct system, and the abnormal non-degenerative bile duct clusters in the liver are called Meyenburg clusters. Thus, BH is a congenital benign tumor-like lesion, as well as a disease in the category of fibrous polycystic lesions, including congenital hepatic fibrosis, Caroli disease, autosomal dominant polycystic liver disease (PLD), and congenital choledochal cyst (CCC) [46].

It has been reported that around 27% of BH patients are complicated with congenital hepatic fibrosis, 27% with FNH, and 20% with hepatic cysts; however, the incidence of BH is 41–100% in polycystic liver disease and approximately 100% in polycystic kidney disease. And 16.9% of the simple cystic liver cases are complicated by BH. Furthermore, multiple BH (>10 lesions) increases the risk of complication of FNH, hemangioma, congenital hepatic fibrosis, polycystic kidney, and cholangiocarcinoma. Though BH is proposed to be hereditary, no evidence has confirmed any BH-related autosomal dominant genetic variation.

5.2.1.2 Clinical Features

The majority of patients are middle-aged women with an average age of 42 years old, ranged 40–85 years old, and the average age of patients with giant BH is 69 years old. Clinical manifestations correlate to the size of the lesion, and most patients present no specific symptoms or signs. However, patients with giant BH have abdominal pain due to the compression of hepatic envelope, and a few patients present obstructive bile duct-related symptoms, including jaundice, cholangitis, fever, abdominal pain, or even portal hypertension, due to the mucous secretion and the complication of bile duct stones. B-mode ultrasonography showed small hypo- or hyperechoic cystic lesions or hyperechoic region between cystic lesions. CT demonstrates multiple small hypodense cystic lesions with no enhancement after administration of venous contrast agent. Dilatation of multiple intrahepatic bile ducts can be seen in liver parenchyma. Enhanced CT shows scattered round hypodense areas with dilatation of intrahepatic bile ducts, which is similar to the image of cholangiocarcinoma. In MRI, the lesions are round cystic masses with clear boundaries and thread-like contoured enhancement, which is hyposignal on T1-weighted images and hypersignal on T2-weighted images [47, 48]. And magnetic resonance cholangiopancreatography (MRCP) shows multiple hyperdensity lesions without communication between the cyst and the normal bile ducts.

5.2.1.3 Gross Features

The lesions in multiple BH are small, often 0.1–0.5 cm in diameter, and locate superficially under the Glisson's capsule. They are diffuse, gray-white micronodules that are solid and tender in nature. In some cases, the nodules colored in yellow-white are distributed in the whole liver and appear like "stars." Solitary BH lesions with clinical manifestation

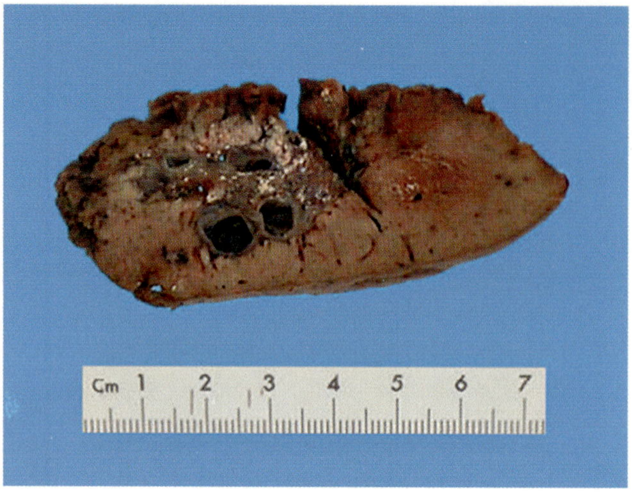

Fig. 5.14 Biliary hamartoma. The lesion was multilocular and no envelope

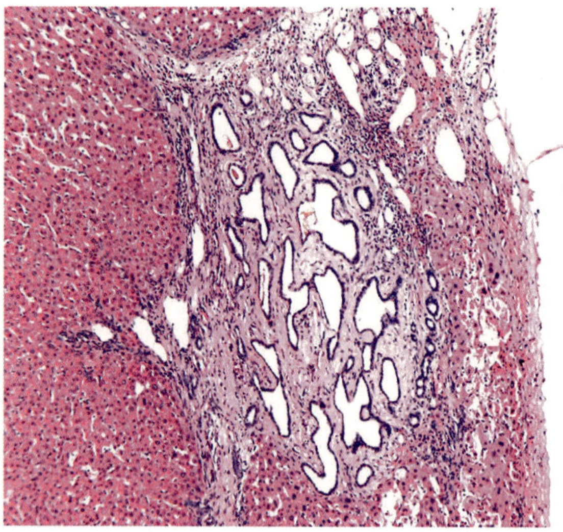

Fig. 5.15 The tumor is composed of cystic dilated small bile ducts

can be large. Martin et al. [47] reported 15 cases of BH, and the lesions were 2.7–21.6 cm in diameter with micro-lesions in the surrounding area, indicating that the giant lesions derived from micro-lesions via dilatation. On the section, BH lesions were small cystic cavities with smooth wall, and the cystic wall was 0.1–0.8 cm in thickness, and the cavities are multilocular with fibrous septa (Fig. 5.14), so they are also known as multicystic biliary hamartoma (MCBH).

5.2.1.4 Microscopic Features

BH is a portal lesion, characterized by small bile duct plates closely located adjacent or in the portal area (Fig. 5.15) or in dense arrangement, with compression to the surrounding liver tissue (Fig. 5.16). The small bile ducts are immature in shape, with angled bend or branches, as well as various cystic dilatation and intraductular communication (Fig. 5.17), and contain bile thrombus, blood, or acidic proteinic secretion. The thin walls of bile ducts are lined with simple squamous epithelium or simple cuboidal epithelium, similar to the epithelium of bile ducts, with no nuclear atypia (Fig. 5.18). The cystic dilatated bile ducts open at the peritubular glands with or without mucous secretion (Fig. 5.19). The small bile ducts are embedded in dense fibrous stroma which is often with collagen degeneration or hyaline degeneration, and there is a fibrous ring around the lesions with clear boundary. It suggests canceration when the glands are in dense arrangement, expansive growth, or invasion of the surrounding liver tissue [47–50].

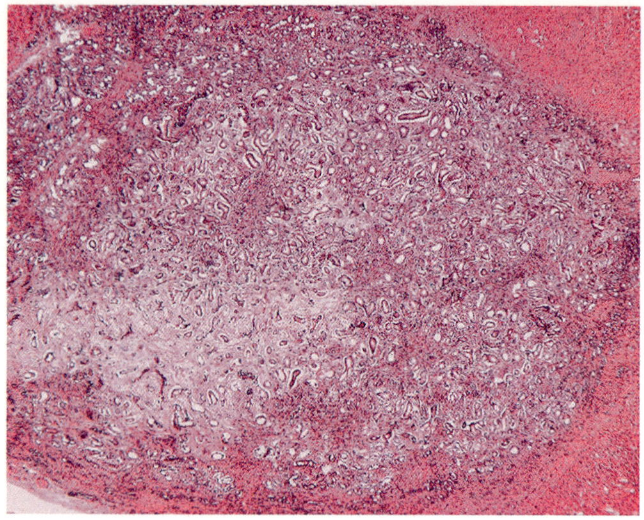

Fig. 5.16 Small bile ducts were dense hyperplasia with uniform shape and abundant fibrous stroma

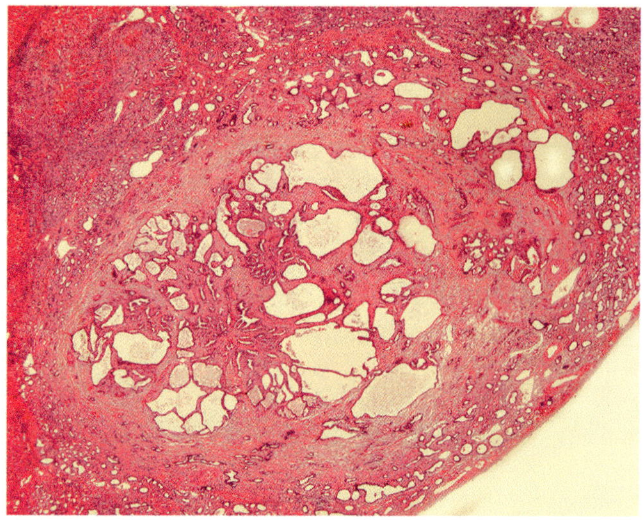

Fig. 5.17 Cystic dilatation of the bile duct and intraductular communication

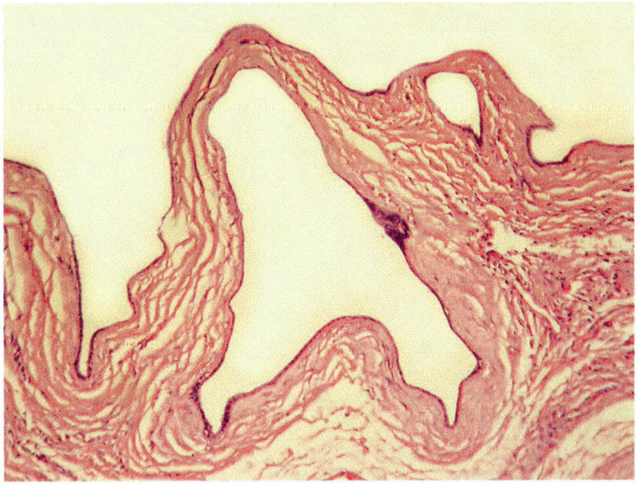

Fig. 5.18 Lumen lined with simple squamous epithelium or simple cuboidal epithelium with high dilatation

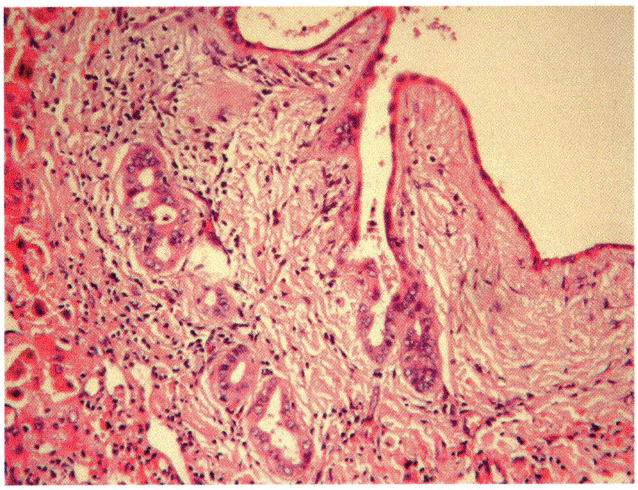

Fig. 5.19 Cystic dilatated bile ducts open at the peritubular glands

5.2.1.5 Immunohistochemistry

CK19 and CA19-9 are positive and CK20 is negative.

5.2.1.6 Differential Diagnosis

1. Ciliated hepatic foregut cyst (CHFC). The cystic wall of CHFC has four layers, pseudostratified ciliated columnar epithelium, subepithelial connective tissue, smooth muscle, and outer layer of fibrous tissue, while the wall of MCBH doesn't have ciliated epithelium.
2. Congenital intrahepatic bile duct dilatation (Caroli disease (CD)). Caroli disease is characterized by segmental cystic or multicystic dilatation of intrahepatic bile ducts, while MCBH is derived from bile duct hamartoma or abnormal bile ducts, often combined with congenital hepatic fibrosis.
3. Mucinous cystic neoplasm. It belongs to the category of biliary cystadenoma, with mucous epithelium-covered cystic wall underneath which is ovarian-like stroma. This is a tumor with potent canceration of biliary cystadenocarcinoma and should be carefully differentiated from MCBH.

Other diseases which should be differentiated from include bile duct adenoma, well-differentiated intrahepatic cholangiocarcinomas, metastatic adenocarcinoma, congenital hepatic fibrosis, and FNH, which are detailed in related sections.

5.2.1.7 Treatment and Prognosis

BH is a benign lesion, however, more than ten cases have been reported to develop into be complicated by intrahepatic cholangiocarcinoma, [51] especially in multiple BH which may cancerate via heperplasia, metaplasia, or dysplasia. Moreover, it has been observed the combination of BH and intrahepatic cholangiocarcinoma with a transitional region between them in histological examination. Thus, BH should be treated with surgery principally.

5.2.2 Simple Hepatic Cysts

5.2.2.1 Pathogenesis and Mechanism

According to the causes, mechanism, origin, histology, and relation with the bile duct, simple hepatic cysts (SHC) have various classifications. For example, hepatic cysts are divided into congenital and acquired groups. The former includes bile duct hamartoma, congenital hepatic fibrosis, solitary cyst, polycystic liver, Caroli disease, and common bile duct cyst. The latter includes parasitic, traumatic, and inflammatory tumors (such as cystadenoma, cystadenocarcinoma, teratoma) and miscellaneous cysts (such as endometrial cyst), and traumatic and inflammatory cysts also belong to the category of pseudocysts.

SHC are congenital, non-hereditary intrahepatic cystic lesions, often referred to as the liver cyst, also known as solitary cyst of the liver. They are commonly seen and accounting for more than 95% of hepatic cysts. SHC are sporadic, with no familial heredity, and may derive from the persistent dilatation and fusion of the residual bile duct plates formed in embryonic phase or biliary hamartoma in which the epithelial hyperplasia of small bile ducts induces obstruction and accumulation of secretion, and SHC are also considered as retention cysts which are present at birth. Most SHC are not complicated by cysts in other organs. However, in the Eastern Hepatobiliary Surgery Hospital, Second Military Medical University, a 46-year-old woman was found to have a 5.3 cm × 4.2 cm cyst in the right posterior lobe of the liver,

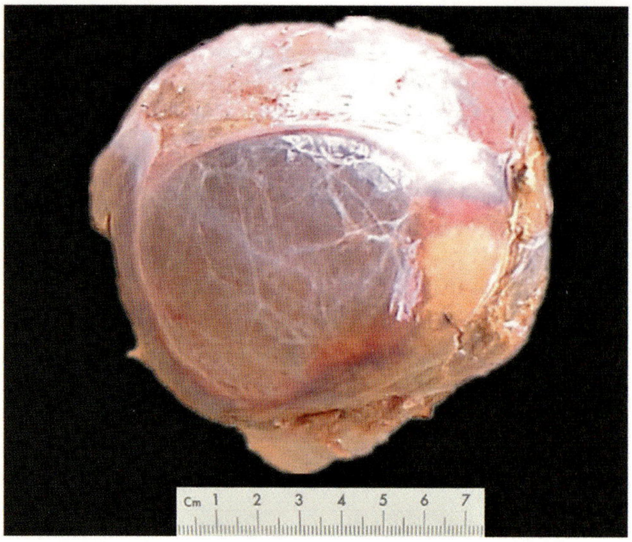

Fig. 5.20 Simple hepatic cysts, the cyst wall was thin and bright

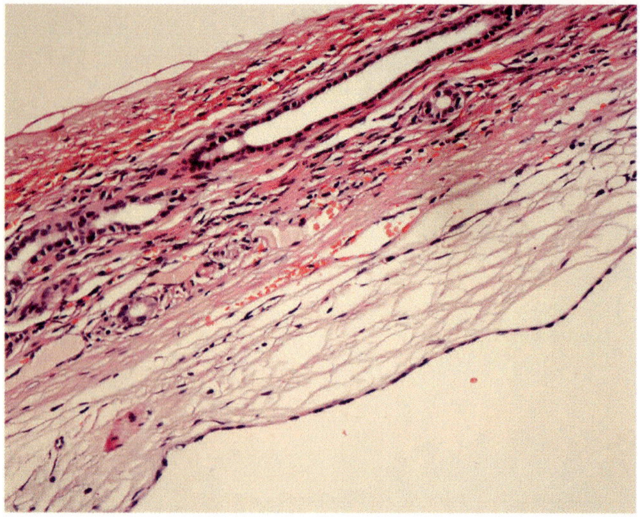

Fig. 5.21 The inner layer of the capsule wall was covered with a single layer of short cubic epithelium, and the lower layer was fibrous tissue

a 1.2 cm × 0.8 cm cyst in the right ovary, and two cysts in the spleen, the sizes of which are 7.4 cm × 4 cm and 4 cm × 2 cm, respectively, and were all excised during the surgery. This case suggests that SHC can be complicated by cysts in other organs resulting in multiple origin cysts or a subtype of the multicystic diseases.

5.2.2.2 Clinical Features

More than 200 cases of SHC have been diagnosed in the Department of Pathology, Eastern Hepatobiliary Surgery Hospital, Second Military Medical University, with the male to female ratio of about 1:2 and age range of 5–87 years old with an average age of 53.5, and the male to female ratio is 1:4. Patients with small lesions may have no obvious clinical symptoms and were identified in physical examination or during abdominal surgery. Larger lesions may lead to slight upper abdominal discomfort, abdominal distention, hepatomegaly, and compression-related symptom. And complications of SHC are very common, including inferior vena cava thrombus [52], Budd-Chiari syndrome [53], fever and elevated white blood cells in intracystic infection, acute abdomen due to cystic rupture and reversion, jaundice in cyst-induced obstruction of the bile duct, and so forth. CT images show round hypodensity cysts with clear and smooth boundaries and should be differentiated from the image of parasitic diseases when both of them show calcification in the cystic walls [54].

5.2.2.3 Gross Features

Typical SHC are solitary monolocular cysts, several millimeters larger than 20 cm in diameter. In a few cases, the SHC are 40 cm in diameter, or multiple cysts, or even solitary polylocular cysts. The cystic walls are thin and smooth (Fig. 5.20). The content in the cysts is several milliliters to more than 10 liters in volume, and the fluid is often clear and canary yellow or mucous, while in certain cases the content is coffee or purulent due to hemorrhage or infection. If the cysts communicate with micro-bile ducts, the intracystic fluid may contain bile.

5.2.2.4 Microscopic Features

The inner layer of the cystic wall is lined with simple low cuboidal epithelium, similar to the epithelium of bile ducts, with or without mucin, and the outer layer of the cystic wall is dense fibrous tissue, containing proliferated mucous glands and capillaries (Fig. 5.21), with intrahepatic biliary hamartoma in some cases.

5.2.2.5 Immunohistochemistry

Epithelium is positive in the immunohistochemistry examination of CEA and EMA.

5.2.2.6 Differential Diagnosis

SHC are generally easily differentiated from tumorous lesions. However, it is difficult to differentiate SHC from malignant cystic tumors or liver abscess when hemorrhagic or purulent fluid is obtained via puncture. In extremely rare cases, canceration of SHC is observed, such as squamous carcinoma, adenocarcinoma (cystadenocarcinoma), and mixed adenosquamous carcinoma (mucoepidermoid carcinoma), and much attention should be paid to sampling and microscopic observation.

5.2.2.7 Treatment and Prognosis

Fukunaga et al. [55] reported one case of a 25-year-old male patient with typical images of SHC without treatment [55].

But the cyst gradually enlarged and was complicated by calcification during the next 11 years' follow-up, and the cystic wall was obviously thickened with papillary nodules on the inner wall. The cyst was excised via surgery and was diagnosed as biliary cystadenoma. Therefore, large cysts may be complicated by reversion, bleeding, rupture, compression on the bile duct, hyperplasia, or canceration and need surgical treatments [56–58].

5.2.3 Polycystic Liver Disease

5.2.3.1 Pathogenesis and Mechanism

Polycystic liver disease (PLD) demonstrates multiple cysts with varying sizes distributed in the whole liver, and the cystic wall was lined with biliary epithelium. In perspective of histogenesis, PLD belongs to the category of noncommunicating cysts, without communication with biliary tree. And the genesis of PLD involves malformation of embryonic bile duct plates of intrahepatic biliary tree, persistent segmentation, and cystic dilatation of the residual embryonic bile duct plates. Meanwhile the disconnection of the plates and distal bile ducts leads to retention of secretion and increased pressure in the ducts, and the cysts are gradually enlarged ending with PLD.

PLD is also known as autosomal dominant polycystic liver disease (ADPKD), classified into two types. One is polycystic kidney-related ADPKD in which ADPKD is complicated by autosomal dominant polycystic kidney disease (ADPKD). The other one is isolated polycystic liver disease (PCLD) without ADPKD. Among the 28 cases of PLD receiving surgery in Eastern Hepatobiliary Surgery Hospital, Second Military Medical University, 24 patients (85.7%) were complicated by polycystic kidney disease with familial cystic diseases in 32% of them.

There are four identified PLD-related genes, among which PKD1 and PKD2 gene mutation exist in almost all ADPKD patients [59]. PKD1 gene is located on chromosome 16 (16p13.3), encoding polycystin PC1, and PKD2 gene is located on 4q22.1, encoding polycystin PC2. A great many reports on genetic mutation of ADPKD patients are found at home and abroad [60, 61], and no high frequency mutations of PKD1 and PKD2 genes have been discovered among their many mutations. Furthermore, about 20% of PLD patients have mutations of PRKCSH and SEC63 genes [62], encoding hepatocystin and SEC63 proteins [63], respectively. Since a proportion of PLD patients are without the mutations of PRKCSH and SEC63 genes, it is necessary to investigate the relation between other genes and PLD.

5.2.3.2 Clinical Features

The progression of PLD is slow and occult. No significant symptoms or signs in the early stage of PLD until the patients grow to middle or elderly ages, and the onset age of PLD is advanced from generation of generation. Among the 28 cases of PLD diagnosed in the Department of Pathology, Eastern Hepatobiliary Surgery Hospital, Second Military Medical University, the male to female ratio is 1:4.6 with an average age of 51.9 years old. And it has been noticed that the numbers and volumes in female patients are larger, and PLD in women with multiple births or replacement treatment of estrogen are severer, suggesting the relation between estrogen and PLD, and estrogen may be one of the factors facilitating the development of PLD [64, 65]. Anjia Yang et al. (1995) reported a case of familial polycystic kidney and polycystic liver diseases, with ten patients among 12 people in three generations, and six patients had both polycystic liver disease and polycystic kidney disease. The age of onset was around 45 years in the first generation, 20–48 years in the second generation, and 5–13 years in the third generations. Clinical manifestations are related to the size of the cysts, and abdominal distention, abdominal pain, and hepatomegaly are the most common symptoms. And the compression of cysts on the adjacent organs or tissues results in the failure of these organs and other related symptoms. For example, compression of cysts on the hepatic duct or common bile duct causes jaundice, compression on the gastrointestinal ducts causes decreased appetite, and compression on inferior vena cava and hepatic vein results in ascites and lower extremity edema. In these cases, differential diagnosis should be made between PLD and malignant tumors. The clinical manifestations in the late phase of PLD as well as the complications are predominantly induced by hepatomegaly.

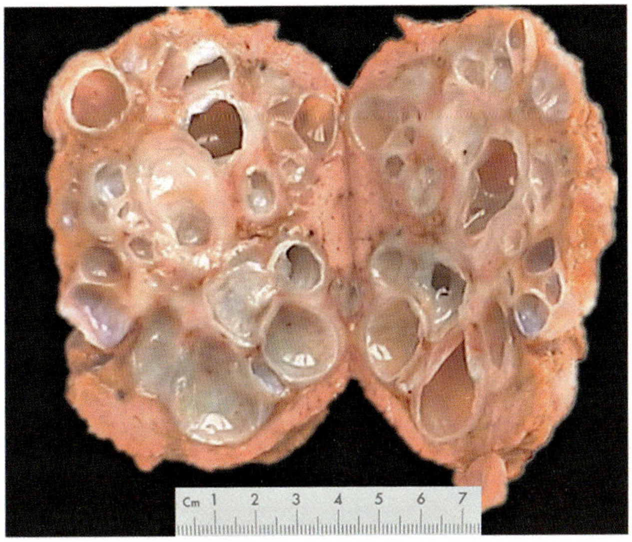

Fig. 5.22 Polycystic liver disease, the liver section with cysts of varying sizes, clear liquid inside

5.2.3.3 Gross Features

The lesions involve the whole or certain lobes of the liver, presenting as vesicular cysts in varying sizes (Fig. 5.22). On the section, the cyst wall is very thin and multilocular cavity with dark brown or clear fluid content can be seen.

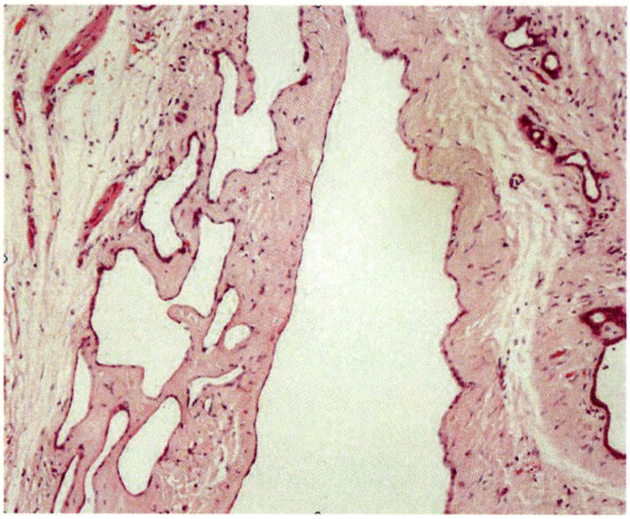

Fig. 5.23 Multiple cavities of varying sizes in the lesion, covered with a single layer of flat or cuboidal epithelium, and hyperplastic small bile duct could be seen in the cystic wall

5.2.3.4 Microscopic Features

The inner layer of the cystic wall is covered by simple squamous epithelium or simple cuboidal epithelium, with positive CK staining, while the outer layer is fibrous tissue. The intercystic space is occupied by liver tissue, and no bile is observed in the cystic cavity due to its disconnection with bile ducts. And biliary hamartoma can be observed in the surrounding liver tissue (Fig. 5.23).

5.2.3.5 Differential Diagnosis

PLD should be differentiated from multiple simple hepatic cyst and lymphangioma in the liver parenchyma. The latter is rare but similar to the lesions of PLD, as they are both multiple cysts, several millimeters to several centimeters in diameter, with or without other organ involvement. The key to identify a lymphangioma is the lymph in the cystic cavity with simple endothelium on the cystic wall which is D2-40 positive and no complication of multicystic kidney.

5.2.3.6 Treatment and Prognosis

Surgical treatments include cystic drainage and sclerotherapy, laparoscopic cyst fenestration, liver resection, and liver transplantation [66].

5.2.4 Caroli Disease

5.2.4.1 Pathogenesis and Mechanism

Caroli disease (CD) was first reported by a French researcher Jaequc Caroli in 1958, also known as congenital segmental cystic dilatation of intrahepatic bile duct, characterized by multicystic dilatations in the large intrahepatic biliary tree, especially the left and right hepatic ducts, segmental bile ducts, and branches. The dilatated bile ducts are communicated with branches of the intrahepatic bile ducts and belong to communicated cavernous dilatation of bile ducts. CD is now considered as an autosomal recessive genetic disease, and Caroli syndrome (CS) refers to the combination of CD and congenital hepatic fibrosis. The incidence of CD is 1/6000–1/400000 in newborns, who may have other congenital disorders. And an autosomal recessive genetic disease has an incidence rate of 1/20000 in newborns, closely related to Caroli syndrome. A case of a 2-month-old male infant has been reported to have Caroli disease accompanied by a rare disease called vein of Galen malformation [67]. Furthermore, mutation of PKHD1 gene was discovered in the whole exome sequencing in familial cases of Caroli disease [68].

5.2.4.2 Clinical Features

CD mainly occurs in children or adolescent, and the proportion of patients with the onset age under 10 years old is about 60%. The predilection age range is 21–49 years, and 75% of the patients are male. Caroli disease is classified into two subtypes. Type I is simple CD, with multicystic dilatations of intrahepatic bile ducts, often combined with intrahepatic stones of bile ducts, and has clinical manifestations such fever, abdominal pain, and recurrent biliary infection. Type II is CD with diffuse or periportal fibrosis and heperplasia of fibrous tissue surrounding the portal area with proliferated small bile ducts, and early occurred hepatosplenomegaly, portal hypertension, and esophageal variceal rupture and bleeding are also observed. The clinical manifestations of CD are often nontypical, including symptoms and signs caused by inflammation and stones due to dilatation and bile retention of the intrahepatic bile ducts, with a wide range of onset age. Patients of simple CD may have decreased appetite and body weight, recurrent right abdominal pain, and fever, with or without jaundice, and patients accompanied by cholangitis present deepened jaundice. In a few cases, recurrent jaundice is the main symptom. And in patients with periportal fibrosis, clinical manifestations are mainly portal hypertension, splenomegaly, and upper gastrointestinal hemorrhage.

5.2.4.3 Pathological Features

The main histological features include: (1) hyperplasia of small portal bile ducts, with dilated ductular lumen and hyperplasia of fibrous tissue in the wall, (2) branches of portal vein in the portal area with fibrous bridges between portal areas, and (3) normal hepatic lobules. Chronic inflammation of biliary mucosa, caused by bile retention and biliary stones in the cystic dilatated bile ducts, often results in biliary epithelial hyperplasia, metaplasia, or dysplasia, and the cystic wall appears thick and rough, thus forming cystic lesions (Fig. 5.24). Under microscope, obvious hyperplasia of the inflammatory fibrous tissue can be observed, with involvement of hyperplasia of fibrous tissue and small bile ducts surrounding the portal area, similar to the changes in sclerosing cholangitis and early phase of liver cirrhosis. Canceration occurs in 7–14% of CD cases, 100 times the risk of healthy people, which is also observed in our pathological work (Fig. 5.25), thus is considered as a precancerous lesion of cholangiocarcinoma.

5.2.4.4 Treatment and Prognosis

Type I CD can be treated with surgical resection, and type II CD can be treated by liver transplantation.

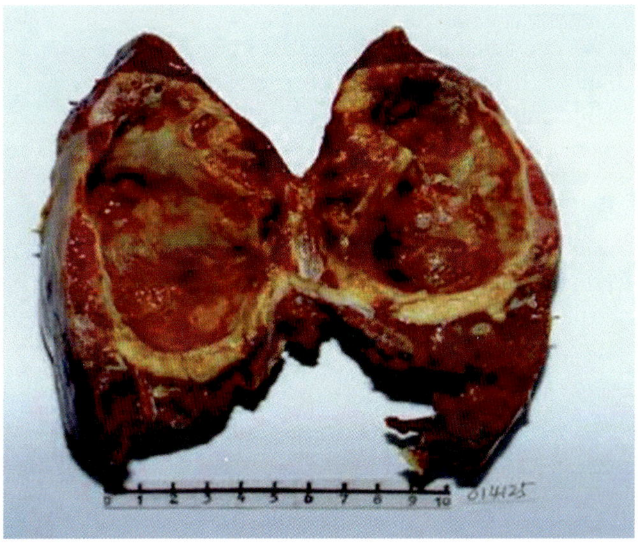

Fig. 5.24 Caroli disease bile duct dilatated into a large cystic cavity, inner wall rough, and thickening

5.2.5 Congenital Choledochal Cyst

5.2.5.1 Pathogenesis and Mechanism

Congenital choledochal cyst (CCC) is characterized by cyst or fusiform dilatation of the common bile duct, with or without dilatation of intrahepatic bile ducts, also known as dilatation of the common bile duct, which is the most common congenital abnormality and most common disease of congenital hepatobiliary cysts, with an incidence rate of 1/1000–1/190000 and a male to female ratio of 1:3–1:4. It is generally believed that the incidence of CCC in the Asian population is significantly higher than that in European and American populations.

5.2.5.2 Clinicopathologic Features

CCC is commonly discovered in infants and children under the age of 10, but its age range covers any ages. More than 200 cases of CCC have been diagnosed in our Department of Pathology, Eastern Hepatobiliary Surgery Hospital, Second Military Medical University, in the last 5 years, with a male to female ratio of 1:3, and the average age of the patients was 51 years old ranged 3–76 years. The clinical manifestations include abdominal pain, jaundice, and upper abdominal mass, which are known as a triad. Pathologically, dilatation of the common bile duct or extrahepatic bile ducts is observed, sometimes forming a diverticulum (Fig. 5.26). Large cysts may perforate or rupture spontaneously [69, 70]. Intrahepatic bile duct cyst containing thick bile can also be observed with a thickened wall consisting of dense collagen fibers, scattered smooth muscular fibers, abnormal glands, and inflammatory cells. And epithelium can rarely be seen in the wall of intrahepatic bile duct cyst.

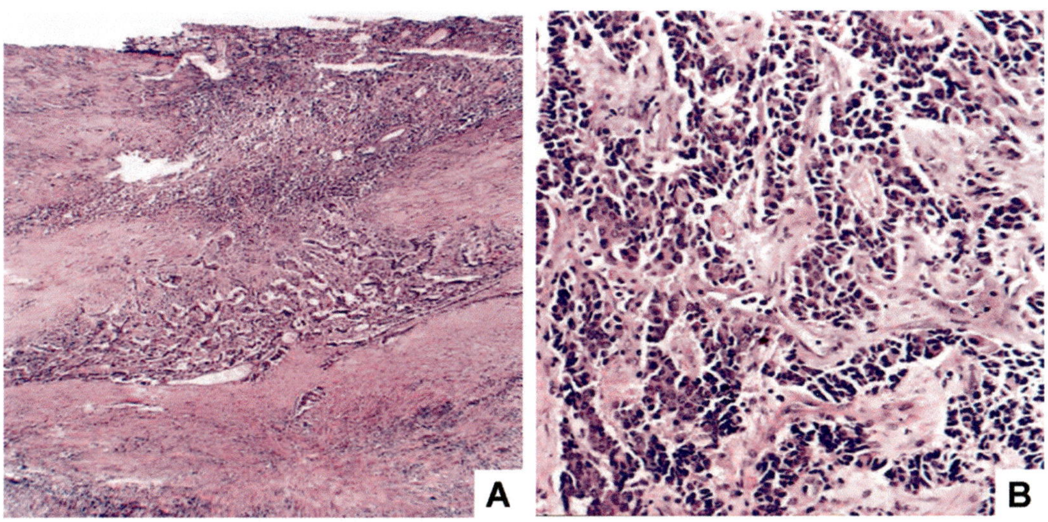

Fig. 5.25 Canceration of Caroli disease. (**a**) Small piece of cancer in the center of the cyst wall; (**b**) poor differentiation of cancer cells, beam and cable-like arrangement, invasive growth

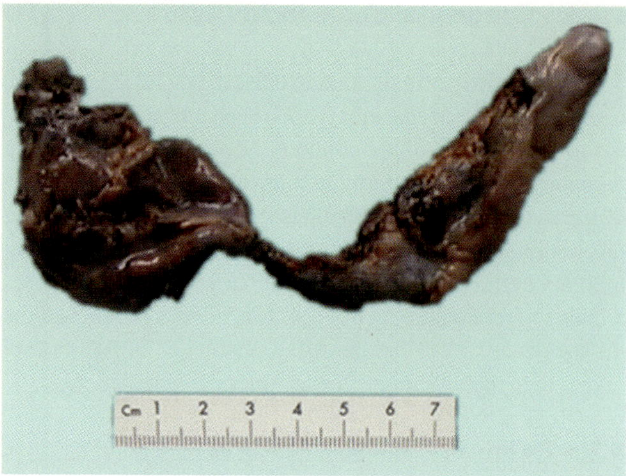

Fig. 5.26 Congenital choledochal cyst, cystic dilatation of the common bile duct, the diameter of bile duct was significantly increased

The classical and widely used classification is proposed by Todani and divided CCs into five types:

Type Ia	cystic dilatation of the common bile duct
Type Ib	segmental dilatation of the common bile duct
Type Ic	fusiform dilatation of common bile duct
Type II	diverticulum of common bile duct formed by outward convex of the bile duct wall
Type III	prolapsed cyst at the end of the common bile duct
Type IVa	combination of the cyst of the common bile duct and dilatation of intrahepatic bile duct
Type IVb	multiple dilatation of extrahepatic bile ducts
Type V	single dilatation of intrahepatic bile duct or multiple cysts (Caroli disease).

In Eastern countries, type IV and type V are the most common CCs. The risk of canceration of CCs is 2.5–15%, and secondary chronic inflammation increases the risk of canceration of CCs by more than 20 times.

5.2.5.3 Treatment and Prognosis

Due to the secondary repeated infections, biliary cirrhosis, bile duct perforation, or canceration complicated to CCs, timely surgical treatments are recommended once the diagnosis of CCs is made. The principle of surgery is to reconstruct the bile drainage into the intestine to prevent retrograde cholangitis and excise the dilatated common bile duct to prevent canceration.

5.2.6 Congenital Hepatic Fibrosis

5.2.6.1 Pathogenesis and Mechanism

Congenital hepatic fibrosis (CHF) was named by Kerr in 1961 and is an important type of hepatic fibrous cystic diseases. The mechanism involves the developmental malformation of biliary plates, and damage occurs mainly in the interlobular bile ducts. CHF is an autosomal recessive hereditary disease, and a domestic report in China concerned a pair of siblings, brother and sister, who both had CHF. CHF is commonly complicated by congenital intrahepatic biliary dilatation (Caroli disease) and polycystic kidney disease, and other complicated diseases include medullary sponge kidney, Ivemark familial dysplasia, Meckel syndrome, vaginal atresia, and less common adult diseases such as polycystic kidney disease and tuberous sclerosis [71, 72]. Al Sarkhy et al. [73] reported a case of 4-year-old boy with Prader-Willi syndrome and CHF [73], suggesting that CHF may be related to the rare hereditary disease induced by abnormal chromosome 15. In addition, Kinugasa et al. [74] reported a case of CHF complicated with HCC [74], while Paradis et al. [75] reported a case of CHF with multiple hepatocellular adenomas [75].

5.2.6.2 Clinical Features

CHF mainly occurs in perinatal, newborn, infant, and juvenile phases, and most patients are aged 1.8–14 years old with an average of 15 years. Patients with symptoms are most 3–6 months old, and males are slightly more than females. The clinical manifestation primarily includes liver cirrhosis and portal hypertension (70%), and hepatosplenomegaly can be found in infant patients, and later hematemesis, hematochezia, esophageal varices, etc. The major clinical feature for CHF is normal hepatic function in the patients. CHF can be divided into four types: portal hypertension type, cholangitis type, mixed type, and occult type.

5.2.6.3 Gross Features

CHF clinically manifests enlarged, hard liver, without visible vesicles or with microvesicles formed by dilatated bile ducts; thus, it is also known as microcystic hepatic disease, communicated with intrahepatic biliary tree, and is a type of communicating cysts.

5.2.6.4 Microscopic Features

Histological change of CHF is the damage on the interlobular bile ducts, including:

1. A large amount of fibrous tissue hyperplasia surrounding the portal area, forming a broad fibrous septa inter portal areas, the portal areas expanded, with no or mild inflammation.
2. Large amounts of different forms of proliferated small bile ducts in the fibrous septa.
3. The septa or fibrous bundles stretch or segment the lobules, with no pseudolobuli, and the structure of lobules maintains normal (Fig. 5.27).

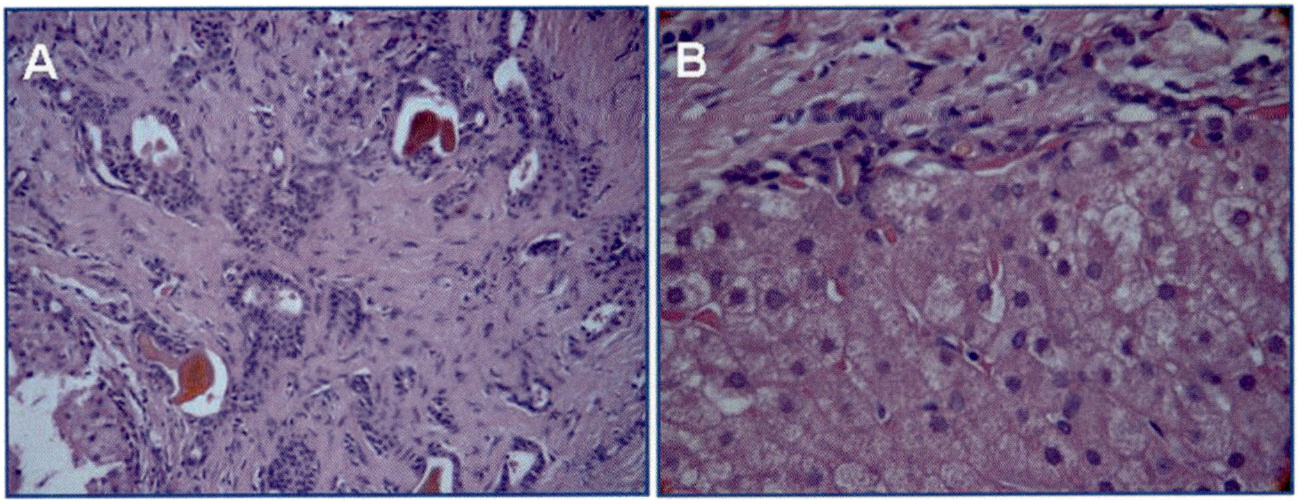

Fig. 5.27 Congenital hepatic fibrosis. (**a**) Interstitial substance small bile duct hyperplasia with cholestasis; (**b**) liver cells have no obvious inflammation or necrosis, portal area fibrosis (Cite from Abdul Wahab A [76])

4. The central veins remains in the center of the hepatic lobules, suggesting the microcirculation of hepatic lobules remains normal.

5.2.6.5 Treatment and Prognosis

The prognosis is related to the severity of portal hypertension in CHF patients, and the fatality rate induced by complications of CHF reaches 50%, among which sepsis, gastrointestinal hemorrhage, or severe nephropathy are important prognostic factors. Due to the commonly seen cholangitis, there is risk of intrahepatic cholangiocarcinoma in the patients of CHF, who often need shunting or devascularization due to portal hypertension, with relatively good prognosis if portal hypertension is well controlled. For patients with severe liver fibrosis and portal hypertension, liver transplantation is the best therapy.

Supplementary: Hepatobiliary Fibrocystic Disease

Hepatobiliary fibrocystic disease (HFD) refers to a group of congenital hereditary diseases, characterized by biliary dilatation and liver fibrosis of intra- and extrahepatic bile ducts and portal areas. Aforementioned biliary hamartoma (microbile duct), polycystic liver disease (microbile duct), congenital hepatic fibrosis (microbile duct), Caroli disease (micro, medium, or large bile duct), and congenital biliary duct cyst (extrahepatic large bile duct) are all members of HFD, sharing the common pathogenesis of malforma.

The development of biliary system includes intrahepatic and extrahepatic parts, both of which converge into interlobular bile ducts in the portal areas. In the early phase of fetal development, biliary plates are bilayered cylindrical structures. In ordinary conditions, in the ninth week of fetal development, hepatoblasts are located around intrahepatic portal veins and branches like sleevelet, forming the primary biliary plates which are the blastema of the development of intrahepatic biliary system. At the twelfth week in fetal development, the reconstruction of biliary plates begins, the primary biliary plates are replaced by ducts circled by interstitial cells, and the epithelium of bile ducts is replaced by cuboidal or columnar epithelium, stretching into the hepatic lobules forming intralobular bile ducts, and further construct the portal ductular system with portal vein and hepatic arteries. By 1 month after birth, the reconstruction of biliary plates has finished, and the residual biliary plates degenerate and disappear. Otherwise, the development of biliary system stagnates, and more embryonic biliary plates retain to form malformation of biliary plates, manifesting large amounts of ductular or cystic dilatation of proliferated small bile ducts in the portal areas with irregular lumen and surrounding fibrous tissue. In malformation of small bile ducts, CD10, CD7, and MUC-1 staining are positive. On the other hand, congenital cysts of the common bile duct manifest malformation of extrahepatic major bile ducts. As to the proliferated small bile ducts in FHD, it should be noted that liver masses predominant in HFD be differentiated from tumors according to clinical, imaging, pathological evidences [77].

5.2.7 Ciliated Hepatic Foregut Cyst

5.2.7.1 Pathogenesis and Mechanism

Ciliated hepatic foregut cyst (CHFC) is a congenital hepatic cyst originating from the embryonic foregut, commonly seen in the spleen. It was first reported by Friedreich (1857) as ciliated hapatic cyst and later was given the name of CHFC by Wheeler and Edmondson. In the perspective of histogenesis, CHFC was developed from residual embryonic foregut and differentiate into bronchial tissue in the liver, forming

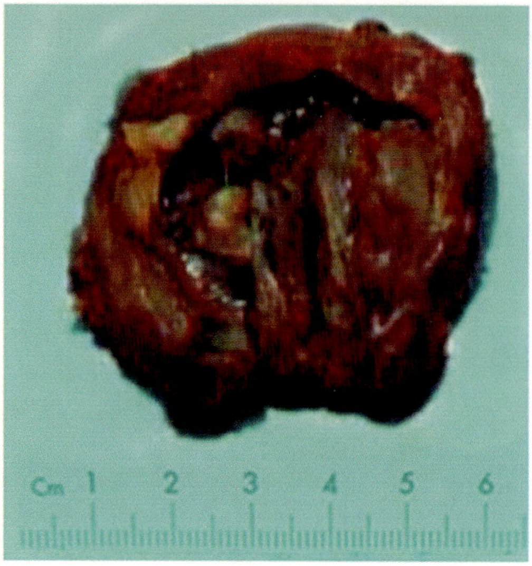

Fig. 5.28 Ciliated hepatic foregut cyst, multilocular cyst with smooth inner wall

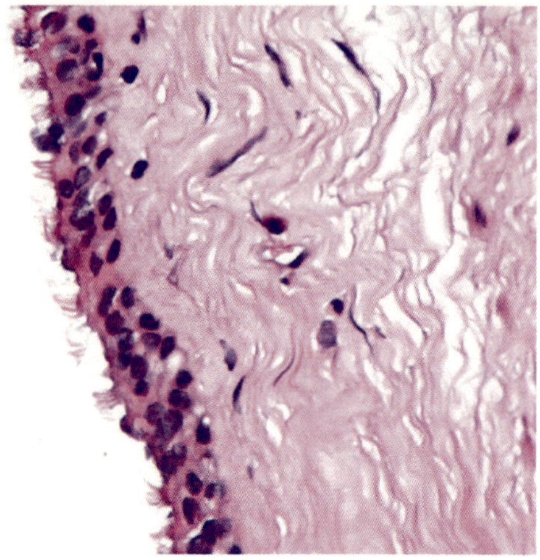

Fig. 5.29 The cyst wall was covered with pseudostratified ciliated columnar epithelium with cilia that appears on the apical

CHFC. The epithelium of CHFC is similar to bronchial mucosa, and Clara cells with positive CD10 have also been observed and reported. By 2014, more than 100 cases of CHFC have been reported in English literature, and around 100 cases of CHFC have been reported in Chinese literature [78].

5.2.7.2 Clinical Features

The patients of CHFC have a male to female ratio of 1.1:1, with an average age of 50 years old aged from 3 months to 82 years. Most of them are discovered accidentally and sometimes manifest upper abdominal pain, obstructive jaundice, and portal hypertension. The level of serum CA19-9 elevates in patients with large cysts. And the cysts in children manifest large masses, due to its communication with bile ducts leading to retention of bile in the cysts. Ultrasound B examination displays hypoechoic lesions with clear boundaries. CT images demonstrate hypodensity with no enhancement after administration of contrast reagent. And CHFC exhibits hyperintensity on T2-weighted images and hyperintensity in most cases on T1-weighted images in MRI. In one third of the cases, the radiation intensity of the lesions varies according to the different mucin concentrations and calcium levels in the cysts [79].

5.2.7.3 Gross Features

The lesions of CHFC are often located in the middle of the left lobe of the liver superficially, restricted under the liver capsule. A patient may have single or multiple cysts, and monolocular cysts are more commonly seen with mucous content. The lesions are usually small with an average volume of 3.6 cm in diameter, while some lesions are larger than 10 cm in a few cases. Monolocular cystic masses are predominant, often 1–4 cm in diameter with an average of 3.6 cm, and the content of the cysts is bile-like fluid, with thin and smooth inner layered walls, and valve-like strips can be observed regionally (Fig. 5.28). And in a domestic case of CHFC, the 8-year-old boy had a 30 cm in diameter lesion and was treated via fenestration and drainage for the cyst.

5.2.7.4 Microscopic Features

The cystic wall of CHFC can be divided into four layers from top to bottom: (1) pseudostratified ciliated columnar epithelium with slender and evenly arranged cilia on the top of the cells and a few amount of goblet cells in the epithelium (Fig. 5.29), and the cilia is positive in actin, CK, CEA, and EMA staining; (2) lamina propria, which is a loose connective tissue beneath the epithelium; (3) smooth muscular layer; and (4) the outer layer of fibrous tissue, which contain thick-walled vessels and proliferated small bile ducts. The content of the cysts includes neutral or acidic mucus and cellular debris.

5.2.7.5 Differential Diagnosis

CHFC should be differentiated from simple hepatic cyst, biliary cystadenoma, and parasitic cyst.

5.2.7.6 Treatment and Prognosis

The clinical course of CHFC is normally benign, while 3% CHFC may develop into invasive squamous carcinoma [80–82], and the size of the lesions is the major factor related to canceration of CHFC, which occurs mostly in adults (21–51 years old). The patients of CHFC can have a history of HBV/HCV infection. Squamous metaplasia of the epithelium of CHFC is positive in CK5/6 staining, based on which the risk of development of squamous carcinoma in CHFC cases is about 3%. Surgical resection is recommended for the treatment of CHFC, especially for those lesions larger than 4–5 cm in diameter [83].

5.2.8 Epidermoid Cyst

Epidermoid cyst is a congenital disease, derived mainly from residual embryonic foregut, similar to other hepatic cysts both clinically and in imaging in some cases. The histological features are keratinized squamous epithelium in the inner layer of the cystic walls, which suffers the risk of developing squamous carcinoma, and lower layer of fibrous connective tissue [84]. It should be differentiated from cystic tumors such as hepatic foregut cyst, cystadenoma, and cystadenocarcinoma.

5.2.9 Endometrial Cyst

Endometrial cyst, also known as endometrioma, may derive from coelomic metaplasia of the peritoneum on the surface of the liver, or ectopic implantation of the caducous Müllerian cells in embryonic development, or postoperative ectopic implantation in patients with endometriosis. Hepatic endometrial cysts are discovered in females aged 47 years old (30–73 years), and approximately 20 cases of this disease have been reported in the literature [85]. It mainly manifests repeated intermittent abdominal pain, partially related to menstrual cycles, and most patients have a history of abdominal surgery or endometriosis in other parts of the body. Ultrasound B examination demonstrates thick-walled cystic masses with septa or irregular echoes in the cysts, and different results may be observed before, during, or after menstrual period.

Hepatic endometrial cysts are 8.3 cm in diameter on average (ranged 2–17 cm). And one case of a 45-year-old female patient was diagnosed as hepatic endometrial cyst in our Department of Pathology, Eastern Hepatobiliary Surgery Hospital, Second Military Medical University. The cyst was about 5 cm in diameter and filled with thick chocolate content (Fig. 5.30). Under microscope, the inner layer of the cystic wall was lined with endometrial tissue containing endometrial glands and stroma in the secretory phase (Fig. 5.31). Furthermore, the epithelium and stroma are positive in estrogen and progesterone receptor staining, and the epithelium is CK7 positive while the stroma is CD10 positive.

Patients with endometrial cyst should be given preoperative comprehensive gynecological examinations, due to the possibility of complicating pelvic endometriosis, to exclude endometrial cysts in other parts of the body, such as the ovary and the peritoneum. It has been reported that endometrial cysts have a high risk of canceration; thus, early surgical resection of the lesions with a certain surgical margin is recommended [86].

5.2.10 Peribiliary Cysts

Peribiliary cysts were first reported by Nakanuma in 1984, occur predominantly in medium or elderly aged male patients with an average age of 57 years, and rarely discovered in children. The incidence of multiple peribiliary cysts in autopsy is about 0.26%. A large amount of peribiliary glands are located in the fibrous connective tissue outside the wall of portal or intrahepatic bile ducts. In the background of liver cirrhosis

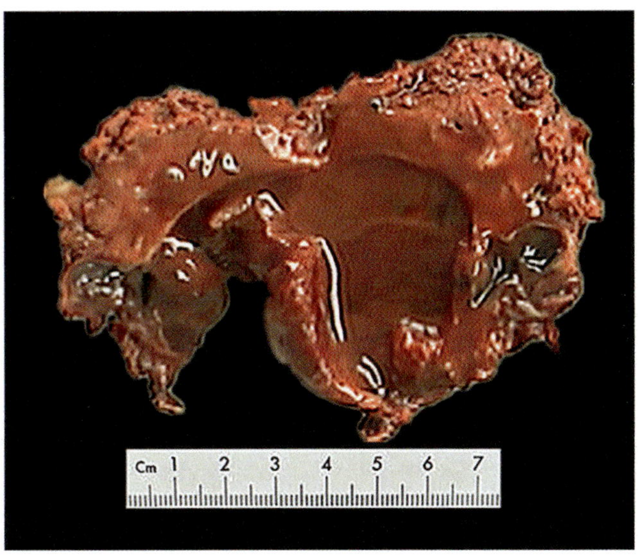

Fig. 5.30 Endometrial cyst was irregular cystic, filled with chocolate content, clear boundaries with liver tissue

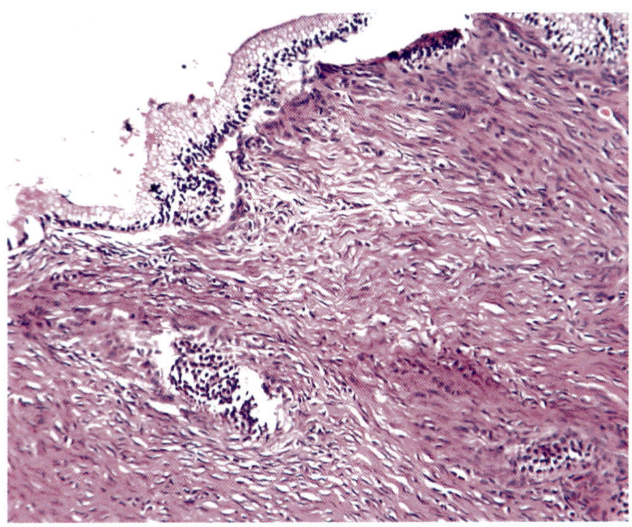

Fig. 5.31 Cyst was covered with endometrioid epithelium

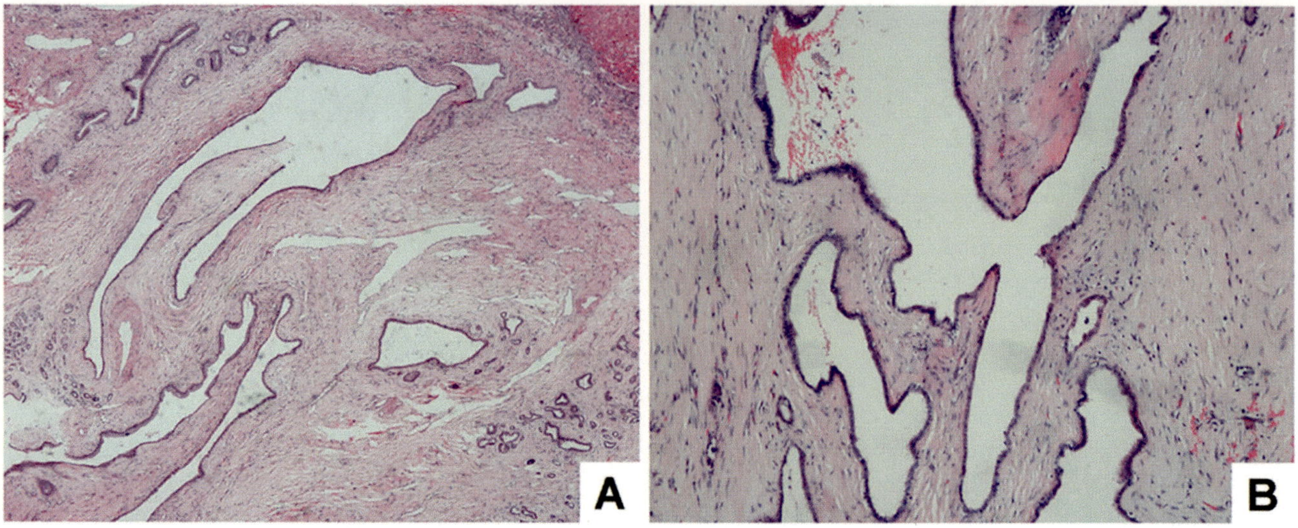

Fig. 5.32 Peribiliary cysts, cystic dilatation peritubular glandular in lesion, inner was lined with low columnar or flattened cuboidal mucous secretory epithelium

[87], hepatolithiasis, portal vein thrombosis, portal hypertension, portal tumor [88], and polycystic liver disease, occlusion of peribiliary glands leads to retention cysts, due to biliary ischemia and inflammation. Some large cysts even compress major intrahepatic bile ducts, hepatic duct, or common bile duct, resulting in stenosis of these ducts and obstructive jaundice, which is similar to cholangiocarcinoma, or even cause secondary mucinous cystadenoma and canceration occasionally. The ultrasound B images exhibit slender intercystic septa in cases of multiple cysts, which are diffenrent from dilatated bile ducts. And reports also suggested the possibility of secondary peribiliary cysts in HCC patients.

In gross appearance, the lesions are multiple cysts in different sizes (0.1–2 cm in diameter), characterized by the string-of-beads distribution along the portal area or major intrahepatic bile ducts, compressing the adjacent intrahepatic bile ducts, with smooth inner wall and serous fluid content. The cysts do not communicate with the biliary system. Under the microscope, the cystic wall is lined with low simple columnar epithelium, simple cuboidal epithelium, or flattened epithelial mucous secretory epithelium, and the lower layer consists of loose fibrous connective tissue, which cluster the peritubular glands. And there is transition between peritubular glandular epithelium and peritubular cystic epithelium (Fig. 5.32). In addition, peritubular glands with atypia are probably the precancerous lesions of cholangiocarcinoma.

5.2.11 Cyst of the Accessory Liver

Cyst of the accessory liver is a segment of hepatic tissue completely separated from the natural liver, existing in the adjacent hepatic ligaments or attaching to other organs, such as the gallbladder, or in the the thoracic cavity or umbilical hernia [89–91]. It has the hepatic lobular structure and the synthetic and secretory function of the bile but has no bile ducts, so the secreted bile may accumulate and form a cyst in the accessory liver. A cyst of the accessory liver can be 10 cm in diameter and may rupture or cancerate, and surgical resection is beneficial with good prognosis, according to the literature. And Rougemont et al. [91] reported two cases of neonatal umbilical hernia, and multilocular mesothelial cysts of the accessory liver were found in the excised hernias.

5.2.12 Alimentary Duplication Cyst

Alimentary duplication cyst is extremely rare with only two cases reported. One case concerned an infant 1 day post birth with a giant abdominal mass and was excised via surgery. During surgery, a monolocular cyst of 5 cm in diameter with brown viscous fluid content was observed, and it was derived from the right lobe of the liver connected to the liver tissue with almost one fourth of the cyst. And microscopic examination revealed that the cystic wall was lined by intestinal villous columnar epithelium, and the mucous glands contained parietal cells with two submucosal muscular layers, indicating it was gastric mucosa.

5.2.13 Biloma

Biloma is a common complication of surgical or interventional treatments, divided into traumatic, iatrogenic, and spontaneous biloma according to the causes. The bile leaks

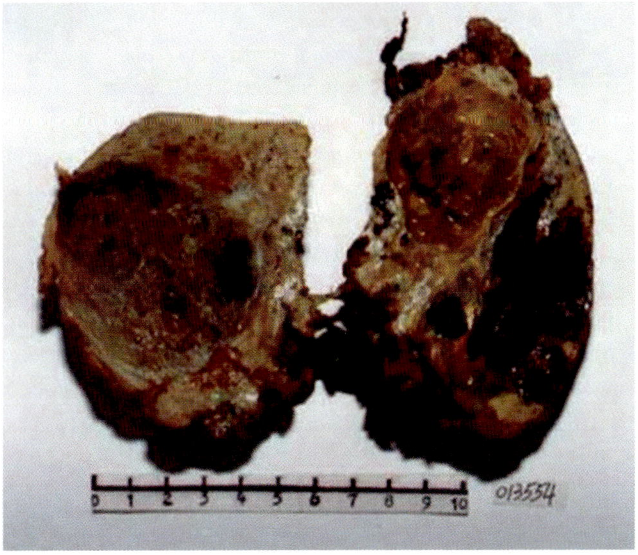

Fig. 5.33 Biloma cyst was located under the liver capsule, and biliary necrotic content in it

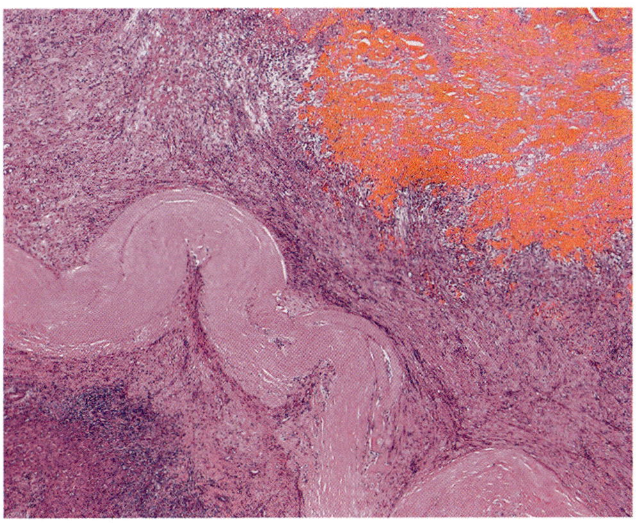

Fig. 5.34 Cavity content was biliary necrotic content (*upper right corner*), surrounded by inflammatory granulation tissue and fibrous connective tissue, and a small amount of liver tissue in peripheral (*lower left corner*)

into the hepatic parenchyma via injured bile duct and forms an intrahepatic encapsulated cavity, also known as bile cyst. The gross appearance of biloma is a cystic mass, 2–19 cm in diameter, and the biliary liquefied necrotic content can be more than 1000 ml in volume, with a thick and rough wall (Fig. 5.33). Under the microscope, the content consists of bile, hemorrhagic necrotic tissue, and inflammatory granulation tissue, and the cystic wall is composed of inflammatory fibrous connective tissue (Fig. 5.34). Larger bilomas often compress the common bile duct resulting in obstructive jaundice. When the fistula between the cyst and the bile duct is closed, the inner cystic wall can be endothelialized with autocrine capacity, and the secretion accumulates and the cyst is enlarged gradually and even ruptures into the abdominal cavity. When the fistula still communicates the cyst and the bile duct and a balanced pressure is maintained, it is called a pseudobiloma. Spontaneous biloma can sometimes be found in elderly people, due to the thin and weak wall of the bile duct. The treatments include conservative treatment, endoscopic or percutaneous drainage, and biliary stenting or surgical intervention with good prognosis [92].

5.2.14 Mesothelial Cyst

Wen-Ming Cong and Xin-Yuan Lu
Department of Pathology, Eastern Hepatobiliary Surgery Hospital, Second Military Medical University,
Shanghai, China

Mesothelial cyst is a rare congenital disease derived from the residue of embryonic cavity, often with no obvious clinical symptoms or abnormal serologic testing [93], only discovered in medical imaging. Patients with large mesothelial cysts present significant symptoms. A report of fetal abdominal cystic lesion at 24-week pregnancy was discovered and became much larger at 2-month post birth in the child, causing vomiting and abdominal distension, which disappeared after resection [94]. The lesions are cyst containing serous fluid in gross appearance, and the cystic wall consists of cuboidal mesothelial cells which are positive in calretinin staining in microscopic observation. And laparoscopic or open resection is the optimal treatment with good effect [95].

5.2.14.1 Supplementary: Cystic Fibrosis

Cystic fibrosis (CF) is the most common autosomal recessive disorder in Caucasians and has an incidence of 1/2500 in Caucasian newborns. The main cause of CF is the disorder of cystic fibrosis transmembrane conductance regulator (CFTR), the gene of which is located on chromosome 7q31–7q32 encoding a chloride channel regulator. The protein consists of 1480 amino acids and forms a phosphorylation-mediated chloride channel on the top of the epithelial cell membrane in exocrine gland duct. The mutation of CFTR gene results in dysfunction of the CFTR protein, leading to poorer transportation of the chloride channel and CF. Current researches have reported over 1900 genetic mutations of CFTR [96], and the first Chinese CF patient was reported to have deletion of 30 base pairs on the second exon in CFTR gene in1995.

CF is a systemic disease, manifesting as dysfunction of exocrine glands, with hyperplasia of mucous glands, increased sodium chloride in sweat, and overproduction of viscous secretions accumulated in ducts and acini, causing cystic distention, secondary infection, and fibrosis. CF involves the entire exocrine glands, including tracheal and bronchial glands, pancreas, intestinal glands, and salivary glands, and damage to the respiratory tract is the most significant. Liver is also involved in some cases. And the abnormal increase of chloride and sodium ion in sweat is one of the diagnostic criteria.

CF mainly occurs in infants, with hepatic involvement in one third of the CF patients, and patients with liver cirrhosis account for 15–20%. They often present no obvious clinical symptoms or have a fever or cough in some cases. And the development of CF is slow. Abnormal increase of serum hyaluronic acid (HA) is observed with an average concentration of 56.1 μg/L (ranged 26-355 μg/L), and the enlarged liver can be palpated at 15 cm below the right costal margin. Due to dysfunction of bile duct epithelial cells, CFRT-related hepatic disease is characterized by fibrosis of the bile duct, the pathological changes of which include:

1. Fatty liver (40–60%), macrovesicular or microvesicular fatty degeneration of liver
2. Focal biliary cirrhosis, portal inflammation, and fibrosis, with dilated bile ducts and acidic content, and 5–20% of them develop into multi-lobular cirrhosis
3. Portal hypertension (5–10%)
4. Intrahepatic bile duct stones (10–30%)
5. Small gallbladder (30%)
6. Stones in the common bile duct (10–13%)
7. Sclerosing cholangitis (1%)

Arumugam et al. reported a case of CF in a 3-year-old boy, characterized by giant hepatomegly with the inferior boundary at iliac crest which was first considered as a liver tumor. Hepatic nodular regenerative hyperplasia can also be seen in CF patients.

According to current reports, drugs treating CF, such as Bronchitol, have already gained good therapeutic effect in clinical trials, and clinical trials of several CFTR targeted drugs including PTC124, VX-770, and VX-809 have been initiated. For CF patients in the late phase of hepatic diseases, liver transplantation is an alternative treatment.

5.3 Other Tumor-Like Lesions

5.3.1 Mesenchymal Hamartoma

5.3.1.1 Pathogenesis and Mechanism

Mesenchymal hamartoma (MH) was first reported by Edmondson in 1956, accounting for 8% of all liver tumors with more than 200 cases reported so far around the world. MH is mainly composed of spindle-shaped mesenchymal cells, myxoid stroma, small bile ducts, lymphatic ducts, and hepatic cells and was previously speculated that MH may derive from the primary mesenchymal tissue in the Glisson's sheath or is related to abnormal embryonic development of biliary plates. MH is also considered to derive from myofibroblasts, according to the positive results of α-SMA and desmin staining, or supposed to originate from hepatic stellate cells, based on the electron microscopic observation of the slender membranous protrusions which is the feature of hepatic stellate cells [97]. MH may have complex translocations between chromosome 11, 17, and 19, known as mesenchymal hamartoma of the liver break point 1 (MHLB1).

Different opinions on the nature of MH nature have been put forward. WHO classification (2010 edition) described it as a benign tumor-like lesion with pre-birth occurrence, while some studies suggest MH is a true neoplasm based on evidences including the similarities of balanced translocation between chromosome 11 and 19, ultrastructure and histological features between MH and undifferentiated embryonal sarcoma, heteroploid of DNA in flow cytometry (FCM) detection, and the finding that undifferentiated embryonal sarcoma originated from MH. We have also observed the coexistence of MH and undifferentiated embryonal sarcoma with transition; thus, we suggest that MH is a tumor-like lesion with malignant potential.

A recent study by Lin et al. [19] discovered androgenetic-biparental mosaicism (ABM) in MH using genome-wide allelic gene imbalance detection method, suggesting the involvement of placental mesenchymal dysplasia (PMD) in the pathogenesis of MH [98]. Kapur et al. [110] detected chromosome 19q microRNA cluster (C19MC) in two sporadic cases of MH and three cases of MH combined with ABM (the latter normally expresses in the male patients), suggesting that chromosomal rearrangement or diploid in single male parent can cause abnormal activation of C19MC in liver mesenchyma, resulting in MH [99].

5.3.1.2 Clinical Features

Newborns or infants under 2 years old account for 80–85% of the patients with MH. A report of MH in a newborn described a neonatal surgical resection of 3.5 cm MH. And MH is the third common liver tumor after hepatic blastoma and infantile hemangioendothelioma. Isaacs [112] reviewed 194 cases of fetal and neonatal (< 2 months) liver tumors in the literature and reported that the first three common hepatic tumors are hemangioma (60.3%), mesenchymal hamartoma (23.2%), and hepatoblastoma (16.5%) [100].

Among MH patients, 60% were male, occasionally young or elderly (17–53 years old). In the Department of Pathology, Eastern Hepatobiliary Surgery Hospital, Second Military Medical University, five cases of hepatic MH have been diagnosed, with a male to female ratio of 2:3, aged 18 months to 38 years old, and the average age was 16 years old (Table 5.3). The most common clinical symptoms are abdominal distention, progressive enlargement of the upper abdominal

Table 5.3 Clinical pathological features of five liver mesenchymal hamartoma

Case no.	Age	Gender	Location in the liver	Tumor size (cm)	With liver cirrhosis
Case 1	2 years	Female	Right lobe	13 × 10 × 5.5	Yes
Case 2	18 months	Male	Right lobe	7 × 4 × 3.6	No
Case 3	2 years	Female	Right lobe	14.5 × 9.5 × 4.5	No
Case 4	38 years	Male	Right lobe	4 × 4 × 3, 1.2 × 1.2 × 1	Yes
Case 5	38 years	Female	Right lobe	11.7 × 7.5 × 4.5	No

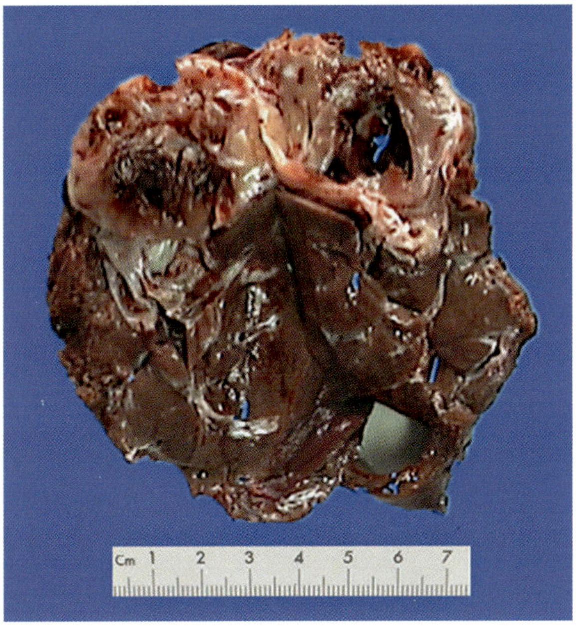

Fig. 5.35 Mesenchymal hamartoma, the section was multilocular

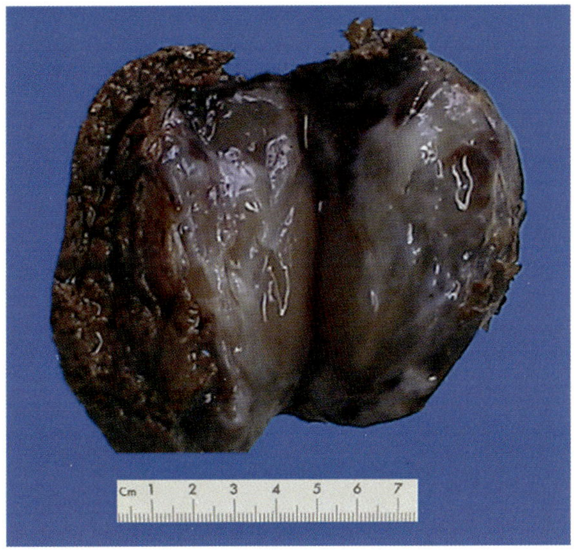

Fig. 5.36 The lesion was solid mucinous mass

mass, abdominal pain, and dyspnea, increased in individual cases, and the serum AFP is elevated in a few cases, even up to 108 g/L, but the liver function is normal. Heart failure and hemorrhage of upper digestive tract are occasionally observed, due to the arteriovenous fistula caused by vascular reconstruction or portal hypertension, respectively. Ultrasound B showed a large echoless polycystic or solid mass with clear boundary in the liver parenchyma. And CT scanning displays a polycystic or solid mass which has a capsule, septa, few vessels, and no calcification.

5.3.1.3 Gross Features

Table 5.3 shows five cases of MH. The size of the lesions is 5.5–14.5 cm in diameter with an average of 10.3 cm, and 80–100% of them are in parenchyma of the right lobe of the liver. The tumor is always solitary, large in size, with a smooth surface. And 59% of the masses are typically multilobular cysts (Fig. 5.35), a few millimeters to 14 cm in diameter, with a smooth or rough cystic wall, containing liquid which appears clear, light yellow, dark red, or glue-like, and the cyst is surrounded by gray-yellow-colored mucous tissue and gray-white fiber bundles. Solid masses account for 41% of the lesions, usually with mucoid degeneration (Fig. 5.36) and a clear boundary.

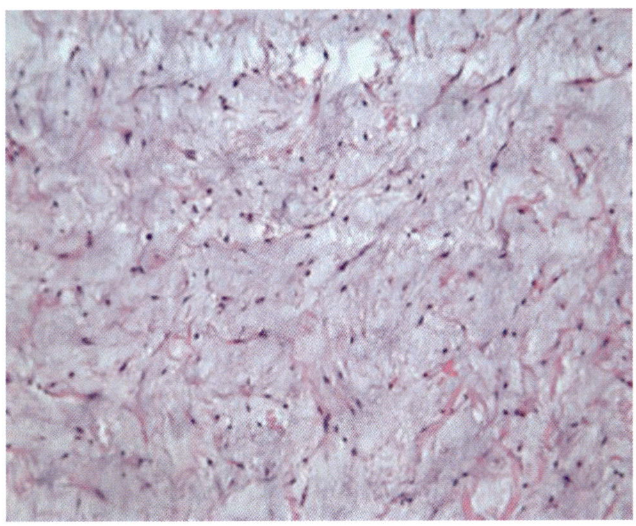

Fig. 5.37 Fibrous projections connect and cross with each other forming a mesh structure

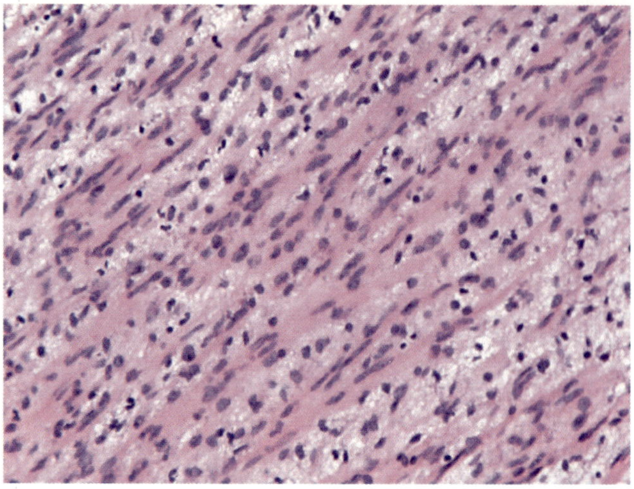

Fig. 5.38 Spindle-shaped cells arranged closely in fascicles

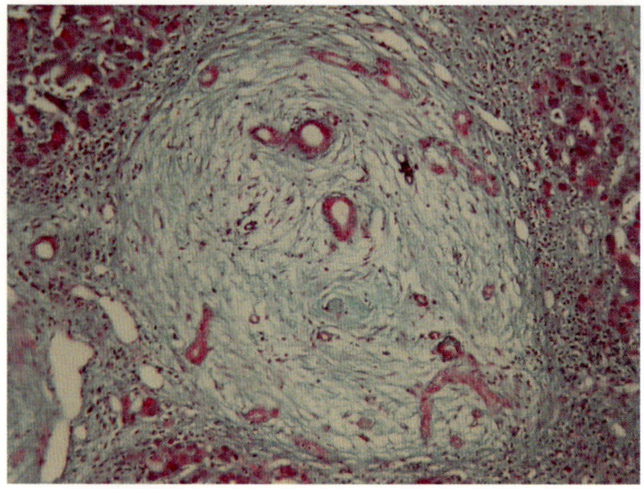

Fig. 5.39 Hyperplasia of small bile ducts in edema and mucinous degeneration of fibrous stroma, with residual liver cell islands around (Masson staining)

5.3.1.4 Microscopic Features

Loose myxoid fibrous matrix is observed in the center of the lesion, interspersed with fusiform stellate cells or mesenchymal cells, characterized by oval and elongated nucleus and slender fibrous cytoplasmic projections, with no atypia, and the fibrous projections connect and cross with each other forming a lace-like or mesh structure (Fig. 5.37), while the cells in some regions are arranged closely to form interwoven celluar bundles (Fig. 5.38). In addition, edema and mucinous degeneration of fibrous stroma in the lesion are often observed, with messy hyperplasia of small bile ducts or bile duct bundles, peritubular glands, small blood vessels, lymphatic vessels, and residual liver cell islands (Fig. 5.39). Some of the involved bile ducts exhibit cystic dilatation, and more than 85% of the MH present extramedullary hematopoietic foci. Large amounts of collagen fibers and spindle cells are usually seen in the peripheral region of the bile ducts, characterized by increased amounts of interstitial tissue and cells arround the glands, with a clear boundary in most cases.

5.3.1.5 Immunohistochemistry

The spindle cells are positive in vimentin, desmin, CD34, S-100, and SMA stainings, suggesting the involvement of Ito cells in MH in the liver, and the proliferated small bile ducts and periductular glands are CK7/CK19 positive.

5.3.1.6 Differential Diagnosis

MH should be differentiated from gastrointestinal duplication cyst, mesenteric lymphangioma, mesenteric cystic teratoma, etc. Cystic MH should be identified from liver cystic mass, such as biliary cystadenoma and hepatic hydatid cyst. In addition, solid or cystic MH should be differentiated from inflammatory pseudotumor, infantile hemangioendothelioma, undifferentiated embryonal sarcoma, etc., and masses in infants with elevated serum AFP should be discriminated between MH and hepatoblastoma identification.

5.3.1.7 Treatment and Prognosis

Surgical resection provides the patients of MH with an excellent prognosis, and no recurrence was reported [101]. However, cases of canceration derived from MH have been reported. Ramanujam et al. (1999) reported one case of an 18-month boy who received a surgical resection of MH in the left lobe of the liver without the notice of the lesion in the right lobe of the liver which developed into malignant mesenchymoma when the patient was 6 years old. Lauwers et al. (1977) reported one case of a 15-year-old girl who developed an undifferentiated sarcoma originating from MH. All these reports suggest the importance of active radical resection in the treatment of hepatic MH, and the patients without radical resection should receive a long-term follow-up.

5.3.2 Inflammatory Pseudotumor

5.3.2.1 Pathogenesis and Mechanism

Inflammatory pseudotumor (IPT) was first described by Pack and Baker in 1953, accounting for about 8% of extrapulmonary IPT, with liver as the second common good location after the lung, characterized by nodular changes due to local hyperplasia of fibrous connective tissue and inflammatory infiltration in the liver. IPT occurs mostly in children and adolescents, and the causes include infection (bacteria, para-

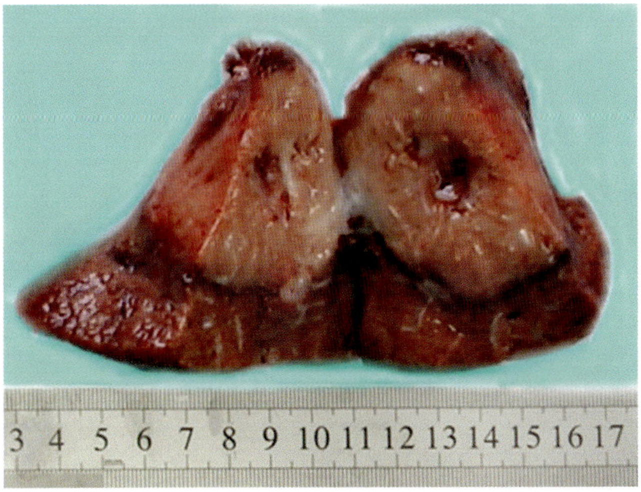

Fig. 5.40 Inflammatory pseudotumor. Lesion was *gray-white* or *yellowish-gray*, tough, mucinous, and clearly bounded

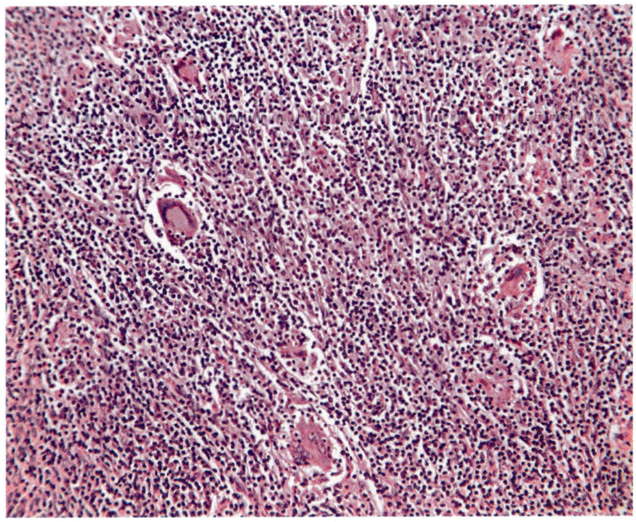

Fig. 5.41 Fibrohistiocytic type characterized by collagen connective tissue hyperplasia and inflammatory cell infiltration

sites, HHV-8, EBV), autoimmune disease, radiotherapy, or chemotherapy [102]. In addition, Crohn disease, gastrointestinal stromal tumor, congenital neutropenia, and pregnancy can also be complicated by IPT. And WHO hepatobiliary tumor classification (2010 edition) defines IPT as a benign, non-tumorous, and nonmetastatic mass, composed of fibrous tissue and proliferated myofibroblasts, with significant infiltration of inflammatory cells, especially plasma cells [103].

Furthermore, elevated serum IgG4 is discovered in a few cases of IPT; thus, hepatic IPT is also known as "IgG4-related to IPT." The disease mainly occurs in middle-aged and elderly people, and its histological features include infiltration of a large number of lymphocytes and IgG4-positive plasma cells, fibrosclerosis, and obstructive phlebitis, which are the same with that in IgG4-positive diseases (such as sclerosing cholangitis) [104].

5.3.2.2 Clinical Features

More than 200 cases of IPT have been diagnosed in Eastern Hepatobiliary Surgery Hospital affiliated to the Second Military Medical University, with a male to female ratio of 1.8:1 and a mean age of 49 (15–77) years old. Clinical and imaging features of IPT were similar to that of malignant tumors, and the most common symptoms include abdominal pain, fever, and weight loss. Some of the patients have increased peripheral white blood cell counts, anemia, and increased erythrocyte sedimentation rate (ESR), with elevated serum AFP occasionally. Ultrasound B examination shows relatively hypoechoic lesions with a clear boundary and heterogeneous echo inside the mass. CT examination shows masses with hypodensity.

5.3.2.3 Gross Features

The lesion was solitary and the average size is 3.6 cm in diameter (ranged 0.2–15 cm). Some lesions of IPT reach 25 cm in diameter as reported. The section of the lesions exhibit gray-white or yellowish-gray, hard, clearly bounded masses without true fibrous capsules (Fig. 5.40).

5.3.2.4 Microscopic Features

IPT basically consists of fusiform myofibroblasts/fibroblasts, fibrous connective tissue, and plasma cells, as well as varying numbers of lymphocytes, eosinophils, neutrophils, and foamy macrophages, with or without formation of lymphoid follicles. Other microscopic appearances include small thick-walled vessels with fibrinoid degeneration, luminal stenosis or occlusion, perivascular loose fibrous myxoid matrix, and focal coagulation necrosis in the center of the lesion. Pathogens may be found in tissue culture. Histological classifications of hepatic IPT are not consistent with each other. Zen et al. [105] briefly divided IPT into two histological types described as follows [105]:

1. Fibrohistiocytic type. This type contains dense collagen fiber bundles which are thread-like or disorderly arranged, dispersed with fat fusiform myofibroblasts/fibroblasts without atypia. And yellow granulomatous inflammation and multinucleated tissue-type giant cells (Fig. 5.41) are commonly observed with pigment particles in their foam-like cytoplasms. Besides, nodular deposition of eosinophilic contents can also be found in the lesions. Thickened wall and luminal stenosis due to organization of thrombus in hepatic vein lead to the formation of noninflammatory venous occlusion. And small bile ducts are infiltrated with inflammatory cells without sclerosing cholangitis. This type resembles the so-called xanthogranulomatous IPT.
2. Lymphoplasmacytic type. This type is characterized by diffuse infiltration of chronic inflammatory cells, mainly

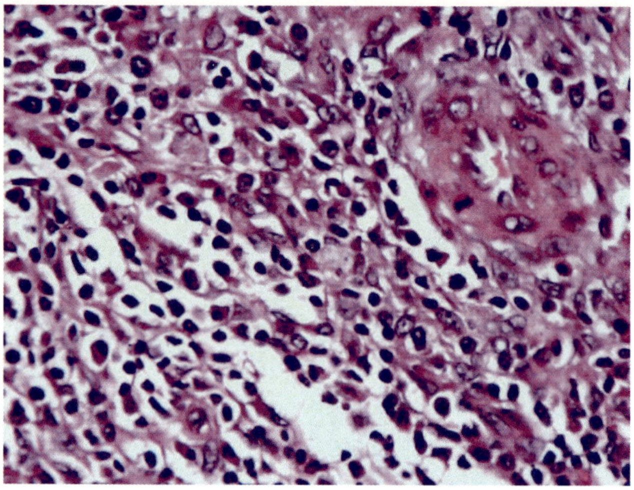

Fig. 5.42 Multinucleated giant cells and a large number of inflammatory cell infiltration

plasma cells and lymphocytes (Fig. 5.42). And Russell bodies are also discovered in the lesions. The inflammatory cells may infiltrate the peripheral nerve tissue and surround the bile ducts, resulting in cholangitis and edema of the peribiliary matrix. Lymphoplasmacytic-type IPT can contain diffusedly distributed IgG4-positive plasma cells and may belong to a special type of IgG4-related diseases. This type resembles the so-called plasmagranulomatous IPT.

5.3.2.5 Immunohistochemistry

Myofibroblasts were vimentin, SMA, desmin, CD30, and ALK (nuclear membrane) positive. ALK gene shows positive result in fluorescence in situ hybridization detection, while it shows negative results in detection in nodular fasciitis, desmoid tumor disease, and gastrointestinal stromal tumors. And CD21 and CD35 examinations show negative results. Assessment on IgG-/IgG4-positive percentage of plasma cells can also be carried out to define lesions of IPT.

5.3.2.6 Differential Diagnosis

IPT and inflammatory myofibroblastic tumor (IMT) are different diseases with different pathological features and should be differentiated from each other. The clinical and pathological characteristics of IMT are described in the next chapter. In addition, IPT should not be used to define disease with definite causes, such as organization of chronic liver abscess. Malignant inflammatory fibrous histiocytoma may contain a large number of inflammatory cells but can be differentiated from IPT due to the predominant content of neutrophils and foamy histiocytes. Lesions with a large number of lymphocytes and the formation of lymphatic follicle-like structure should be identified to exclude lymphoma which presents obvious atypia of lymphocytes. And IPT with SMA-positive spindle cells should be differentiated from leiomyosarcoma. The latter contains few inflammatory cells in the stroma and a high molecular weight protein, caldesmon, which is highly specific for smooth muscle but shows negative result in reactive myofibroblasts and can provide an evidence for differentiation. As to fibrosarcoma, it contains fusiform cells in characteristic "herringbone" arrangement, with negative SMA and actin examination. When IPT contains numerous polyclonal plasma cells, it should be differentiated from extramedullary plasmacytoma (EMP) and lymphoplasmacytic lymphoma, both of which are composed of monoclonal plasma cells and immunohistochemistry of EMP results in positive monoclonal IgG kappa or lambda light chain staining, and vimentin-positive myofibroblasts and tissue cells are absent. Futhermore, epithelioid cells occurring in IPT must be identified to exclude IPT-like follicular dendritic cell tumor. Patients with chronic hepatitis B may present elevated serum AFP, related to the damage of IPT to the surrounding liver cells, or other factors such as liver cirrhosis, especially when the IPT-like interstitial reaction occurs in tissues of HCC and cholangiocarcinoma, and the few tumor cells hide within inflammatory fibrous tissue; it should be carefully differentiated based on comprehensive evidences including the clinical history.

5.3.2.7 Treatment and Prognosis

A few cases concerning malignant hepatic tumors 6–7 years after surgery of IPT in the liver and postoperative recurrence of IPT have been reported, but it is unknown whether they are multiple primary lesions in the liver. Clinical treatment for the undefined lesions or large lesions with obvious symptoms in the patients is surgical resection. The patients of hepatic IPT treated in our hospital have reported no postoperative recurrence or metastases.

5.3.3 Inflammatory Myofibroblastic Tumor

Wen-Ming Cong
Department of Pathology, Eastern Hepatobiliary Surgery Hospital, Second Military Medical University,
Shanghai, China

Inflammatory myofibroblastic tumor (IMT) was once included in the classification of IPT, and the description of IPT in classification of tumors in the digestive system (2010 edition) was similar to the description of IMT in WHO classification of soft tissue tumors (2013 edition). It is probably true that some cases of IMT are actually IPT according to the descriptions in the literature. However, it is now recognized that IMT is a unique mesenchymal tumor with special molecular variation. Fusiform muscle fibroblasts may exhibit different degrees of atypia, and tumor cells were scattered in the

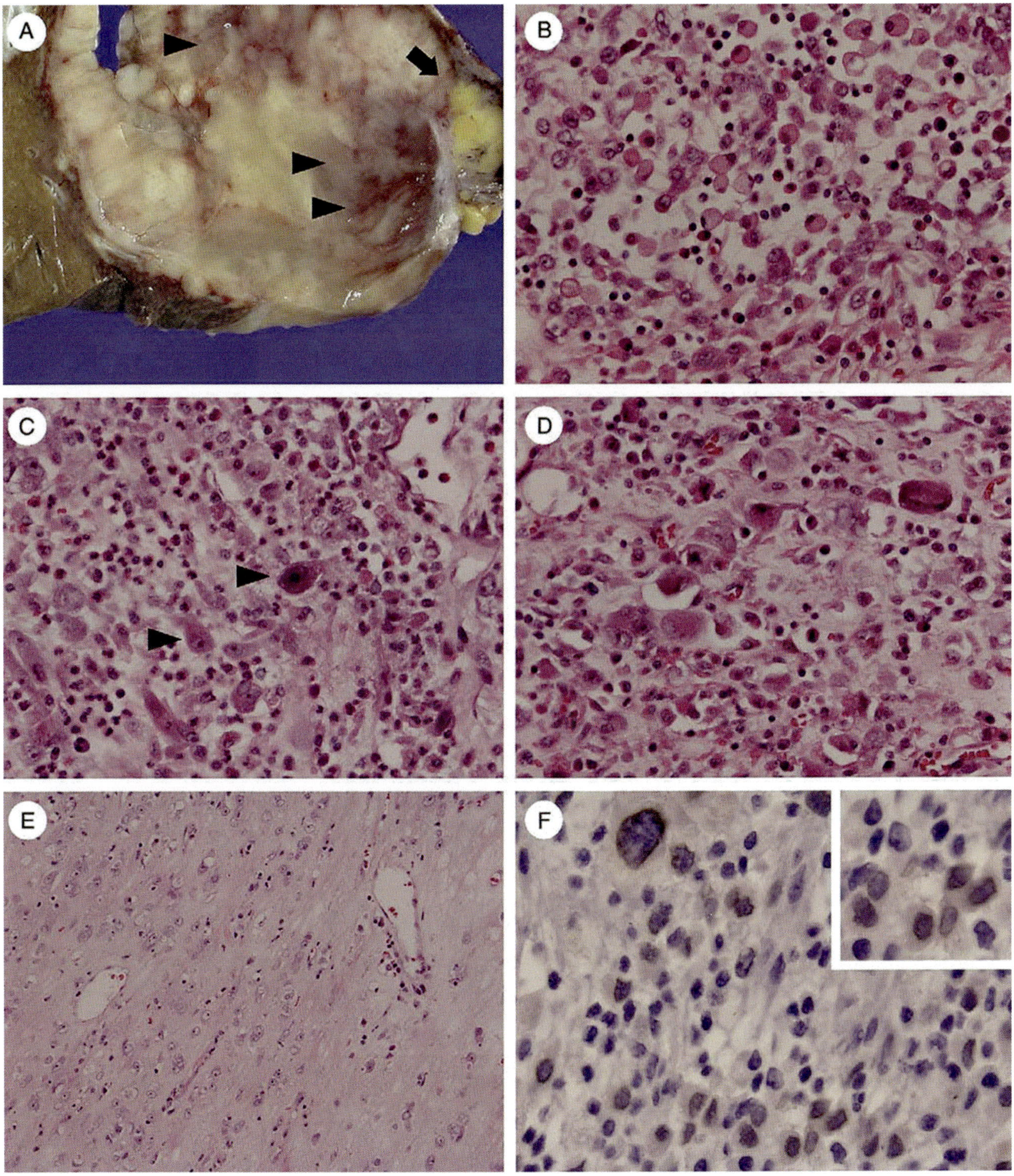

Fig. 5.43 Lymphoplasmacytic-type infiltration of inflammatory cells, mainly lymphocytes and plasma cells, with cholangitis

lesion with a circular or polygonal contour, abundant eosinophilic cytoplasm, a large eccentric vesicular nuclei, and a prominent nucleoli (Fig. 5.43) [106]. WHO classification of soft tissue tumors (2013 Edition) defined IMT as a borderline tumor with malignant potential [107], based on the finding that 50–70% of the children or young cases of IMT have rearrangements on chromosomal 2p23, involving anaplastic lymphoma kinase (ALK) and fusion of TIC, TMP3, TMP4, CLTC, and RANBP2 genes [108]. Overexpression or rearrangement of ALK gene occurs in 87.5–100% of IMT, and

Table 5.4 Clinical, pathological, and genetic properties in IPT and IMT

Factors	IPT	IMT
Pathogenesis	Infection/inflammation	Infection/self-immunology
Classification	Tumor-like lesion	Borderline tumor
Predilection site	Lung and liver	Mesentery, omentum majus, retroperitoneum, pelvis, soft tissues of the abdomen
Average age	37 years old	10 years old
Gender	More men than women	More women than men
IgG4-related sclerosis	Relevant	Irrelevant
Rearrangement of chromosome 2p23	None	With
Gross features	Single, nodular, off-white	Mutinodular, whirlpool-like
Microscopic typing	Fibrocyte type	Mucoid type
		Spindle cell type
	Lymphoplasmacyte type	Fibrous type
Cellular atypia	None	With
Expression of ALK gene	None	87.5~100%
ALK gene fusion	None	Frequent
IgG4-positive plasmocyte	Commonly seen	None
Recurrence	Rare	25%
Metastasis (lung, brain, liver, bone)	None	2%

some IMT cases may exhibit local postoperative recurrence (25%) [109] and metastasis (2%) [110]. Although WHO classification of soft tissue tumors (2013 Edition) defined IPT as a synonym for IMT, but in the classification of tumors in the digestive system (2010 Edition), it was suggested that IMT should be carefully differentiated from IPT to exclude misdiagnosis. Thus, taking into account the differences of IPT and IMT in clinical, pathological, and genetic variation (Table 5.4), histological features and concepts of them should be distinguished clearly.

5.3.4 Pseudolymphoma

5.3.4.1 Pathogenesis and Mechanism

Hepatic pseudolymphoma was first reported by Snover et al. in 1981, also known as reactive lymphoid hyperplasia, or nodular lymphoid disease, characterized by polyclonal lymphocyte proliferation and formation of active follicular germinal centers. Forty-six cases of hepatic pseudolymphoma have been reported by 2012 [111], and pseudolymphoma was also seen in the kidney, thyroid, breast, spleen, and other organs. The etiology and pathogenesis of pseudolymphoma are still unknown [112], while chronic infection or inflammation in its clinical course is shown to be relevant with immune response. Reports in the literature show it can be found in primary biliary cirrhosis, viral hepatitis, diabetes, autoimmune thyroiditis, or Sjögren syndrome (an exocrine gland-targeted autoimmune disease), suggesting that it may be related to autoimmune diseases, drug-induced damage, or malignant tumor [113].

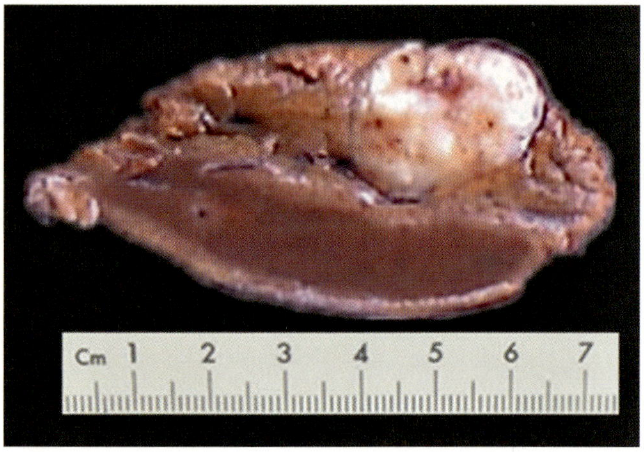

Fig. 5.44 Pseudolymphoma solitary nodule with a clear boundary and no envelope

5.3.4.2 Clinical Features

Six cases of hepatic pseudolymphoma have been diagnosed in the Department of Pathology, East Hepatobiliary Surgical Hospital, Second Military Medical University, with a male to female ratio of 2:1, an average age of 40 years old (ranged 20–50 years), and the average tumor diameter of 4 cm (ranged 1.8–8.5 cm). The patients manifest no special clinical symptoms or signs, and the lesions are often accidentally discovered. Ultrasound B inspection exhibits hypoechoes, and precontrast CT demonstrates hypodensity. MRI shows hypointensity on T1-weighted images and hyperintensity on T2-weighted images.

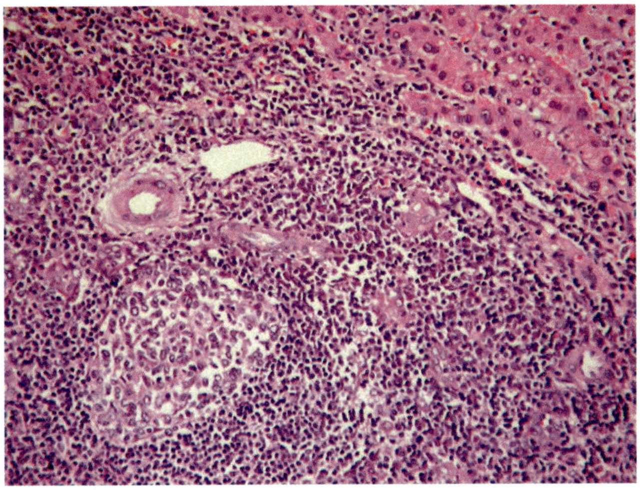

Fig. 5.45 Hyperplasia of lymphocytes to form lymphoid follicles with germinal centers

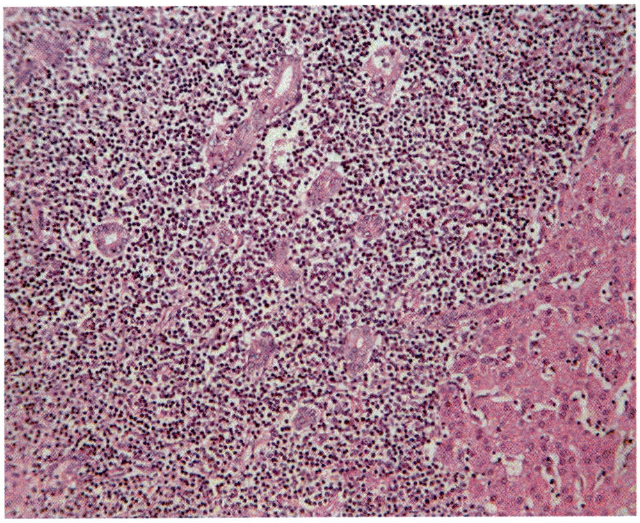

Fig. 5.46 Lymphocytes were uniform in morphology and no atypia, proliferated small bile ducts and a variety of inflammatory cells in lesion, with clear boundaries

5.3.4.3 Gross Features

Hepatic pseudolymphoma is commonly solitary nodule (84%), hard in texture, with a clear boundary and no envelope (Fig. 5.44).

5.3.4.4 Microscopic Features

Lesions consist of lymphoid follicles with germinal centers (Fig. 5.45), and the lymphocytes are diffusely distributed and uniform in morphology, with little cytoplasm and a round nucleus, and no atypia was observed. Other cells include different numbers of immuneblast lymphocytes, plasma cells, and histiocytes. And residual liver cell cords and proliferated small bile ducts are also observed in the tissue (Fig. 5.46), suggesting these are inflammatory hyperplastic lesions. In addition, small thick-walled blood vessels with hyaline degeneration, clear boundaries, and no invasion of the surrounding liver tissue can also be observed.

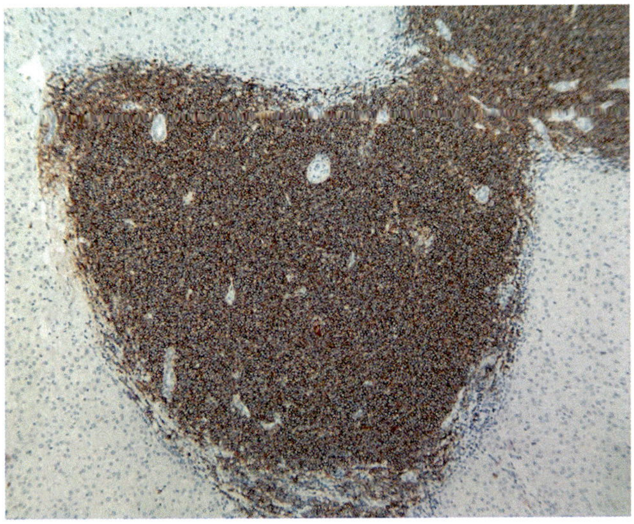

Fig. 5.47 B lymphocytes in germinal centers were positive in CD20 staining

5.3.4.5 Immunohistochemistry

The number of T cells and B cells are equal, indicating they are polyclonal. PCNA staining results in weak positive or negative. Bcl-2, IgG4, ALK, and SMA staining are negative. The germinal centers are mainly composed of B cells (Fig. 5.47), with peripheral T cells. In addition, no gene arrangements have found in situ hybridization of immunoglobulin protein kappa and lambda light chains and rearrangement analysis of IgH and TCR gene, suggesting hepatic pseudolymphoma is polyclonal.

5.3.4.6 Differential Diagnosis

Hepatic masses with predominant composition of lymphocytes should be distinguished from lymphoma, and the latter contains cells with poor adhesion ability, obvious atypia, and mitosis, and invasive growth along the hepatic sinus and immunohistochemistry and gene rearrangement analysis demonstrate it as monoclonal.

5.3.4.7 Treatment and Prognosis

There have been case reports of malignant lymphoma in the lung and stomach derived from pseudolymphoma. Therefore, when it is difficult to determine the nature of the lesions based on clinical evidences, surgical resection is a proper choice.

5.3.5 Pseudolipoma

5.3.5.1 Pathogenesis and Mechanism

Up to now, more than 20 cases of hepatic pseudolipoma have been reported in the literature. Its etiology is still unknown. Possible causes include abdominal surgery or poor physical conditions, which lead to poor local blood supply to the liver and degeneration of fat tissue in the omentum or abdomen. The degenerated fat tissue is then encapsulated by fibrous tissue before it is reversed and compressed into the space of the liver and the diaphragmatic muscle. Another possible mechanism involves the dislocation of embryonic omentum appendix and attachment into hepatic Glisson's capsule, with the lesion separated from the liver parenchyma. Thus, because of the special relationship between hepatic pseudolipoma and hepatic Glisson's capsule, the disease is also known as pseudolipoma of Glisson's capsule.

5.3.5.2 Clinical Features

Eight cases of hepatic pseudolipoma have been diagnosed in the Department of Pathology, East Hepatobiliary Surgical Hospital, Second Military Medical University in the past 30 years, and the patients were mainly elderly men, with a male to female ratio of 1:1 and an average age of 44.2 (25–76) years old. The lesions were generally found incidentally during physical examination or abdominal surgery. Some of the patients had a history of abdominal surgery. CT images display hypodense masses under Glisson's capsule on the surface of the right anterior lobe or right posterior lobe of the liver with hyperdensity in the center, with or without calcification.

5.3.5.3 Gross Features

Lesions are mostly seen in the right lobe of the liver, often solitary, encapsulated adipose masses, ovary or round in shape, 0.4–2 cm in diameter, and rarely larger than 2cm in size. The section is yellow or gray-white with elasticity.

5.3.5.4 Microscopic Features

The lesion is composed of mature adipose tissue. The central part is often accompanied by necrosis, calcification or ossification, and hyaline degeneration of capsular membrane, with few vessels in the capsule.

5.3.5.5 Differential Diagnosis

Pathological diagnosis is not difficult, but attention should be paid to differentiate it from true lipoma. Lipoma is often located within the liver parenchyma, with no adipose necrosis or calcification. Differentiation from adipose cell dominant angiomyolipoma should be made.

5.3.5.6 Treatment and Prognosis

When there are difficulties in differentiation from true tumors, surgical resection is the proper treatment with good prognosis.

5.3.6 Solitary Necrotic Nodules

5.3.6.1 Pathogenesis and Mechanism

Solitary necrotic nodules (SNN) were first proposed by Shepherd and Lee in 1983 and are rare inflammatory tumor-like lesion. The pathogenesis is still unknown, and no definite pathogens can be found in most of the lesions. And "nutrient vessels" were found in the tissue surrounding SNN in 1985, suggesting this may be the results of fibrosclerosis of small cavernous hemangioma. Some patients have a history of trauma, schistosomiasis, and sclerosing hemangioma.

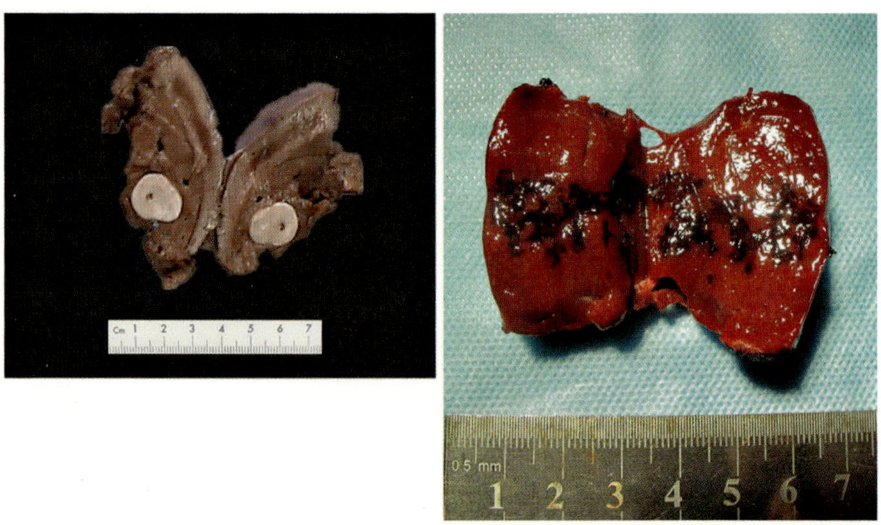

Fig. 5.48 Solitary necrotic nodules. A single pale *yellow* nodule with superficial small liquid cavity and clear boundary

5.3.6.2 Clinical Features

More than 250 cases of hepatic SNN have been diagnosed in the Department of Pathology, East Hepatobiliary Surgical Hospital, Second Military Medical University, and the ratio of male to female was 1.77:1. The average age of the patients was 46.4 (5–76 years). The patients are predominantly middle-aged or elderly male. No significant clinical symptoms or signs in most patients, and the lesions are more often found in medical imaging examination. The patients generally have no history of chronic hepatopathy, with a minority with the history of HBV infection. In patients with extrahepatic tumors, SNN is often misdiagnosed as metastasis tumor in the liver. Ultrasound B type examination shows hypoechoic lesions, and CT showed hypodense round nodules, with clear boundary and no infiltration. Plain and dynamic-enhanced MRI exhibits a higher diagnostic accuracy, while liver puncture biopsy is still difficult for the diagnosis [114].

5.3.6.3 Gross Features

The lesions are often solitary oblong nodules, mostly found in superficial parenchyma of the right posterior lobe of the liver near Glisson's capsule, with an average diameter of 2.4 (0.3–5 cm). The section exhibits pale or grayish-yellow, homogeneous, non-hemorrhage, and non-necrotic lesions, and small superficial liquid cavities are often seen and are one of the characteristics. Lesions show a clear boundary with a slender fibrous capsule (Fig. 5.48).

5.3.6.4 Microscopic Features

Histological features vary according to different causes for different lesions. And the lesions can be generally divided into four layers:

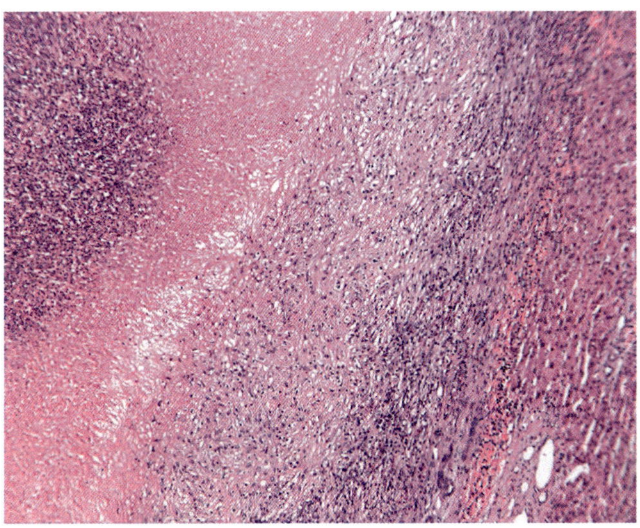

Fig. 5.49 Homogeneous necrotic tissue in the center of lesion, and outer layer is inflammatory fibrous zone

1. The central blue-stained necrotic tissue with cell debris, no live cells, and no definite pathogens
2. The peripheral homogeneous, coagulation necrosis without certain structure
3. Inflammatory fibrous tissue capsule with hyaline degeneration, varying numbers of eosinophils, and other inflammatory cells
4. Lymphocytic infiltration at the interface of the envelope and the adjacent liver tissue, with congestion in the peripheral hepatic sinus, proliferation of thick-walled blood vessels, and small bile ducts (Fig. 5.49)

In some SNN cases, lesions can be observed to exhibit multifocal fusion with a clear boundary and normal live cells and hepatolobules in the surrounding areas.

5.3.6.5 Differential Diagnosis

For patients with a history of malignant tumors, SNN is often misdiagnosed as a metastasis or hepatic tumor, due to the coagulative necrosis tissue in the lesion, and it is often more difficult to make a diagnosis via liver puncture of microtissue, and the lesion should be differentiated from tumor necrosis, including the observation of the morphology of the necrotic tissue, and tumor necrosis is often cord shaped. Increasing sample volume may be beneficial to find the residual tumor cells. SNN is different from acute liver abscess. The latter showed multifocal suppurative inflammation, and there are a large amount of degenerated and necrotic neutrophils, and the formation and organization of a thick fibrous envelope can be observed in cases with a longer course.

5.3.6.6 Treatment and Prognosis

Patients with SNN generally do not require special treatment. For cases difficult to define the nature of the lesions, surgical resection is a proper choice. Imura et al. [115] reported one case with a hepatic mass which grew from 3 cm to 8.5 cm in diameter, and the serum CA19-9 of the patient increased persistently during 7 month's follow-up [115]. Repeated liver biopsy failed to confirm the diagnosis and surgical resection was conducted. The postoperative pathological diagnosis was SNN and serum CA19-9 of the patient dropped to normal level.

5.3.7 Peliosis Hepatis

5.3.7.1 Pathogenesis and Mechanism

Hepatic peliosis hepatis (PH) was first named by Schoenlank in 1916 and reported by Zak for the first time in 1950. The pathogenesis is probably the damage to the liver microvascular system due to a variety of causes, leading to blocked output flow, and highly expansion of the liver parenchyma due to

Table 5.5 Surgical cases of PH in Eastern Hepatobiliary Surgery Hospital

Case No.	Age (years)	Gender	Location in the liver	Tumor size (cm)	Medical history
Case 1	29	Male	Left lobe	16 × 11 × 9	Abdominal mass
Case 2	36	Male	Right lobe	5.2 × 4.6	Hepatitis/liver cirrhosis
Case 3	42	Female	Right lobe	6 × 4	Physical examination
Case 4	49	Female	Right lobe	1.4 × 1	Post-breast cancer
Case 5	40	Female	Right lobe	0.6 × 0.4	Physical examination

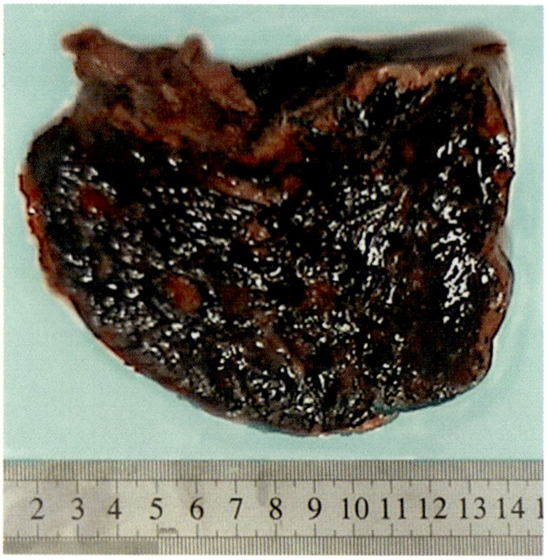

Fig. 5.50 Peliosis hepatis. Large mass containing blood in the cavities (Case 1), cite from Pan W

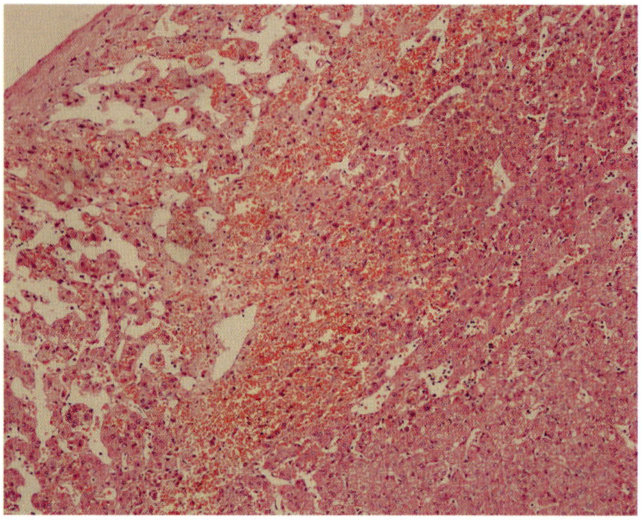

Fig. 5.51 Cavities containing blood were in various sizes and communicated with hepatic sinus

local hyperemia and hemorrhage in the regional liver sinus, forming multicystic hyperemia lesions. More than 20 cases of PH have been reported in China. And the possible causes of PH include long-term use of androgens and anabolic hormones, drugs for the treatment of leukemia (such as 6-thioguanine, mercaptopurine, 2-chloro-3'-deoxyadenosine), chemotherapy for colonic carcinoma (capecitabine combined with oxaliplatin), or oral contraceptive medication. And the lesion can be reduced in size after the drug withdrawal of the oral contraceptive medication. PH is also seen in patients with some chronic wasting diseases, such as tuberculosis, malignant tumors, long-term use of immunosuppressive agents after liver or renal transplantation (such as azathioprine), and AIDS. And infection by Bartonella henselae in diseases such as cat scratch disease may result in bacillary peliosis. In addition, purpura can occur in other organs, such as the lung, spleen, and lymph nodes. There are reports of PH complicated by hereditary hemorrhagic telangiectasia, suggesting the relation between PH and this autosomal-dominant genetic disease [116]. In our department, obvious purpuric change surrounding the hepatic focal nodular hyperplasia was observed in two cases with surgical resection of the lesions.

5.3.7.2 Clinical Features

Five cases of surgically excised PH have been diagnosed in the Department of Pathology, East Hepatobiliary Surgical Hospital, Second Military Medical University, with a male to female ratio of 2:3 and average age of 39.2 years (29–49), including one case with hepatitis B-related cirrhosis and suspected HCC, one case with breast cancer surgery, and suspected breast cancer of liver metastasis (Table 5.5). HP can occur at any age with the elderly as the majority. Except the above diseases, patients with PH often manifest no symptoms or signs. Only a minority of them present hepatomegaly and mild elevation of transaminase level, occasionally accompanied by spleen purpura or abdominal bleeding due to rupture of large HP [117]. Liver failure is observed in a few cases with massive hepatocellular damage, serious complications, and diffuse liver purpura. Coli purpura patients may have a fever, weight loss, anorexia, diarrhea, abdominal distention and pain, hepatosplenomegaly, and other manifestations. One report concerned one case of HP patients with pyelonephritis induced by *Escherichia coli*, acute liver failure, and intraperitoneal hemorrhage as the first symptoms. Ultrasound examination shows multiple hypoechoic areas with different sizes. CT images display multiple intrahepatic lesions with peripheral hypodensity and focal hyperdensity, suggesting the presence of blood. Clinical differentiation should be made mainly from multiple liver abscesses, adenoma, focal nodular hyperplasia, nodular regenerative hyperplasia, hemangioma, and metastasis of malignant tumor [118].

5.3.7.3 Gross Features

Lesions can be divided into mononodular type and multinodular type. The HP cases in our hospital were all mononodular type. The lesions were generally 0.1–1 cm in diameter or up to 16 cm in a certain case (Fig. 5.50). Lesions of multinodular type are located in the whole liver, characterized by diffuse, slightly rounded cystic cavities or blots containing blood with different sizes in liver parenchyma (involving both the right and the left lobes), with fibrosis or organization in some obsolete lesions.

5.3.7.4 Microscopic Features

Lesions are composed by numerous oval cavities containing blood in various sizes, with or without the endothelial cell lining, and communicate with the adjacent hepatic sinus or central veins, and intraluminal thrombus may be found (Fig. 5.51). In bacillary peliosis, round cells similar to histoid cells can be discovered in the loose and edema matrix, with slightly purple granular cytoplasm, and special staining indicates microorganisms. And infiltration of inflammatory cell is observed in the interstitial tissue. Yanoff divided hepatic peliosis into two types in 1964, namely, vein type and hepatic parenchymal type, but it has been rarely mentioned because of its little clinical significance.

5.3.7.5 Differential Diagnosis

PH should be differentiated from hepatic angiosarcoma or hemangioma, and misdiagnosis of common dilation and congestion of the hepatic sinus as PH should be avoided.

5.3.7.6 Treatment and Prognosis

Symptomatic treatment. For drug-induced lesions with mild symptoms, drug withdrawal results in spontaneous decrease of the lesions in size. Erythromycin and doxycycline have good effect on bacillary peliosis, and surgical resection or hepatic artery ligation is suitable for localized lesions which rupture and cause bleeding. Severe PH may induce hepatic failure or hypovolemic shock and death due to the rupture and bleeding of PH lesions. If the lesion size is limited, close observation without any treatments is an alternative, and if the lesion size increases, microwave coagulation and radiofrequency ablation therapy may be helpful. Since huge lesions are at high risks of bleeding, hepatic artery embolization or surgical resection should be demonstrated [119], and liver transplantation is also a choice in treating PH.

In addition, Cha et al. [120] reported five cases of hepatic lipopeliosis occurred after liver transplantation. Lipopeliosis is a purpura-like change, mainly caused by liver cell necrosis due to preservation injury. Fat content in the necrotic liver cells overflows into the liver sinusoids, resulting in fat globule-filled hepatic sinusoid [120]. And a later report demonstrated the nodular lesions with fat content in the images of lipopeliosis.

5.3.8 Sarcoidosis

5.3.8.1 Pathogenesis and Mechanism

Sarcoidosis, also known as sarcoid pseudotumor or sarcoidoma, was described as early as in 1877. The incidence of sarcoidosis is (10~20)/10 million people, and the highest incidence is reported in Nordic and African Americans, especially in women, and Japan has the lowest incidence rate [121]. Sarcoidosis is a systemic chronic noncaseating granulomatous disease involving multiple systems. The lung and lymph nodes (> 90%) are the most common organs, and the liver ranks the third. Nearly two thirds of the patients with sarcoidosis have lesions in the liver. Other organs include the skin, salivary gland, spleen, heart, muscle, bone, eyes, and nervous system. Among the 14 types of hepatic granulomatous lesions in 202 cases, according to the statistics provided by Institute of Hepatology, University of Southern California, USA, the most common type was hepatic sarcoidosis, accounting for 28.3%.

The exact etiology of sarcoidosis remains unclear, and pathogens have not been found in tissue culture, special staining, and serological examination. It has been presumed that individuals with genetic susceptibility suffer immunological response involving cellular and humoral immune systems, induced by factors including special, environmental, and occupational pathogen. During the process, host macrophages are activated by various antigens to produce IL-1. T lymphocytes are activated by second contact with those antigens and produce IL-2 and a variety of lymphokins, stimulating proliferation of T lymphocytes and local aggression of macrophages in the lesion, resulting in a series of pathological changes. It has been reported that DNA and RNA of mycobacterium were isolated from the lesions, and growth of acid fast bacilli was detected in the serum of the patients. And DNA of mutated human herpesvirus 8 was discovered in the lesions recently, suggesting the relation of these factors to the pathogenesis of sarcoidosis. And whether HIV is the cause of sarcoidosis remains to be further studied. Genes including angiotensin-converting enzyme (ACE), BTNL2, HLA-DR [122], and MHC-2 may associate with the susceptibility, phenotype, and prognosis of sarcoidosis, and pri-

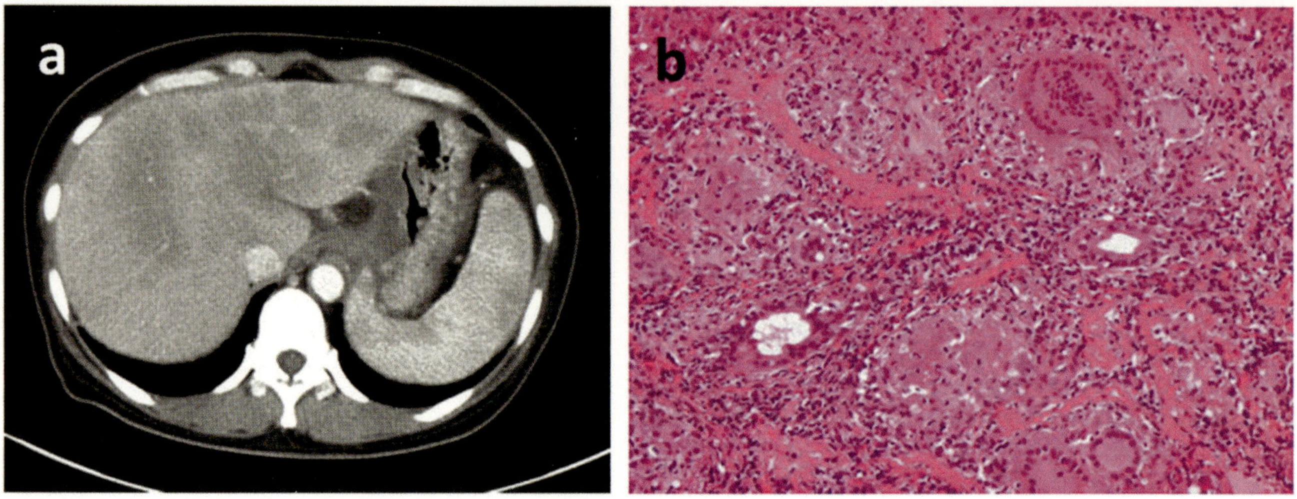

Fig. 5.52 (**a**) Enhanced CT showed multiple low attenuation lesions in the liver; (**b**) liver biopsy showed noncaseating granuloma in portal area (Cite from Ara N) [124]

mary biliary cirrhosis complicated by hepatic sarcoidosis has also been reported [123].

5.3.8.2 Clinical Features

The diagnosis of sarcoidosis consists of three elements: clinical manifestations, imaging, and noncaseating necrotizing granuloma. The patients are generally aged 20–40 years old, patients aged less than 20 years, and over 60 years account for less than 1%, with male to female ratio of approximate 1:1. It has an occult clinical course, and 50% of the patients with sarcoidosis manifest no symptoms for a long time. Its clinical manifestations are relevant to the involved organs, and 5–30% of the patients exhibit hepatosplenomegaly, nausea, vomiting, abdominal pain, and jaundice. Laboratory testing indexes for the diagnosis of sarcoidosis include complete blood count (CBC), electrolytes, urea nitrogen and creatinine, liver enzymes, alkaline phosphatase, serum calcium, urine (urine calcium and creatinine), immunoglobulin, and angiotensin-converting enzyme (ACE). And 40% of the patients have abnormal liver function with elevated levels of ALP (2–30 times higher than normal level) in most of the cases, while 50–80% of the patients have higher levels of ACE than normal, even up to 28–30 times, related to the degree of disease activity. CT scan shows multiple hypodense lesions, sometimes similar to the image of lymphoma (Fig. 5.52a).

5.3.8.3 Gross Features

Diffusely distributed multiple nodules in the whole liver are observed, with large fusion lesions of 0.1–5 cm in diameter. Involvement of extrahepatic bile duct or portal lymph nodes can also be observed.

5.3.8.4 Microscopic Features

The diagnosis of sarcoidosis can be made via liver puncture biopsy in 60–75% of the patients. Epithelioid granulomas often appear in the portal area and its surroundings, and the typical sarcoid granulomas consists of Langhans multinucleated macrophages in the center of the lesion, peripheral epithelioid cells, outer layer with a small amount of inflammatory cells (lymphocytes, plasma cells addicted to eosinophile cells), and fibroblasts (Fig. 5.52b). Bile accumulation is found in the liver cells. No damage or fibrosis of hepatic lobules is observed in the early stage of the lesions, and hepatocirrhosis pseudolobuli can be seen in the late stage of the disease.

Inclusion bodies in the multinucleated giant cells exhibit in three forms: (1) asteroid body, starfish shaped, often found in the spherical vesicles, 5–20 μm in diameter, and positive in anti-ubiquitin (UB) antibody staining; (2) Schaumann bodies, with a diameter of 25–200 μm, round or oval in shape, concentric laminated, and more commonly seen in sarcoidosis in the lymph node; and (3) homogeneous vesicle, single or multiple.

5.3.8.5 Immunohistochemistry

Epithelioid histiocytes and multinucleated giant cells exhibited positive results in SACE, alpha-1-AT, and lysozyme staining, and the lymphocytes are positive in CD4, CD45RO, and CD68 staining and negative in CD20 staining. Fibrinoid necrosis instead of non-caseous necrosis can be shown in the center of a granuloma.

5.3.8.6 Differential Diagnosis

The basic features of sarcoidosis is onset in young or middle-aged people, multiorgan involvement, without a clear etiology and noncaseating epithelioid granuloma; the latter can be observed in many hepatic diseases, such as histoplasmosis, schistosomiasis, cytomegalovirus (CMV) infection, Rickettsia infection (Q fever), lymphoma, or drug-induced hepatitis. Therefore, the diagnosis of sarcoidosis is primarily based on the exclusion of other granulomatous diseases and identification of sarcoidosis in other parts of the body. In addition, elevated serum ACE can also appear in patients with TB. And clinical manifestations in some patients of sarcoidosis are similar to that of primary biliary cirrhosis, such as chronic cholestasis, portal hypertension, or liver cirrhosis, except the absence of anti-mitochondrial antibody in serum.

5.3.8.7 Treatment and Prognosis

Granuloma in early sarcoidosis can heal completely without a scar, but a few patients (less than 1%) can develop liver fibrosis and cirrhosis. Granulomatous cholangitis, similar to primary biliary cirrhosis or primary sclerosing cholangitis, can cause destruction of portal area resulting in portal hypertension, Budd-Chiari syndrome, gastroesophageal varices, etc., and the oppression on hepatic bile ducts by enlargement of portal lymph nodes contributes to obstructive jaundice. Thus, early and proper interventions are generally with good prognosis. For patients with systemic sarcoidosis, periodic examination on the liver is recommended, regardless of whether there is liver cirrhosis. Systemic corticosteroid therapy is usually the first choice, and clinical symptoms in 25–40% of the patients alleviate after 2–3 months' treatment. And azathioprine, methotrexate, or hydroxychloroquine can be used in case of ineffective corticosteroid therapy. Other alternative drugs include immunosuppressant and infliximab. Studies have shown that hepatic sarcoidosis can be treated by ursodeoxycholic acid, which significantly improve the index of liver function and alleviate symptoms such as itching and fatigue [125].

Supplementary, Pathological diagnostic criteria in Diagnosis and Treatment of Sarcoidosis (1994) by Respiratory Disease Branch of Chinese Medical Association include:

1. Lesions are mainly small and homogeneous granulomatous nodules composed of epithelioid cells, with clear boundaries.
2. Non-caseous necrosis in the nodules and focal fibrinoid necrosis in the center of the nodules can be observed occasionally.
3. Multinucleated giant cells (foreign body giant cells and Langhans giant cells) as well as a few lymphocytes are distributed in the nodules. Infiltration of a large amount of lymphocytes can be seen around the nodules, which is replaced by fibrous tissue in the late phase of the disease. Fusion nodules can be seen in lesions with large amounts of small nodules which usually maintain their original nodular contour.
4. Inclusion Schaumann bodies, double refraction crystals, and stellate bodies are more commonly seen than tubercles, especially Schaumann bodies. And large amounts of double refraction crystals under polarizing microscopy are suggestive of sarcoidosis.
5. Silver staining shows massive hyperplasia of reticular fibrous tissue in the nodules and around the nodules (reticular fibers and nodule in the center of tubercles are often complete).
6. Special staining fails to show *Mycobacterium tuberculosis* (oil polyperimetry inspection), fungus, or other pathogens.
7. Small thin-walled blood vessels in the nodules.

Terminology in the diagnosis of sarcoidosis:

Diagnosed as sarcoidosis: with typical pathological and clinical features
Cannot exclude sarcoidosis: granulomatous lesions with atypical pathological features, with or without typical clinical features
Localized sarcoid reaction: basically consistent with the histological features of sarcoidosis, complicated by other diagnosed diseases, such as malignant tumors

5.3.9 Nodular Extramedullary Hematopoiesis

5.3.9.1 Pathogenesis and Mechanism

Hepatic nodular extramedullary hematopoiesis (NEMH) is one of the most common types of extramedullary hematopoiesis, exhibiting hepatic tumor or space-occupying lesions. The liver is one of the hematopoietic sites in the early stages of fetal development, and hepatic hematopoiesis has been observed in the fetus since the sixth month of pregnancy, while bone marrow is the only normal site for hematopoiesis after birth which lasts a lifetime. Under pathological conditions, in the embryonic phase, tissue that once made blood will be reactivated to form hematopoietic foci again, namely, extramedullary hematopoiesis. Mechanism of extramedullary hematopoiesis involves two main hypotheses. One is hematopoiesis of atavic mesenchymal cells which consist of hematopoietic organs in the embryonic phase and are reactivated to compensate the deficiency of medullary hematopoiesis. The other is the homing and reconstruction of hematopoietic foci of hematopoietic stem cells in the peripheral circulation, which are relocated in the organs with hematopoietic function in embryonic phase and consist of new hematopoietic foci under pathological conditions. Extramedullary hematopoiesis can be induced by damage to the bone marrow in the case of some lesions, such as bone marrow fibrosis and aplastic anemia, or destruction of large amounts of blood cells, such as hemolytic anemia caused by

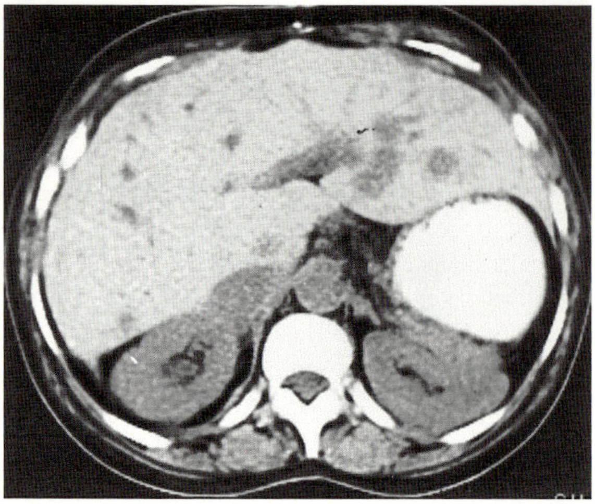

Fig. 5.53 Nodular extramedullary hematopoiesis. CT showed multiple hypodense regions in the liver parenchyma (Cite from Lemos L [127])

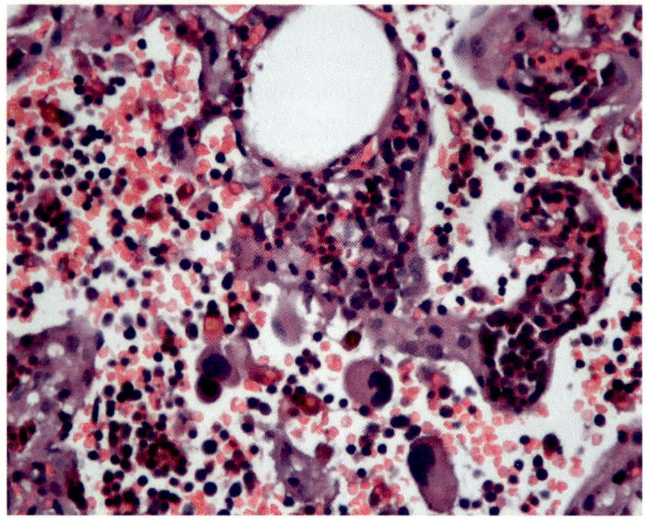

Fig. 5.54 Extramedullary hematopoiesis. A large number of diffuse distribution erythroid, granulocytic, and megakaryocytic cells

various factors. Besides the liver, extramedullary hematopoiesis can also occur in the retroperitoneum, adrenals, kidneys, pelvis, falx cerebri, spleen, lung, lymphoid tissue, mediastinum, and brain tissue. Up to now, less than 20 cases have been reported at home and abroad, almost all of which were primarily diagnosed as metastatic liver cancer or multiple hepatic abscesses.

5.3.9.2 Clinical Features

NEMH is often seen in patients with chronic mediterranean anemia, hereditary spherocytosis, leukemia, myelofibrohyperplasic syndrome, aplastic anemia, etc. [126]. The patients commonly manifest hepatosplenomegaly and abnormal liver function. Nucleated red blood cells in peripheral blood smear and active hyperplasia shown in bone marrow examination are helpful to the diagnosis. CT revealed multiple hypodense regions in the liver parenchyma with homogeneous density and clear boundaries in patients with NEMH (Fig. 5.53), and enhanced CT scan showed significant homogeneous enhancement of the lesions in arterial phase, nearly isodensity in venous phase, and mild hypodensity in delayed phase, with no signs of envelope or edema around the lesions. ^{59}Fe (iron) citrate imaging is helpful to the diagnosis, and NEMH can be diagnosed by liver biopsy.

5.3.9.3 Gross Features

Multiple lesions, which can be as large as 14.5 cm × 12.5 cm [128].

5.3.9.4 Microscopic Features

The lesions consist of myeloid hematopoietic cells in different stage of maturation in clusters, including erythroid, granulocytic, and megakaryocytic cells (Fig. 5.54). The nucleated red blood cells aggregate into groups with rich eosinophilic cytoplasm and a large and round nuclear which is located in the center with hyperchromatic chromatin. The megakaryocytes contain atypical multilobular nucleus, with positive F-VII in immunohistochemistry and positive Diff-Quik staining. Hemosiderin deposition often occurs in the liver cells of patients with hemolytic anemia, and when liver cells and tissue cells contain large amounts of black or brown pigment in the cytoplasm, Prussian blue staining can be used to confirm the iron particles, which is helpful in the diagnosis.

5.3.9.5 Immunohistochemistry

Hematopoietic cells are F-VII positive.

5.3.9.6 Differential Diagnosis

NEMH should be mainly differentiated from metastatic tumors. And atypical megakaryocytes, almost absent in HCC, should not be mistaken as cancer cells.

5.3.9.7 Treatment and Prognosis

The patients of NEMH should be treated with symptomatic therapy and generally do not need surgical treatment.

5.3.10 Cystic Echinococcosis

5.3.10.1 Pathogenesis and Mechanism

The four main types of *Echinococcus* cause cystic echinococcosis (CE), namely, *Echinococcus granulosus*, *Echinococcus multilocularis*, *Echinococcus oligarthrus*, and *Echinococcus vogeli* Rausch and Bernstein. The former two have been reported in China, and the most commonly seen CE is induced by *Echinococcus granulosus* larvae (also known as *Echinococcus granulosus* disease). The scientists of our country have sketched the gene map of 151.6 MB sequence of *Echinococcus granulosus* in 2013 [129], including 11,325 coding genes. And alveolar echinococcosis (AE, also known as *Echinococcus multilocularis*), induced by *Echinococcus multilocularis* larvae, accounts for only 3.3% of the hepatic CE, mainly distributed in Northwestern China and the Qinghai-Tibet Plateau.

CE is mainly found in countries and regions with developed animal husbandry. In China, most patients with CE are found in Northwestern regions including Xinjiang, Inner Mongolia, Tibet, and Qinghai [130], and sporatic cases of CE patients, who have contacted or kept pets, have been reported in cities, such as Shanghai. Adult *Echinococcus* parasite in canine animals, such as dogs and wolves, are the final hosts, and human, cattle, sheep, horses, and pigs are the intermediate hosts for larvae (*Echinococcus*). An adult *Echinococcus* generally has three segments, namely, the scolex, somite, and gestational segment. The scolex is fixed in the crypt of the intestinal villi of the proximal small intestine, via 28–40 hooks on the rostellum and 4 suckers. The hooks are arranged alternately with large ones and small ones. The gestational segment, which contains 200–800 oncosphere ova discharged along with the host feces, is hyperactive in movement and can crawl across the lawn or plant in the form of peristalsis, resulting in contamination of animal fur and the surrounding environment by the ova, including pastures, barns, vegetables, soil, water source, and so on.

After the intermediate hosts (cattle, sheep) swallow *Echinococcus* eggs and gestational segments, onchospheres hatch and go into the intestinal wall into the blood circulation and arrive in the liver, lungs, and other organs, later developing into *Echinococcus* tapeworms in 3–5 months with a diameter of 1–3 cm [131]. Protoscolices grow into new *Echinococcus* during dispersion in the intermediate hosts and develop to adults in the final hosts. As for human beings, who are one of the intermediate hosts of *Echinococcus granulosus*, *Echinococcus* eggs are delivered into the mouths of people via contaminated foods and drinks such as meat, vegetables, fruits, dairy products, and drinking water or by contacting the fur of animals with egg adhesion, and then larvae, namely, onchospheres, hatch out of the eggs in the duodenum, which drill through the intestinal mucosa into the mesenteric vein and then the portal vein system and finally into the liver. About 75% of onchosphere larvae will stay in the hepatic portal area and develop into *Echinococcus*, resulting in CE, and the rest of the larvae will circulate into other organs such as the lung and brain causing CE at these sites.

5.3.10.2 Clinical Features

CE involves people of all age. There are 58 cases of CE diagnosed in the Department of Pathology, East Hepatobiliary Surgical Hospital, Second Military Medical University. The male to female ratio is 1:1, and the average age is 38.7 years old (ranged 7–76 years). The symptoms and signs are determined by the sizes, number, and location of cysts. For patients with a history of living in animal husbandry areas or epidemic regions, or close contact with dogs, sheep, or cattle, and manifesting upper abdominal cystic masses with slowly increasing sizes during a long period with good conditions in general, the diagnosis of CE may be the primary consideration. On average, the diameters of the cysts half a year after the initial infection reach 0.5–1.0 cm and increase by 1–5 cm per year with large ones reaching the size of tens of centimeters. For sporadic cases in urban with or without a history of pet keeping, the latent period of CE can be several years or even decades. And the diagnostic accuracy of testing for CE, including *Echinococcus* antigen intradermal test (Casoni test), indirect agglutination test, and complement fixation test, is over 90%, and larvae with complete structure can be observed on the smear of punctured fresh cystic fluid. Type-B ultrasonic inspection reveals a bilayer structure of the cyst. And according to the images of ultrasonic examination, classification of the cysts has been proposed by WHO [132], including cystic lesion (CL), monocyst (CE1), polycysts (CE2), cysts with collapsed inner cyst (CE3), cysts with consolidation (CE4), and cysts with calcification (CE5). CL, CE1, and CE2 echinococcosis are in growth stage with high activity, and CE3 is in transition stage with decreased developmental capacity, while CE4 and CE5 are echinococcosis with no activity or developmental capacity.

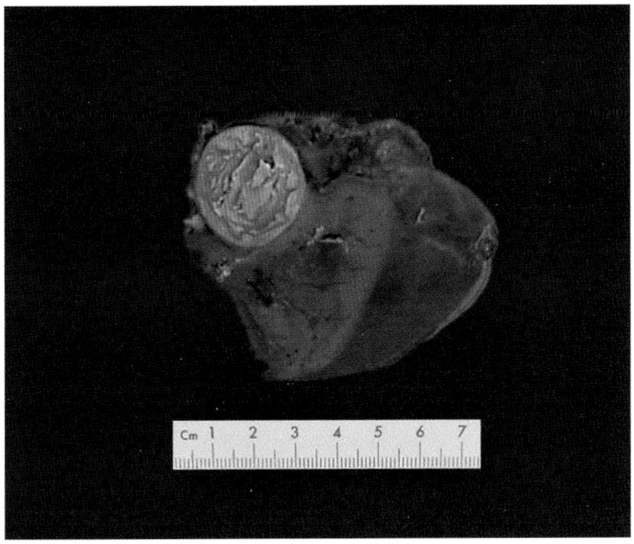

Fig. 5.55 Cystic echinococcosis multicystic structure

5.3.10.3 Gross Features

Unilocular CE, accounting for 75% of CE, are mostly found in the right lobe of the liver, often two or three cysts and 1.5 to 20 cm in diameter with an average of 3 cm. The outermost layer of the cyst is a fibrous capsule, also called capsula externa, and the sublayer is milky-white vermicelli-like internal capsule, composed of smooth cuticle, about 1 mm

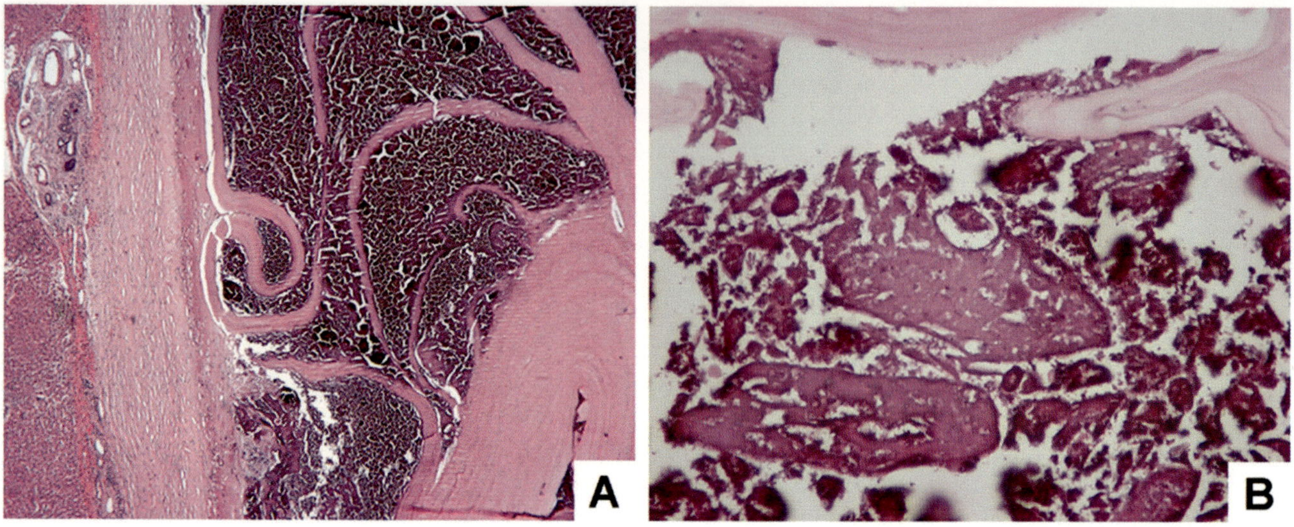

Fig. 5.56 (**a**) There is fibrous capsule, cuticle, germinal layer, and its contents from outside to inside; (**b**) daughter cyst at high magnification

thick (Fig. 5.55) and filled with hydatid fluid, which is colorlessly transparent or milky-white, and the fluid is with varying volumes from a dozen to tens of thousands milliliter containing a large number of daughter cyst, granddaughter cyst, and protoscolex. And once a cyst ruptures into the abdominal cavity, thoracic cavity, or biliary tracts, it will cause secondary CE at these sites.

5.3.10.4 Microscopic Features

Oncosphere is rounded and saccate in shape, which gets the name for its three pairs of hooks. Its internal capsule consists of the stratum corneum and germinal layer; the outer stratum corneum is a red-stained lamellar layer, composed of secretion produced by cells in the germinal layer, which is the underneath layer close to the stratum corneum with composition of *Echinococcus* bodies (Fig. 5.56). The germinal cells may continue sprout formation to generate germinal vesicles containing large quantities of larval scolex, which will dissociate to form a daughter cyst, and the latter generates a granddaughter cyst following similar process. The internal capsule is coated with fibrous tissue which gives it a clear boundary from the liver tissue.

5.3.10.5 Differential Diagnosis

The shape and structure of AE adults are similar to *Echinococcus granulosus*, but their bodies are smaller, though the shape and size of the eggs are difficult to distinguish from *Echinococcus granulosus*. Different from the clinical and pathological features of CE, almost all AE occurred in the liver and demonstrate vesicle-like masses constructed by a large number of small grape-like vesicles instead of large solitary vesicles. Under the microscope, AE have no internal capsula, and the vesicle clusters are surrounded by fibrous hyperplasia with infiltration of eosinophils, lymphocytes, plasma cells, and macrophages, forming *Alveococcus* nodules. According to the status of *Alveococcus* proliferation, pathological grading of AE is proposed as follows. Grade I of recessive AE is mainly composed by fibrous connective hyperplasia, suggesting decrease of parasite vigor. Grade II of proliferation AE is mainly composed by vesicles with visible internal or external colonization of gemmation, suggesting high *Alveococcus* vitality.

5.3.10.6 Treatment and Prognosis

CE may undergo spontaneous or collision rupture, and the patients may even suffer sudden death because of anaphylactic shock in severe cases. Occasionally, CE complicated by hepatocellular carcinoma is reported. Besides, AE can also disseminate along the blood and lymphatic vessels with high mortality. Surgical treatment remains to be the main therapy for AE, and the principles include excision of internal capsule, prevention of the overflow of the cystic fluid, elimination of the extracapsular residual cavity, and prevention of infection. In addition to surgery therapy, chemotherapy, radiation intervention, etc. are also options for early treatment with good effect. Percutaneous puncture treatment is alternative in some cases [133]. Hepatic alveolar echinococcosis is generally found in middle and advanced stages in clinical practice, and the cases with radical resection of the lesions account for less than 30%.

Liver transplantation has become the optimal treatment approach for these patients. According to a foreign report of 45 cases of liver transplantation in patients with echinococcosis of the liver, the 5-year overall survival rate and disease-free survival rate were 71% and 58%, respectively [134]. And domestic reports presented a good curative effect of liver transplantation in these patients [135]. Those patients who have inactive simple CE4 and CE5 cysts without any symptoms are suggested to be closely observed and followed up.

5.3.11 Liver Abscess

Liver abscess is the process of inflammation of liver parenchyma and stroma, including suppurative and amebic abscess. Ninety-five cases of liver abscess have been diagnosed in the Department of Pathology, East Hepatobiliary Surgical Hospital, Second Military Medical University, with a male to female ratio of 2:1, and the average age was 46.3 (ranged 3–76) years old.

1. Bacterial abscess

The main pathogen of bacterial abscess is pyogenic bacterium and predominantly consists of *Escherichia coli*, *Streptococcus*, *Escherichia coli*, *Staphylococcus aureus*, *Klebsiella* pneumonia, etc., while liver abscess due to infection of anaerobic bacteria accounts for one third with a mortality rate of 30–75%. In addition, fungal infection has also been reported, such as cases infected by *Cryptococcus neoformans*. There are seven main pathways of infection: (1) via bile duct (e.g., suppurative cholangitis), mostly common, accounts for 43%, (2) via hepatic artery (e.g., septicemia), (3) via portal vein (e.g., suppurative portal vein), (4) direct spreading (e.g., subdiaphragmatic abscess), (5) post-traumatic infection, (6) nosocomial infection, and (7) cryptogenic abscess in a few cases in which definite pathogen cannot be determined. Generally, biliary liver abscess is multiple small abscesses, distributed along the biliary tracts, while hematogenous liver abscess is multiple or solitary large abscesses. And it is difficult to differentiate liver abscess from HCC or metastatic tumors due to the multifarious performance of liver abscess in imaging [136].

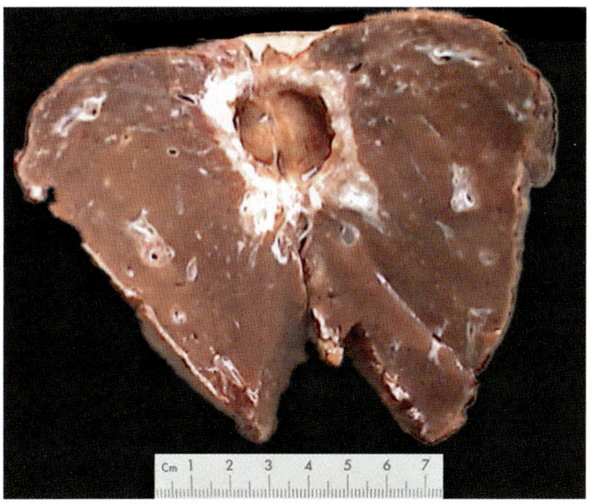

Fig. 5.57 Liver abscess cavity in the center of the lesion, and thick fibrous wall was formed surrounding the cavity

In general, 73% of the liver abscess is a single lesion with an average diameter of 6.8 cm. An acute abscess is purulent, consisting of degenerative necrotic neutrophils and liquefactive necrotic cells in liver parenchyma, surrounding by inflammatory congestive hemorrhage, without fibrous encapsulation. In chronic abscess, a thick fibrous connective encapsulation is observable around the lesion (Fig. 5.57), and the necrotic tissue in the abscess may undergo gradual organization (Fig. 5.58) and calcification, with significant infiltration of eosinophilic granulocytes within encapsulation. Chronic abscess is different from inflammatory pseudo-tumor in the liver, because the latter consists of various compositions with plasma cells as the predominant content and necrotic tissue is few and insignificant.

Liver abscess caused by different pathogens should be treated with corresponding strategies. Active conservative

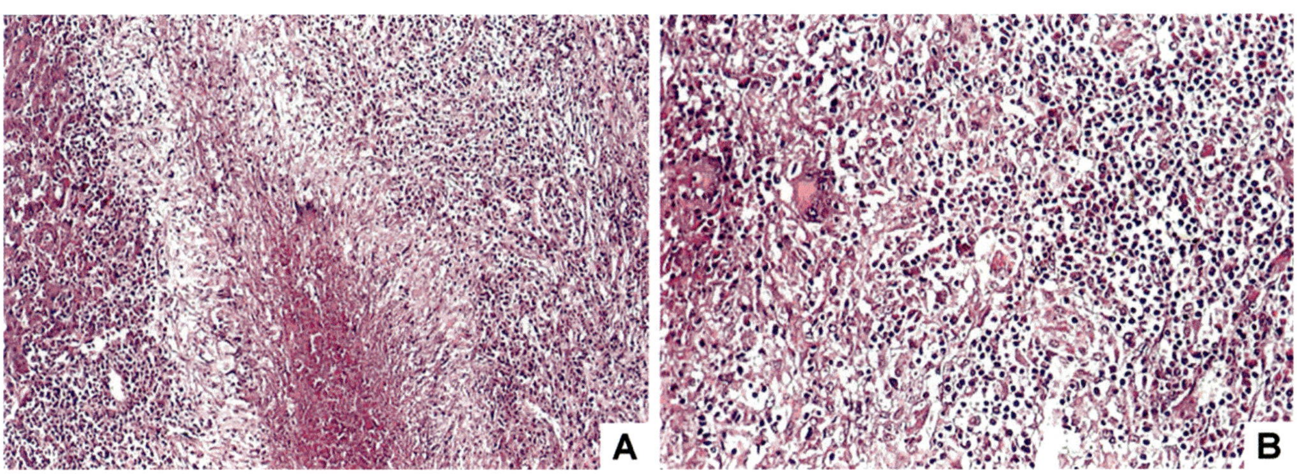

Fig. 5.58 (**a**) Most of the abscess was organization; (**b**) many nuclear giant cells and a large number of inflammatory cells at high magnification

treatment should be given to acute focal inflammation in the liver with no formation of abscess or with only multiple small abscesses. And systemic antibiotics and supporting therapy should be combined with the treatment of the primary lesions, which contribute to the control and absorption of the inflammation. For patients with a large abscess which risks rupture, who have obvious clinical manifestations, but the antibiotic treatment is ineffective or the diagnosis cannot be determined, surgical drainage is an option.

2. Amebic abscess

Amoeba echinococcosis is a zoonotic intestinal protozoal disease, which is a common complication of intestinal amebiasis, caused by the invasion of protozoa into the small veins of intestine wall which circulate into the liver via portal vein, resulting in lytic necrosis of liver cells to form typical chocolate-like abscess. Lesions located in the right lobe of the liver account for 80~90%, mostly single large cystic masses with a medium of 6.9 (ranged 5~29) cm in diameter [137], and *Amoeba* trophozoites can be found in the necrotic tissue at the margin of the abscesses. The *Amoeba* trophozoites are slightly rounded, with clear cell membrane, small and round nuclei, and cytoplasm with vacuolization or red blood cells via phagocytosis (Fig. 5.59). The punctured fluid is "chocolate sauce" pus in the amebic liver abscess, consisting of degenerative and necrotic liver cells, red blood cells, bile, and residual necrotic tissue, clinically manifested as acute abdomen. The abscess can develop secondary bacterial infection [138]. The first choice for treatment is anti-amebic drugs (metronidazole as the preferred drug), and drainage should be considered when necessary.

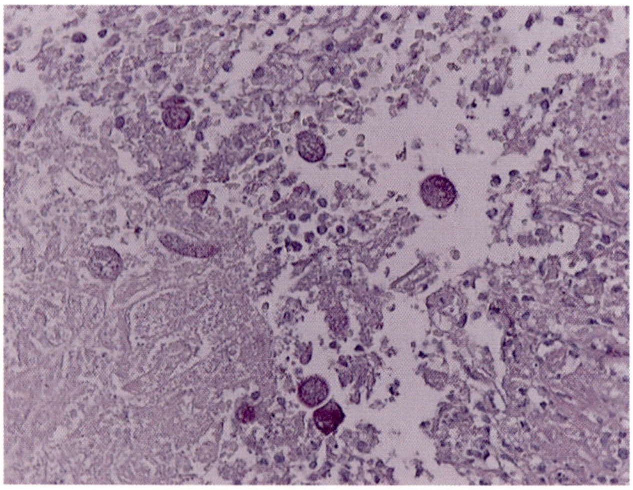

Fig. 5.59 Amebic abscess. *Amoeba* trophozoites in the necrotic tissue (Cite from Papavramidis TS)

3. Tuberculosis

Liver tuberculosis is an infectious disease caused by *Mycobacterium tuberculosis*, due to blood spread of pathogen in the pulmonary lesions into the liver via hepatic artery in most cases, or the *Mycobacterium tuberculosis* located in each part of digestive tract can transport into the liver via portal vein. In addition, the pathogen can be delivered into the liver via lymphatic system or direct infiltration from adjacent organs. Liver tuberculosis is a part of systemic tuberculosis, usually secondary to pulmonary tuberculosis, and more than 50% of the patients with lung tuberculosis have liver tuberculosis. Secondary liver tuberculosis occurs in 70–100% of disseminated pulmonary tuberculosis, and isolated hepatic tuberculosis has also been reported.

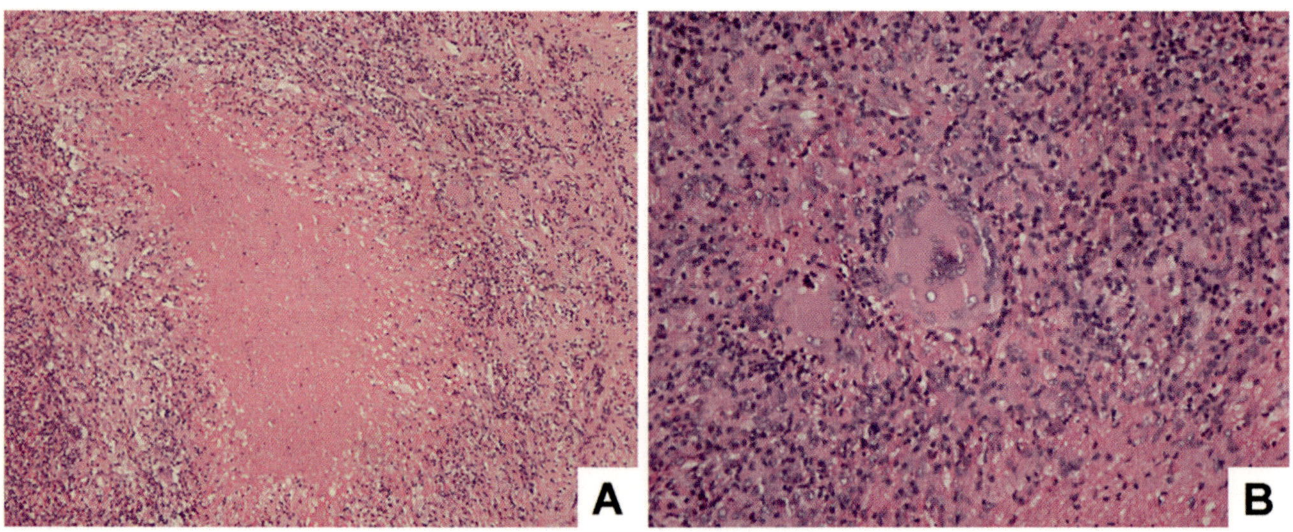

Fig. 5.60 Tuberculosis. (**a**) Caseous necrosis in center of the lesion; (**b**) a large number of inflammatory cells in the lesion, including multinucleated histiocytes

5.3.11.1 Clinical Features

Fever is the most common symptom, followed by abdominal pain and hepatomegaly, while anomaly in the liver function tests is nonspecific. Imaging demonstration shows various changes in different types and phases of the disease. However, in patients with significant symptoms, diagnosis is not difficult, while in atypical symptoms or asymptomatic cases, missed diagnosis or misdiagnosis may be made.

Different types of liver tuberculosis are discovered according to the various conditions related to the immunity, disease progression, invasion sites, and number of lesions following infection of the pathogen [139], including (1) miliary type (nodules), which is most common and multiple scattered small nodules; (2) tuberculoma or tuberculous abscess (nodular), circular- or multinodular fusion-shaped masses which are more than 1 cm in diameter; and (3) intrahepatic bile duct type (tuberculous cholangitis).

5.3.11.2 Microscopic Features

Scattered granuloma are seen with caseous or fibrinoid necrosis in the center of typical tuberculous granuloma, forming tuberculous abscess surrounded by horseshoe-shaped Langhans giant cells, and the peripheral epithelioid cells are infiltrated by a large number of inflammatory cells including lymphocytes and eosinophils (Fig. 5.60). Fusion tuberculous granuloma is sometimes seen with a fibrous capsule to form a tumor-like lesion (tuberculoma). Positive results in acid fast staining or bacterial culture are obtained in a few cases [140]. Furthermore, liver tuberculosis should be differentiated from cancer, abscess, and metastatic tumor in the liver and other granulomatous lesions caused by other reasons.

5.3.11.3 Treatment and Prognosis

The treatment for liver tuberculosis is the same with standard antituberculosis treatment, and combined chemotherapy of four antituberculosis drugs remains to be the basis of the treatment. The drugs in the quadruple therapy, isoniazid, rifampicin, pyrazinamide, and ethambutol, should be taken for 2–4 months, followed by another 6–12 months administration of isoniazid and rifampicin. For patients with tuberculous abscess in the liver, antituberculosis drugs should be administrated as well as percutaneous liver puncture and drainage of pus or surgical resection which receives good therapeutic effect. As to patients with biliary obstruction caused by abscess compression, stent or drainage will relieve the obstructive symptoms. Surgical resection should be considered in cases with large lesions or undetermined diagnosis.

4. Botryomycosis

5.3.11.4 Pathogenesis and Mechanism

Rivolta described botryomycosis in horses for the first time in 1870, which contains the grape-like granules in the lesions. The first report on human botryomycosis was described by Opie in 1913. The pathogenesis has been clearly illustrated that botryomycosis is a local granulomatous lesion caused by a chronic bacterial infection, mainly *Staphylococcus* infection or other bacteria such as *Streptococcus*, *Pseudomonas aeruginosa*, *Escherichia coli*, *Proteus hauser*, etc. It is commonly discovered in the skin and subcutaneous tissue of patients in all ages. Rapid progressions of the disease are sometimes found in patients with diabetes, immunoglobulin deficiency, cutaneous allergy, AIDS, or hormone therapy. Reports on the disease in patients with normal immune system have also been witnessed [141]. Visceral botryomycosis can be divided into primary and secondary types. The latter refers to dissemination of skin botryomycosis into visceral organs. Among the over 100 cases of botryomycosis reported up to date, deep visceral organ involvement accounts for less than 30%, including the lung, kidney, bone, lymph nodes, brain, prostate, etc. And only two cases of pri-

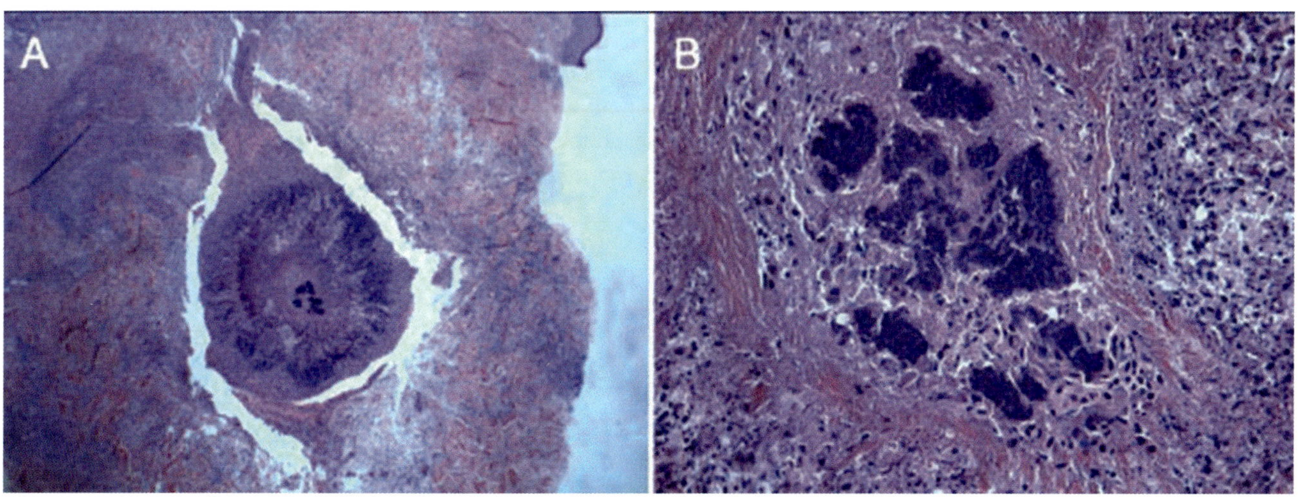

Fig. 5.61 Botryomycosis Splendore-Hoeppli phenomenon (Cite from Barreiros HM)

mary botryomycosis have been reported by Omar et al. and Schlossberg et al., respectively. Leong et al. [142] reported a case of a 14-year-old girl with primary lung botryomycosis which disseminated into multiple organs including the liver [142]. The girl was healthy before the onset of the disease and manifested cough and expectoration without clear causes. The CT inspection demonstrated hypodensity in the right lobe of the lung, with involvement of the pleura, thoracic wall, diaphragm, liver, vertebral rib combinations, etc., and a biopsy showed lung botryomycosis. The lesion in the right lobe of the lung disappeared completely after 3 months of antibiotic therapy.

5.3.11.5 Clinical Features

The two patients of liver botryomycosis were all males at the age of 50 and 68, manifesting upper right abdominal pain, weight loss, lethargy, fever, and other symptoms. The CT images show multiple hepatic hypodense lesions with large ones reaching the size of 5.8 cm × 4.6 cm, which are suspected as malignant lesions or metastatic tumors clinically.

5.3.11.6 Pathological Features

Microscopic observation shows fibrous lesions containing multiple small abscesses, with gram-positive or gram-negative cocci clusters displaying eosinophilic translucent crystalline particles in round, oval, or lobulated shapes (considered as a kind of antigen-antibody precipitates or conjugates of debris of plasma cells, macrophages, lymphocytes, and eosinophils and eosinophil granule major basic protein). In the center, colony of parasites, fungi, or bacteria can be observed, with peripheral eosinophilic matrix or external membrane accompanied by red plague-like matrix, also known as Splendore-Hoeppli phenomenon (Fig. 5.61), which is an important evidence for the diagnosis of the disease and should be differentiated from the granules in actinomycetes disease, foot disease, and fungi. Specific staining and culture of tissue and blood help to identify the pathogens.

5. Actinomycosis

Actinomycetes are opportunistic pathogens causing progressive, suppurative, and granulomatous lesions, occurring mostly on the face and neck (56.8%) or in the abdomen (22.3%) or chest (15%) and at other sites (5.9%). Actinomycosis is characterized by formation of fistula extending into the surrounding tissue and discharge of pus with sulfur-like granules. Liver actinomycosis accounts for 10–15% of all actinomycosis, and there have been more than ten cases of the disease derived mainly from the appendix and large intestine and invasion of the actinomycetes into the liver via portal vein up to now. Masses in the actinomycosis are easily misdiagnosed as liver abscesses or liver tumors [143]. Furthermore, high-mobility group box chromosomal protein 1 (HMGB1) has been reported as a novel serum cytokine, which has a major role in the pathogenesis of liver actinomycosis and can be used as a key indicator for the differentiated diagnosis [144].

In the literature, more than ten cases of liver actinomycosis have been reported, among which one case concerned a hard cellular liver abscess with a diameter reaching 11 cm and no encapsulation. The contents were gray-yellow or light yellow sticky pus and hard sulfur-like bacterial granules in the cavity. And the microscopic observation demonstrated granulomatous changes with proliferation of inflammatory fibrous tissue and formation of abscess accompanied by large amounts of lymphocytes, plasma cells, and neutrophils. The typical characterization was the vision of irregular granular colonies (sulfur granules) made of a large number of filamentous bacteria in a diameter of 100–300 μm, and the homogeneous central region in the granules was surrounded by rod-like bodies in a radiation arrangement [145]. And the peripheral acidic proteins were observable and were known as Splendore-Hoeppli phenomenon. The separation and culture of actinomycetes are difficult, and they are gram-positive stained, magenta in PAS staining, and black in methenamine silver staining. Conservative antibiotics and surgical resection are the main therapies.

6. Cryptococcosis

Cryptococcus neoformans, as a conditional pathogenic fungus, would infect deep tissues in immunocompromised patients. So far, there have been more than ten cases of liver cryptococcosis leading to multiple masses in the liver, complicated by lymphadenectasis in the portal area and abdominal cavity, which had been suspected as liver tumors and received surgical resection or open exploration. Under the microscope, the lesions are characterized by non-caseous necrotic granuloma with colloid changes, infiltration of massive multinucleated giant cells surrounded by fibrous tissue hyperplasia and chronic inflammatory cell infiltration, and formation of local small abscesses. *Cryptococcus* spores are unicellular, round, or oval, vacuolated, and 5-12 μm in size, and the germinated fungus is gourd-like shaped. Substantial *Cryptococcus* spores and mucinous degeneration of the tissue constitute the colloid lesions. The spores cannot be stained in HE sections, so specific staining is helpful for the diagnosis. Ink staining would show transparent *Cryptococcus* in the black background of the cytoplasm in the multinucleated giant cells, and PAS (glycogen) staining shows the purple-red cell wall and cytoplasm. GMS (Gomori's methenamine silver) staining exhibits the black cell wall, while MC (mucin carmine) staining shows a bright red capsule. Alcian blue stains the fungus as light blue with a dark blue-stained capsule, and MGG (May-Grunwald Giemsa) staining shows a purple-red fungus, while acid fast staining exhibits negative results. Hence, specific staining should be taken into consideration in diagnosing suspected infection of special pathogens. Treatment methods include antifungal drugs and surgical resection.

5.3.12 Malacoplakia

5.3.12.1 Pathogenesis and Mechanism

Malacoplakia is a rare inflammatory granulomatous disease, characterized by dense inclusion bodies within histiocytes. Its first description was provided by Michaelis and Gutmann in 1902, and the name of malacoplakia was proposed by von Hansemann a year later. Over 300 cases have been reported on malacoplakia in the literature so far with more than 20 cases came from China. Seventy-five percent of all the malacoplakia are located on the urinary tract, and other situations include adrenal gland, testis, epididymis, prostate, retroperitoneal sites, uterus, vagina, breast, lung, lymph nodes, muscle, skin, etc. Particularly, liver malacoplakia is rarely seen. The Russian scholar named Moldavski (1984) first reported a case of liver malacoplakia, and the first English report on the disease was provided by Robertson et al. (1991). To this day, there are only seven cases reported in the foreign literature, while gallbladder malacoplakia is more often seen than its liver counterparts [146].

Causes of the disease are still unclear. Based on the finding that partially digested bacterial components exist in the cytoplasm of macrophages in malacoplakia, it is speculated that it is an inflammatory disease caused by decreased lysosomal function of the macrophages after infection of bacteria, such as *Escherichia coli*, *Klebsiella pneumoniae*, *Pseudomonas aeruginosa*, etc. Another speculation is supported by other researchers that the pathogenic basis is the dysfunction of lymphocytes. Since malacoplakia can be discovered in conditions such as immunosuppressive therapy, malignant tumors, or decreased immune function due to other systemic diseases, it can be complicated by lymphoma, systemic lupus erythematosus, tuberculosis, sarcoidosis, diabetes, alcohol liver disease, etc.

5.3.12.2 Clinical Features

Liver malacoplakia are more commonly seen in female patients with a male to female ratio of 1:3 and an average age of 45 (ranged 34–68) years old, and the clinical manifestations include fever, nausea, anorexia, weight loss, abdominal pain, etc.

5.3.12.3 Gross Features

The lesions are multiple brown nodules with a sunken center and a diameter of approximate 0.5 cm. Boucher et al. (1994) reported a case of liver malacoplakia with a mass of 8 cm in diameter in the liver.

5.3.12.4 Microscopic Features

Observation shows granulomatous lesions mainly composed of macrophages (also known as von Hansemann histiocytes), with infiltration of plasma cells, lymphocytes, and neutrophils. The macrophage cytoplasm contains acidic granules, sometimes vacuoles, and one or more dense round and basophilous calcified bodies in hawkeye or ring-like shapes and 5~20 μm in diameter, which are also called as Michaelis-Gutmann (MG) bodies and the characteristic diagnostic indicator. Significant fibrosis can also be observed in the portal area.

According to the histological characteristics, the pathological process of malacoplakia can be divided into three phases. Phase I is the early stage of the disease characterized by infiltration of plasma cells and histiocytes in the hydropic interstitial without MG bodies. Phase II is the typical stage with MG bodies visible in the histiocytes and slight infiltration of a few lymphocytes and plasma cells. Phase III is the fibrous stage with fibroblasts and collagen appearing between the lesions of histiocytes [147].

5.3.12.5 Specific Staining

MG bodies are positive stained in PAS, von Kossa calcium staining, and Prussian iron staining.

5.3.12.6 Electron Microscopic Observation

MG bodies are concentric and transparent layered with a dense center and a thin margin, the compositions of which include incompletely digested bacteria encapsulated by phagocytic lysosomes and deposition of hemosiderin and calcium phosphate salts.

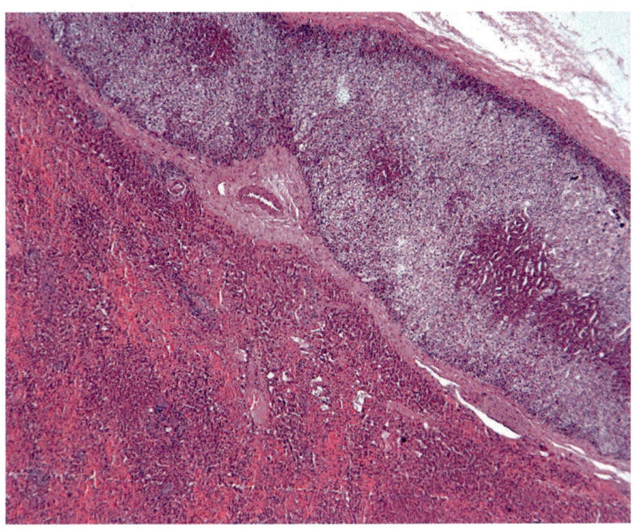

Fig. 5.62 Ectopic adrenal tissue in the liver

5.3.12.7 Differential Diagnosis

Malacoplakia is an inflammatory tumor-like lesion; however, its tumor-like nodules are misleading and difficult to differentiate them from malignant or metastatic tumors, which should be diagnosed by pathological examination. In addition, it should be carefully differentiated from liver abscess, histocellular tumor, and granulosa cell tumor. Tissue culture is often important for defining pathogens.

5.3.12.8 Treatment and Prognosis

Malacoplakia is a benign and self-limited disease, but invasion of vital organs or severe complications can cause death. Satisfactory curative effect can be achieved by the combination of anti-inflammatory treatment and surgical resection.

5.3.13 Ectopic Tissues

Ectopic tissues of the pancreas, spleen, gallbladder, and adrenal gland (Fig. 5.62) can occasionally be discovered in the liver parenchyma, known as heterotopias. The pathogenesis is speculated that these tissues lost their way during congenital embryonic development, or post-traumatic plantation of the tissues in the liver, as there are several cases reporting ectopic spleen tissue in the liver after spleen injury. Another report concerns a solid tumor mass of 17 cm in diameter in the liver proved to be pancreatic tissue, and microscopic observation showed normal exocrine pancreatic tissue, including atrophic pancreatic duct and glands with no atypia, and the wall of the dilatated cyst was lined with tall columnar epithelium. The origin pancreas is normal in situ. Cases of intrahepatic ectopic pregnancy have also been reported occasionally. Of course, liver tissue can also be found in thoracic cavity, abdominal cavity, intestinal lumen, gallbladder, etc., and cases of canceration or even metastasis of the ectopic liver tissue have also been reported. Differentiation of the lesions from metastasis of the tumor of the in situ tissue should be paid close attention in pathological diagnosis [148, 149].

5.3.14 Larva Migrans

Larva migrans was proposed by Beaver et al. In 1952, and apart from toxocariasis, other worms, such as *Gnathostoma hispidum* and *Paragonimus szechuanensis*, have also been found in human body in the form of larva causing larva migrans. The disease can be divided into cutaneous larva migrans (CLM) and visceral larva migrans (VLM), and the two types of the disease can coexist in the same patient. CLM refers to the process of invasion of the larva into the human skin and long-term migration in the skin leading to skin damage and migrant lesions.

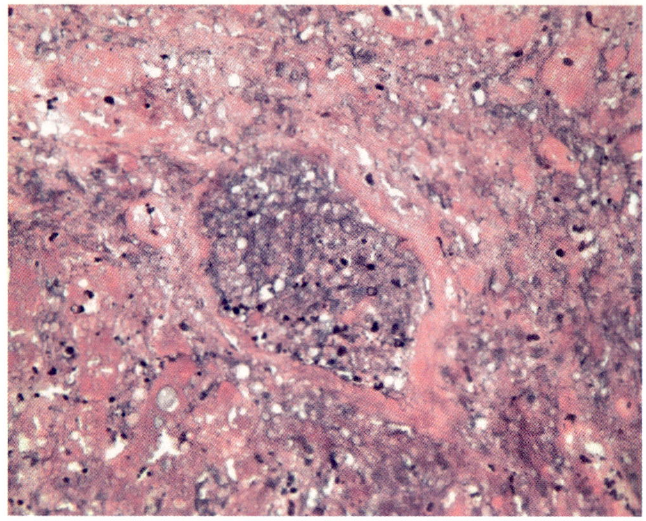

Fig. 5.63 Hepatic infarction coagulation necrosis of the liver tissue, and thrombi can be found in the lesion

VLM refers to the viscera larva migrans inside the body, during the process of invasion of the worm larva into the lung, liver, brain, eye, and other visceral organs leading to lesions. And common worms include *Toxocara canis*, *Toxocara cati*, *Paragonimus szechuanensis*, *Gnathostoma hispidum*, *Angiostrongylus cantonensis*, etc. Patients with liver VLM are often children, manifesting fever, significantly increased eosinophilic granulocytes, hepatomegaly, and so on. The lesions in the liver can be multifocal or massive, and the imaging of the lesions demonstrated hypodense nodules with vague boundaries and an enhanced margin in CT scan, which are difficult from primary liver tumors, metastatic tumors, liver abscess, or cystic lesions. A positive result of serum *Toxocara canis* antibody testing is the evidence of the diagnosis of VLM.

Histologically, liver VLM exhibits eosinophilic granuloma, consisting of large amounts of eosinophilic granulocytes, various inflammatory cells, giant cells, and epithelioid cells with a necrotic center in the lesions and leading to the formation of multiple eosinophilic abscesses. Anthelmintic treatment is the common effective treatment, with decreased volume and number of the lesions, and surgical resection is an option for large lesions.

5.3.15 Hepatic Infarction

Hepatic infarction is the necrosis of focal liver tissue due to the obstruction of hepatic arteries. However, the duplicate blood supply from hepatic artery and portal vein in the liver makes hepatic infarction uncommon. In general, blood obstruction in focal liver tissue without any effective collateral circulation established will develop into ischemia and necrosis of the focal tissue. For an instance, in situations such hepatic trauma, perinatal hypertension syndrome, antiphospholipid syndrome, ischemic hepatitis, portal vein embolization, liver surgeries, drug induced liver injury, diabetes, hypertension, etc., thrombosis is prone to obstruct the hepatic artery or cause hepatic artery embolization or inflammatory stenosis of liver arterial branches, leading to sharply decreased blood in the liver without establishment of collateral circulation and resulting in hepatic infarction. As to atypical cases, it is difficult to differentiate hepatic infarction from liver abscess and liver tumors. Anemic infarction lesions, shaped in wedges or irregular structure, are often located in the margin of the liver with distinct boundaries. Under the microscope, liver infarction exhibits nongranulomatous lesions, with patched coagulation necrosis of the liver tissue and visible hepatocellular contour, and thrombus can sometimes be found in the lesions or the surrounding liver tissue (Fig. 5.63) [150].

Table 5.6 Common causes and characteristics of liver granuloma

Causes	Characteristics
Autoimmune	Noncaseating epithelioid granuloma
Sarcoidosis	
Primary biliary cirrhosis	Noncaseating epithelioid granulom near the portal area
Infectious	Epithelioid cell granulomas containing acid fast bacilli, giant cell enclosed by lymphatic and tissue cells
Mycobacterium tuberculosis	
Mycobacterium avium	
Mycobacterium leprae	Foamy macrophages assembling in hepatic parenchyma and portal area, positive acid-fast stain
Brucella	Infiltration of foam cells in the portal area and lobules, with a large amount of acid fast bacilli
Rickettsia	Non-caseating granuloma
Francisella	Fat vesicles enclosed by fibrin ring
Listeria monocytogenes	Microabscess enclosed by macrophages
Bartonella	Small granulomatous microabscess
Gram-negative coccobacilli	Stellate abscess
Histoplasma	Epithelioid granuloma
Schistosome	Tissue and epithelioid cells surrounded by infiltration of macrophages and lymphocytes
Leishmania	Deposition of eosinophils and fibrosis and collagen in the portal area and around hepatic sinusoid, with eggs in the center
Hepatitis C	Fibrousrings or epithelioid granuloma
	Epithelioid granuloma
Drug and chemical	Eosinophilic granuloma
Malignant tumor	Non-necrotizing granuloma

5.3.15.1 Supplementary: Hepatic Granuloma

Granuloma is a lesion with a clear boundary consisting of chronic inflammatory cell clusters, and granulomas in the liver parenchyma are not rare, accounting for 2.4–15% of the tissue obtained via liver puncture biopsy. And 66% of the cases are secondary lesions, while 28% of the cases are primary liver disorders, and idiopathic cases account for 6%. Large granuloma can be larger than 1 cm in diameter. Chunhua Liu et al. (2009) reported one case of giant liver granulomas, a 9.5 cm × 8.8 cm lesion in the right lobe and a 2.5 cm × 3.2 cm lesion in the left lobe of the liver showed in CT scan [151]. Further biopsy confirmed the lesions as inflammatory granulomas; however, the cause remains undetermined. After methylprednisolone pulse therapy, the patient's symptoms disappeared, and the two lesions decreased in size significantly.

Granulomas can be divided into four types according to their histological features:

1. Inflammatory granulomas are consisted by proliferated fibrous tissue and lymphocytes, eosinophils, neutrophils, and tissue cells. In some cases, a certain type of cells can be the predominant components, such as eosinophilic granuloma which is mainly comprised of eosinophilic granulocytes [152].
2. Epithelioid granulomas are mainly comprised of epithelioid histiocytes containing a giant round or oval nucleus, surrounded by lymphocytes and sometimes plasma cells. The epithelioid histiocytes fuse to form multinucleated giant cells, containing 6–50 or more nuclei, and lesions consisting of cells with nuclei in horseshoe-shaped arrangement are known as Langhans cell-type granulomas.
3. Lipogranuloma is a reactive change of chronic inflammatory cells corresponding to extracellular lipids, characterized by giant macrophages containing lipid droplets, and is common in fatty liver and alcoholic liver disease.
4. Granuloma which is composed of substantial multinucleated histiocytes with phagocytic foreign contents in the cytoplasm is known as giant cell granuloma containing foreign bodies.

In addition, Coash et al. made a summary of the causes and characteristics of the liver granulomas, and the causes can be divided into autoimmune, infectious, drug- and chemical-induced, and malignant tumor categories (Table 5.6) [140]. And causes cannot be defined after careful examination in 3–37% of the patients, and these cases should be classified into idiopathic liver granulomas.

References

1. Cong WM, Wu MC, Chen H, et al. Focal nodular hyperplasia of the liver: report of 2 cases. J Clin Hepatol. 1991;7(2):112.
2. Kondo F. Benign nodular hepatocellular lesions caused by abnormal hepatic circulation: etiological analysis and introduction of a new concept. J Gastroenterol Hepatol. 2001;16(12):1319–28.
3. Vilgrain V, Uzan F, Brancatelli G, et al. Prevalence of hepatic hemangioma in patients with focal nodular hyperplasia: MR imaging analysis. Radiology. 2003;229(1):75–9.
4. Fukukura Y, Nakashima O, Kusaba A, et al. Angioarchitecture and blood circulation in focal nodular hyperplasia of the liver. J Hepatol. 1998;29(3):470–5.
5. Rebouissou S, Bioulac-Sage P, Zucman-Rossi J. Molecular pathogenesis of focal nodular hyperplasia and hepatocellular adenoma. J Hepatol. 2008;48(1):163–70.
6. Li AJ, Zhou WP, Wu MC. Diagnosis and treatment of hepatic focal nodular hyperplasia: report of 114 cases. Chin J Surg. 2006;44(5):321–3.
7. Chen LL, Ji Y, Xu JF, et al. Focal nodular hyperplasia of liver: a clinlcopathologic study of 238 patients. Chin J Pathol. 2011;40(1):17–22.
8. Zhang X, Gu WQ. Focal nodular hyperplasia: a review of new progress in the diagnosis and therapy. Chin J Hepatobiliary Surg. 2013;19(6):473–6.
9. Bioulac-Sage P, Cubel G, Balabaud C, et al. Revisiting the pathology of resected benign hepatocellular nodules using new immunohistochemical markers. Semin Liver Dis. 2011;31(1):91–103.
10. Finley AC, Hosey JR, Noone TC, et al. Multiple focal nodular hyperplasia syndrome: diagnosis with dynamic, gadolinium-enhanced MRI. Magn Reson Imaging. 2005;23(3):511–3.
11. Chandler TM, Heran MK, Chang SD, et al. Multiple focal nodular hyperplasia lesions of the liver associated with congenital absence of the portal vein. Magn Reson Imaging. 2011;29(6):881–6.
12. Kuo YH, Wang JH, Lu SN, et al. Natural course of hepatic focal nodular hyperplasia: a long-term follow-up study with sonography. J Clin Ultrasound. 2009;37(3):132–7.
13. Maillette De Buy Wenniger L, Terpstra V, Beuers U. Focal nodular hyperplasia and hepatic adenoma: epidemiology and pathology. Dig Surg. 2010;27(1):24–31.
14. Ghabril M, Vuppalanchi R. Drug-induced nodular regenerative hyperplasia. Semin Liver Dis. 2014;34(2):240–5.
15. Force J, Saxena R, Schneider BP, et al. Nodular regenerative hyperplasia after treatment with trastuzumab emtansine. J Clin Oncol. 2014.
16. Louwers LM, Bortman J, Koffron A, et al. Noncirrhotic portal hypertension due to nodular regenerative hyperplasia treated with surgical portacaval shunt. Case Rep Med. 2012;2012:965304.
17. Turk AT, Szabolcs MJ, Lefkowitch JH. Portal hypertension, nodular regenerative hyperplasia of the liver, and obstructive portal venopathy due to metastatic breast cancer. Case Rep Pathol. 2013;2013:826284.
18. Liu JJ, Li MT, Li Q, et al. Nodular regenerative hyperplasia of the liver: a report of 22 cases and literature review. Chin J Clin (Electronic Edition). 2011;5(24):7377–81.
19. Lin F, Chen BF, Zhang RD, et al. Nodular regenerative hyperplasia of liver: a case report. Chin J Hepatol. 2011;19(9):709–10.
20. Albuquerque A, Cardoso H, Lopes J, et al. Familial occurrence of nodular regenerative hyperplasia of the liver. Am J Gastroenterol. 2013;108(1):150–1.
21. Sood A, Cox 2nd GA, Mcwilliams JP, et al. Patients with nodular regenerative hyperplasia should be considered for hepatocellular carcinoma screening. Hepatol Res. 2014;44(6):689–93.
22. Alhosh R, Genyk Y, Alexopoulos S, et al. Hepatopulmonary syndrome associated with nodular regenerative hyperplasia after liver transplantation in a child. Pediatr Transplant. 2014;18(5):E157–60.
23. Sood A, Castrejon M, Saab S. Human immunodeficiency virus and nodular regenerative hyperplasia of liver: a systematic review. World J Hepatol. 2014;6(1):55–63.
24. Dhiman RK, Chawla Y, Vasishta RK, et al. Non-cirrhotic portal fibrosis (idiopathic portal hypertension): experience with 151 patients and a review of the literature. J Gastroenterol Hepatol. 2002;17(1):6–16.
25. Di Tommaso L, Sangiovanni A, Borzio M, et al. Advanced precancerous lesions in the liver. Best Pract Res Clin Gastroenterol. 2013;27(2):269–84.
26. International Working P. Terminology of nodular hepatocellular lesions. Hepatology. 1995;22(3):983–93.
27. Park YN. Update on precursor and early lesions of hepatocellular carcinomas. Arch Pathol Lab Med. 2011;135(6):704–15.
28. Chang O, Yano Y, Masuzawa A, et al. The cytological characteristics of small cell change of dysplasia in small hepatic nodules. Oncol Rep. 2010;23(5):1229–32.
29. Cong WM, Wu MC. Quantitative analysis of DNA content in hepatocellular carcinoma by image analysis technique. Chin J Oncol. 1988;10(5):367–9.
30. Cong WM, Wu MC, Zhang XZ. Quantitative studies on the DNA content and morphological features of liver cell dysplasia. Chin J Cancer Res. 1989;1(3):21–3.
31. International Consensus Group for Hepatocellular Neoplasiathe International Consensus Group for Hepatocellular N. Pathologic diagnosis of early hepatocellular carcinoma: a report of the international consensus group for hepatocellular neoplasia. Hepatology. 2009;49(2):658–64.
32. Dong H, Cong WM, Xian ZH, et al. Using loss of heterozygosity of microsatellites to distinguish high-grade dysplastic nodule from early minute hepatocellular carcinoma. Exp Mol Pathol. 2011;91(2):578–83.
33. Kojiro M. Diagnostic discrepancy of early hepatocellular carcinoma between Japan and West. Hepatol Res. 2007;37(Suppl 2):S121–4.
34. Roncalli M. Hepatocellular nodules in cirrhosis: focus on diagnostic criteria on liver biopsy. A Western experience. Liver Transpl. 2004;10(2 Suppl 1):S9–15.
35. Kojiro M. Focus on dysplastic nodules and early hepatocellular carcinoma: an Eastern point of view. Liver Transpl. 2004;10(2 Suppl 1):S3–8.
36. Kojiro M. 'Nodule-in-nodule' appearance in hepatocellular carcinoma: its significance as a morphologic marker of dedifferentiation. Intervirology. 2004;47(3–5):179–83.
37. Gligorijevic J, Djordjevic B, Petrovic A, et al. Expression of CD34 in cirrhotic liver – reliance to dedifferentiation. Vojnosanit Pregl. 2010;67(6):459–62.
38. Gong L, Wei LX, Ren P, et al. Dysplastic nodules with glypican-3 positive immunostaining: a risk for early hepatocellular carcinoma. PLoS One. 2014;9(1):e87120.
39. Jin GZ, Yu WL, Dong H, et al. SUOX is a promising diagnostic and prognostic biomarker for hepatocellular carcinoma. J Hepatol. 2013;59(3):510–7.
40. Zhou WX, Liang ZY, Liu TH. Clinicopathological observation on hepatocellular dysplastic nodules. Med J Peking Union Med Coll Hosp. 2012;3(1):68–71.
41. Wang MR. Heterogeneity of fatty liver misdiagnosed as primary liver cancer: case report. Chin Clin Oncol. 2010;15(12):1150–1.
42. Uenishi T, Yamamoto T, Ishihara K, et al. Focal fatty change in the medial segment of the liver occurring after gastrectomy: report of a case. Osaka City Med J. 2008;54(1):47–51.

43. Sirasanagandla SR, Kumar N, Nayak SB, et al. Accessory liver lobe attached to the wall of the gallbladder: a cadaveric case report. Anat Sci Int. 2013;88(4):246–8.
44. Liu QY, Wang Y, He Y, et al. Accessory lobe of right liver intruding into thoracic cavity: case report. Chin J Med Imag Technol. 2009;25(2):300.
45. Ruiz Hierro C, Vazquez Rueda F, Vargas Cruz V, et al. Focal nodular hyperplasia on accessory lobe of the liver: preoperative diagnosis and management. J Pediatr Surg. 2013;48(1):251–4.
46. Quentin M, Scherer A. The "von Meyenburg complex". Hepatology. 2010;52(3):1167–8.
47. Martin DR, Kalb B, Sarmiento JM, et al. Giant and complicated variants of cystic bile duct hamartomas of the liver: MRI findings and pathological correlations. J Magn Reson Imaging. 2010;31(4):903–11.
48. Gong J, Kang W, Xu J. MR imaging and MR Cholangiopancreatography of multiple biliary hamartomas. Quant Imaging Med Surg. 2012;2(2):133–4.
49. Zen Y, Terahata S, Miyayama S, et al. Multicystic biliary hamartoma: a hitherto undescribed lesion. Hum Pathol. 2006;37(3):339–44.
50. Tohme-Noun C, Cazals D, Noun R, et al. Multiple biliary hamartomas: magnetic resonance features with histopathologic correlation. Eur Radiol. 2008;18(3):493–9.
51. Karahan OI, Kahriman G, Soyuer I, et al. Hepatic von Meyenburg complex simulating biliary cystadenocarcinoma. Clin Imaging. 2007;31(1):50–3.
52. Musielak MC, Singh R, Hartman E, et al. Simple hepatic cyst causing inferior vena cava thrombus. Int J Surg Case Rep. 2014;5(6):339–41.
53. Long J, Vaughan-Williams H, Moorhouse J, et al. Acute Budd-Chiari syndrome due to a simple liver cyst. Ann R Coll Surg Engl. 2014;96(1):109E–11E.
54. Peng B. Simple hepatic cyst calcification: case report. Med J West China. 2012;24(8):1628.
55. Fukunaga N, Ishikawa M, Ishikura H, et al. Hepatobiliary cystadenoma exhibiting morphologic changes from simple hepatic cyst shown by 11-year follow up imagings. World J Surg Oncol. 2008;6:129.
56. Zhu JY, Qiu BA, Guo XD, et al. Clinical effects of laparoscopic fenestration on the treatment of simple hepatic cyst. Prog Mod Biomed. 2014;10:1901–3.
57. Zhang WB, Chen J, Yan CH, et al. Comparison of the treatment of simple hepatic cysts by ultrasound guided percutaneous ethanol injection. J Prac Med. 2014;30(8):1312–4.
58. Jin HM, Chen JQ, An LE, et al. Minimally invasive technique in the treatment of simple hepatic cyst. J Tianjin Med Univ. 2011;17(3):395–7.
59. Harris PC, Torres VE. Polycystic kidney disease. Annu Rev Med. 2009;60:321–37.
60. Hafizi A, Khatami SR, Galehdari H, et al. Exon sequencing of PKD1 gene in an Iranian patient with autosomal-dominant polycystic kidney disease. Iran Biomed J. 2014;18(3):143–50.
61. Yu CW, Yang Y, Zhang SZ, et al. Identification of mutations in PKD1 and PKD2 genes in two Chinese families with autosomal dominant polycystic kidney disease. Chin J Med Genet. 2011;28(5):485–9.
62. Waanders E, Venselaar H, Te Morsche RH, et al. Secondary and tertiary structure modeling reveals effects of novel mutations in polycystic liver disease genes PRKCSH and SEC63. Clin Genet. 2010;78(1):47–56.
63. Qian Q. Isolated polycystic liver disease. Adv Chronic Kidney Dis. 2010;17(2):181–9.
64. Alvaro D, Barbaro B, Franchitto A, et al. Estrogens and insulin-like growth factor 1 modulate neoplastic cell growth in human cholangiocarcinoma. Am J Pathol. 2006;169(3):877–88.
65. Chapman AB. Cystic disease in women: clinical characteristics and medical management. Adv Ren Replace Ther. 2003;10(1):24–30.
66. Wang LJ, Deng YL, Zhu ZJ, et al. Liver transplantation for the treatment of seven cases of massive polycystic liver disease. Chin J of Organ Transplant. 2010;9:569–70.
67. Grieb D, Feldkamp A, Lang T, et al. Caroli disease associated with vein of Galen malformation in a male child. Pediatrics. 2014;134(1):e284–8.
68. Hao X, Liu S, Dong Q, et al. Whole exome sequencing identifies recessive PKHD1 mutations in a Chinese twin family with Caroli disease. PLoS One. 2014;9(4):e92661.
69. Zhang YN, Zhang ZX. Diagnosis and treatment for spontaneous perforation of choledochal cyst in infant. J Hepatobiliary Surg. 2010;18(1):39–40.
70. Huang HJ, Jiang Y, Wu BQ. A case of spontaneous rupture of congenital common bile duct cyst. J Hepatopancreat Surg. 2012;24(6):519–20.
71. Wu X, Li ZB, Liu HH, et al. Clinical and pathological features of 35 patients with congenital hepatic fibrosis. Chin J Gastroenterol Hepatol. 2013;22(6):529–32.
72. Ren H, Ma XM, Zhang JB, et al. Clinical analysis of 16 cases of congenital hepatic fibrosis with Caroli disease. People's Mil Surg. 2013;2:211–3.
73. Al Sarkhy A, Hassan S, Alasmi M, et al. Congenital hepatic fibrosis in a child with Prader-Willi syndrome: a novel association. Ann Saudi Med. 2014;34(1):81–3.
74. Kinugasa H, Nouso K, Kobayashi Y, et al. Hepatocellular carcinoma occurring in hepatobiliary fibropolycystic disease. Hepatol Res. 2011;41(3):277–81.
75. Paradis V, Bioulac-Sage P, Balabaud C. Congenital hepatic fibrosis with multiple HNF1alpha hepatocellular adenomas. Clin Res Hepatol Gastroenterol. 2014;38(6):e115–6.
76. Abdul Wahab A, Al-Mansoori M, El-Hawli M, et al. Unexplained cyanosis revealing hepatopulmonary syndrome in a child with asymptomatic congenital hepatic fibrosis: a case report. J Med Case Rep. 2013;7:120.
77. Holzinger F, Z'graggen K, Buchler MW. Mechanisms of biliary carcinogenesis: a pathogenetic multi-stage cascade towards cholangiocarcinoma. Ann Oncol. 1999;10(Suppl 4):122–6.
78. Kwon JH, Kim MJ, Kim YH, et al. Monosegmental hepatobiliary fibropolycystic disease mimicking a mass: report of three cases. Korean J Radiol. 2014;15(1):54–60.
79. Saravanan J, Manoharan G, Jeswanth S, et al. Laparoscopic excision of large ciliated hepatic foregut cyst. J Minim Access Surg. 2014;10(3):151–3.
80. Wilson JM, Groeschl R, George B, et al. Ciliated hepatic cyst leading to squamous cell carcinoma of the liver – A case report and review of the literature. Int J Surg Case Rep. 2013;4(11):972–5.
81. Zhang X, Wang Z, Dong Y. Squamous cell carcinoma arising in a ciliated hepatic foregut cyst: case report and literature review. Pathol Res Pract. 2009;205(7):498–501.
82. Vick DJ, Goodman ZD, Ishak KG. Squamous cell carcinoma arising in a ciliated hepatic foregut cyst. Arch Pathol Lab Med. 1999;123(11):1115–7.
83. Guerin F, Hadhri R, Fabre M, et al. Prenatal and postnatal ciliated hepatic foregut cysts in infants. J Pediatr Surg. 2010;45(3):E9–14.
84. Odemis B, Koksal AS, Yuksel O, et al. Squamous cell cancer of the liver arising from an epidermoid cyst: case report and review of the literature. Dig Dis Sci. 2006;51(7):1278–84.
85. Hsu M, Terris B, Wu TT, et al. Endometrial cysts within the liver: a rare entity and its differential diagnosis with mucinous cystic neoplasms of the liver. Hum Pathol. 2014;45(4):761–7.

86. Sanchez-Perez B, Santoyo-Santoyo J, Suarez-Munoz MA, et al. Hepatic cystic endometriosis with malignant transformation. Cir Esp. 2006;79(5):310–2.
87. Seguchi T, Akiyama Y, Itoh H, et al. Multiple hepatic peribiliary cysts with cirrhosis. J Gastroenterol. 2004;39(4):384–90.
88. Miura F, Takada T, Amano H, et al. A case of peribiliary cysts accompanying bile duct carcinoma. World J Gastroenterol. 2006;12(28):4596–8.
89. Jiang WS, Li DM, Zhang ZH, et al. A ease of accessory liver. Chin J Clin Anat. 2007;25(6):668.
90. Wang BS, Liu JS, Li L, et al. One case of ectopic liver in thoracic cavity. Chin J Clinic (Electron Ed). 2011;5(19):5840–1.
91. Rougemont AL, Sartelet H, Oligny LL, et al. Accessory liver lobe with mesothelial inclusion cysts in an omphalocele: a new malformative association. Pediatr Dev Pathol. 2007;10(3):224–8.
92. Chao CT. Sclerotherapy as a palliative treatment for spontaneous huge biloma. Intern Emerg Med. 2014;9(5):597–8.
93. Silva AR, Fragoso AC, Oliveira M, et al. Laparoscopic excision of a hepatic mesothelial cyst. Cir Pediatr. 2009;22(4):229–32.
94. Komori K, Hoshino K, Shirai J, et al. Mesothelial cyst of the liver in a neonate. Pediatr Surg Int. 2008;24(4):463–5.
95. Vijayaraghavan R, Chandrashekar R, Aithal S, et al. Mesothelial cyst of the spleen in an adult: a case report. BMJ Case Rep. 2010.
96. Wilschanski M. Novel therapeutic approaches for cystic fibrosis. Discov Med. 2013;15(81):127–33.
97. Shintaku M, Watanabe K. Mesenchymal hamartoma of the liver: a proliferative lesion of possible hepatic stellate cell (Ito cell) origin. Pathol Res Pract. 2010;206(7):532–6.
98. Lin J, Cole BL, Qin X, et al. Occult androgenetic-biparental mosaicism and sporadic hepatic mesenchymal hamartoma. Pediatr Dev Pathol. 2011;14(5):360–9.
99. Rosado E, Cabral P, Campo M, et al. Mesenchymal hamartoma of the liver – a case report and literature review. J Radiol Case Rep. 2013;7(5):35–43.
100. Park JY, Choi MS, Lim YS, et al. Clinical features, image findings, and prognosis of inflammatory pseudotumor of the liver: a multicenter experience of 45 cases. Gut Liver. 2014;8(1):58–63.
101. Miettinen M, CDM F, Kindblom LG, et al. Mesenchymal tumors of the liver. In: Bosman FT, Carneiro F, Hruban RH, et al., editors. WHO classification of tumours of the digestive system. Geneva: WHO Press; 2010.
102. Hastir D, Verset L, Lucidi V, et al. IgG4 positive lymphoplasmacytic inflammatory pseudotumour mimicking hepatocellular carcinoma. Liver Int. 2014;34(6):961.
103. Parra-Herran C, Quick CM, Howitt BE, et al. Inflammatory myofibroblastic tumor of the uterus: clinical and pathologic review of 10 cases including a subset with aggressive clinical course. Am J Surg Pathol. 2014.
104. Fletcher Cdm BJ, Hogendoorn P, et al. World health organization classification of tumours of soft tissue and bone. Lyon: WHO Press; 2013.
105. Zen Y, Fujii T, Sato Y, et al. Pathological classification of hepatic inflammatory pseudotumor with respect to IgG4-related disease. Mod Pathol. 2007;20(8):884–94.
106. Yamamoto H, Yamaguchi H, Aishima S, et al. Inflammatory myofibroblastic tumor versus IgG4-related sclerosing disease and inflammatory pseudotumor: a comparative clinicopathologic study. Am J Surg Pathol. 2009;33(9):1330–40.
107. Chang SD, Scali EP, Abrahams Z, et al. Inflammatory pseudotumor of the liver: a rare case of recurrence following surgical resection. J Radiol Case Rep. 2014;8(3):23–30.
108. Chen ST, Lee JC. An inflammatory myofibroblastic tumor in liver with ALK and RANBP2 gene rearrangement: combination of distinct morphologic, immunohistochemical, and genetic features. Hum Pathol. 2008;39(12):1854–8.
109. Yang CT, Liu KL, Lin MC, et al. Pseudolymphoma of the liver: report of a case and review of the literature. Asian J Surg. 2013;S1015–9584(13):00070–5.
110. Kapur RP, Berry JE, Tsuchiya KD, et al. Activation of the chromosome 19q microRNA cluster in sporadic and androgenetic-biparental mosaicism-associated hepatic mesenchymal hamartoma. Pediatr Dev Pathol. 2014;17(2):75–84.
111. Takahashi H, Sawai H, Matsuo Y, et al. Reactive lymphoid hyperplasia of the liver in a patient with colon cancer: report of two cases. BMC Gastroenterol. 2006;6:25.
112. Isaacs Jr H. Fetal and neonatal hepatic tumors. J Pediatr Surg. 2007;42(11):1797–803.
113. Park HS, Jang KY, Kim YK, et al. Histiocyte-rich reactive lymphoid hyperplasia of the liver: unusual morphologic features. J Korean Med Sci. 2008;23(1):156–60.
114. Teixeira Martins RJ, Guilherme Tralhao J, Cipriano MA, et al. Solitary necrotic nodule of the liver: a very challenging diagnosis! BMJ Case Rep. 2014.
115. Imura S, Miyake K, Ikemoto T, et al. Rapid-growing solitary necrotic nodule of the liver. J Med Investig. 2006;53(3–4):325–9.
116. Alessandrino F, Felisaz PF, La Fianza A. Peliosis hepatis associated with hereditary haemorrhagic telangiectasia. Gastroenterol Rep (Oxf). 2013;1(3):203–6.
117. Zuang ZX, Wang W, Zhu Z, et al. Spontaneous rupture and hemorrhagic shock in 1 cases of giant hepatic purpura. Chin J Bases Clin Gen Surg. 2012;19(2):219.
118. Liu C, Pasupathy A, Weltman M. Multifocal peliosis hepatis simulating metastatic malignancy. Dig Liver Dis. 2014;46(9):862–3.
119. Pan W, Hong HJ, Chen YL, et al. Surgical treatment of a patient with peliosis hepatis: a case report. World J Gastroenterol. 2013;19(16):2578–82.
120. Cha I, Bass N, Ferrell LD. Lipopeliosis. An immunohistochemical and clinicopathologic study of five cases. Am J Surg Pathol. 1994;18(8):789–95.
121. Valeyre D, Prasse A, Nunes H, et al. Sarcoidosis. Lancet. 2014;383(9923):1155–67.
122. Iannuzzi MC. Advances in the genetics of sarcoidosis. Proc Am Thorac Soc. 2007;4(5):457–60.
123. Grunewald J, Idali F, Kockum I, et al. Major histocompatibility complex class II transactivator gene polymorphism: associations with Lofgren's syndrome. Tissue Antigens. 2010;76(2):96–101.
124. Arai T, Akita S, Sakon M, et al. Hepatocellular carcinoma associated with sarcoidosis. Int J Surg Case Rep. 2014;5(8):562–5.
125. Bakker GJ, Haan YC, Maillette De Buy Wenniger LJ, et al. Sarcoidosis of the liver: to treat or not to treat? Neth J Med. 2012;70(8):349–56.
126. Wang HQ. One case of liver internal marrow hematopoietic tissue hyperplasia. China Mod Med. 2011;18(5):130–1.
127. Lemos LB, Baliga M, Benghuzzi HA, et al. Nodular hematopoiesis of the liver diagnosed by fine-needle aspiration cytology. Diagn Cytopathol. 1997;16(1):51–4.
128. Shakeri R, Rahmati A, Zamani F. Solitary huge intrahepatic mass (extramedullary hematopoiesis). Arch Iran Med. 2013;16(5):315–6.
129. Zheng H, Zhang W, Zhang L, et al. The genome of the hydatid tapeworm Echinococcus granulosus. Nat Genet. 2013;45(10):1168–75.
130. Xie TH, Lv HL, Zhao YY. Correlation between CT findings and clinical pathological changes of hepatic hydatid cyst. J Pract Med. 2013;29(13):2107–10.
131. Rinaldi F, Brunetti E, Neumayr A, et al. Cystic echinococcosis of the liver: a primer for hepatologists. World J Hepatol. 2014;6(5):293–305.

132. International classification of ultrasound images in cystic echinococcosis for application in clinical and field epidemiological settings. Acta Trop. 2003; 85(2):253–261.
133. Li YS, Tang QK. Puncture drainage guided by ultrasound for liver cystic echinococcosos (III). J Hepatobillary Surg. 2008;16(3):195–6.
134. Koch S, Bresson-Hadni S, Miguet JP, et al. Experience of liver transplantation for incurable alveolar echinococcosis: a 45-case European collaborative report. Transplantation. 2003;75(6):856–63.
135. Ji XW, Zhang JH, Yu XY. Liver autotransplantation for the treatment of end-stage hepatic alveolar echinococcosis: a report of one case. Chin J Dig Surg. 2011;10(4):299–301.
136. Kim JW, Shin SS, Heo SH, et al. Hepatic abscess mimicking hepatocellular carcinoma in a patient with alcoholic liver disease. Clin Mol Hepatol. 2013;19(4):431–4.
137. Cordel H, Prendki V, Madec Y, et al. Imported amoebic liver abscess in France. PLoS Negl Trop Dis. 2013;7(8):e2333.
138. Papavramidis TS, Sapalidis K, Pappas D, et al. Gigantic hepatic amebic abscess presenting as acute abdomen: a case report. J Med Case Rep. 2008;2:325.
139. Chaudhary P. Hepatobiliary tuberculosis. Ann Gastroenterol. 2014;27(3):207–11.
140. Coash M, Forouhar F, Wu CH, et al. Granulomatous liver diseases: a review. J Formos Med Assoc. 2012;111:3–13.
141. Barreiros HM, Cunha H, Bartolo E. Photoletter to the editor: botryomycosis in an immunocompetent woman. J Dermatol Case Rep. 2013;7(1):29–30.
142. Leong YL, Liaw YS, Chang YL, et al. Primary pulmonary botryomycosis with multiple adjacent organ involvement mimicking mucosa-associated lymphoid tissue lymphoma. J Formos Med Assoc. 2005;104(10):744–7.
143. Ma L, Lu Q, Ling WW, et al. One case of liver cancer were misdiagnosed as hepatocellular carcinoma. Chin J Med Imaging Technol. 2013;29(4):671–2.
144. Wu CX, Guo H, Gong JP, et al. The role of high mobility group box chromosomal protein 1 expression in the differential diagnosis of hepatic actinomycosis: a case report. J Med Case Rep. 2013;7:31.
145. Badea R, Chiorean L, Matei D, et al. Accidentally ingested foreign body associated with liver actinomycosis: the diagnostic value of imaging. J Gastrointestin Liver Dis. 2013;22(2):209–12.
146. Vaiphei K, Singh P, Verma GR. Gallbladder malakoplakia in type 2 diabetes mellitus: a rare entity. BMJ Case Rep. 2012.
147. Botros N, Yan SR, Wanless IR. Malakoplakia of liver: report of two cases. Pathol Res Pract. 2014;210(7):459–62.
148. Ultrasonic diagnosis of 1 case of ectopic pregnancy. Chin J Ultrason. 2013;22(9):799–799.
149. Kang EJ, Choi YJ, Kim JS, et al. Bladder and liver involvement of visceral larva migrans may mimic malignancy. Cancer Res Treat. 2014;46(4):419–24.
150. Wu Z, Lu Y, Zhang XG, et al. Liver infarction: analysis of two cases. J Hepatobiliary Surg. 2002;10(4):288–90.
151. Liu CH, Zhou SM. Giant hepatic granuloma: report of one case. Chin J Clin Hepatol. 2009;25(1):77.
152. Mukund A, Arora A, Patidar Y, et al. Eosinophilic abscesses: a new facet of hepatic visceral larva migrans. Abdom Imaging. 2013;38(4):774–7.

Benign Tumors of the Liver and Intrahepatic Bile Duct

6

Wen-Ming Cong, Yuan Ji, Qian Zhao, Xin-Yuan Lu, Xia Sheng, Long-Hai Feng, and Yu-Yao Zhu

6.1 Hepatocellular Tumors

6.1.1 Hepatocellular Adenoma

Yuan Ji
Zhong-shan Hospital, Fudan University, Shanghai, China

6.1.1.1 Pathogenesis and Mechanism

Hepatocellular adenoma (HCA) is a benign tumor derived from hepatocytes, the incidence of which is 3–4/100,000 in Europe and North America; most of the patients are female with administration of oral contraceptives, and women account for 85% of all the patients [1]. In Western countries, contraceptives have been considered as a key cause for HCA, and studies have shown that HCA will decrease in sizes in patients who have a history of taking some of the oral contraceptives after they stop them [2]. Androgen is another potential cause for HCA [3]. Hereditary metabolic diseases, hepato-glycogenosis [4], maturity-onset diabetes of young type 3 (MODY3) [5], familial adenomatous polyposis (FAP), and hemoglobin deposition are all associated with the onset of HCA. Several researches have proposed abroad that obesity is also a key factor with an impact on the genesis of HCA [6, 7]. In addition, the relationship between alcohol and HCA should also be paid more attention. However, the epidemiological situation of the disease in China is different from that in the Western countries. According to the statistics from the Department of Pathology, East Hepatobiliary Surgery Hospital, Second Military Medical University, among the 189 cases with surgical resection of HCA, middle-aged male patients account for 70% of all the patients, and 50% of the patients are overweight or obese, while female patients rarely have a history of oral contraceptive administration [8], suggesting the difference in the pathogenesis and prevalence populations of HCA between China and Occidental countries which deserves further study.

6.1.1.2 Clinical Features

In China, HCA is discovered predominantly in males with a male to female ratio of about 2:1 and an average age of 37.9 (ranged 13–71) years old. Most of the female patients have no history of long-term oral contraceptives. Most HCA patients manifest no clinical symptoms, while a few of them have abdominal pain, abdominal distention, nausea, abdominal mass, abnormal serum liver function tests, etc. with AFP levels within the normal range. Rupture of the tumor can be found in 20–25% of the patients which may lead to shock, and as tumor increases in sizes to be >5 cm, the risk of tumor rupture and hemorrhage increases. It has been reported that 7% of the HCA cases will develop into HCC in the literature [9].

HCA imaging is corresponding to its histological classification, including three types as following:

1. HNF1α-inactivated HCA: Intratumoral hemorrhage or much fat content in HCA exhibits typical hyperintensity on T_1-weighted magnetic resonance imaging and iso-, hypo-, or hyperintensity on T_2-weighted images [10], but shows enhancement to a certain extent in arterial phase and no enhancement in venous or delayed phase after venous administration of gadolinium chelate. HCA with diffused fatty degeneration is difficult to be differentiated from benign nodular fatty degeneration and HCC containing large amounts of fat based on the imaging results.
2. β-Catenin-activated HCA: The performance of the lesions shows homogeneous or heterogeneous mass with rich blood supply, without any identifiable intratumoral fat. And heterogeneous intensity is shown on MRI

W.-M. Cong (✉) • Q. Zhao • X.-Y. Lu • X. Sheng • L.-H. Feng
Y.-Y. Zhu
Department of Pathology, Eastern Hepatobiliary Surgery Hospital, Second Military Medical University, Shanghai, China
e-mail: wmcong@smmu.edu.cn

Y. Ji
Zhong-shan Hospital, Fudan University, Shanghai, China

W.-M. Cong (ed.), *Surgical Pathology of Hepatobiliary Tumors*, DOI 10.1007/978-981-10-3536-4_6

T_2-weighted images which can be iso-, hypo-, or hyperintensity.

3. Inflammatory HCA: The lesions demonstrate liver masses with rich blood vessels with continuous enhancement in venous and delayed phase, and MRI T_2-weighted images show obvious hyperintensity. A few cases (11%) exhibit tiny fat infiltration in the lesion. The sensitivity, specificity, positive and negative predictive values of T_2-weighted hyperintensity, and enhanced scan in delayed phase for the diagnosis of HCA are 85.2%, 87.5%, 88.5%, and 84%, respectively.

6.1.1.3 Gross Features

HCA is usually a mass with a clear boundary (Fig. 6.1), and a few HCA cases involve multiple lesion, with the size of the lesion varying from several millimeters to 26 cm in diameter and most lesions encapsulated in a thin or no fibrous envelope, near to which can observe supplying vessels. The section of the mass is often gray-red, soft, and homogeneous in texture (Fig. 6.1a), while cholestasis (Fig. 6.1b), congestion, hemorrhage, necrosis, fibrosis (Fig. 6.1c), etc. can also be found. The boundary between the lesion and the surrounding liver tissue is distinct, while the latter often appears in no pathological changes. Fatty degeneration and glycogen storage are found in a few cases (Fig. 6.1d).

6.1.1.4 Microscopic Features

HCA is a type of benign tumor due to proliferation of hepatocytes, and the tumor cells are similar to normal liver cells without obvious atypia that karyoplasmic ratio is not

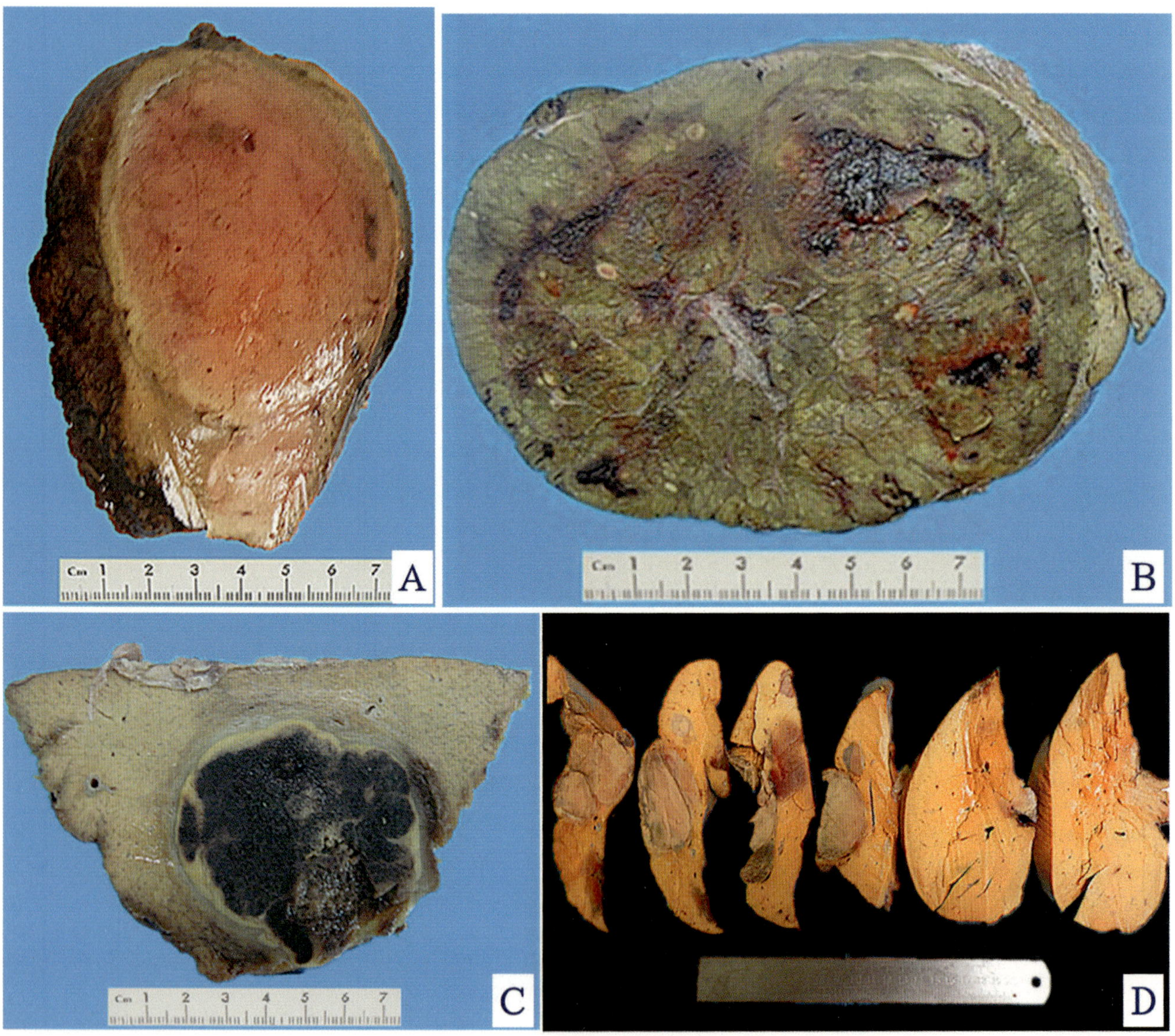

Fig. 6.1 (**a**) The section of a huge mass is *gray-red*, soft, and homogeneous in texture. (**b**) A huge mass with a *gray-green* section. (**c**) HCA with hemorrhage. (**d**) Mutiple HCA of a case of glycogen storage; the section of surrounding liver tissue is *yellow*

increased and nuclear division is rarely seen under the microscope. Fatty degeneration and hyaline degeneration can be found in the tumor cells, the cytoplasm of which contains lipofuscin and bile particle. The disorderly trabecular arrangement of the tumor cells is often 1–2 hepatocytes thick, with visible pseudoglandular structure occasionally and interstitial thin-walled veins; orphan arterioles have no concomitant bile ducts. The lesions are often accompanied by bleeding, necrosis, fibrosis, purpura, and other changes. The surrounding liver tissue is without cirrhosis, with fatty degeneration in some cases. Glycogen storage appears in a few cases with a pale hepatocellular cytoplasm, a clear membrane, and a lucent nuclear.

HCA can be divided into four different molecular types according to WHO classification, and each molecular type of HCA has corresponding clinical, imaging, pathological, and moleculobiological characteristics.

1. HNF1α mutation-inactivated HCA (H-HCA). H-HCA accounts for 35–40% of all the HCA cases. HNF1α (hepatocyte nuclear factor 1 α) gene is a tumor suppressor gene located on chromosome 12q24, encoding HNF1 protein, associated with the differentiation of the liver cells. H-HCA mutations include somatic type (90%) and germ line cell type (10%), both resulting in the production of a nonfunctional protein HNF11α which facilitates fatty degeneration and hepatocellular proliferation. Approximately 90% of the patients are young females with a history of oral contraceptives, while germ line cell type H-HCA are primarily seen in patients complicated by MODY-3 or young patients with familial adenomatous polyposis rather than a history of oral contraceptives. From the perspective of the characteristics of morphological pathology, H-HCA generally is a lobulated mass, with single or multiple lesions. Under the microscope, the boundary is clear and the arrangement of the liver plates is regular. The liver cells are enlarged with a small and anachromasis nucleus, obvious fatty degeneration, and no atypia or infiltration of inflammatory cells (Fig. 6.2). No dilation of the hepatic sinusoid. Some cases showed abundant lipofuscin (Fig. 6.3) with normal or fatty degenerated liver cells around the tumor. FABP is a gene positively regulated by HNF1A, encoding liver fatty acid-binding protein (L-FABP) positively expressed in normal liver tissue but markedly decreased in H-HCA. Immunohistochemical staining showed β-catenin stained on the cell membrane, almost complete negative or low expression of L-FABP, and intensive positive expression in the surrounding normal liver cells. L-FABP is a diagnostic marker of H-HCA with both 100% specificity and sensitivity. HCA does not express C-reactive protein (CRP) or serum amyloid A (SAA). GS stained the perivascular region, while focal GS positive expression can be found in the surrounding liver tissue. Focal expression of CD34 is also observed (Fig. 6.4) [11]. The risk of malignant transformation for H-HCA is lower than that of other types of HCA.

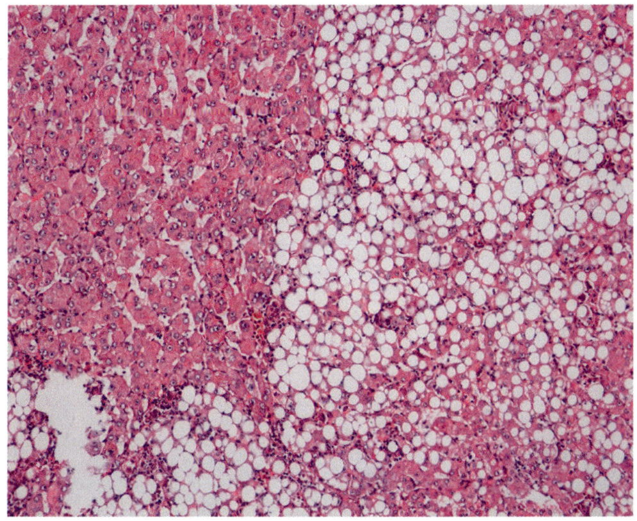

Fig. 6.2 HNF1α mutation-inactivated HCA (H-HCA). The boundary is clear, hepatic cells with obvious fatty degeneration and no atypia, without infiltration of inflammatory cells

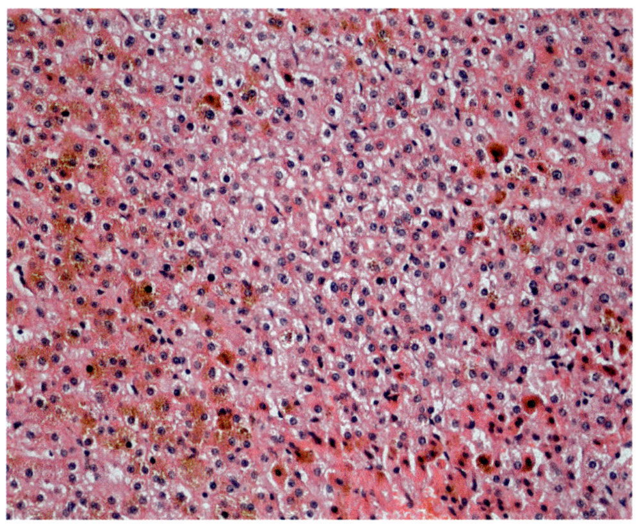

Fig. 6.3 HNF1α mutation-inactivated HCA (H-HCA) abundant lipofuscin in the tumor tissue

2. β-Catenin mutant-activated HCA (B-HCA). B-HCA often occurs in males, which is associated with glycogen storage disease and male hormone use. This type accounts for 10–15% of all the HCA cases with malignant potential. To date, the Wnt pathway associated with beta-catenin takes part in the genesis of adenomas. No HNF1α mutation has been found in B-HCA, but it can have both mutations of gp130 and GNAS, and about 50% of β-catenin mutant

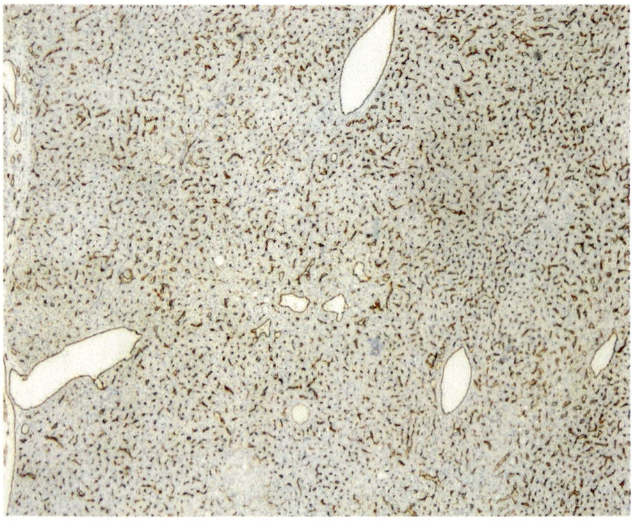

Fig. 6.4 Immunohistochemistry expression of CD34. Focal-patchy-diffused positive, negative in some area

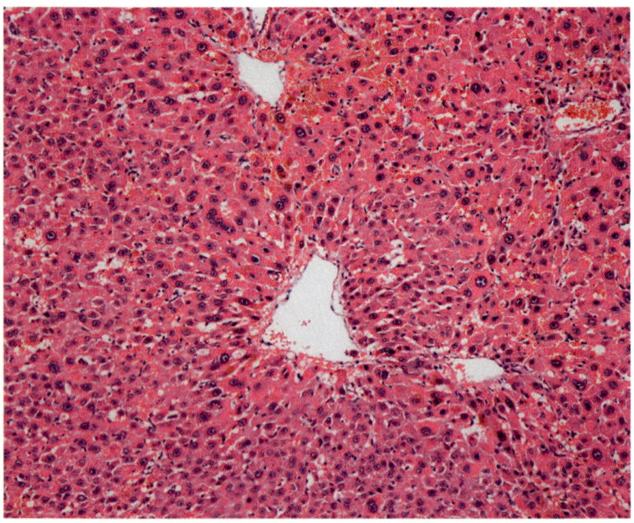

Fig. 6.5 β-Catenin mutant-activated HCA (B-HCA). B-HCA had no fatty degeneration or infiltration of inflammatory cells, while the liver cells are atypia

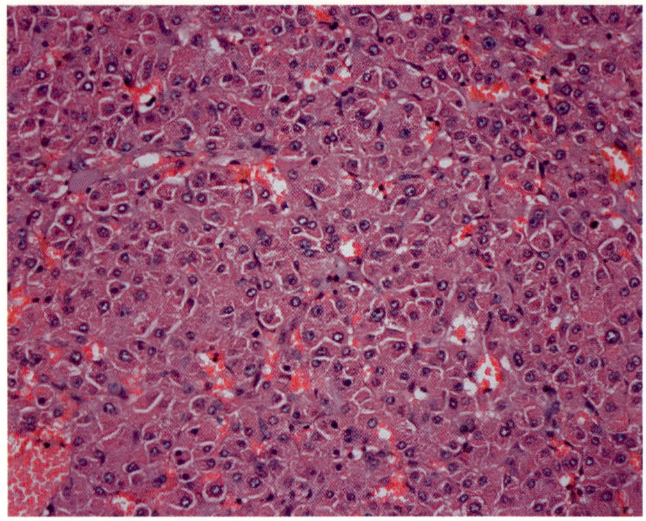

Fig. 6.6 β-Catenin mutant-activated HCA (B-HCA). B-HCA had no fatty degeneration or infiltration of inflammatory cells, while the liver cells are atypia

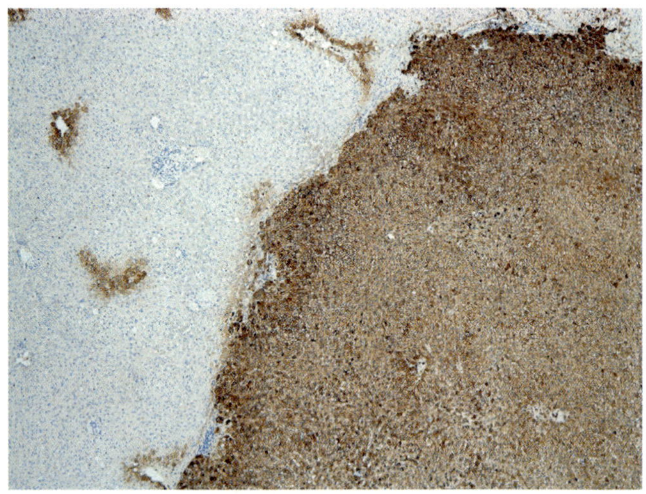

Fig. 6.7 β-Catenin mutant-activated HCA (B-HCA). GS was diffuse and homogeneous positive in the cytoplasm

adenomas are inflammatory ones. B-HCA is often solitary nodules, while in cases with glycogen deposition disease, the multiple lesions are observed. Histologically, B-HCA often had no fatty degeneration or infiltration of inflammatory cells (Figs. 6.5 and 6.6), while the liver cells are atypia, enlarged cellular volumes, and irregular nuclei, and the liver plates thicken to form pseudoglandular structure, which sometimes makes it difficult to distinguish it from well-differentiated HCC. Immunohistochemical staining showed high expression of β-catenin and glutamine synthetase (GS) in B-HCA. β-Catenin was nucleus positive and often observed in only a small number of nuclei which needs careful investigation. GS was diffuse and homogeneous positive in the cytoplasm (Fig. 6.7), which is different from the map-like expression pattern of FNH. Though the combination of β-catenin and GS antibodies would increase the specificity for the diagnosis of B-HCA (100%), its sensitivity is relatively poor (75%–85%) [12]. Considering potential malignant transformation of B-HCA, molecular pathological screening of β-catenin mutation is necessary in HCA cases with no overexpression of β-catenin target genes or HNF1α mutation.

3. Inflammatory hepatocellular adenoma (I-HCA). I-HCA is the most common type of HCA, accounting for 40–55% of all HCA cases and also known as vascular expansion type of hepatic adenoma, which is closely related to obesity, alcohol consumption, and liver steatosis, and almost all I-HCA cases are found in young and middle-aged women with a history of oral contraceptives. The tumor is vulnerable to rupture and hemorrhage, generally with no nuclear atypia and low risk of malignant transformation, which can be divided into two subtypes.
   (1) Inflammation with β-catenin activation: Sixty percent of the inflammation-type HCA cases contain gp130 (IL-6ST) somatic frameshift mutation, which is responsible for binding to IL-6 to activate the downstream inflammatory signal pathway of STAT3. And when gp130 mutation occurs, it will automatically activate the downstream inflammatory signaling pathways leading to inflammation without the ligand IL-6 [13]. β-Catenin staining is positive or GS staining shows diffusely positive.
   (2) Inflammation without β-catenin activation: A small part (10%) of inflammation-type HCA may contain both β-catenin gene and gp130 mutations with mild malignant potential [14]. β-Catenin staining shows positive stained cell membrane and GS stains perivascular region.

Fifty percent of the patients demonstrate elevated serum C-reactive protein and accelerated erythrocyte sedimentation rate, and fever and anemia can be observed in rare cases which can be eliminated after resection of the tumors. In general, I-HCA can be solitary or multiple with clear boundaries to the surrounding tissue. The tumor is soft and its cross section is heterogeneous, with no central scar. Histological characteristics of I-HCA include proliferation of liver cells, significant expansion or purpura of the liver blood sinus, focal or diffuse infiltration of inflammatory cells in the tumor (Figs. 6.8 and 6.9), visible fiber interval, dysplasia of the bile ducts, and solitary arteries (Fig. 6.10). In addition, various degrees of the fatty degeneration can be found in the liver cells. Immunohistochemistry showed overexpression of CRP (Fig. 6.11) or SAA. The proliferated bile ducts can sometimes be distinguished with expression of CK7 (Fig. 6.12) or CK19 immunohistochemical staining.

4. Undifferentiated HCA. This type of HCA accounts for less than 10% of all the cases, without any mutations or histological or immunohistochemical characteristics involved in the previously discussed types, and no explicit predisposing factors or clinical features have been determined currently.

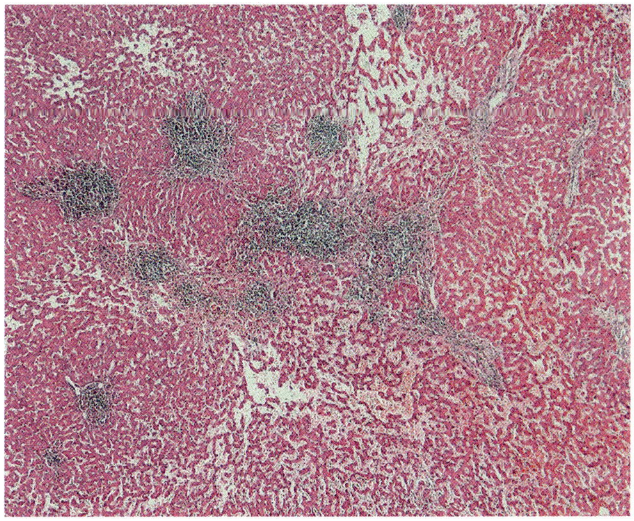

Fig. 6.8 Inflammatory hepatocellular adenoma (I-HCA) proliferation of liver cells, significant expansion of the liver blood sinus, and focal infiltration of inflammatory cells in the tumor

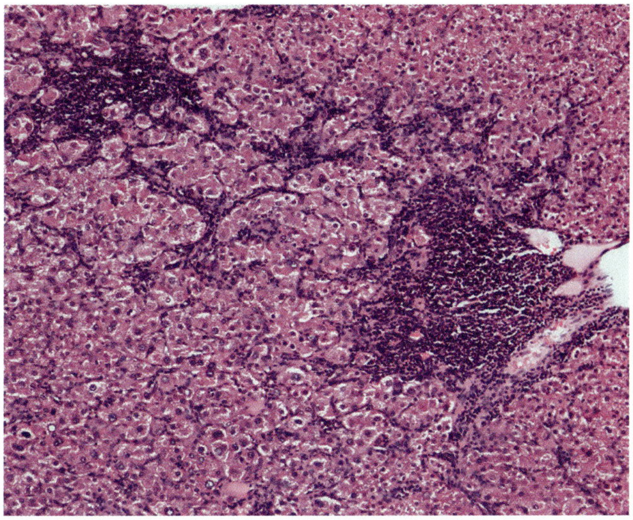

Fig. 6.9 Inflammatory hepatocellular adenoma (I-HCA). High power of Fig. 6.8

It is worth noting that molecular pathological changes of Chinese HCA patients can be different from that in the Western countries. In the Department of Pathology of East Hepatobiliary Surgery Hospital of Second Military Medical University, we studied three HCA marker genes including HNF1α, β-catenin, and gp130 in 36 cases of HCA [15], and the gene sequencing showed that all HCA contained HNF1α mutation with a significantly higher mutation rate by 35–40% than that reported in Europe. Furthermore, we also found several new hot spots of HNF1 gene mutation which were not included in the European reports. However, no mutations

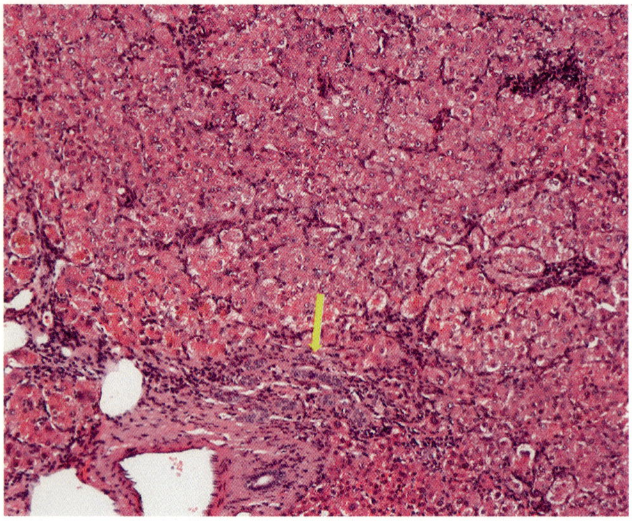

Fig. 6.10 Inflammatory hepatocellular adenoma (I-HCA). Visible fiber interval and dysplasia of the bile ducts in the tumor

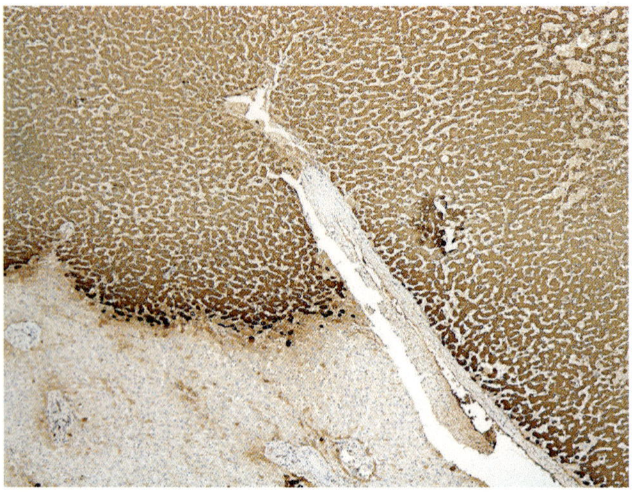

Fig. 6.11 Inflammatory hepatocellular adenoma (I-HCA). Immunohistochemistry showed overexpression of CRP

of β-catenin or gp130 genes in the HCA tissues have been found in our experience with negative β-catenin nuclear staining in immunohistochemical investigation. Varying incidences of inflammation type of HCA with β-catenin activation have been reported abroad, ranged 0–17%. In addition, the canceration rate of Chinese HCA cases is reported lower than that in Western countries [17]. Therefore, we should put more efforts into the researches on the tumor molecular pathology of Chinese HCA cases to determine molecular markers for molecular typing.

6.1.1.5 Differential Diagnosis

Differential diagnosis of HCA and focal nodular hyperplasia and fibrolamellar hepatocellular carcinoma is shown in Table 6.1.

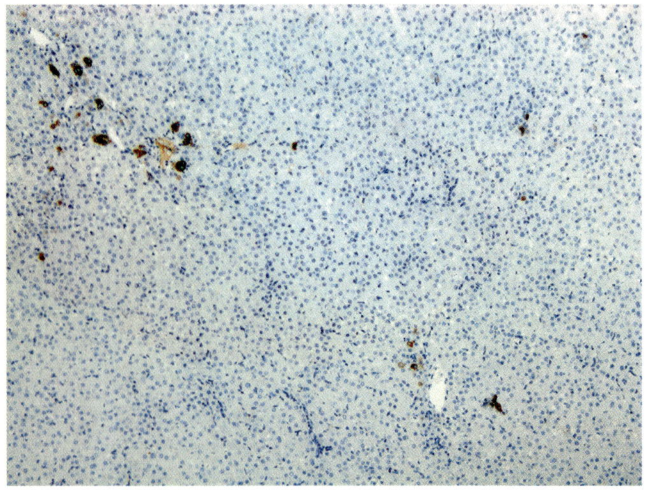

Fig. 6.12 Inflammatory hepatocellular adenoma (I-HCA). CK7 showed the proliferated bile ducts

6.1.1.6 Treatment and Prognosis

The major complications of HCA are tumor rupture and malignant transformation. The occurrence of rupture and hemorrhage is directly related with tumor size. For adenomas larger than >5 cm in diameter, the risk of rupture and bleeding is higher. The risk of malignant transformation of hepatic adenomas is about 7%, predominantly found in males with β-catenin mutation. So far, no uniform standards for the treatment of hepatic adenoma have been determined. Nauh et al. [19] proposed the principles for the diagnosis and treatment of hepatic adenoma and suggested indications for surgery, including: ① adenoma with a maximum diameter > 5 cm, ② male, and ③ female, adenoma with a maximum diameter <5 cm, with manifestation of B-HCA. Indications for follow-up by MRI include: female, MRI shows typical features of H-HCA or I-HCA and adenoma in small volumes. And if MRI shows no typical images of H-HCA or I-HCA, a biopsy should be conducted for screening of β-catenin mutation to evaluate the risk of malignant transformation.

6.1.2 Hepatic Adenomatosis

Wen-Ming Cong and Yu-Yao Zhu
Department of Pathology, Eastern Hepatobiliary Surgery Hospital, Second Military Medical University, Shanghai, China

6.1.2.1 Pathogenesis and Mechanism

Hepatic adenomatosis was first described by Flejou et al. [20] in 1985, and no consistent standard for the tumor number of hepatic adenomatosis has been determined. Some scholars suggested that hepatic adenomatosis can be diag-

Table 6.1 Comparison of focal nodular hyperplasia (FNH), hepatocellular adenoma (HCA), and fibrolamellar hepatocellular carcinoma (FLC)

Items	FNH	HCA	Highly differentiated HCC
Incidence	0.6–3% [1]	Lower than the incidence of FNH by 3–10 times	0.5–5.8% of the incidence of HCC
Predilection age	39 years on average	38 years on average	25 years on average
Male/female ratio	1.6 : 1	2.3 : 1	~ 1 : 1
Clinical symptoms	Few	None or sudden abdominal pain	None or abdominal discomfort or jaundice
Hepatitis	Few	Few	Few
Serum AFP	Negative	Negative	Negative
Mass number	Single or multiple (10%)	Single (70%)	Single
Mass size	<5 cm in diameter	>5 cm in diameter	>10 cm in diameter
Boundary	Clear	Clear	Clear
Transection	40.5% cases with stellate scar or nodular	Homogeneous, mostly without stellate scar	Nodular, 75% cases with stellate scar [18]
Hemorrhage and necrosis	Rare	Tumor rupture and hemorrhage	Necrosis, calcification
Hepatocells in the mass	No atypia	No or mild atypia	Obvious atypia, large cells with eosinophilic cytoplasm
Vessel	Vascular malformation with thick vessel wall	Often thin-walled vessels	Thin-walled vessels
Fiber bundles	Radial	Often none	Parallel or lamellar
Bile ductule	Obvious hyperplasia	Often none, Observable in cases with vascular expansion	None
Kupffer cell	Observable	Decrease	Disappear
Surrounding liver tissue	No cirrhosis or fibrosis	No cirrhosis or fibrosis	No cirrhosis or fibrosis

nosed according to the number of more than ten and the involvement of left and ring lobes of the liver without any history of steroid medication or glycogen storage disease [21, 22]. However, we support the diagnostic criteria proposed by Wesley et al. [23] in 2008 including more than four tumor lesions because of the scarcity of more than four tumors in hepatic adenomatosis. Despite the low incidence, there have been 177 reported cases of hepatic adenomatosis [24]. Many studies suggested the major difference of hepatic adenomatosis from hepatocellular adenoma that the former is mainly found in young or middle-aged females with oral contraceptive medication.

6.1.2.2 Clinical Features

The disease is more common in young and middle-aged women with an average age of 32 years old. However, Babaoglu et al. [25] reported one case of a 7-year-old female patient who had about 20 nodules with varying sizes, the maximum one was 7 cm in diameter, which were confirmed as hepatic adenomatosis via liver biopsy. She was the youngest patient that has ever been reported. Most cases exhibit no clinical symptoms, though abdominal pain and fever can be found in cases with intratumoral hemorrhage, and severe pain, shock, and even death can be observed in cases with tumor rupture into the abdominal cavity. Imaging often shows multiple intrahepatic lesions consistent to the nature of hepatic adenoma.

6.1.2.3 Pathological Features

Histopathology of single nodule in hepatic adenomatosis is identical to that of simple hepatocellular adenoma, the relevant description of which has been discussed in the first section of this chapter.

6.1.2.4 Molecular Pathology

Iwen et al. [26] reported one case associated with juvenile patient with diabetes type 3 and hepatic adenomatosis who was found to have Q495X mutation, which was suggested to repress the expression of wild HNF1A gene, resulting in the genesis of the disease. His father had the same mutation but only suffered from impaired glucose tolerance, suggesting the necessity of liver examination for diabetes patients without autoimmune antibodies and oral glucose tolerance test (OGTT) for adenomatosis patients without diabetes. Furthermore, OGTT screening is beneficial in the early diagnosis of diabetes in the patients' lineal relatives with HNF1A mutation.

6.1.2.5 Differential Diagnosis

Hepatic adenomatosis should be differentiated from multiple hepatic focal nodular hyperplasia, liver cirrhosis, liver metastasis of tumor, liver dysplastic nodules, and liver multiple well-differentiated hepatocellular carcinoma.

6.1.2.6 Treatment and Prognosis

Hepatic adenomatosis belongs to benign tumors with severe potential complications, such as malignant transformation, tumor rupture, and hemorrhage. At present, the treatment of the disease is still in discussion with much controversy. For patients in whom the tumor cannot be completely excised, surgical resection of huge lesion can be conducted to remove part of the lesions, relieve symptoms, and prevent complications, followed by close follow-up subsequently. And in suspected malignant cases or cases with significant symptoms, surgical resection can be adopted. There have been cases in which liver transplantation was adopted, with good therapeutic effects in most of these cases, while reports of deaths due to postsurgical complications or HCC in transplanted liver have also been discovered [27].

6.2 Bile Duct Tumors

Intrahepatic bile duct benign tumors and tumorlike lesions account for 1.9–2.4% of bile duct epithelial tumors. Although benign tumors of bile duct are relatively rare, they are occasionally cancerous and should be differentiated from malignant and metastatic tumors both clinically and pathologically. Therefore, it is necessary to give enough attention to them.

6.2.1 Bile Duct Adenoma

6.2.1.1 Pathogenesis and Mechanism

Intrahepatic bile duct adenoma (BDA), also known as benign cholangioma, is a type of low-incidence bile duct benign lesions. However, the biological characteristics of BDA are still not clear. Currently, it is believed that BDA is a post-damage repair process, including inflammation due to injury of liver cells and reactive hyperplasia of small bile ducts, and it is not relevant to bile duct hamartoma or hepatic cysts. Another hypothesis of the genesis of BDA involves peribiliary glands and thus can be called peribiliary gland hamartoma, because both of them have the same immunohistochemistry phenotype. However, due to the finding of K-ras mutation in BDA cases, it is also regarded as a true-type tumor.

6.2.1.2 Clinical Features

The average age of the patients was 55 years old (1.5–99 years), with men accounting for 59.39% and without specific symptoms or signs, most of which are found by chance in examinations or abdominal surgeries for other diseases. Enhanced MRI images demonstrate mild arterial enhancement and continuous enhancement in portal venous phase, and the apparent diffusion coefficient shown on diffusion-weighted MRI is more than twice that of the background of liver parenchyma [28]. Eight cases of BDA diagnosed in the Department of Pathology, Eastern Hepatobiliary Surgery Hospital, Second Military Medical University, with an average age of the patients of 56 years old (37–74 years), including six males, and four accidental discoveries of BDA lesions were made in HCC surgeries which received resection during the operations.

6.2.1.3 Gross Features

The tumors are often solitary small nodules, accounting for 82.9%, while about 10% of the cases involve multiple lesions, predominantly located in the subcapsular region or can also be present in the deep liver parenchyma, white or gray, round or oval in shape, hard in texture, with clear boundaries and no true envelopes. The average diameter of the nodules in about 90% cases is 0.6 (0.5–1) cm or occasionally even up to 9.2 cm. The eight cases of BDA diagnosed in the Department of Pathology, Eastern Hepatobiliary Surgery Hospital, Second Military Medical University, were all solitary lesions with an average diameter of 0.98 (0.2–3.8) cm [29] (Figs. 6.13 and 6.14).

6.2.1.4 Microscopic Features

The lesions of BDA is composed of small bile ducts with similar sizes and narrow lumens, in a curved shape or a solid cords, mostly containing no concentrated bile (Fig. 6.15), showing no cystic cavity or dilation. The epithelial cells of the bile ducts are cuboidal or low columnar with no atypia and rich cytoplasm which is slightly basophilic, and the nuclei are small and round in uniform sizes showing no mito-

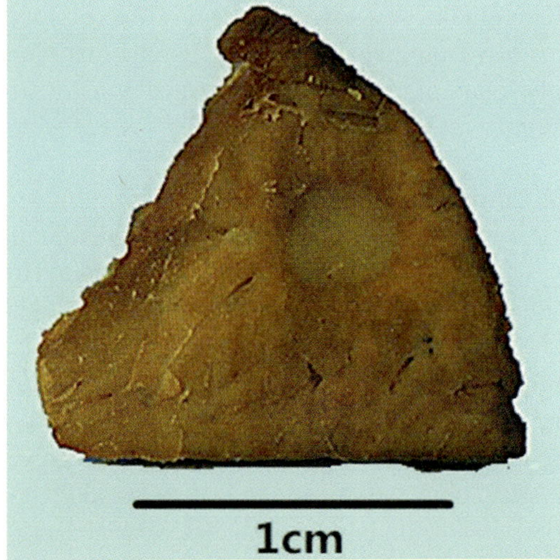

Fig. 6.13 Intrahepatic bile duct adenoma. A *yellow* round lesion with clear boundary and no envelope

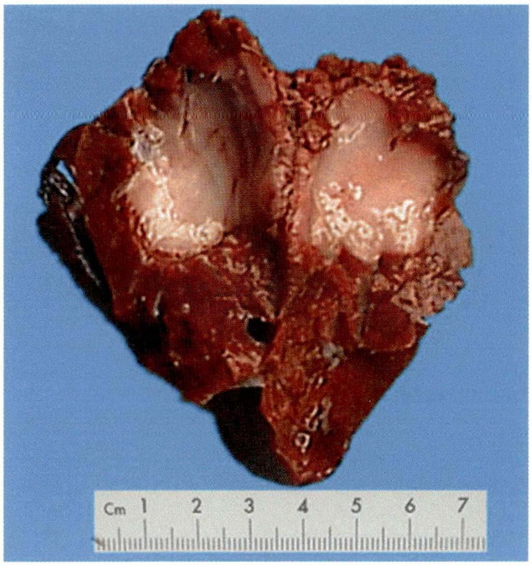

Fig. 6.14 Intrahepatic bile duct adenoma. A *gray-white* round lesion with clear boundary, it is a canceration case

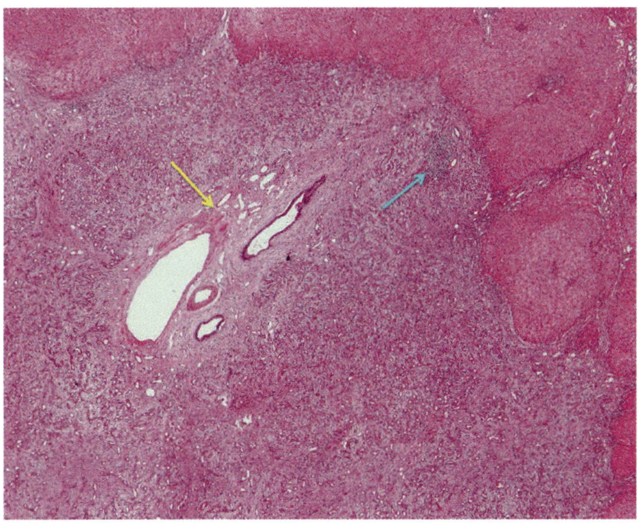

Fig. 6.15 Intrahepatic bile duct adenoma. Dense prolification of small bile ducts, remaining portal area, and focal lymphocyte infiltration (*yellow arrow*); the boundary is clear

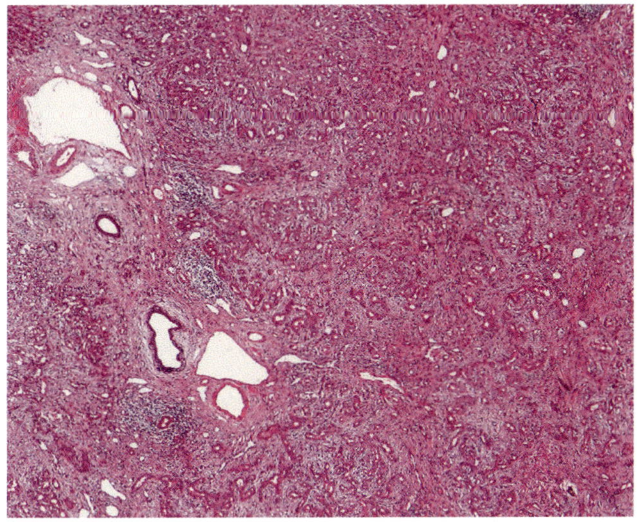

Fig. 6.16 Intrahepatic bile duct adenoma. High power of Fig. 6.16

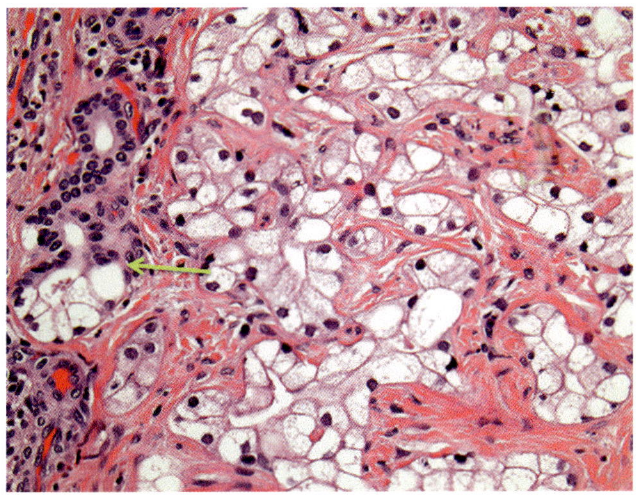

Fig. 6.17 Clear cell-type BDA. Substitution of normal bile duct epithelium by hyaline cells (*yellow arrow*)

sis, even with visible focal mucinous metaplasia of glandular epithelium and moderate chronic inflammation mainly containing fibrous tissue and lymphocytes rather than ovarian interstitial tissue, and the fibrous interstitial tissue was loose and edematous or with hyaline degeneration. Residual normal bile ducts can be seen around the proliferated bile ductules in the portal area (Fig. 6.16), and no capsules are found surrounding the lesions while the boundary is clear showing no invasion into the surrounding liver tissue varying amounts of fat.

Albores-Saavedra J et al. [32] and Wu et al. [30] reported four cases of clear cell-type BDA, 0.8–2.8 cm in diameter, with abundant clear cytoplasm in the tumor cells which arranged in shapes of small tubules, fine beam cable, or small nests, and more than 99% of the tumor cell cytoplasm was translucent, hyperchromatic nucleus were round or oval, and the substitution processes of normal bile duct epithelium by hyaline cells can been seen (Fig. 6.17).

Three cases of BDA with acidophilic degeneration in tumor cells have been reported [31, 33, 34], with the tumor diameter of 0.3–1.8 cm. Acidophilic degeneration refers to the generation of abundant fine granular eosinophilic cytoplasm in epithelial cells due to increase in the number of mitochondria under the microscope [33] (Fig. 6.18). The scarce bile duct tumors with acidophilic degeneration are mainly seen in intrahepatic bile duct papillary tumors and intrahepatic biliary cystadenocarcinoma, so whether BDA with acidophilic degeneration is a type of precancerous lesions for the aforementioned bile duct tumors should be

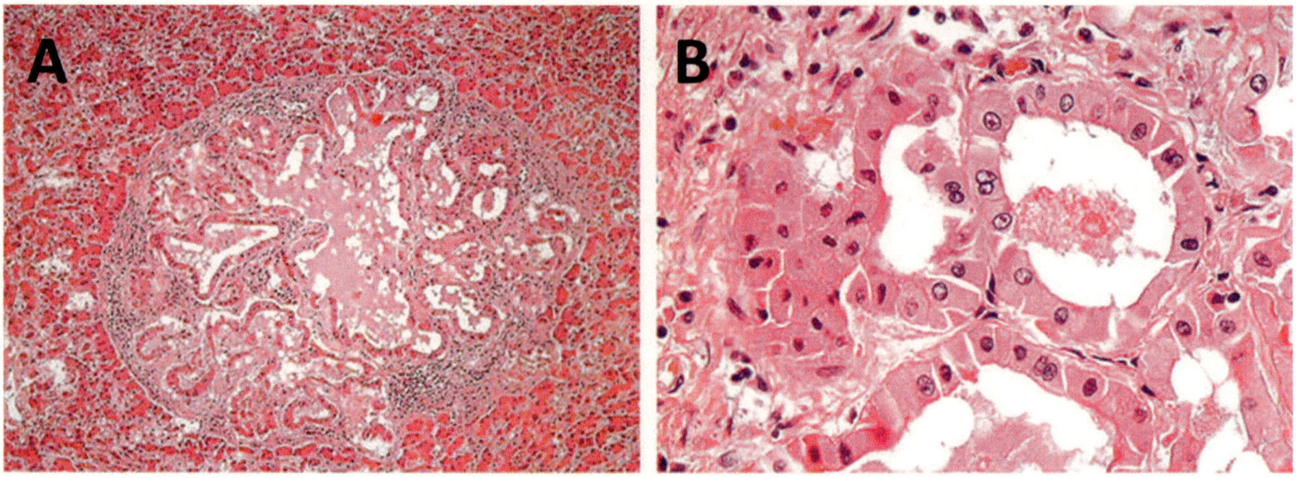

Fig. 6.18 BDA, with acidophilic degeneration. A,B: H&E staining showed abundant eosinophilic cytoplasm

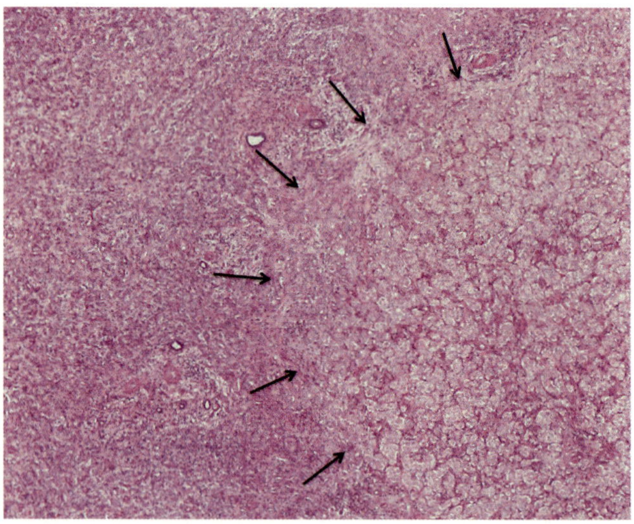

Fig. 6.19 Canceration with transition between cancerous tissue (*right*) and BDA (*left*)

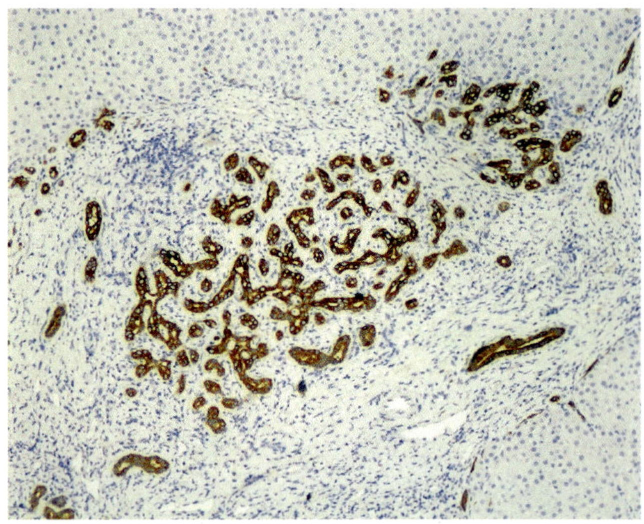

Fig. 6.20 CK19 immunohistochemical staining in BDA. CK19-positive expression in tumor gland duct (*blue arrow*), the normal interlobular bile ducts (*red arrow*)

discussed further. And comprehensive consideration on the nature of BDA should be made according to the size and cellular and nuclear morphology of the lesions.

Among the eight cases of BDA diagnosed in the Department of Pathology, Eastern Hepatobiliary Surgery Hospital, Second Military Medical University, four cases have concomitant HCC, one case with high-grade intraepithelial neoplasia, and one case canceration with transition between cancerous tissue and BDA (Fig. 6.19).

6.2.1.5 Immunohistochemistry

EMA, CEA, CK, and CK19 (Fig. 6.20) staining are positive, while CK20 and hepatic cell marker staining should be negative. BDA also expresses CD10 and 1F6 antigen as peripheral glands do, and 1F6 is not expressed in the normal interlobular bile ducts. CD10 staining exhibits continuous stains on the luminal surface of the apical cells in the clear cell-type BDA and outlines the irregularly shaped lumen (Fig. 6.21).

6.2.1.6 Differential Diagnosis

BDA in liver parenchyma should mainly be differentiated from well-differentiated intrahepatic cholangiocarcinoma and metastatic adenocarcinoma, needing careful identification especially in the frozen biopsy. The author has encountered one case of a 71-year-old male patient receiving a surgical resection of gastric cardia adenocarcinoma, and a 0.2 cm gray-white nodule was found in the left lobe of the liver which was suspected as metastasis and excised during the operation. Later pathological examination confirmed is an intrahepatic BDA. Studies have shown that EZH2 and p16

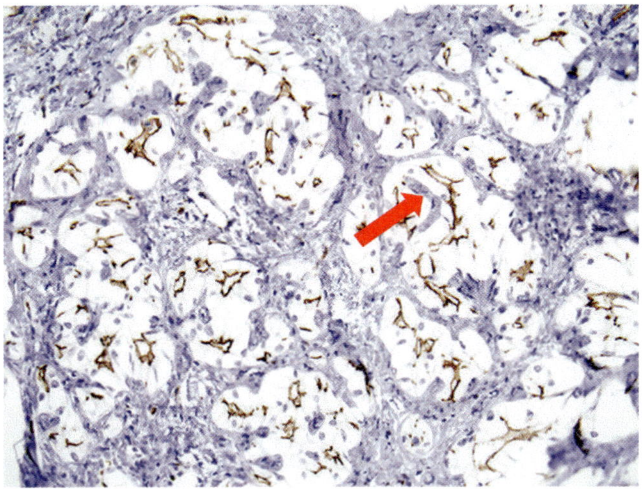

Fig. 6.21 Clear cell-type BDA. CD10 staining exhibits continuous stains on the luminal surface of the apical cells in the clear cell-type BDA

Table 6.2 Differentiation of BDA and biliary hamartoma

Features	BDA	Biliary hamartoma
Pathogenesis	Reactive hyperplasia of bile ducts	Development labyrinth of bile duct plates
Number of nodules	Solitary	Multiple
Diameter of nodules	>0.5 cm	<0.5 cm
Texture of nodules	Solid	Cyst
Bile duct epithelium	Cubic or short columnar	Flat or cubic
Distribution of lesions	Random or beneath hepatic capsule	Surrounding or intra-portal area
Cystic dilatation	None	Yes
Arrangement of glandular ducts	Dense	Loose
Bile in the lumen	None	Yes
With polycystic disease	None	Yes in most of the cases
Carcinogenesis	In some cases	In all cases

(INK4a) can be used as markers of immunohistochemistry to distinguish ICC and BDA, because EZH2 is expressed in all ICC but not expressed in BDA, while p16 (INK4a) is expressed in 12% ICC and 81% BDA [36]. CD10 is expressed in benign tumors of bile duct but not expressed in malignant tumors, indicating that CD10 can be adopted as a marker for the identification of the nature of intrahepatic bile duct transparent cell tumors to tell whether a tumor is malignant or benign [37]. In addition, BDA and bile duct hamartoma are both benign intrahepatic bile duct proliferative lesions which are difficult to differentiate [35]. Main points of the differentiation for them are shown in Table 6.2.

6.2.1.7 Treatment and Prognosis

BDA grows slowly and may undergo hyaline degeneration to form scars. Despite the nature of benign lesions, canceration of BDA has already been reported in some cases. To date, BDA is recognized as precancerous lesions which may develop into bile duct carcinoma, so once diagnosed, surgical resection should be considered. For distal bile duct adenoma, endoscopic resection and argon plasma coagulation can be conducted for the treatment. And endoscopic resection in situ is suitable for the treatment of common bile duct adenoma.

6.2.2 Biliary Cystadenoma

6.2.2.1 Pathogenesis and Mechanism

Biliary cystadenoma (BCA) was reported by Hueter in 1887 for the first time, and Keen reported the first BCA resection in 1892. An epidemiological study published in 1993 has shown that 5–10% of the population may have cystic lesions in the liver, and the occurrence rate of bile duct cystic lesions was less than 5% the rate of intrahepatic cysts. And 90% bile duct cystic lesions arise in the intrahepatic while only 10% occur in extrahepatic biliary system.

The etiology of BCA remains unclear; Wheeler and Edmondson speculated that it may be a tumor formed during the development of ectopic bile ducts in the embryo. The patients may have hepatic cysts, polycystic liver abnormalities, or abnormal hepatic bile ducts. Comparison between mucous membrane of the gallbladder in adult BCA and fetus showed that the columnar epithelium in the former was similar to that in the embryonic development both under light microscope and electron microscope, mesenchymal vimentin staining was positive, and the latter only appeared in the fetal gallbladder tissue at 15th week of gestation, suggesting that BCA may derive from the ectopic embryonic gallbladder tissue. Another hypothesis for the genesis involves ectopic ovarian tissue or residual tissue of congenital embryonic foregut. In addition, due to endocrine cells found in about 50% of bile duct cysts, it has been also suggested that BCA may originate from intrahepatic peritubular glands.

6.2.2.2 Clinical Features

More than 85–90% of the patients are middle-aged or elderly women. An American report by Devaney et al. (1984) concerned a group of 52 cases of BCA patients, aged from 2 to 87 years old, and the average age was 45 years old, including 51 cases of mucinous type. Seventy-eight cases of BCA have been diagnosed in the Department of Pathology, Eastern Hepatobiliary Surgery Hospital, Second Military University, with 55 cases of females (70.5%). The average age was 49.3

(26–77) years old, and the majority of the patients had no symptoms or only manifested nonspecific symptoms such as abdominal pain. Some patients came to the hospital because of abdominal tumor rupture and bleeding, secondary infection, obstructive jaundice, etc., and some had ascites as the first symptom due to rupture of BCA. Cases of BCA with pleural effusion have also been reported [48].

More than half of the patients have varying degrees of elevated serum CA19-9 [(838.4 + 2485.7) U/ml, reference value of 0–37 U/ml], mild elevation of serum alkaline phosphatase (ALP), γ-glutamyl transfer peptidase (γ-GT) and CEA, and negative serum AFP detection, all of which can turn normal after complete resection of the tumors. Despite controversy, cystic fluid obtained via puncture for tests of CA19-9 and CEA level were reported to be adopted to differentiate bile duct cystic lesions from cysts and abscess. However, due to the risk of rupture of the lesions leading to ascites or pleural effusion and the major difficulty in differentiation of benign tumor and malignant ones, cyst puncture biopsy should be conducted with much cautiousness.

ERCP cholangiopancreatography often shows filling defects [51]. B-ultrasound examination shows irregular thickening of the cyst wall and several thickened septa inside the cavity, with papillary projections and nodules on the inner wall of the cyst. CT images display several hypodense circular regions inside the cystic mass. And MRI images show typical irregular thick-walled multilocular lesions.

6.2.2.3 Gross Features

BCA occurs mainly in the liver, which can be located in the liver parenchyma, underneath the capsule, or even into the bile duct in the form of polyp, or involves both intra- and extrahepatic bile ducts, characterized by solitary multilocular cystic lesions (Fig. 6.22), and in some cases BCA are unilocular cysts with a smooth inner wall, while cases of multiple cysts are rare. Mucoid BCA contains transparent mucus or has a soapy section, and serous BCA is microcystic similar to cystadenoma of the pancreas. Both types of BCA can occur with intraductal papillary tumors. Among the 78 cases of BCA diagnosed in the Department of Pathology, Eastern Hepatobiliary Surgery Hospital, Second Military Medical University, 60 cases are multilocular, with an average diameter of 8.4 cm, and the maximum diameter was 34 cm in one case (Fig. 6.23). Sixty-nine cases concerned the intrahepatic bile duct, five cases extrahepatic bile duct, and four cases hilar bile duct, while one case involved both the left lobe of the liver and extrahepatic bile ducts. In cases with cystic papillary hyperplasia on the inner cystic wall, gray-white granular papilla can be observed, with clear, yellow-brown mucinous, jelly or bloody cystic fluid and complete fibrous capsules.

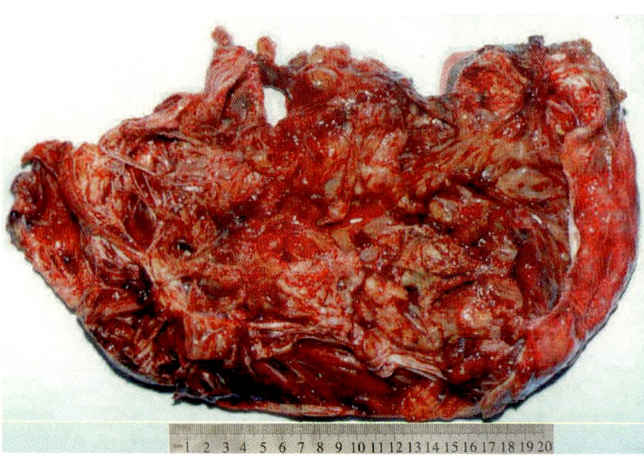

Fig. 6.22 Biliary cystadenoma. The tumor was huge, cystic, and solid

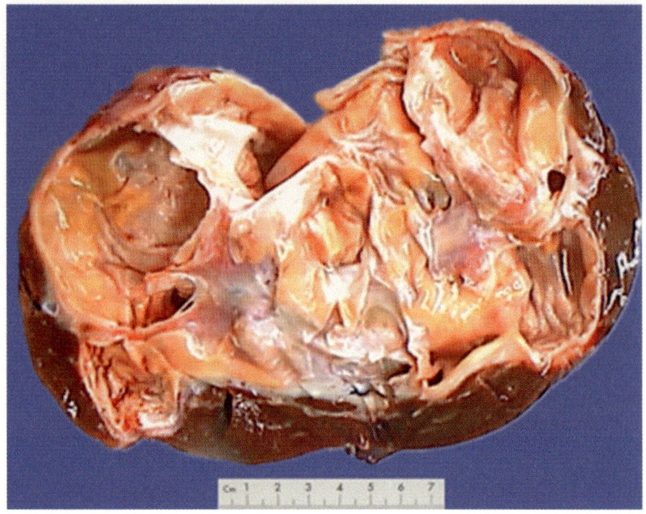

Fig. 6.23 Biliary cystadenoma. A multilocular cystic lesion

6.2.2.4 Microscopic Features

1. Mucinous BCA. Columnar, cuboidal, or flattened epithelial cells are lined on the basement membrane of the cyst wall, which secretes mucus, with pale eosinophilic cytoplasm, nucleus located in the basal part, and no atypia (Fig. 6.24). Sometimes there will be focal intestinal epithelial metaplasia or absence of the lining epithelium (Fig. 6.25). The tumor cells were arranged into tubules. Bile duct papillary cystadenoma can be diagnosed according to the existence of papillary hyperplasia. Borderline lesions are indicated if dysplasia of epithelial cells is observed, such as increased nuclear volume, increased chromatin, multilayer arrangement, absence of cellular polarity, and mitotic activity. Lesions with highly graded atypical hyperplasia have a tendency of canceration, and junctional zone of normal mucosal epithelium-highly graded atypical lesion-cystadenocarcinoma can be found in canceration cases. Among the 78 cases of BCA diag-

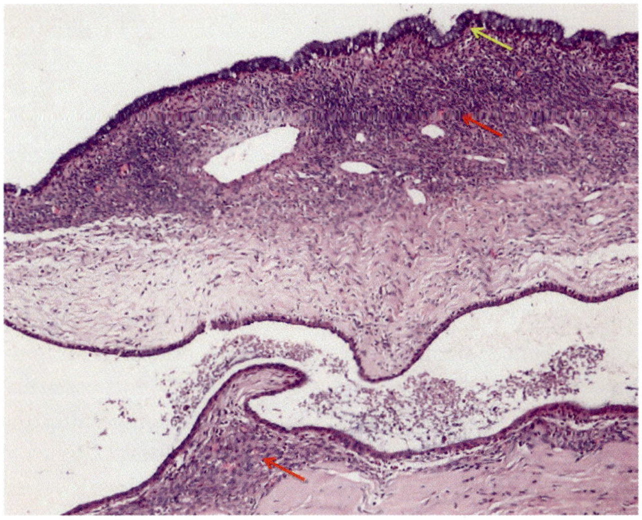

Fig. 6.24 Intrahepatic biliary cystadenoma. Cuboidal epithelial cells are lined on the surface of the cyst wall; the lower layer was the ovarian-type stroma

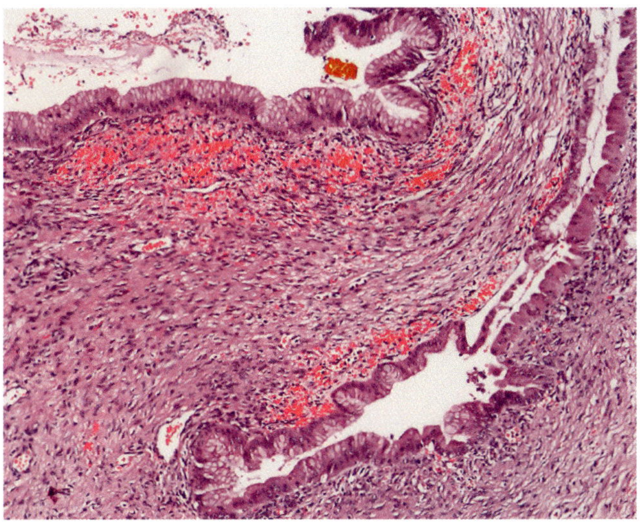

Fig. 6.25 Intrahepatic biliary cystadenoma. Intestinal epithelial metaplasia of the lining cells, ovarian-type stroma, and few hemorrhages were seen in the cyst wall

nosed in the Department of Pathology, Eastern Hepatobiliary Surgery Hospital, Second Military Medical University, 30 cases involved low- or high-grade intraepithelial neoplasia, 3 cases involved canceration, and statistical analysis showed patients with portal or extrahepatic bile duct tumors, or male patients had higher proportions of intraepithelial neoplasia or canceration (Table 6.3). It is worth noting that two cases of hilar BCA had canceration. The cystic wall of BCA was composed of dense fibrous tissue with potential secondary changes, such as macrophages containing foam or pigments, hyaline degeneration, hemosiderin deposition, cholesterol fracture, focal calcification, etc. Spindle cells with round nucleus are found between the basement membrane and

Table 6.3 Relationship of location and gender with intraepithelial neoplasia or carcinogenesis

Factors		Intraepithelial neoplasia or carcinogenesis		*P* value
		Yes	No	
Gender	Male	16	7	*P*=0.002
	Female	17	38	
Location	Extrahepatic or portal	7	2	*P*=0.022
	Intrahepatic	26	43	

the lower part of the outer layer of fibrous connective tissue, which can go on differentiation to smooth muscle cells, fibroblasts, or adipose tissue and are termed as ovarian-type stroma. About 85% of mucinous BCA cases can have ovarian-type stroma, but only in females, while BCA cases with absence of ovarian-type stroma often concern male patients and only a few females. And among the 78 cases diagnosed in the Department of Pathology, Eastern Hepatobiliary Surgery Hospital, Second Military Medical University, 37 cases of ovarian-type stroma are all women.

2. Serous BCA. The cyst wall is lined with a single layer of cuboidal epithelium with bright cytoplasm because of the rich glycogen, and mucous staining shows negative. The lower layer below the basement membrane is connective tissue with hyaline degeneration, and the interstitial tissue is composed of varying amounts of smooth muscle, fat, mucous glands, capillaries, and inflammatory cells rather than spindle cells.

6.2.2.5 Immunohistochemistry

Glandular epithelium was positive for CA19-9, low molecular weight CK, CEA, and EMA, similar to that of the normal bile duct and the pancreatic and ovarian tumors. Approximately 5% of BCA may have neuroendocrine differentiation; immunohistochemistry shows positive for synaptophysin (Syn) and chromogranin A (CgA) staining. Ovarian-type stroma was positive for vimentin, actin, desmin, and SMA, suggesting differentiation of smooth muscle, and expression of ER and PR, which may explain the reason of female predomination in BCA patients. Reports demonstrated that BCA often occurred in patients with hormone therapy, and tumor volume increased during pregnancy [53, 54].

6.2.2.6 Differential Diagnosis

1. Differentiation should be made between BCA and various kinds of cystic lesions in the liver, such as bile duct hamartoma, cystic mesenchymal hamartoma, liver hydatid cysts, post-traumatic cysts, liver abscess, polycystic liver

disease, bleeding cysts, embryonal sarcoma, HCC with cystic necrosis, metastatic tumors, biliary cystadenocarcinoma, teratoma, etc., all of which are without overlying epithelial ovarian-type stroma. Serum CA19-9 is synthesized by normal pancreatic and biliary ductal epithelium and thus will increase mildly in BDC which may be mistaken as a malignant tumor.
2. Mucinous papillary BCA should be particularly distinguished from intraductal papillary mucinous tumors. Females account for the majority of all BCA patients, often with multilocular cysts and the mucous confined in the cystic cavity, while IPNB has no obvious gender difference in incidence, and the mucus can be found in all bile ducts. Both tumors are intraductal papillary neoplasms, demonstrating papillary protruding growth of epithelial cells from the cyst wall under the microscope; however, BCA cysts do not have communication with the normal bile duct system, while IPNB may involve multiple bile ducts and exhibit transition of bile duct epithelial cells. Microscopically, ovarian-like stroma can be found in BCA but not in IPNB. Furthermore, both have malignant potential, and IPNB is more prone to recurrence and residue due to crisp nature and easy defluvium of the tumor tissue and larger involvement [52].
3. BCA and biliary cystadenocarcinoma are both rare liver-occupying lesions, but are common bile duct cystic lesions, with similar imaging manifestations and clinical manifestation which are difficult to distinguish. According to the studies by Sang et al. [49]. (2011) and Wang et al. [50], some clinical indicators can be used for the differentiation (Table 6.4).

6.2.2.7 Treatment and Prognosis

BCA grows slowly; however, up to 25% of the BCA may develop into biliary cystadenocarcinoma in a few years as pointed out by some scholars, and 33% of mucinous cystadenocarcinoma tissues contain residual benign cystadenoma tissue or transition of severe atypical epithelial hyperplasia and carcinoma tissue. Therefore, BCA is considered to be a precancerous lesion for biliary cystadenocarcinoma and should receive active surgical resection. In addition, ovarian-like stroma may also develop into cystadenocarcinoma or sarcoma [55–60].

The patients with complete resection of BCA have a good prognosis, but partial resection is potentially complicated by recurrent or residual cancer. Patients of about 132 cases reported in English literature during the recent 20 years of follow-up underwent surgical resection, with only 3 cases of recurrence after operation. There are reports on increased risks of recurrence in incomplete resection cases. Sun Zengpeng [61] reported 15 cases of BCA, with no recurrence in 12 cases receiving complete resection during the follow-up period, while patients with partial resection in 3 cases had recurrence 5 months, 12 months, and 18 months after the operations, respectively. Shen Hua [62] reported 11 cases of BCA, with 2 cases of canceration. One patient received puncture and drainage, developed recurrence and metastasis 2 years later, and died 3 months later, while the other patient was without recurrence. Therefore, puncture of liver cystic masses which is unclear in nature is with a considerable risk. Romagnoli et al. [63] reported one case of BCA with injury of intrahepatic bile duct, during the surgery due to the deep location of the tumor, and it was then treated via liver transplantation, obtaining satisfactory curative effect.

Table 6.4 Clinical indicators for differentiation of BCA from bile duct cystadenocarcinoma

Indicators	BCA	Bile duct cystadenocarcinoma
Average age (years)	44.2	57
Gender ratio	Largely female (>85%)	Male and female (~1:1)
Average tumor diameter	13 cm	8.3 cm
Average serum CA19-9	838.4 U/ml	337.9 U/ml

6.2.3 Intraductal Papillary Neoplasms of the Bile Ducts

According to the fourth edition of the WHO's *Neoplasms of Digestive System* in 2010, intraductal papillary neoplasms of the bile ducts (IPNB) include papilloma or papillary adenoma and papillomatosis, among which papillary tumors with mucous secretion are known as intraductal papillary mucinous biliary neoplasm (IPMN), and multiple bile duct papillary tumors are called biliary papillomatosis.

6.2.3.1 Pathogenesis and Mechanism

With the gradually deepening knowledge on IPNB in recent years, more and more reports on the disease have been found, and there are more than 100 cases reported in the literature both abroad and at home since 1958 when the first case was reported by Caroli.

Studies from Taiwan, China, and South Korea showed that cholelithiasis and clonorchiasis are two major risk factors of this disease, which has highly malignant tendency. It takes 6–8 years for bile duct stones to develop into IPNB, while it takes 1–2 years for the development of a carcinoma into invasive cancer, the benign-to-malignant development of which is consistent with the general canceration process of adenoma, similar to the process of colorectal adenoma-adenocarcinoma. In addition, this tumor also involves inflammatory reaction, cell damage and repair, and dysplasia [64, 65]. IPNB often shares gene mutation spectrum with cholangiocarcinoma, including KRAS, TP53, p16, and SMAD4. It has been reported in the literature that 40–80% IPNB contain components of tubular adenocarcinoma, mucinous adenocarcinoma, or invasive carcinoma, indicating a high malignant risk for IPNB canceration. A total of 29 cases of IPNB have been diagnosed in the Department of Pathology, Eastern Hepatobiliary Surgery Hospital, Second Military Medical University, among which 27 patients are with low- or high-grade intraepithelial neoplasia or carcinogenesis.

The histogenesis of IPNB is still unknown and there are a variety of views. Nakanuma et al. [67] suggested that IPNB probably originated from peribiliary gland cells, while Cardinale et al. considered periductal stem or progenitor cells surrounding the bile duct as the origination, and the genesis includes a sequence of processes including reaction to risk factors such as inflammation, mutations in stem or progenitor cells, and gradual development of dysplasia into invasive cancer.

6.2.3.2 Clinical Features

According to an epidemiological survey in 2012 [66], the male to female ratio of IPNB patients was 1.06:1, with an average age of 60 (ranged 40–77) years old, and the majority of the patients are 50–70 years old. The most common clinical symptoms are recurrent abdominal pain, jaundice, and fever, and acute cholangitis is commonly seen in mucoid cases, while patients with non-mucoid IPNB are often asymptomatic. Some patients are complicated by hepatolithiasis, ulcerative colitis, Caroli disease, choledochal cyst, and polyposis coli. Twenty-nine cases have been diagnosed in the Department of Pathology, Eastern Hepatobiliary Surgery Hospital, Second Military Medical University, concerning 13 males and 16 females, with the average age of 59.7 (38–79) years old, including five cases with biliary stones and one case of colorectal cancer and liver metastasis. Imaging study demonstrates intraductal masses and dilatation of bile duct, and dilatation of both proximal and distal bile ducts has certain significance in diagnosis of IPNB. Laboratory examination results are often indicative of the general performance of the bile duct obstruction, such as an increase in ALT, AST, total bilirubin, conjugated bilirubin, γ-glutamyl transferase, and alkaline phosphatase. About 74.4% of the patients have elevated total serum bilirubin, 40–80% have elevated serum levels of CA19-9 which is much higher in mucous cases, and about 25% of patients have increased serum CEA.

6.2.3.3 Gross Features

IPNB usually consists of diffuse or multicentric papillary clusters which are ecru in color, connected to the bile duct mucosa via peduncles and mostly found in the left hepatic lobe, involving the whole biliary tree or even the extrahepatic bile ducts, cystic duct, and main pancreatic duct. The tumor, crisp, soft, and easy to fall off, mainly generated from epithelial growth on the surface, protruding into the lumen, and may cause complete obstruction of the bile ducts. The surrounding liver tissue is green in color due to cholestasis or presents biliary cirrhosis. Among the 29 cases of IPNB diagnosed in the Department of Pathology, Eastern Hepatobiliary Surgery Hospital, Second Military Medical University, 19 cases involved intrahepatic bile ducts, and 10 cases involved the hilar or extrahepatic bile ducts. The cross section of the tumors exhibited obvious dilatation of the bile ducts filled with gray-white or gray-red floccule, tumor thrombus-like tissue (Fig. 6.26), bile duct polyp, or cauliflower mass in the lumen.

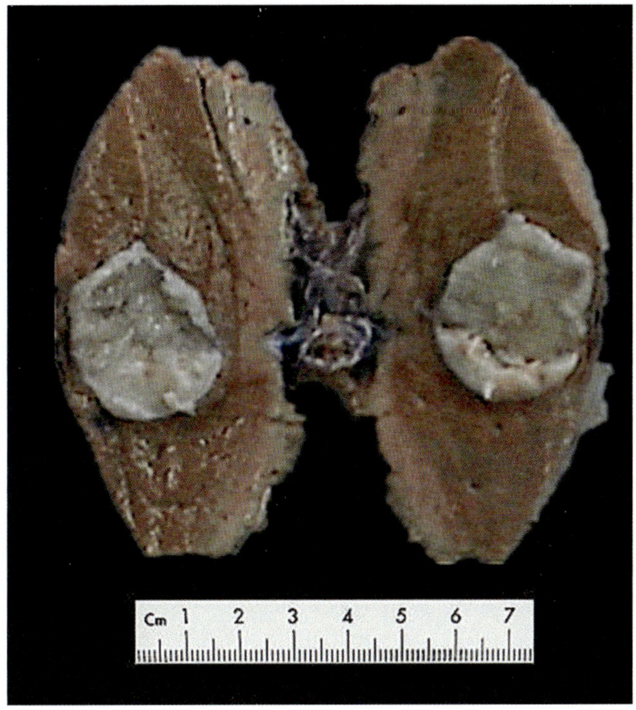

Fig. 6.26 Intraductal papillary neoplasms of the bile ducts. The bile ducts filled with *gray-white* polyp tissue

6.2.3.4 Microscopic Features

Histologically, IPNB shows multiple papillary-villous hyperplasia of biliary epithelium, which grows in branches from fibrous vascular axis protruding into the lumen and lined with cuboidal or columnar epithelium on the surface. The cells are with pale eosinophilic cytoplasm (Figs. 6.27 and 6.28) and arranged in multilayers with darker staining nuclei during dysplasia (Figs. 6.29 and 6.30). And as the degree of dysplasia increases, the cell layers and cells with mitosis multiply, with a visible transition between the lesion and the epithelium of normal bile duct (Fig. 6.31). The bile ducts dilate significantly, surrounded by normal bile ducts with acute or chronic inflammation of epithelium, which may detach due to ulcer, and duct wall thickens because of fibrous

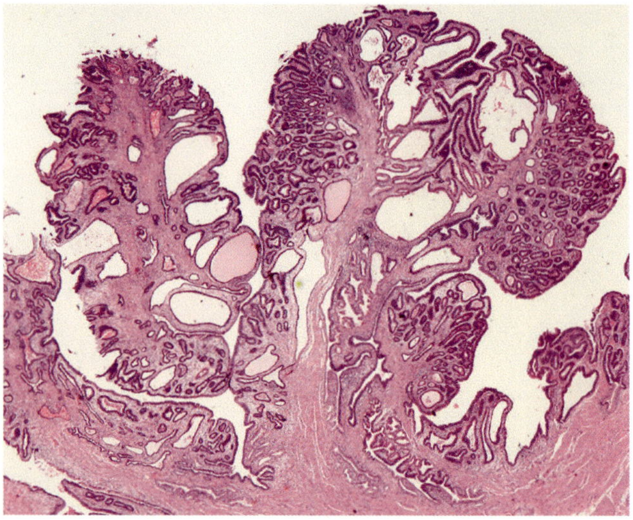

Fig. 6.27 Intraductal papillary neoplasms of the bile ducts. IPNB shows papillary hyperplasia, which grows in branches from fibrous vascular axis protruding into the lumen

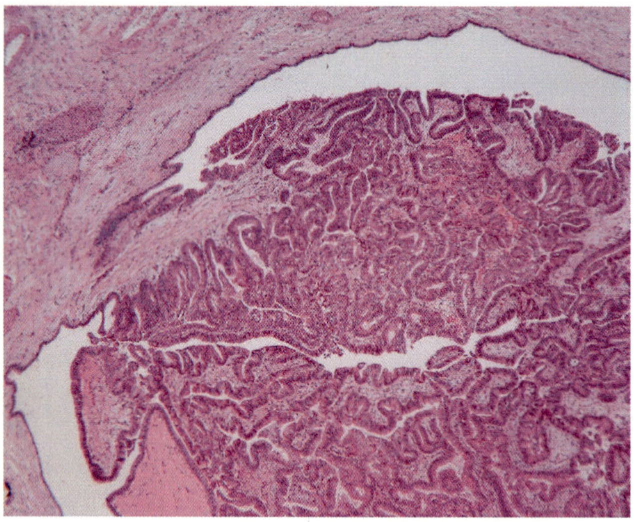

Fig. 6.28 Intraductal papillary neoplasms of the bile ducts

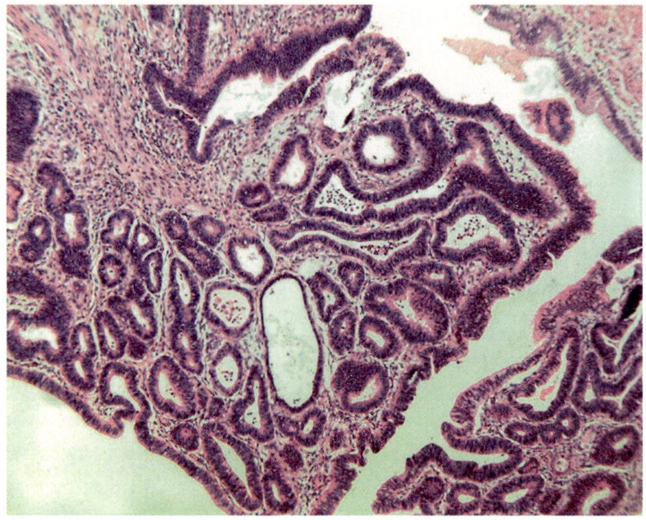

Fig. 6.29 Intraductal papillary neoplasms of the bile ducts with high-grade intraepithelial neoplasia. The tumor cells are arranged in multilayers with darker staining nuclei. High power of Fig. 6.28

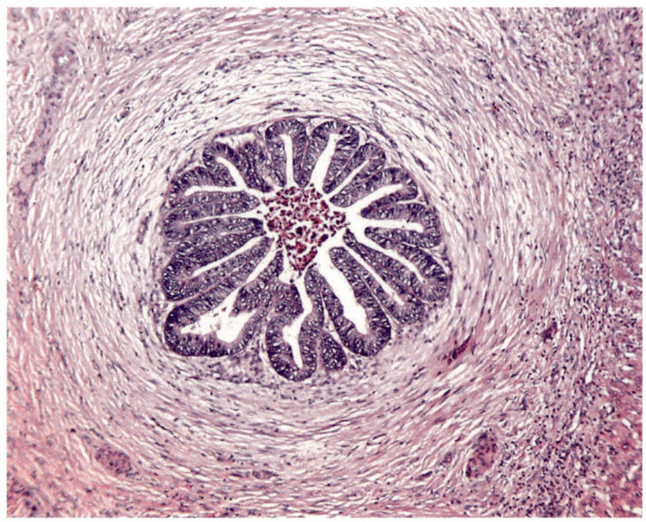

Fig. 6.30 Intraductal papillary neoplasms of the bile ducts with high-grade intraepithelial neoplasia. The small bile duct branch cells are arranged in multilayers with darker staining nuclei; the lumen is narrow with necrosis

tissue hyperplasia. Most of the lesions protrude into the lumen which may be filled up, and infiltration into basal bile duct wall can be observed when canceration occurs (Fig. 6.32). Mucus secretion is found in one third cases of IPNB (IPMN). IPNB is prone to be malignant; thus, multiple sections are needed for careful examination. According to different degrees of dysplasia and infiltration, it can be divided into four stages: IPNB with low-grade intraepithelial neoplasia; IPNB with high-grade intraepithelial neoplasia; intraductal carcinoma of bile duct in situ, T_1; and infiltrating carcinoma of the bile duct, T_2 or higher. The 29 cases of IPNB diagnosed in the Department of Pathology, Eastern Hepatobiliary Surgery Hospital, Second Military Medical University, included 8 cases with low-grade intraepithelial neoplasias, 14 cases with high-grade intraepithelial neoplasia, and 5 cases with canceration.

According to the tumor tissues and the morphological characteristics, IPNB can be divided into the following four types:

1. Pancreatobiliary type. The tumor is similar to the pancreas duct and ductular epithelium with columnar cells which have basophilic cytoplasm and round nuclei (Fig. 6.33). Immunohistochemistry staining often shows MUC1 positive and MUC2 negative. It is the most com-

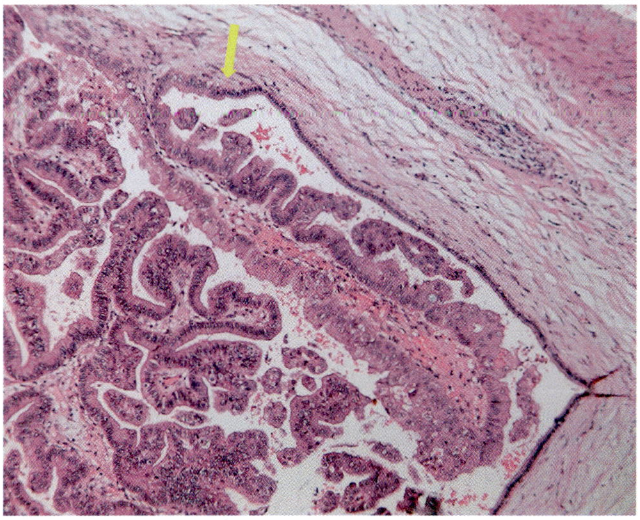

Fig. 6.31 Intraductal papillary neoplasms of the bile ducts. Transition between the lesion and the epithelium of normal bile duct

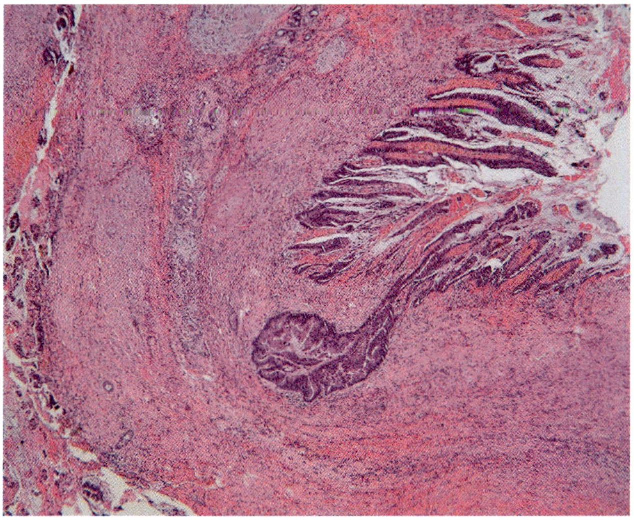

Fig. 6.32 Intraductal papillary neoplasms of the bile ducts with canceration. Papillary hyperplasia of biliary epithelium infiltration into basal bile duct wall

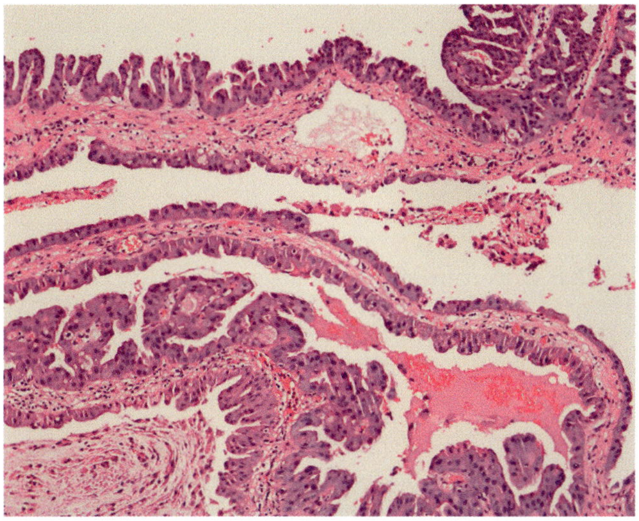

Fig. 6.33 Intraductal papillary neoplasms, pancreatobiliary type. The tumor is similar to the pancreas duct and ductular epithelium with columnar cells

mon type which tends to undergo malignant transformation to form tubular adenocarcinoma.

2. Intestinal type. The tumor has similarity to the features of intestinal villous tumors (Fig. 6.34), and immunohistochemistry staining shows that the tumor cells stably expressed MUC2 and MUC5AC, while no expression of MUC1 was detected. It is less likely to undergo malignant transformation which results in colloid (mucinous) invasive carcinoma.

3. Oncocytic type. The tumor cells have rich cytoplasm which is strongly eosinophilic (Fig. 6.35), and immunohistochemistry staining shows stable expression of MUC5AC and focal expression of MUC1 and (or) MUC2 in the cells. It has less tendency of malignant transformation.

4. Gastric type. The tumor consists of columnar epithelial cells, similar to the gastric pit structure (Fig. 6.36), and immunohistochemistry staining shows MUC5AC expression and no expression of MUC1 or MUC2.

Papillomatosis was reported by Caroli in 1959 for the first time, and more than 150 cases have been reported till now. The lesions grow in multiple foci, with involvement of the whole intrahepatic biliary tree in severe cases, and both intra- and extrahepatic bile ducts can be involved. Furthermore, lesions in different regions may be at different stages in the developmental course and can be divided into mucus biliary papillomatosis (MBP) and non-mucus biliary papillomatosis (NMBP). Generally, it is believed that BP has a highly malignant tendency and is an important type of precancerous lesions. Its canceration rate is as high as 41–83%, and radical surgical resection or liver transplantation should be preferred for the treatment [68].

6.2.3.5 Immunohistochemistry

Almost all of the IPNB lesions express biomarkers of bile duct epithelium and gastrointestinal epithelium, such as CK7, CK20, and MUC5AC, suggesting the combination of its retaining bile duct epithelial immunophenotypes and

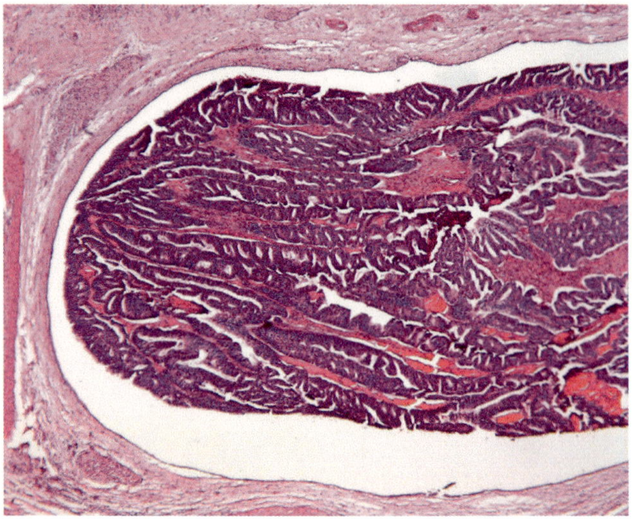

Fig. 6.34 Intraductal papillary neoplasms, intestinal type. Columnar tumor cells have similarity to the features of intestinal villous tumors

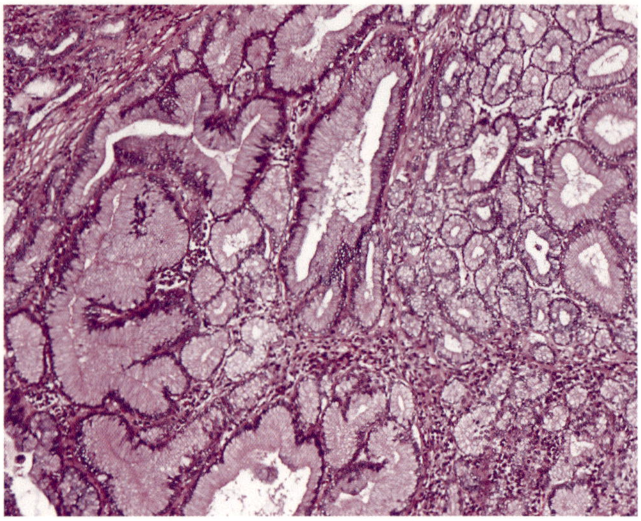

Fig. 6.36 Intraductal papillary neoplasms, gastric type. The tumor consists of columnar epithelial cells, similar to the gastric pit structure

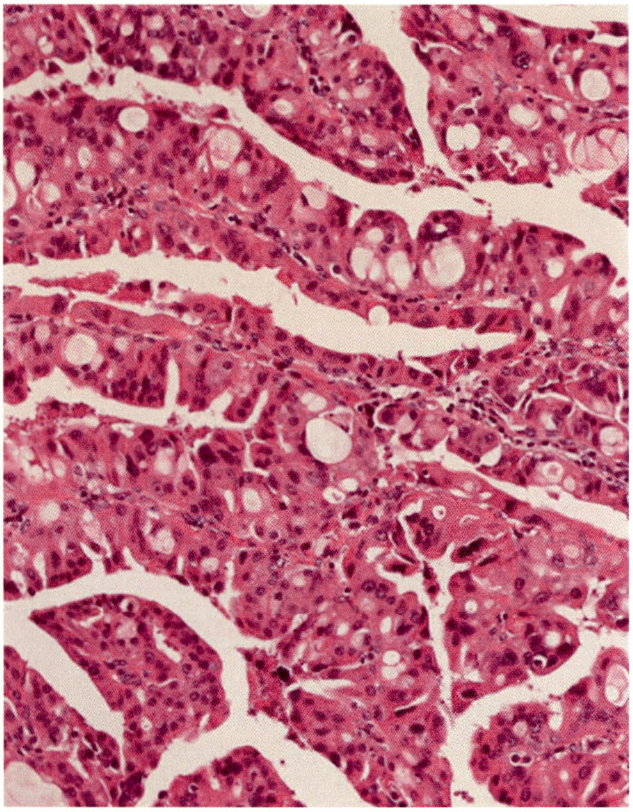

Fig. 6.35 Intraductal papillary neoplasms, oncocytic type. The tumor cells have rich cytoplasm which is strongly eosinophilic

obtaining MUC1 immunophenotypes of the gastrointestinal epithelium in the genesis of IPNB. The expression of MUC1 usually indicates the infiltrating carcinoma, while mucinous tumors in IPMN are MUC1 negative and MUC2 positive. Sasaki et al. [69] demonstrated that IPNB overexpressed EZH2 and MUC1, and the low expression of MUC6 may indicate the malignant biological behavior of the tumor. Tubulin β-III (TUBB3) is negative in IPNB but positive in about half the number of extrahepatic bile duct carcinoma. Murakami et al. [70] found P53, CD133, and mucus staining were positive in primary tumors and cell line (KBDC)-11 of IPNB.

6.2.3.6 Differential Diagnosis

IPNB should be distinguished from intrahepatic bile duct stones, bile duct cystadenoma or carcinoma, cholangiocarcinoma, etc.

1. Intrahepatic bile duct stones. The clinical symptoms of intrahepatic bile duct stones are similar to that of IPNB, and the latter can be complicated by bile duct stones, while intrahepatic bile duct stones often present simple dilatation of the bile duct, active proliferation of the peripheral glands, interstitial infiltration of lots of inflammatory cells, no papillary hyperplasia of epithelium, and little mucus in the lumen under the microscope. They are benign lesions, but intraepithelial neoplasia and cancer can also be found occasionally. Therefore, careful sample drawing is needed to prevent missed diagnosis.
2. Biliary cystadenoma. IPNB is without ovarian-like stroma, and its cystic dilatation is communicated with bile ducts.
3. Cholangiocarcinoma. Cholangiocarcinoma exhibits no cholangitis or biliary stones in most cases, and visible mucus is not common in it, while the above three manifestations are common in IPNB. Enhancement of IPNB is noted in outflow phase of enhanced CT, rather than persistent or progressive enhancement as in cholangiocarcinoma.

6.2.3.7 Treatment and Prognosis

IPNB may develop into intrahepatic papillary carcinoma or mucinous cholangiocarcinoa and is a defined type of precancerous lesions. Focal resection is for limited localized lesions in one side of the hepatic lobe. However, lesions that are widely distributed cannot be easily removed, and they are often crisp and easy to fall off, resulting in high relapse rate after surgery and poor prognosis. Papillomatosis can also cause a variety of complications, including intrahepatic duct stones, biliary hemorrhage, common bile duct stones, and gallbladder stones. Other common and fatal complications include bacterial cholangitis, obstructive jaundice, sepsis, hepatic failure, and malignant transformation, which need liver transplantation when necessary.

Generally, the growth of IPNB is mainly limited inside the bile duct, and it has a better prognosis than that of common intrahepatic cholangiocarcinoma. Mucous IPNB accounts for 83% of all the cases, and the average postoperative survival period of non-mucinous IPNB is reported longer than that of mucous IPNB, 52.27 + 6.72 months and 30.84 + 8.36 months, respectively. However, biological behaviors of IPNB lesions differ from each other due to their different stages. Rocha et al. [71] demonstrated that different infiltration depths and different canceration degrees of the tumors are influencing factors for patients' survival time. Kim et al. [72] suggested that the biological behavior of pancreatobiliary type was different from other types with a higher risk of lymph node metastasis and recurrence.

6.2.4 Biliary Adenofibroma

Wen-Ming Cong and Yu-Yao Zhu
Department of Pathology, Eastern Hepatobiliary Surgery Hospital, Second Military Medical University, Shanghai, China

6.2.4.1 Pathogenesis and Mechanism

Biliary adenofibroma (BAF) is a very rare tumor, first reported by Tsui et al. in 1993 [73], and is considered as a benign tumor with potential of malignant transformation originating from the bile duct. Only six cases of BAF have been reported in the Chinese and foreign literature (Table 6.5), and one case was diagnosed in the Department of Pathology, Eastern Hepatobiliary Surgery Hospital, Second Military Medical University. Concentrated bile was found in the duct of BAF indicating the connection to the bile duct system, which is a supportive evidence that it derives from hamartomatous bile ducts. Parada et al. [74] detected the chromosome mutation of one case of BAF using cytogenetic methods, finding abnormal chromosome 22, which is common in benign mesenchymal tumors, suggesting that BAF is originated from mesenchymal tissue rather than epithelium.

6.2.4.2 Clinical Features

The average age of the patients is 56.5 (25–79) years old, and the first symptom is often dull pain in the right upper abdomen, with normal laboratory examination and hypervascular masses in CT scanning. The case diagnosed in the Department of Pathology, Eastern Hepatobiliary Surgery Hospital, Second Military Medical University, concerned a 51-year-old patient, who was admitted into the hospital because of upper abdominal pain for 5 months and an occupying lesion in the right lobe of the liver found in CT examination, with normal laboratory examination and no history of hepatitis.

6.2.4.3 Gross Features

The tumor is a spherical mass with an average diameter of 9.9 (3.5–20) cm, and the section shows multiple closely distributed oval thin-walled cavities with a diameter of 1–5 mm accounting for three fourths of the volume of the tumor. The cystic cavity was divided into lobules by slender septa throughout the tumor, and the remaining part of the tumor is

Table 6.5 Reported cases of biliary adenofibroma

Authors	Year	Gender	Age (years)	Diameter (cm)	Malignancy	Recurrence/metastasis	Feature
Tsui et al. [73]	1993	Female	74	7	None	None	Right upper abdominal pain
Parada et al. [74]	1997	Female	49	7.5	None	None	Right hypochondrium pain
Akin and Coskun [75]	2002	Male	25	20, recurrent 14	Yes	Recurrence 3 years postsurgery/lung metastasis	Abdominal distension and right upper abdominal pain
Varnholt et al. [76]	2003	Female	47	16	None	None	Right upper abdominal pain for several months
Xu Li et al. [77]	2009	Female	65	3.5	None	None	Intermittent right upper abdominal pain for 10 years
Alessandra et al. [78]	2010	Male	79	5.5	None	None	Dull abdominal pain

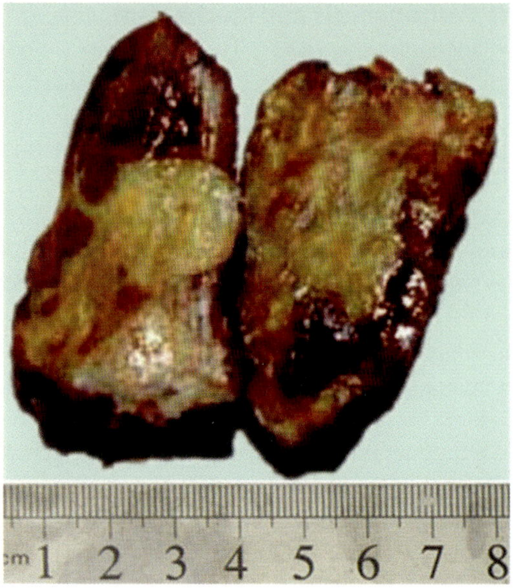

Fig. 6.37 Biliary adenofibroma. The cross section *gray* and *grayish yellow*, and hard in texture, with visible fibrous bands

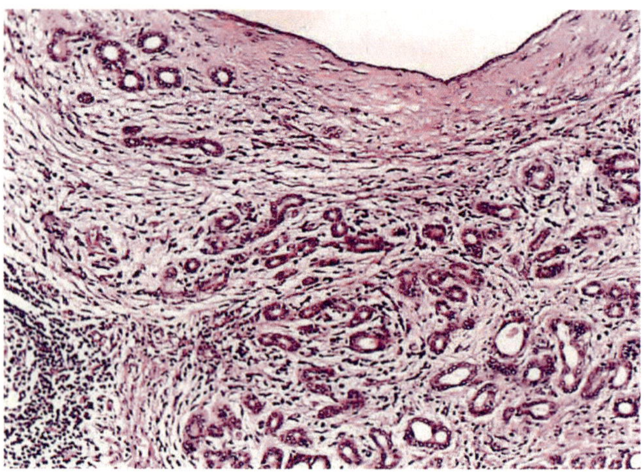

Fig. 6.38 Biliary adenofibroma. The tumor consists of proliferated small bile duct and abundant fibrous stroma

composed of relatively dense stroma. The tumor has a clear boundary with no capsule and paler than the surrounding liver tissue in color, while the latter may exhibit atrophy. One case of BAF was diagnosed in the Department of Pathology, Eastern Hepatobiliary Surgery Hospital, Second Military Medical University, the size of which was 3 cm ×2.4 cm × 1.3 cm, the cross section gray and grayish yellow, and hard in texture, with visible fibrous bands, no hemorrhage or necrosis, multiple small cavities in the lesion, fiber bundles stretching out along the duct wall, no complete capsule, and a clear boundary (Fig. 6.37).

6.2.4.4 Microscopic Features

The tumor consists of small vesicles and tubular or cystic cavity-like structures of varying sizes in loose and separated arrangement, embedded in abundant fibrous stroma (Fig. 6.38). The major cells of the tumor are cuboidal and columnar epithelial cells containing abundant cytoplasm with no atypia, and the cytoplasm of some epithelial cells is both eosinophilic and basophilous. The nucleus is small and round or oval, with small and clear nucleolus. The dilated ducts can be cystic with branches or bending, or small papillary protrusions formed on the ductal wall, and a few ducts contain cell debris, bile embolus, or thin eosinophilic fluid. The epithelial cells do not contain mucus, but can go through apocrine glands which changes occasionally on the inner layer of the ductal wall (Fig. 6.39), or are arranged in multilayers with darker nuclear staining and mild to moderate atypical hyperplasia. The interstitial fibrous tissue contains moderate numbers of cells which are myofibroblast-like and spindle shaped, with sparse and red-dye cytoplasm. The local interstitial tissue can exhibit inflammatory reaction mainly composed of lymphocytes, and densely distributed glandules can be found in sparse interstitial regions, similar to the features of BDA. Residual liver cell islands can be observed in the tumor tissue, with no envelope surrounding the tumor, a clear boundary, and no invasion into the surrounding liver tissue.

6.2.4.5 Immunohistochemistry

The epithelial cells are CK5.2, CK7, CK19, EMA, CEA and D10 positive, 1F6, desmin, SMA, mucus staining negative, and interstitial VI and SMA positive. P53 staining positive suggests potential for malignant transformation. Interstitial fibrous tissue staining demonstrates positive VI and SMA and negative NSE and S-100.

6.2.4.6 Differential Diagnosis

1. Bile duct adenoma parts of the lesions may be similar to BDA, but BDA does not contain any bile, and it often presents tubular lumen of bile ducts rather than cystic cavities, which is narrow, closely arranged, and compressed by the matrix. BDA is usually 1–20 mm in diameter, and positive D10 and 1F6 are shown in immunohistochemistry staining positive.
2. Biliary cystadenoma (BCA) is often a huge multilocular cystic mass, and the BAF sac and BCA are similar, but a BCA lesion is generally a solid one, less than 5 mm in diameter. And epithelial mucus staining is positive in BCA but negative in BAF, and the latter does not contain ovarian-like stroma.
3. Well-differentiated cholangiocarcinoma, congenital choledochal cysts, liver benign cystic mesothelioma, and biliary hamartoma should also be taken into consideration during differentiation.

6.2.4.7 Treatment and Prognosis

BAF with positive p53 staining has been reported, presenting tetraploid and S phase block, suggesting that it may belong

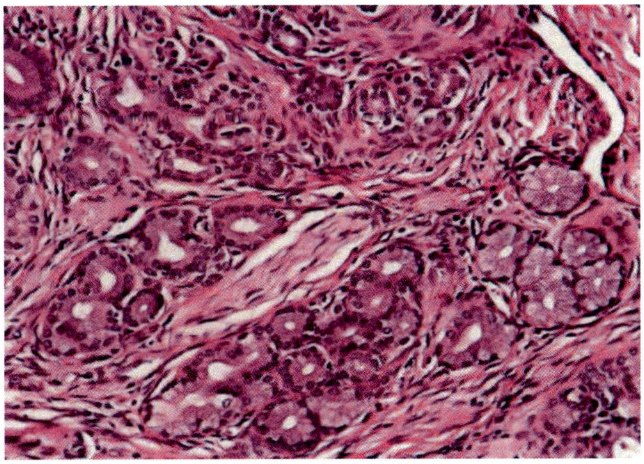

Fig. 6.39 Biliary adenofibroma. Abundant bile ducts and glands hyperplasia, with abundant collagen fibrous stroma

to the precancerous lesions. And if untreated, the epithelial cells in BAF can go on malignant transformation, especially in regions with multilayers of epithelial cells and darker staining. Therefore, complete surgical resection is the recommended treatment. Lesions with no atypia and negative p53 indicate benign and inert biological behaviors; however, there was one reported case of BAF with epithelial malignant components. Therefore, it is necessary to pay attention to the disease.

6.3 Vascular and Lymphatic Tumors

6.3.1 Cavernous Hemangioma

Wen-Ming Cong and Qian Zhao
Department of Pathology, Eastern Hepatobiliary Surgery Hospital, Second Military Medical University, Shanghai, China

6.3.1.1 Pathogenesis and Mechanism

Cavernous hemangioma is a benign vascular tumor composed of thin-walled honeycomb vascular cavities and is the most common benign tumor of the liver, with an incidence rate of 1–7%, accounting for about 74% of benign hepatic tumors. The tumor usually occurs in childhood and is often diagnosed in adulthood, regarded as a type of congenital lesions and related to vascular developmental loss of embryonic liver, or an acquired disease induced by steroids, contraceptive, pregnancy, etc. Recent studies have shown that accumulation of mast cells may be associated with its occurrence. From January 1982 to July 2014, 2732 cases of cavernous hemangioma have been diagnosed in the Pathology Department of East Hepatobiliary Surgery Hospital of Second Military Medical University.

6.3.1.2 Clinical Features

Among 172 cases of excised liver hemangioma, diagnosed in the East Hepatobiliary Surgery Hospital of Second Military Medical University from 2004 to 2006, the ratio of male to female ratio was 1:2.4, with an average age of 44.5 years old. Among them, 83 cases had symptoms, including 68 cases of abdominal pain, 16 cases of back and shoulder discomfort, and 4 cases of abdominal distension. The tumors can be palpated in the hypochondrium region in 25 patients, and the size of tumor increased significantly in 84 cases during the course of the disease, with an average increase of 4.4 cm. Most liver hemangiomas did not cause obvious symptoms or signs despite huge volume and were found only in the physical examination. Some of these patients may have symptoms, mainly chronic abdominal dull pain and postprandial fullness, which were occasionally mistaken as hepatic neoplasms. B-ultrasound examination showed small hemangioma with low to medium echo, and CT images showed hypodensity lesions, while MRI T2-weighted images showed high signal density, the so-called bulb sign.

6.3.1.3 Gross Features

Among 172 cases of excised liver hemangioma, diagnosed in the East Hepatobiliary Surgery Hospital of Second Military Medical University from 2004 to 2006, solitary lesions were found in 94 cases [79], two lesions in 40 cases, and three or more lesions in 38 cases. The tumors were 4–32 cm in diameter, averaged at 10.5 cm. A giant hepatic cavernous hemangioma was found and excised by Mengchao Wu and colleagues in one case with a tumor of 63 cm * 48.5 cm * 40 cm in size and 18 kg in weight. The cavernous hemangioma exhibited expansive growth, lobulated surface, and purple-red or dark red in color, soft, with streak-shaped fibrous coating. The cross section showed spongy or cellular lacunae containing blood components, often accompanied by varying sizes of gray-white fibrous sclerosis nodules. A few cases of hemangioma were found with degeneration, thrombosis, or further fibrosis and calcification, with gray fibrosclerosis nodules, and the hemangioma was called sclerosed hemangioma. Liver cirrhosis in the surrounding liver tissue was also found in patients with chronic hepatitis (Figs. 6.40 and 6.41).

6.3.1.4 Microscopic Features

Lesions of cavernous hemangioma are often uniform, composed of varying sizes of communicating vascular cavities, lined with flattened epithelial cells supported by fibrous tissue on the inner wall of the vessels, and filled with blood, and the vascular wall is often thickened to varying degrees due to fibrosis, also known as sclerosed hemangioma (Figs. 6.42, 6.43, and 6.44). The surrounding liver tissue is often distributed with scattered hemangioma foci or highly dilated vascular clusters.

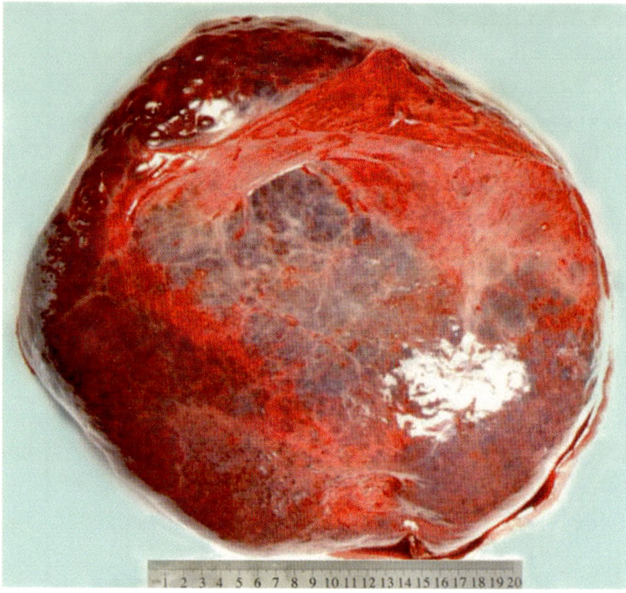

Fig. 6.40 Cavernous hemangioma. The tumor is *purple-red* in color and soft

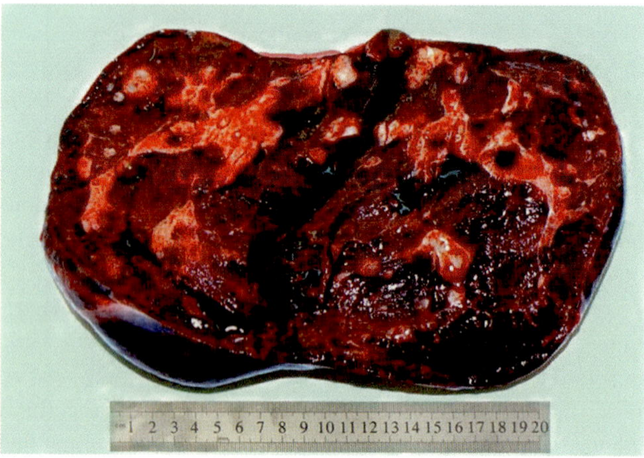

Fig. 6.41 Cavernous hemangioma. The cross section showed spongy, accompanied by *gray-white* fibrous sclerosis nodules

Hepatic hemangioma includes the following rare subtypes. ① Capillary hemangioma, diagnosed in a 58-year-old woman with a surgical resection of a tumor in the left lobe of the liver in our experience, 2.3 cm × 2 cm in size with a dark red section (Fig. 6.45), was clustered with immature capillaries (Fig. 6.46), lined by a monolayer flattened endothelial cells (Fig. 6.47) under the microscope, and CD34 staining showed the immature microvascular lumens (Fig. 6.48). In addition, visible thrombosis and arteries with thickened vascular wall and stenosis can also be seen. ② Infantile hemangioma (IH), also known as infantile hemangioendothelioma, often occurs in 10-day-old to 3-month-old infants after birth, with multiple lesions of infantile skin hemangiomatosis, 0.8–21 cm in diameter, and can be divided into focal (single

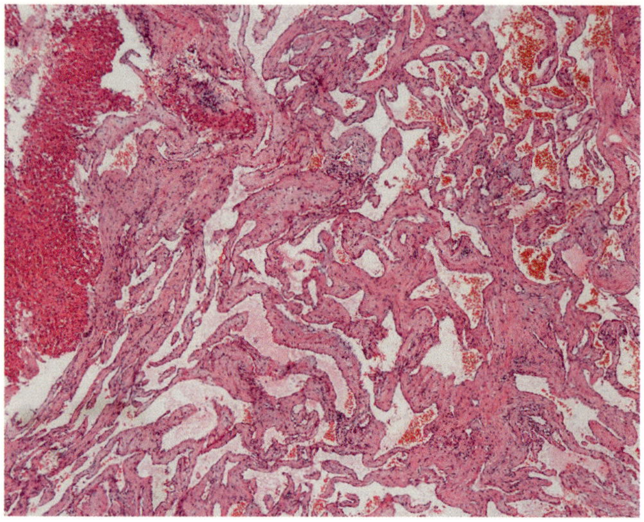

Fig. 6.42 Cavernous hemangioma. The tumor was composed of highly dilated thin-walled vessels, filled with blood

lesion), multifocal (4–20 lesions), and diffuse type (>20 lesions). The morphological characteristics are similar to those of juvenile capillary hemangioma in the soft tissue. In the early stage of the disease, the neocapillaries may contain no or only a few cavities, and the hypertrophic endothelial cells are arranged in the shape of solid plates, while in maturity stage they are similar to adult capillary hemangioma with intensive expression of glucose transporter (GLUT1) and formation of angiosarcoma in a small number of cases [80], and the solitary lesions can be surgically excised, while multiple lesions can be treated by liver transplantation. ③ Hepatic vascular malformation with capillary proliferation (HVMCP), with lesions of 5–11 cm in diameter, typically exhibits as major infarction and hemorrhage center and strip-shaped arrangement of congested blood vessels with thick walls, lined with flat endothelial cells, surrounded by proliferation of peripheral blood capillaries and interstitial mucinous degeneration. Negative GLUT1 staining is shown in vascular endothelial cells and major blood vessels. The prognosis of the tumor which receives surgical resection is good [81].

6.3.1.5 Immunohistochemistry

CD34 and F-VIII positive.

6.3.1.6 Differential Diagnosis

Pathological diagnosis of the disease is not difficult, but misdiagnosis from vascular lesions, such as angiolymphoma, angiosarcoma, and peliosis hepatis, should be avoided.

6.3.1.7 Treatment and Prognosis

Cavernous hemangioma grows slowly with no malignant tendency. Lesions >5 cm in diameter or manifests by obvious symptoms can be treated with surgical resection or hepatic artery ligation, and conservative treatment or observation is

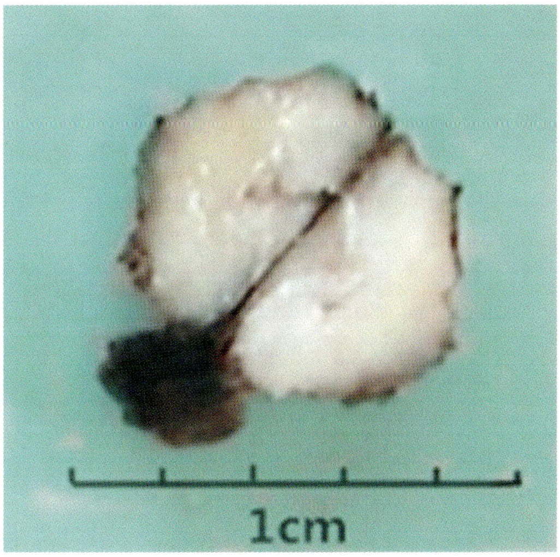

Fig. 6.43 Sclerosed hemangioma

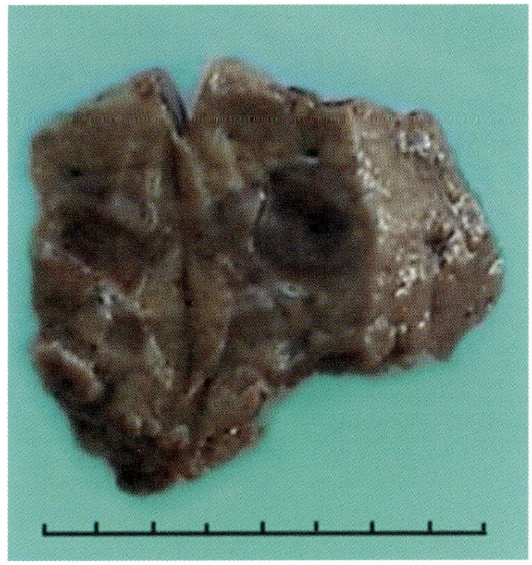

Fig. 6.45 Capillary hemangioma. The cross section showed *dark red* with clear boundary

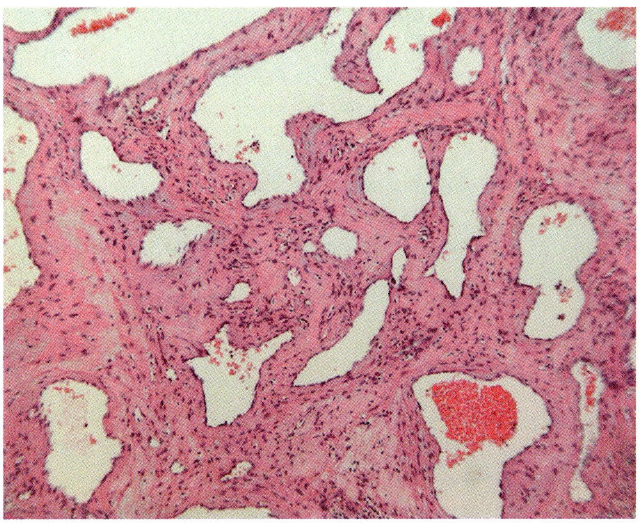

Fig. 6.44 Cavernous hemangioma, sclerosed type. The vascular wall is thickened to varying degrees due to fibrosis

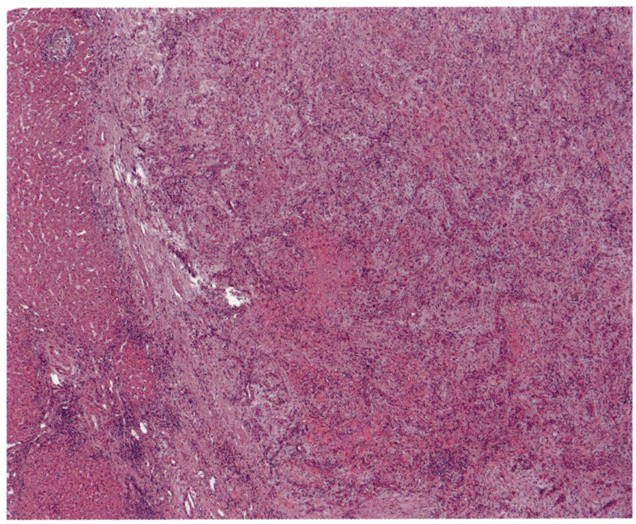

Fig. 6.46 Capillary hemangioma. The tumor was clustered with capillaries; vascular lumens were narrow

suited for small or asymptomatic lesions, while selective hepatic portal occlusion and anatomic technique are extremely important when treating hemangioma located at complex and difficult sites [82]. Successful liver transplantation was reported in a case of giant hepatic cavernous hemangioma (40 cm×30 cm×30 cm) by Zhongshan Medical University. In recent years, interventional technique and radiofrequency ablation have also been applied to the treatment of this disease which shows good curative effects in surgery. The prognosis is good, with no recurrence, and hepatic cavernous hemangioma associated with medication may disappear spontaneously or stop growing or after drug withdrawal.

6.3.2 Hemangioblastoma

Wen-Ming Cong and Yu-Yao Zhu
Department of Pathology, Eastern Hepatobiliary Surgery Hospital, Second Military Medical University,
Shanghai, China

Hemangioblastoma, also called as haemangioblastomas and composed of large thick-walled blood vessels and stromal cells with rich lipid droplets, is a benign vascular tumor originated from mesoderm and commonly found in patients with von Hippel-Lindau disease (VHL). VHL is an autosomal

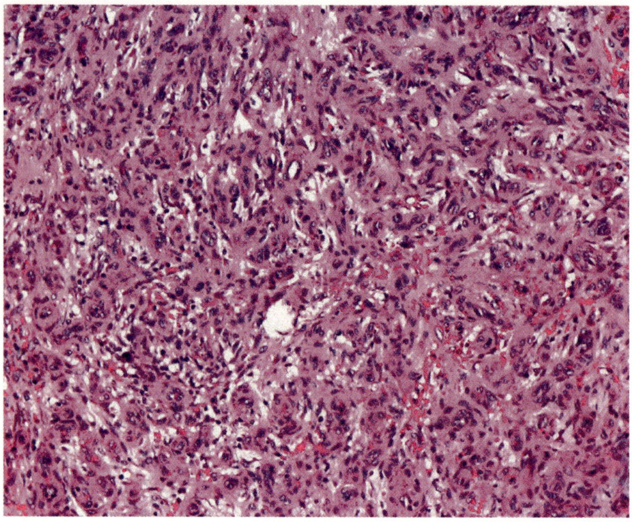

Fig. 6.47 Capillary hemangioma. Immature small vessels lined by endothelial cells showed microvascular lumens

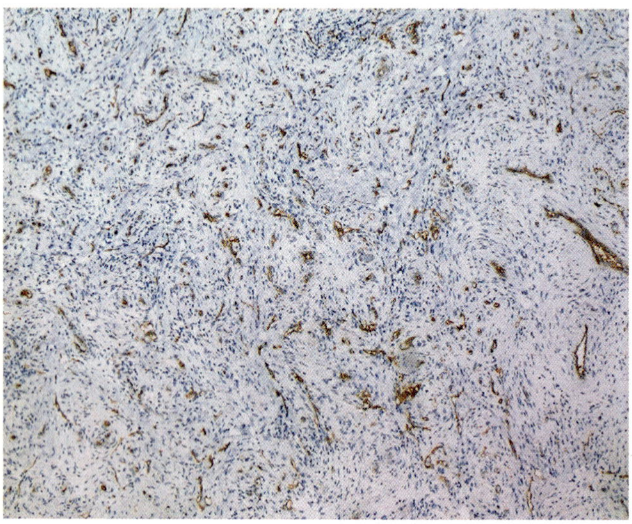

Fig. 6.48 Capillary hemangioma. CD34 staining showed the immature microvascular lumens

dominant cancer predisposition syndrome, mainly involving multiple organs and systems and a variety of hereditary neoplastic syndromes, and hemangioblastoma of central nervous system is the most common tumor, often found in the cerebellum, cerebrum, spinal cord, brain stem, and retina and rarely seen in the liver. Only three cases of liver hemangioblastoma have been reported in the English literature, all of which were combined with VHL [83–85].

Previous reports of VHL involving the liver were often adenoma, cysts, and hemangioma, while liver hemangioblastoma is extremely rare. Ultrasound examination shows a solid hypoechoic mass, and CT shows a hypodense mass, while angiography shows a mass with rich blood vessels. Microscopic observation shows the similarity of the lesion to hemangioblastoma of the central nervous system, consisting of vascular endothelial cells, pericytes, and stromal cells which form atypical capillaries with expansion of vessels and a small amount of red blood cells in the lumen. The stromal cells are rich in adipose tissue, which may form bubbles or bubble-like structures, and increased nuclear chromatin and enlarged nuclei are occasionally found in the stromal cells. When VHL patients are accompanied with liver occupation, hemangioblastoma should be first excluded. Surgical treatment for intracranial hemangioblastomas shows good therapeutic effects, and complete resection is a radical therapy. However, there are also many reported cases concerning hemangioblastoma in the liver or lung after multiple surgeries.

6.3.3 Infantile Hemangioendothelioma

Wen-Ming Cong and Qian Zhao
Department of Pathology, Eastern Hepatobiliary Surgery Hospital, Second Military Medical University,
Shanghai, China

6.3.3.1 Pathogenesis and Mechanism

Infantile hemangioendothelioma (IHE) is the most common benign vascular tumor in the liver; almost all cases concern infants under 1 year old after birth, derived from abnormal development of the central vein and portal vein system. From January 1982 to December 2012, six cases of IHE were diagnosed in the Department of Pathology, Eastern Hepatobiliary Surgery Hospital, of Second Military Medical University, accounting for 0.019% of all liver primary malignant tumors during the same period. IHE is similar to skin capillary hemangioma that if regression occurs after proliferation, maturation, and degradation stages, liver-occupying lesions cannot be formed. This disease can also be a part of Kasabach-Merritt syndrome, characterized by cutaneous and visceral angiomatosis, thrombocytopenia syndrome, and disseminated intravascular coagulation, or accompanied by certain congenital diseases, such as congenital heart disease, 21 trisomy syndrome, deletions in chromosome 6q, and heterotopic left liver in the thoracic cavity. Rapini et al. [86] conducted karyotype analysis in one 3-year-old child with IHE (tumor size, 57 mm × 56 mm × 70 mm), finding interstitial deletion of 13q13.3 to 21.32 on the long arm of chromosome 13, with a deletion range of 27.87 MB containing the RB1 gene, and the patient manifested developmental delay and poor growth.

6.3.3.2 Clinical Features

The patients of IHE include infants within 6 months after birth accounting for 86% and children under the age of 3 years old accounting for 99%. However, there are also reports of adult IHE. Among the six cases of IHE in the Department of Pathology, Eastern Hepatobiliary Surgery Hospital, of Second Military Medical University, the male to female ratio was 5:1, and the average age was 38.8 years (5–61). About 30% of the children cases had angioendothelioma and at the same time in the skin, lymph node, spleen, gastrointestinal tract, pleura, prostate, lung, and bone. Riley et al. [87] reported two cases of IHE with biliary atresia, acute liver failure, and some other congenital diseases, such as diaphragmatic hernia, Down syndrome, large artery transposition, and multi-finger deformity. Forty percent of the patients were primarily diagnosed when their mother manifested abdominal masses. Related clinical manifestations include hepatomegaly, nausea, vomiting, gastrointestinal bleeding, jaundice, hemolytic anemia, thrombocytopenia, liver failure, or even death caused by high-output heart failure because of intrahepatic arteriovenous shunt due to tumor compression. Mild to moderate increase of serum AFP levels can be found in the children patients, which is limited for reference in younger children, because its level in normal newborns reaches 2500 ng/ml and decreases to normal level in adults at 6 months after birth. The performance of the lesions on CT shows hypodensity with a clear boundary, and scattered calcification in the center can be found in 50% cases, while obvious calcification demonstrates wide distribution inside the mass-forming granular clusters. And early filling of the lesions in SPECT scans is of diagnostic value.

6.3.3.3 Gross Features

Intrahepatic solitary or multiple lesions are found in liver IHE. In our hospital, all the six cases diagnosed as IHE concerned solitary lesions of 1.2–6.3 cm in diameter. The cross section of the tumors was brownish-red capillary cavities with rich blood contents or yellow white in cases with necrosis. The boundary was not completely clear between the tumor and the surrounding liver tissue, and local infiltration can be observed (Fig. 6.49).

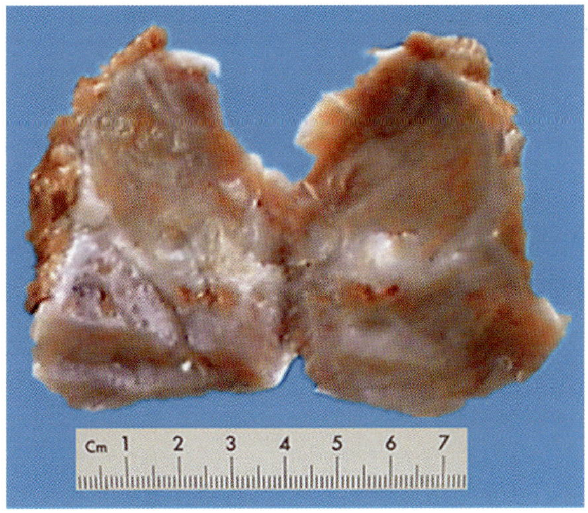

Fig. 6.49 Infantile hemangioendothelioma. The cross section was *yellow white* with unclear boundary

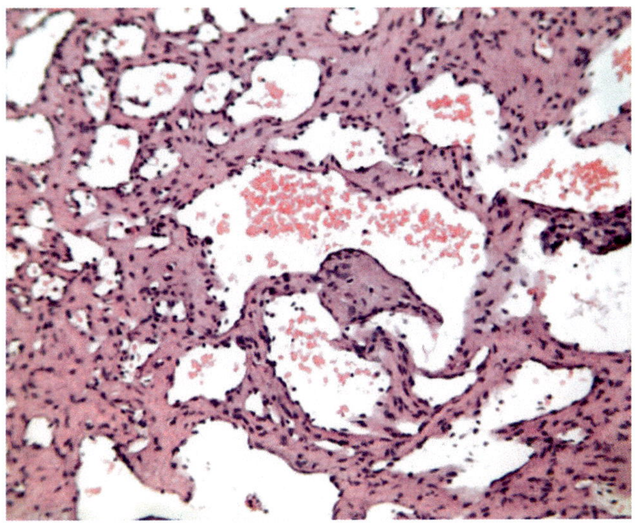

Fig. 6.50 Infantile hemangioendothelioma, type I. Capillary cavities lined with flat endothelial cells

6.3.3.4 Microscopic Features

IHE can be divided into two pathological types:

Type I accounts for about 80% of the tumors. The surrounding structure was composed of dense proliferation of irregular thin-walled capillary cavities, lined with monolayer of fat or flat endothelial cells (Figs. 6.50 and 6.51), which are consistent in morphology and contain small- or medium-sized nuclei and eosinophilic nucleoli, with little nuclear fission. The cavities contain red blood cells, and fewer tumorous interstitial components can be found with visible residue of hepatocytes, bile duct, extramedullary hematopoiesis regions, and no fibrous envelope. The infiltration border was interspersed in the liver between the plates (Fig. 6.52). Moreover, hemorrhage, necrosis, and calcification can also be found in the tumor. Type I IHE can undergo canceration.

Type II accounts for about 20% of the tumors. And five type I and one type II of IHE were found among the six cases diagnosed in our hospital. The latter mainly demonstrated obvious proliferation of vascular endothelial cells, occurrence of pleomorphic endothelial cells arranged in a single layer of nail dendritic shape or multiple layers, or even protrudes to the cavity in tufted morphology. No lumen or ambiguous tubular structure can be found, and some of them may form papillary structures. The cells are with significant nuclear atypia, hyperchromatic nuclei, and mitosis. The nature of this type IHE is angiosarcoma, with strong infiltrating ability into the surrounding liver tissue.

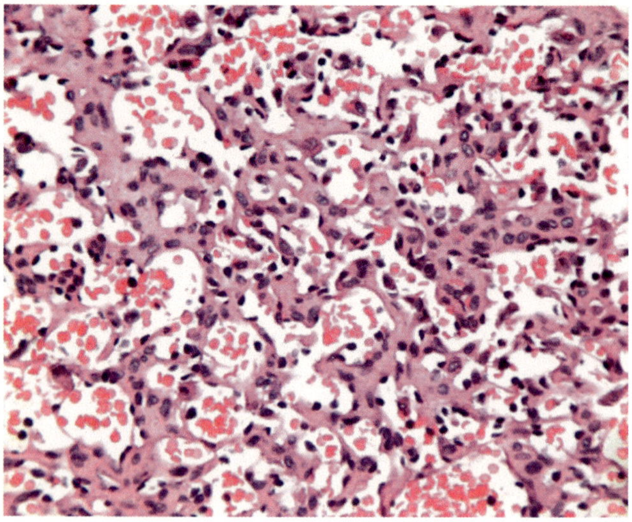

Fig. 6.51 Infantile hemangioendothelioma, type II. Irregular capillary cavities, lined with monolayer of cubic endothelial cells

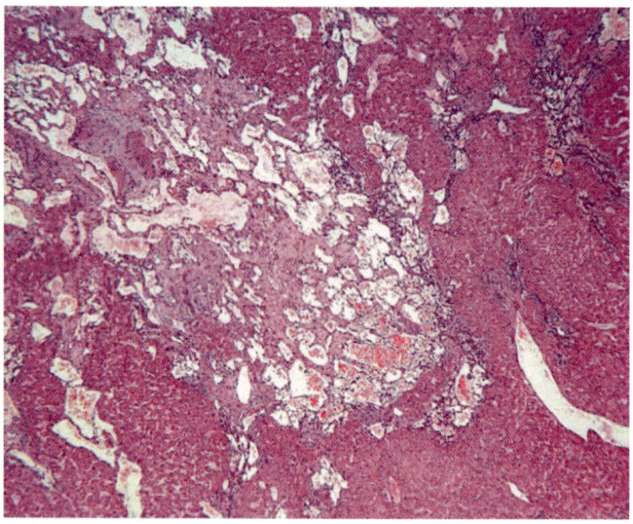

Fig. 6.52 Infantile hemangioendothelioma, type I. The tumor was composed of dense proliferation of irregular thin-walled capillary cavities, no fibrous envelope and infiltration border

6.3.3.5 Immunohistochemistry

Vascular endothelial cells were positive in vimentin, CD34 (Fig. 6.53), CD31, UEA-1, and F-VIII staining and negative in CK staining, and SMA staining displays positive smooth muscle cells within the vascular basement membrane.

6.3.3.6 Differential Diagnosis

According to the age of the patients and characteristics of tumor growth, correct diagnosis can be made, with cautions of differentiation from angiosarcoma, epithelioid hemangioendothelioma, and malignant hemangiopericytoma (Table 6.6). Other tumors that should be differentiated from are primary or secondary tumors of the liver, such as hepatoblastoma, neuroblastoma with liver metastasis, hepatic

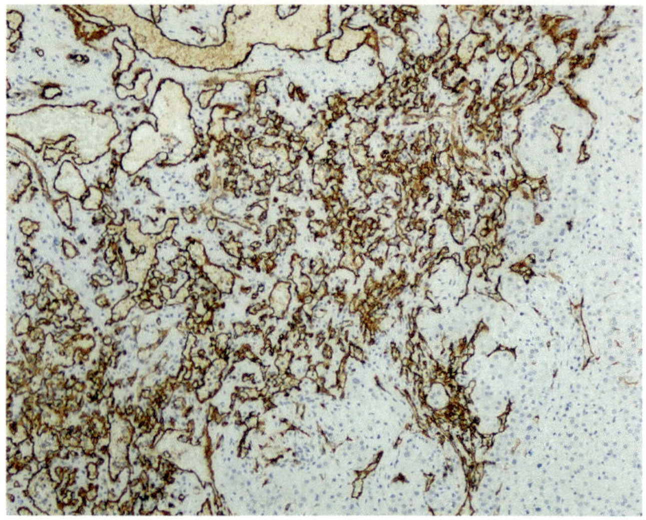

Fig. 6.53 CD34 staining showed active hyperplasia microvessels and "infiltrated border"

mesenchymal hamartoma, cavernous hemangioma of the liver, and teratoma. The final diagnosis depends on the pathological examination.

6.3.3.7 Treatment and Prognosis

Surgical resection is usually preferred. This group of IHE patients with surgical resection had a good prognosis. Sondhi et al. [88] treated one case of huge multiple liver IHE with TACE, finding volume reduction of the primary tumor, after which surgical resection was conducted and the residual tumor was treated via chemotherapy, but this was of poor efficacy and replaced by metronomic therapy of cyclophosphamide and tamoxifen, with complete disappearance of liver lesions.

6.3.4 Lymphangioma and Lymphangiomatosis

Wen-Ming Cong and Qian Zhao
Department of Pathology, Eastern Hepatobiliary Surgery Hospital, Second Military Medical University,
Shanghai, China

6.3.4.1 Pathogenesis and Mechanism

Lymphangioma is a benign tumor consisting of dilated lymphatic vessels containing lymph, once called cavernoma lymphaticum, lymphatic endothelioma, etc. and derived from congenital dysplasia of embryonic lymphatic system, or abnormal formation of lymphatic vessels, resulting in blocked lymphatic flow. Lymphangioma can be involved in the spleen, lung, bone, kidney, gastrointestinal tract, and other parts. Multiple lymphangiomas are known as lymphan-

Table 6.6 Clinical pathology of four primary vascular tumors in the liver

Pathodiagnosis	Gross features	Histological features
Epithelioid hemangioendothelioma	Multiple tumors, clear boundaries, gray-white or brownish yellow, dense and tough, can be accompanied by calcification, can be accompanied by large vascular lumen closure	With vascular differentiation of dendritic cells and (or) in the cytoplasm of vascular cavity epithelioid cells, interstitial myxoid change to dense fibrosis
Angiosarcoma	The boundary is not clear; the cross section is dark red, honeycomb, and with hemorrhage and necrosis, cystic fibrosis, or calcification	The pathological features were diverse, hemangioma, spindle cells, and epithelioid sarcoma morphology
Infantile hemangioendothelioma	Cross section of the tumor was brownish red, rich blood capillary lumen, necrosis and yellowish white, with the surrounding liver tissue dividing line not clear, local infiltration	Type I, lumen lining coated with single layer of endothelial cells, cell morphology consistent, non-nuclear fission; type II, tumor pleomorphic endothelial cells, is a multilayer arrangement, even tufted protrudes to the cavity, cell atypia, irregular nuclei, deep staining, the invasion is strong
Malignant hemangiopericytoma	The tumor boundary is clear, the appearance is light brown, the section has the cystic region, has the hemorrhage necrosis	Hemangiopericytoma consistency, staghorn or slit-like capillaries around the adventitia in the radial growth

giomatosis. Hepatic lymphangioma and lymphangiomatosis are very rare with more than ten cases reported so far, both in the domestic and foreign literature, and seven cases have been diagnosed in the Department of Pathology, Eastern Hepatobiliary Surgery Hospital, Second Military Medical University.

6.3.4.2 Clinical Features

The patients include infants and the elderly as reported in the literature, but children and youth are more common, with a male and female ratio of 1:2 [89]. Seven patients of liver lymphangioma were diagnosed in the Department of Pathology, Eastern Hepatobiliary Surgery Hospital, Second Military Medical University, with five males and two females aged 10–65 years old, and the average age was 31.9 years old. The symptoms and signs were associated with the number and location of the involving organs, generally abdominal distention, hepatosplenomegaly, pleural effusion, ascites, and organ dysfunction. Imaging showed a multilocular cystic mass, with clear or pale red liquid content which can be obtained via puncture. MRI examination is more effective, which can demonstrate lymphangioma as irregular lesions with ambiguous boundaries, and part of them is surrounded by vessels which is called vascular package, producing mass-occupying effects. Liquid-liquid plane can be observed in cystic lymphangioma lesions. Mild or no enhancement is shown in enhanced scan which can be differentiated from the images of other hepatic tumors [90].

6.3.4.3 Gross Features

Solitary lymphangioma is large in volume, often > 10 cm in diameter. The lesions in seven cases of liver lymphangioma, diagnosed in the Department of Pathology, Eastern Hepatobiliary Surgery Hospital, Second Military Medical University, were 3.2–24 cm in diameter with an average of 11.8 cm. The tumor section was gray-white (Fig. 6.54), honeycomb, or multilocular cavities with varying sizes, and local solid fibrous scars can be found with transparent slurry or chylous fluid in the lumen. Lymphangiomatosis contains multiple lesions distributed in the whole liver, and the numbers of lesions vary in cases.

6.3.4.4 Microscopic Features

The lesions are characterized by numerous lymphatic cavities of varying sizes with cystic dilatation in the liver parenchyma, containing eosinophilic lymphatic fluid (serous fluid and small lymphocytes) (Fig. 6.55), surrounded by small bubbles. Red cells can be found in the cavities when there is bleeding (Fig. 6.56), and the walls of them are lined with a single layer of flat endothelial cells (Fig. 6.57) with consistent nuclei and no atypia. Fibrous hyperplasia can be seen in part of tumor tissue forming a more solid region (Fig. 6.58), and the surrounding patches of fibrous connective tissue with residual hepatocyte isles can be observed (Fig. 6.59).

6.3.4.5 Immunohistochemistry

Endothelial cells express CD31, CD34, and F-VIII, and lymphatic marker of podoplanin staining is positive.

6.3.4.6 Differential Diagnosis

Note that it should be differentiated from mesenchymal hamartoma of the liver and hepatic hemangioma.

6.3.4.7 Treatment and Prognosis

Lymphangioma is a benign tumor, but it can cause significant damage to the surrounding liver tissue when active pro-

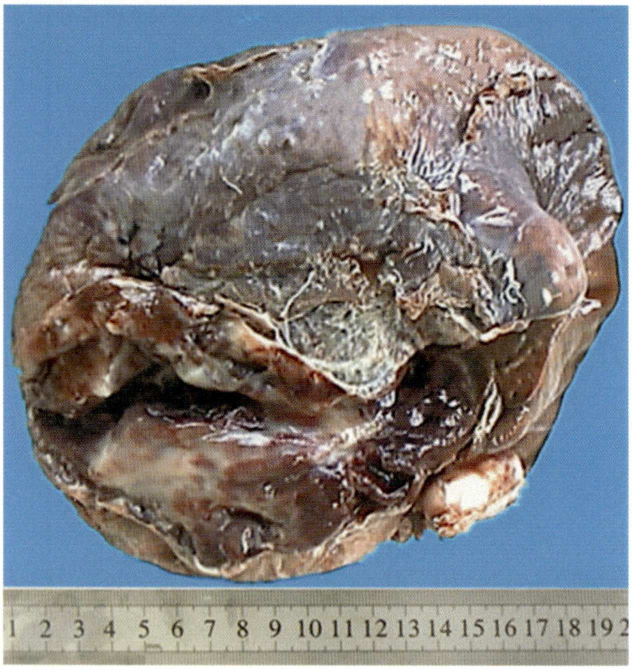

Fig. 6.54 Lymphangioma. Cystic and solid tumor, 14 cm in diameter

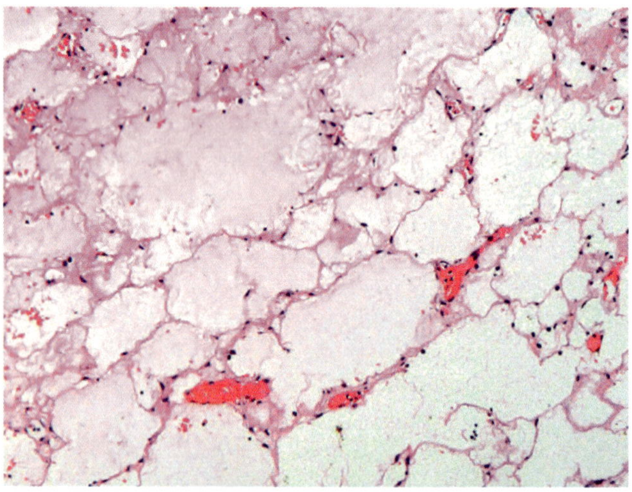

Fig. 6.55 Lymphangioma. Lymphatic cavities with cystic dilatation are lined with a single layer of flat endothelial cells, containing light dye lymphatic fluid

liferation occurs. Ra et al. [91] reported a case of lymphangiomatosis in the liver, which was treated by liver transplantation with recurrence 19 years later. Speculation has been made that it is related to the lymph tube endothelial progenitor cells which were released into the peripheral blood circulation. Thus, it is considered as a low-grade tumor or with metastatic potential. In general, surgical resection is the preferred treatment method, and liver transplantation is another choice. It is worth noting that the use of immunosuppressive agents may result in progression of extrahepatic lymphangiom if lymphangioma involves both the liver and extrahepatic organs [92, 93].

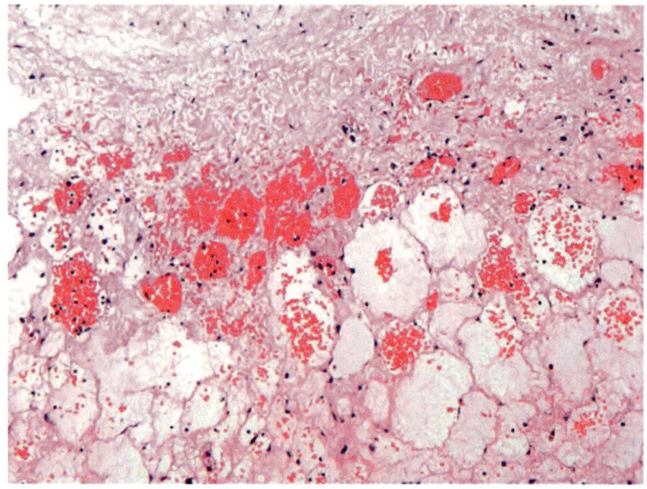

Fig. 6.56 Lymphangioma. Interstitial hemorrhage, red cells can be found in the cavities

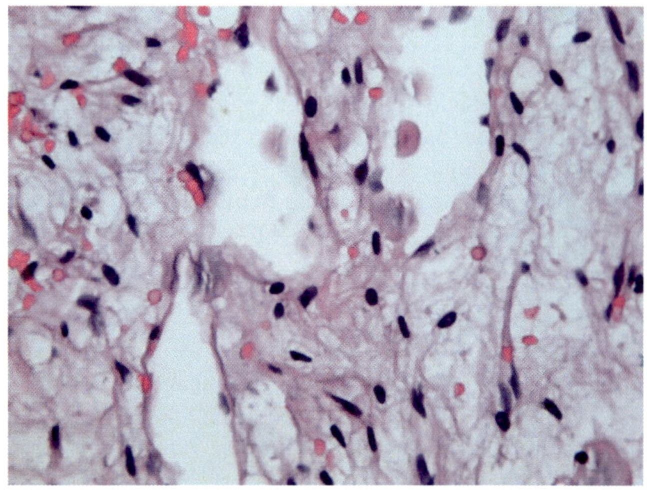

Fig. 6.57 Lymphangioma. Lymphatic cavities lined with a single layer of flat cells

6.4 Muscular, Fibrous, and Adipose Tumors

6.4.1 Leiomyoma

Wen-Ming Cong and Qian Zhao
Department of Pathology, Eastern Hepatobiliary Surgery Hospital, Second Military Medical University, Shanghai, China

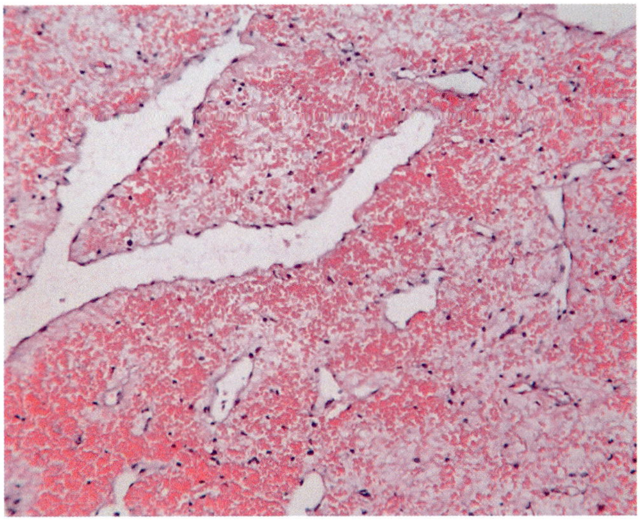

Fig. 6.58 Lymphangioma. Interstitial fibrous hyperplasia with hemorrhage

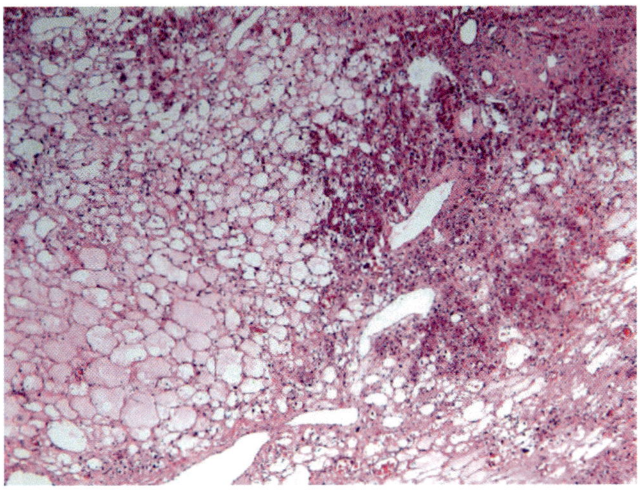

Fig. 6.59 Lymphangioma. The surrounding patches of residual hepatocytes

6.4.1.1 Pathogenesis and Mechanism

Leiomyoma is more accepted to originate from visceral or vascular muscular layer, commonly found in the urinary tract and digestive tract. Demel reported the first case of primary liver leiomyoma in 1926, and a total of about 30 cases have been reported in English literature so far. One case has been diagnosed in the Department of Pathology, Eastern Hepatobiliary Surgery Hospital, of Second Military Medical University. Possible origination of liver leiomyoma is in the blood vessels or biliary tree of the liver, and primary hepatic leiomyoma can be found in posttransplantation patients using immunosuppressant and patients with AIDS. Researches have also shown that EBV infection might be related to the occurrence of the disease.

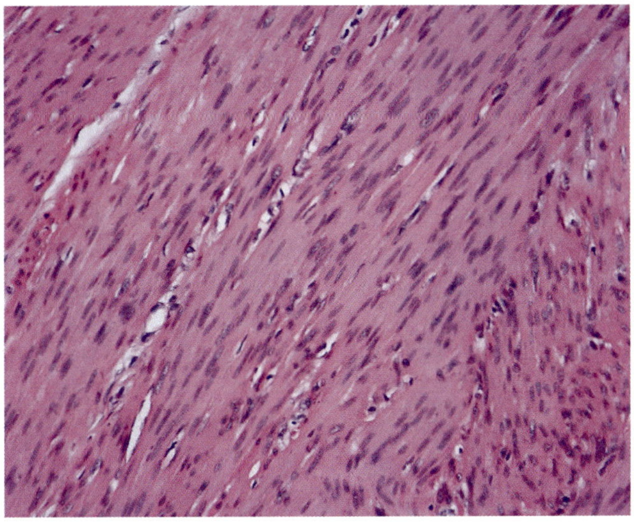

Fig. 6.60 Leiomyoma. The tumor is composed of spindle-shaped smooth muscle cells and shown in interwoven bundle arrangement

6.4.1.2 Clinical Features

Primary hepatic leiomyoma is more commonly seen in adult females, and the male to female ratio is about 1:1.8, with an average age of 41 (1.5–71) years old. No early discomfort is found with no obvious clinical symptoms, and it is often discovered in physical examination. When the tumor grows to a size sufficient to cause oppression or pull on the adjacent organs, symptoms appear such as abdominal fullness, discomfort, or pain. Imaging findings include: ① large tumors with clear boundaries and visible patchy necrosis, ② significant enhancement in arterial phase and more significant enhancement in portal vein phase on CT enhanced scan, ③ multiple abnormal blood vessels which are thickened and circuitous around the tumor, and ④ MR T_2WI showed solid and low signals indicating tumors which is the feature for leiomyoma [94].

6.4.1.3 Gross Features

The average diameter of the tumors was 6.8 (2–12) cm, which are solid masses with cystic degeneration in some cases. The section shows gray-white bundles and the capsule is complete.

6.4.1.4 Microscopic Features

The tumor is composed of spindle-shaped smooth muscle cells with pale staining cytoplasm, rod-shaped nucleus, normal nucleocytoplasmic ratio, no nuclear atypia, and no or occasional nuclear division. The tumor tissue was shown in interwoven bundles or plexiform arrangement (Fig. 6.60). Interstitial tissue may contain mucous secretion, forming myxoid leiomyoma, with a complete capsule and no invasion into the surrounding liver tissue.

6.4.1.5 Immunohistochemistry

Vimentin, SMA, and desmin expressions are positive, and CD-117, CD34, DOG-1, and other GIST markers are negative, which should also be combined with clinical findings and the detection of EBV infection.

6.4.1.6 Differential Diagnosis

It should be differentiated from gastrointestinal stromal tumors, neurofibroma, leiomyosarcoma, and other hepatic tumors.

6.4.1.7 Treatment and Prognosis

There is no report on the recurrence of leiomyoma after surgical resection.

6.4.2 Solitary Fibrous Tumor

Wen-Ming Cong and Long-Hai Feng
Department of Pathology, Eastern Hepatobiliary Surgery Hospital, Second Military Medical University, Shanghai, China

6.4.2.1 Pathogenesis and Mechanism

Solitary fibrous tumor (SFT) is a kind of dendritic cell neoplasm expressing CD34, first reported by Klemperer and Rabin, and is more commonly found in the pleura, also known as localized fibrous mesothelioma previously. The occurrence sites for extrapleural SFT include the upper respiratory tract, nasal cavity, mediastinum, lung, orbit, pelvic peritoneum, mesenterium, peridiydmis, liver, breast, spinal cord, kidney, and adrenal gland. Primary hepatic SFT is rare, and more than 40 cases have been reported by 2013. The origin of the tumor is inconclusive and is more accepted that it originates from the liver submesothelial tissue. For a long period, whether the lesions are benign or malignant remains controversial. Liu et al. [95] regarded it as a borderline tumor, while Fisher [96] classified it into intermediate fibroblastic and myofibroblastic tumors in Atlas of Soft Tissue Tumor Pathology published in 2013, which is not defined as benign fibrous tumor. And in the 2010 WHO's Histological Classification Guideline of Digestive System Tumors, it is grouped into benign hepatic tumors derived from mesenchymal tissue [97].

6.4.2.2 Clinical Features

Two cases of hepatic SFT were diagnosed in the Department of Pathology, Eastern Hepatobiliary Surgery Hospital, Second Military Medical University, from January 2005 to June 2014, including a 49-year-old male and 51-year-old female, both of them had no history of hepatitis. Combined with the reports of 61 cases of primary hepatic SFT in the literature, the patients of the disease are often adults aged from 16 to 85 years old with an average of 55.6 years old, and most of them are females with a male to female ratio of 1:1.47. Nonspecific clinical manifestations mainly involving the digestive system and accounting for 77% include epigastric fullness, nausea and vomiting, abdominal pain, diarrhea, back pain, abdominal distention, painless abdominal mass, hepatomegaly, lower limb edema, and weight loss (or increase). No abnormality was found in laboratory examinations, with normal liver function. Mild to moderate elevation of ALP and (or) γ-GT is found in a few cases, and tumor markers including AFP, CA19–9, and CEA are generally normal. Ultrasound examination shows heterogeneous masses, and CT images demonstrate clearly bounded hypodense lesions, with necrosis and calcification in some cases, and cyclic centripetal progressive enhancement is shown in enhanced CT. MRI shows low signals on T_1WI and high signals or mixed signals on T_2WI, and flaky, arc, or ring enhancement is shown in gadolinium contrast enhancement MRI. PET-CT displays elevated SUV values in the tumor region.

6.4.2.3 Gross Features

The tumors are often solitary, while multiple lesions are rare, and it is located mainly in the left lobe of the liver, or ligamentum teres hepatis as reported, with a mean diameter of 16.6 (0.5–32) cm. In two cases of SFT in the liver, diagnosed in the Department of Pathology, Eastern Hepatobiliary Surgery Hospital, Second Military Medical University, the diameters were 8.7 and 8.1 cm, and the lesions are located in the left and the right lobe, respectively. The tumor body in one case was completely dissociated from the liver parenchyma, with only two thin pedicles connected to the hepatic

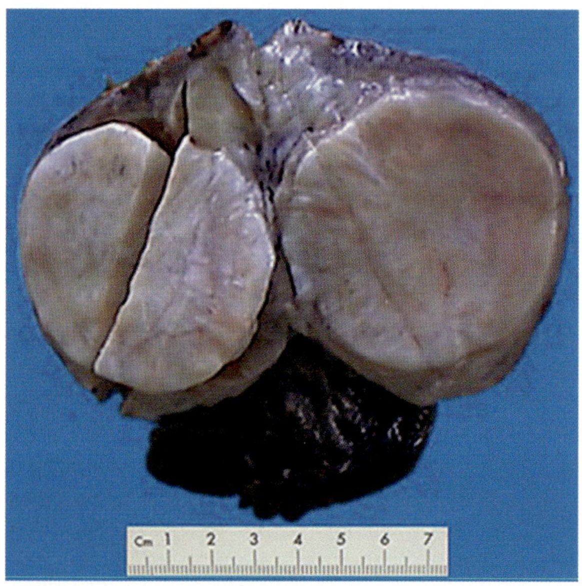

Fig. 6.61 Solitary fibrous tumor. The section is *gray* or *grayish yellow*, showing interwoven fiber bundles

capsule. The surface of the tumors was smooth, and the tumor capsule is complete, and continuity with liver capsule was observed with good tenacity. The section is gray or grayish yellow, showing interwoven fiber bundles (Fig. 6.61), mucoid degeneration, and varying numbers and sizes of cystic cavities.

6.4.2.4 Microscopic Features

Most of the hepatic SFT is benign, composed of spindle fibroblasts with a small amount of eosinophilic cytoplasm, and transparent eosinophilic bodies can be visible in part of the cytoplasm. The nuclei were spindle-like with thin ends, obsolete nucleolus, and no nuclear atypia. The tumor cells were arranged in short seat patterns or disordered distribution in abundant collagen fibrous interstitial tissue. Some tumor cells are found around the expanded vessels forming a hemangiopericytoma-like structure. Cells with nuclear division (< 3/10HPF) and increased nuclear atypia indicate a malignant potential. The WHO classification of soft tissue tumors suggested the characteristics of SFT, including large lesions (≥5 cm or 10 cm), no tumor pedicle, infiltrative borders, abundant cells, moderate or high degree of nuclear atypia, mitotic activity (> 4/10HPF), hemorrhage, and necrosis (Fig. 6.62).

6.4.2.5 Immunohistochemistry

Most of the tumor cells were intensively positive for CD34, Bcl-2 (Figs. 6.63 and 6.64), and vimentin; negative for CK, S-100, HMB45, and EMA and SMA; and partially positive for CD99 and desmin, while malignant tumor cells may lose expression of CD34.

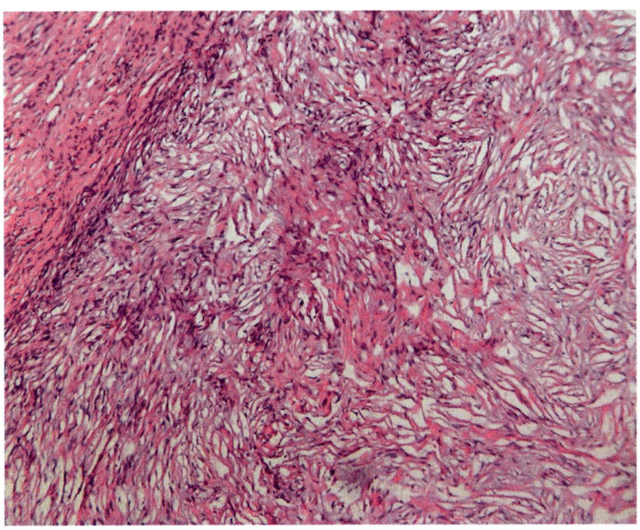

Fig. 6.62 Solitary fibrous tumor. Spindle cells with small *rod-shaped* and no atypia nuclei and no mitosis

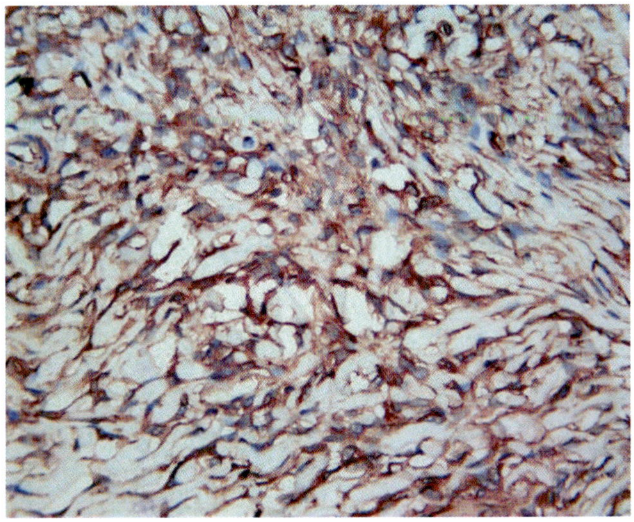

Fig. 6.63 Solitary fibrous tumor. CD34, positive

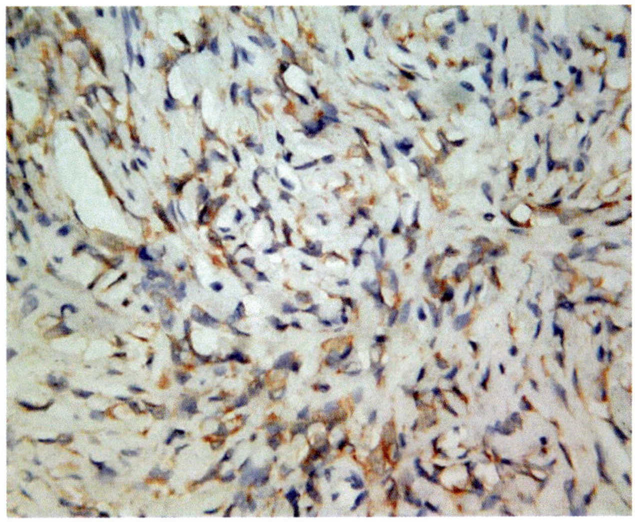

Fig. 6.64 Solitary fibrous tumor. BCL-2, positive

6.4.2.6 Specific Staining

Masson trichrome staining shows dense collagen bundles, and reticular fiber staining shows reticular fibrous septa surrounding tumor cell bundles.

6.4.2.7 Differential Diagnosis

1. Hepatic leiomyoma expresses SMA and desmin, but no CD34.
2. Malignant mesothelioma contains cells with rich polymorphism, active nuclear division, and CD34 negative.
3. Fibrosarcoma contains cells in woven-like arrangement, with obvious nuclear atypia, active mitosis, and invasive growth.
4. Hepatic inflammatory pseudotumor contains a large number of mixed inflammatory cells and fibrous tissue.

5. Gastrointestinal stromal tumors were positive for CD117 staining.
6. Malignant SFT has been reported in five cases of primary malignant liver SFT with postoperative recurrence and extrahepatic multiple organ metastasis since 2000, seriously worsening the prognosis [98–102].
7. Metastatic SFT in the liver is often derived from extrahepatic organs such as the mesenterium, kidney, and spinal cord.
8. Other tumors which should be differentiated from include hemangioperithelioma, synovial sarcoma, and peripheral nerve sheath tumors.

6.4.2.8 Treatment and Prognosis

The prognosis of benign hepatic SFT treated with resection is good.

6.4.3 Angiomyolipoma

Yuan Ji
Zhong-shan Hospital, Fudan University,
Shanghai, China

6.4.3.1 Pathogenesis and Mechanism

Angiomyolipoma (AML) was first reported by Ishak with a case of hepatic AML in 1976, and Cong Wen Ming and colleagues began to report the constitution of thick-walled blood vessels, smooth muscle, and fat in different proportions in AML in 1992 [103]. Once known as hamartoma, it is now known as a true neoplasm, and it derives from perivascular epithelioid cells (PEC), belonging to the family of perivascular epithelioid cell tumors (PEComas). These cells are usually epithelioid, with transparent or eosinophilic red cytoplasm, PAS staining positive, not resistant to diastase digestion, and small nucleoli are often visible, with differentiation characteristics of both melanoma cells and muscular cells. The etiology of hepatic AML is not clear, and there are reports on AML with tuberous sclerosis complex (TSC), accompanied by hamartoma in the kidney or other organs or skin nodules [104, 105].

6.4.3.2 Clinical Features

A total of 244 cases of surgically excised hepatic AML were diagnosed in the Department of Pathology, Eastern Hepatobiliary Surgery Hospital, Second Military Medical University, from January 2001 to November 2012, with 68 males (27.87%) and 176 females (72.13%), with an average age of 44.3 (23–79) years old, and the male to female ratio was 1:2.6 (Fig. 6.65). The reported male to female ratio of hepatic AML patients was about 1:2–5, and the average age was 41.7 (10–86) years old in the literature, and the age of onset was mainly concentrated in the range of 35–55 years old. Hepatic AML cases are mostly solitary, 60% located in the right lobe, 30% located in the left lobe, 20% in both the left and right leaves, and 8% in the caudate lobe.

Most of the patients with hepatic AML are asymptomatic, usually discovered in physical examination. A few patients with larger tumors have upper abdominal discomfort or pain, and other rare manifestations include abdominal mass, hematemesis and melena, fever, fatigue, lack of appetite, and weight loss. If accompanied by renal AML, the patients may manifest corresponding symptoms such as lumbago, and those with nodular sclerosis may have mental retardation and developmental delay [106]. The difference between renal and hepatic AML includes that about half of renal AML are associated with tuberous sclerosis and about 1.15% of the hepatic AML cases are associated with tuberous sclerosis [107]. Wang Jue-ru et al. [108] reviewed the clinical data of 523 cases of hepatic AML and found that most patients had no history of hepatitis suggesting irrelevance with hepatitis, and female patients are without long-term oral contraceptives indicating hepatic AML is not associated with a contraceptive history. No obvious abnormalities are found in biochemical or liver function tests.

Imaging results of AML vary according to different proportions of the three components, blood vessels, vascular smooth muscle, and fat. Ultrasound examination shows high or mixed echoes, and when the mass reflects a strong echo, indicating fat or fatlike component, while a weak echo is reflected, strong patchy or strip-shaped echoes can be detected inside the lesion which is similar to the echo of fat [109, 110]. Signs of blood vessels in fat shown on CT scan are of diagnostic value [111], and enhanced scan shows enhancement in patterns such as "fast in and fast out," "fast in and slow out," or delayed enhancement. The enhancement amplitude of the tumor is often weaker than that of the surrounding normal liver parenchyma in portal venous/delay phase, and some large tumors oppressing the surrounding normal liver parenchyma to form a pseudocapsule show delayed enhancement [112, 113]. MRI images of hepatic AML show high or low signals on T_1-weighted image and heterogeneous high signals on T_2-weighted image. The definition of fat signals on MRI imaging of hepatic AML with much fat is an evidence to differentiate from the majority of liver cancers [114].

6.4.3.3 Gross Features

The tumors often have no capsule, and the diameter is 0.8–36 cm with an average of > 5 cm. The gross appearance of the tumors often varies according to different proportions of the components. Tumors with a majority of muscular cells are often gray-white or gray-brown (Fig. 6.66), accompanied by varying amounts of hemorrhage. Tumors with major content of fat are similar to the appearance of lipoma which is gray in color. And those composed mainly of blood vessels

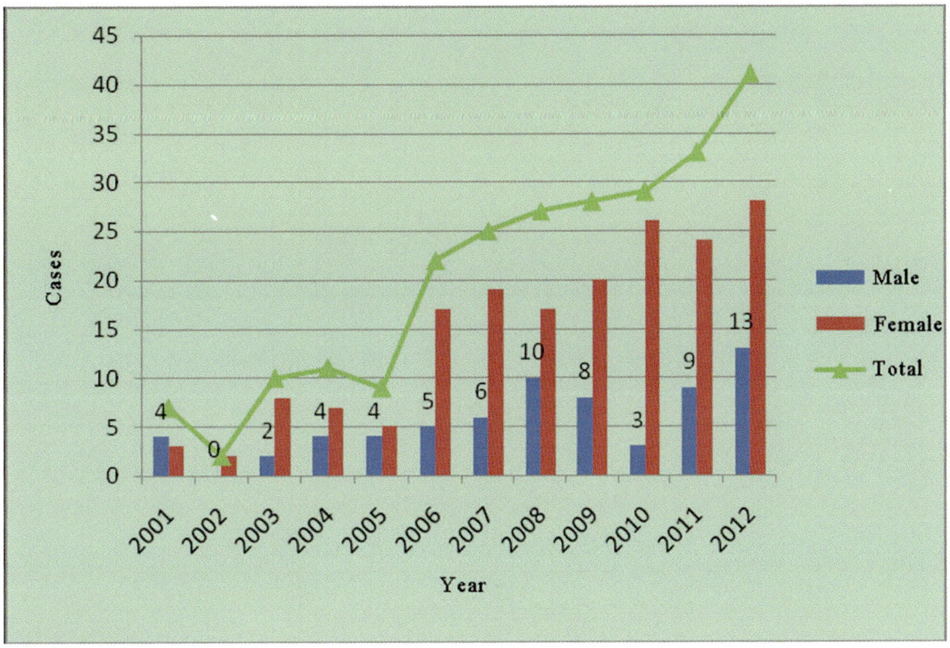

Fig. 6.65 Angiomyolipoma. Surgically treated hepatic AML patients were diagnosed in the Department of Pathology, Eastern Hepatobiliary Surgery Hospital

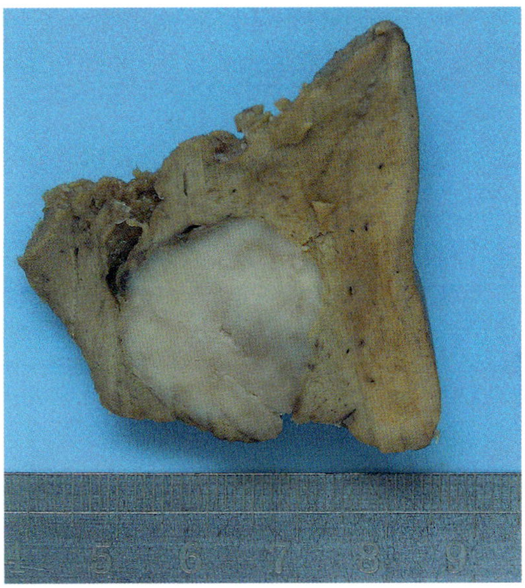

Fig. 6.66 Angiomyolipoma, muscle cell-based type

are grayish red or grayish brown on the cross section, soft in texture. The tumors have clear boundaries with the surrounding liver tissue, and the latter often shows no sclerosis [115].

6.4.3.4 Microscopic Features

Hepatic angiomyolipoma (HAML) contains curved thick-walled blood vessels, muscle cells, and fat cells in different proportions, and much difference is found in different tumors or different regions of the same tumor. According to the varying proportions of the composition, HAML is divided into four types [116–118]:

1. Classical type. Solid patches of myoid cells mixed with slices of fat cells, interspersed with irregular thick-walled blood vessels (Fig. 6.67).
2. Muscle cell type. Mainly composed of muscle cells. And according to various morphological features of muscle cells, this type of HAML can be divided into five subtypes as some scholar suggested: epithelioid cells (Fig. 6.68), intermediate cell type, spindle cell type, monomorphic cell type/eosinophilic cell type, and polymorphic cell type [119] (Fig. 6.69). And epithelioid angiomyolipoma accounts for most of hepatic AML.
3. Fat cell type. The tumor is mainly composed of mature fat cells, which interlace with intermediate muscle cells to form a network (Fig. 6.70).
4. Angiomatous type. The vascular components consist of varying amounts of bending thick-walled blood vessels, often without elastic layer, and the muscle cells are locally distributed. Epithelioid cells and spindle myoid cells often surround the blood vessels to form peripheral vascular sheaths, especially evident in the periphery region of the tumor, and many thin-walled veins or blood vessels diffuse in the whole parenchyma, similar to purpura [120].

The tumors often have no capsule with clear boundaries with the surrounding liver tissue, and "invasive boundary" can also be found (Fig. 6.71), which is not a sign of malignant transformation.

6.4.3.5 Immunohistochemistry

Epithelioid cells of hepatic AML have the ability to synthesize melanin, so they express HMB45 (Fig. 6.72) and A103, but did not express CD34, VIII factor, EMA, keratin, myo-

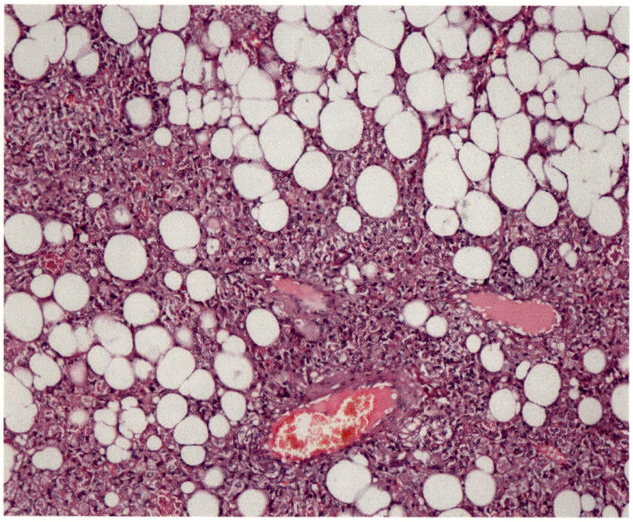

Fig. 6.67 Angiomyolipoma, classical type

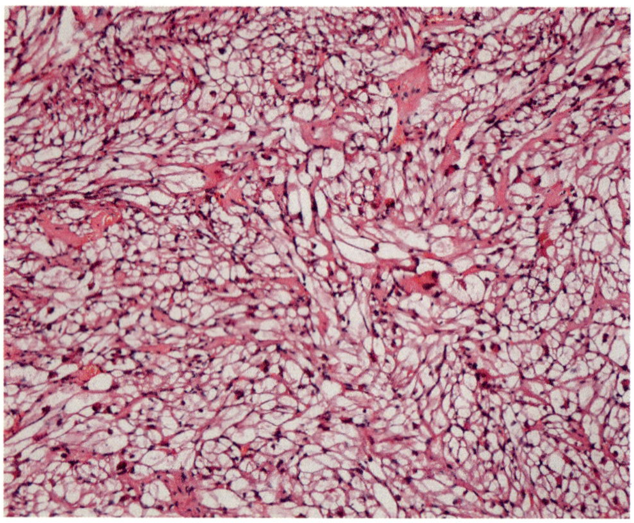

Fig. 6.68 Angiomyolipoma, epithelioid cell type. No vessels and adipocytes

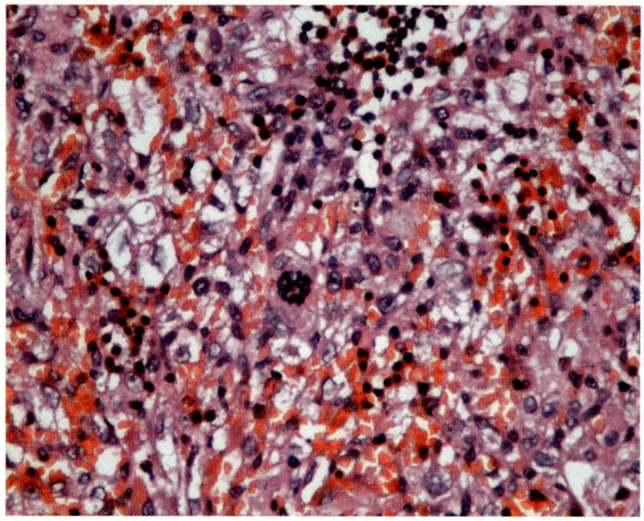

Fig. 6.69 Angiomyolipoma, polymorphic cell type

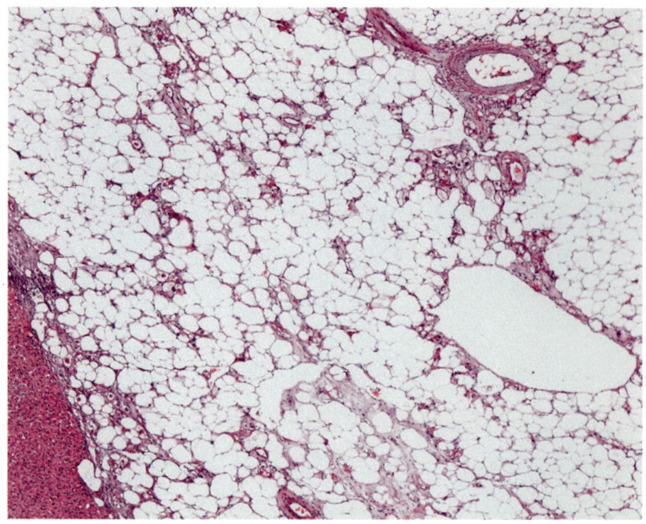

Fig. 6.70 Angiomyolipoma, fat cell type

globin, etc. [122]. Stronger positive HMB45 and A103 are found in the epithelioid and pleomorphic muscle cell type than those in spindle cell type, which often express VI, SMA (Fig. 6.73), and desmin. Muscle cells in intermediate cell type also express vimentin, SMA, and desmin, the positive degrees of which are between those of epithelioid and spindle cell type. Recent reports suggested that cathepsin K demonstrated a higher positive rate in the perivascular epithelioid cell tumors (PEComas), as well as higher specificity [121].

6.4.3.6 Differential Diagnosis

When the tumor is mainly composed of fat, especially in cases with visible lipoblasts, it can be easily misdiagnosed as well-differentiated liposarcoma, and positive HMB45 and SMA detected by immunohistochemistry are very helpful in diagnosis. FISH detection of MDM2 gene status is a choice when necessary. In AML with major spindle-shaped cells, which is easy to confuse with tumors derived from smooth muscle or nongastrointestinal ST, the finding of thick-walled blood vessels and fat is a good indication for AML. AML with epithelioid cells arranged in trabecular structure containing eosinophilic or transparent cytoplasm and pleomorphic cells with visible nucleoli can be easily misdiagnosed as hepatocellular carcinoma. And HMB45 and SMA are beneficial during differential diagnosis. It should also be differentiated from malignant melanoma, metastatic carcinoma, and angiosarcoma of renal cell tumor identification.

6.4.3.7 Treatment and Prognosis

The preoperative diagnosis accuracy of hepatic AML is low with a high misdiagnosis rate, so most scholars advocate sur-

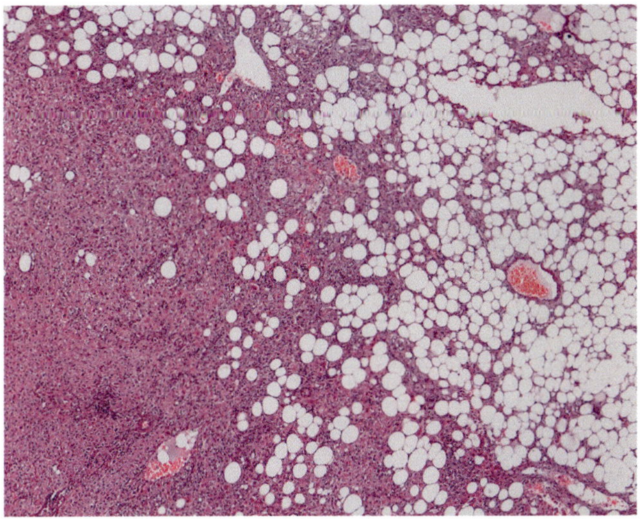

Fig. 6.71 Angiomyolipoma "invasive boundary"

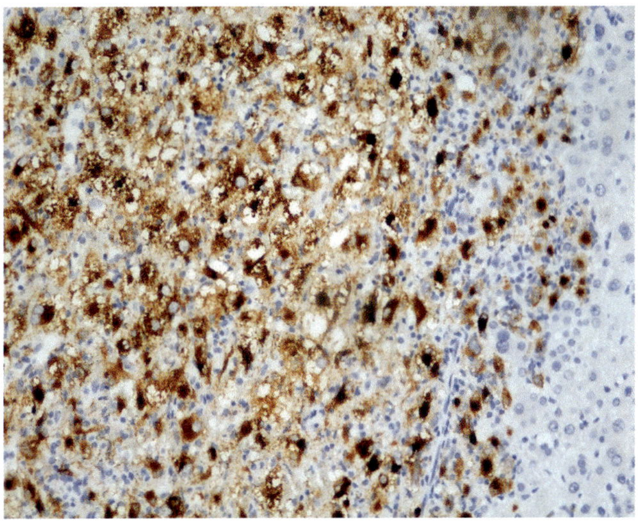

Fig. 6.72 Angiomyolipoma. HMB45 positive

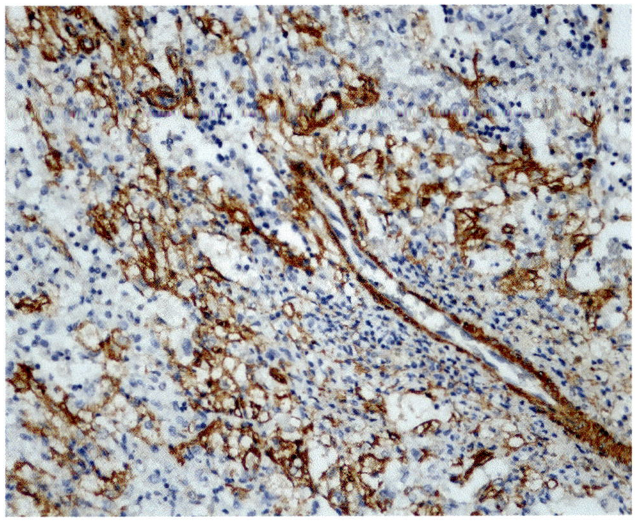

Fig. 6.73 Angiomyolipoma. SMA positive

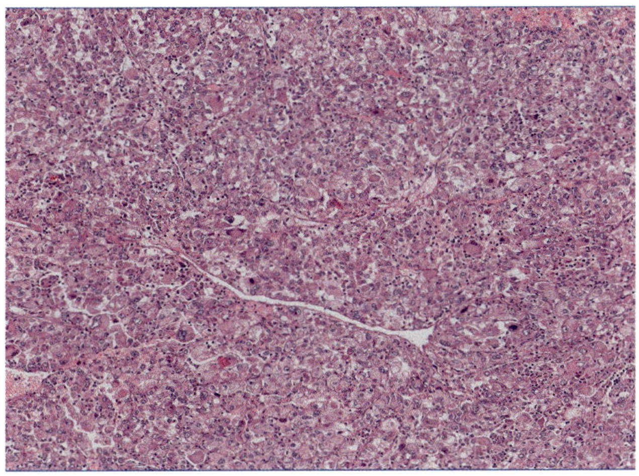

Fig. 6.74 Angiomyolipoma. Mitosis is visible

gical treatment for the patients as soon as possible. Small tumors (e.g., < 5 cm) can be observed during follow-up; however, large tumors (> 5 cm) or small tumors in rapid growth should be treated with surgical resection as soon as possible. It has been reported in the literature that with the passage of time, the tumor size increases to form a giant hepatic tumor, easily affecting liver function, and is at risk of rupture or canceration [122]. You J et al. [106] report one case of multiple hepatic AML, renal AML associated with tuberous sclerosis treated by superselective arterial embolization with a good curative effect. And foreign reports suggested that hepatic AML contains estrogen and progesterone receptors; thus, tamoxifen can be adopted for the treatment and has obtained certain curative effects [123]. Gennatas [124] reported a case of PEComas treated with the mTOR inhibitor everolimus with good therapeutic effects. All these case reports provide valuable experience for the treatment of hepatic AML.

Hepatic AML has long been considered as a benign tumor, but with the development of researches and the accumulation of cases including reports on malignant hepatic AML, hepatic AML is a potentially malignant tumor [125, 126]. However, so far, it lacks reliable morphological criteria to determine whether it is benign or malignant. Malignant hepatic AML described in the literature are often separate cases. To date, the common features of malignant hepatic AML suggested by Folpe [127] include: tumor diameter > 10 cm, tumor necrosis, cellular atypia, visible epithelioid cells, and increased mitosis (Fig. 6.74). Immunohistochemistry shows elevated Ki-67 proliferation index, positive p53, and negative CD117. However, simple invasive growth, vascular deformity, and visible nucleoli are shared by both benign and malignant AML, which are no hints of biological behaviors [128].

In summary, hepatic AML is a type of tumor with malignant potential originating from perivascular epithelioid cells, often contributing no clinical manifestations or specific imaging features. The preoperative diagnostic accurate is relatively low; therefore, early surgical treatment should be recommended once the tumor is discovered. During postoperative pathological diagnosis, careful observation and identification of the morphology of muscle cells should be made, as well as the varying kinds of immunophenotype of different muscle cell types. After surgery, long-term follow-up to observe recurrence or metastasis for the patients is recommended.

6.4.4 Lipoma

Wen-Ming Cong and Qian Zhao
Department of Pathology, Eastern Hepatobiliary Surgery Hospital, Second Military Medical University, Shanghai, China

6.4.4.1 Pathogenesis and Mechanism

Ramchand reported the first case of hepatic lipoma in 1970, and over 20 cases have been reported in the literature up to now. Thirteen cases of surgically excised hepatic lipoma were diagnosed in the Department of Pathology, Eastern Hepatobiliary Surgery Hospital, of Second Military Medical University from 1982 to 2013. Hepatic lipoma is composed of mature adipose cells, suggesting its potential origin of pluripotent stem cells with lipid-storing ability surrounding the hepatic sinusoids. Martin-Benitez et al. [129] suggested the relationship of hepatic lipoma and fatty liver, and insulin resistance may be the possible mechanism of the disease.

6.4.4.2 Clinical Features

The 13 cases of hepatic lipoma excised surgically in our hospital concerned three males and ten females, and the average age was 41.4 (29–58) years old. The patients almost manifested no obvious symptoms, and the lesions were often discovered occasionally during physical examination.

6.4.4.3 Gross Features

The tumor was 6.8 (2–12) cm in diameter, mostly pale yellow or gray-white in a few cases, soft in texture, part of which are encapsulated and lobulated, with a greasy section and a clear boundary (Fig. 6.75).

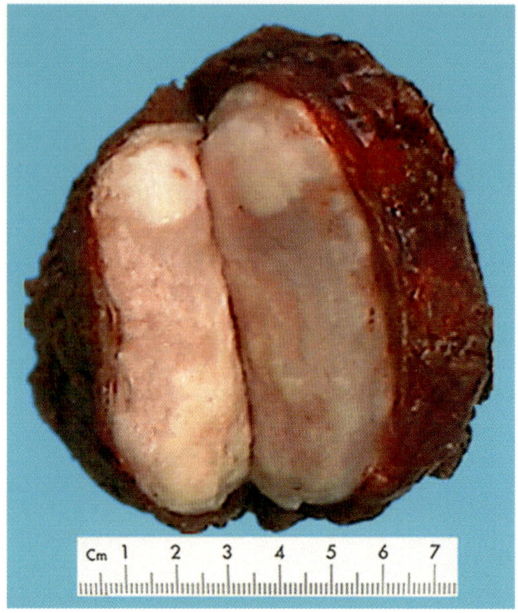

Fig. 6.75 Lipoma. The tumor was *yellow* and *white*, with a greasy section and a clear boundary

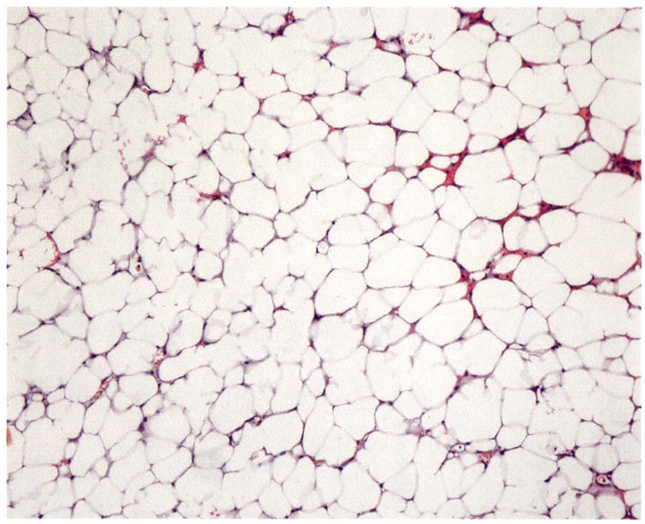

Fig. 6.76 Lipoma. The tumor was composed of mono-differentiation mature fat cells

6.4.4.4 Microscopic Features

The tumor was composed of mono-differentiation mature fat cells, which are consistent in size, and the karyoplasmic ratio is normal, with no mitotic figures (Fig. 6.76).

6.4.4.5 Differential Diagnosis

It should sometimes be differentiated from focal hepatic steatosis, well-differentiated liposarcoma, and lipid-rich type of hepatic angiomyolipoma.

6.4.4.6 Treatment and Prognosis

Focal resection is the main treatment for hepatic lipoma. And for small lipomas with definite diagnosis, temporary observation can be adopted, and surgical resection can be applied when the tumors increase significantly. Aggressive surgical resection if the optimal therapeutic scheme for those cases is difficult to identify from malignant tumors, such as liposarcoma.

6.4.5 Myelolipoma

Wen-Ming Cong and Yu-Yao Zhu
Department of Pathology, Eastern Hepatobiliary Surgery Hospital, Second Military Medical University,
Shanghai, China

6.4.5.1 Pathogenesis and Mechanism

Myelolipoma is a benign lipoma mixed with extramedullary hematopoietic tissue, often found in the adrenal cortex. The cause is unknown; however, there are several viewpoints concerning the pathogenesis of myelolipoma, including development and differentiation of residual embryonic mesenchymal cells, transposition of adrenal myelolipoma, plantation and metaplasia of bone marrow emboli, etc. In present, gene analysis has been conducted on only one patient, finding translocation of chromosomes (3; 21) (q25; p11), suggesting that the tumor belongs to neoplastic lesions [130]。 . Allison et al. [131] suggested the relation between myelolipoma and obesity, gene mutation, and hormone use. Reports on hepatic myelolipoma have been published since the 1970s, and over ten cases both abroad and at home were found in the literature. One case of hepatic myelolipoma was diagnosed in the Department of Pathology, Eastern Hepatobiliary Surgery Hospital, Second Military Medical University, and no association of the hepatic myelolipoma with metabolic and endocrine diseases has been found. However, there are reports of myelolipoma in surgically excised hepatocellular carcinoma.

6.4.5.2 Clinical and Pathological Features

Hepatic myelolipoma is more common in people older than 40 years old in both genders, mostly with no clinical symptoms and found during physical examination, surgery, or autopsy, while some patients manifest recurrent abdominal distension, decreased appetite, hepatomegly, or even rupture and hemorrhage in cases with larger tumors. Individual patients may have a history of up to 10 years' hepatic masses which gradually increased in size. CT examination demonstrates hypodensity which indicates adipose tissue [132]. The tumor is commonly seen in the right lobe of the liver with a diameter of 1–16 cm, light yellow or brown, often with no capsule, exhibiting gray or grayish red and circular nodules on the section with or without hemorrhage and necrosis. The boundary is clear and the tumor is generally solitary lesions, and multiple hepatic myelolipomas have also been reported [133]. The case diagnosed in the Department of Pathology, Eastern Hepatobiliary Surgery Hospital, Second Military Medical University, concerned a 60-year-old male with the tumor located in the right lobe of the liver, and the diameter was 2.3 cm. Microscopic observation showed that the tumor was mainly composed of mature fat cells and hematopoietic cells which were similar to the bone marrow. The latter included granulocyte, erythroid, and megakaryocytic components at different mature stages; however, they are different from the cells in the bone marrow because of the lack of sinusoid in the bone marrow with no capsule in the surrounding area, and tumor tissue and liver tissue are staggered into each other to form an "infiltration border" (Figs. 6.77 and 6.78). Attention should be paid to the differential diagnosis from angiomyolipoma, lipoma, liposarcoma, etc.

6.4.5.3 Treatment and Prognosis

Myelolipomas are benign tumors, and surgical resection is recommended with good effects, especially when symptoms or complications appear. Generally, no other auxiliary treatments are necessary, and there is no report of malignant transformation of myelolipoma.

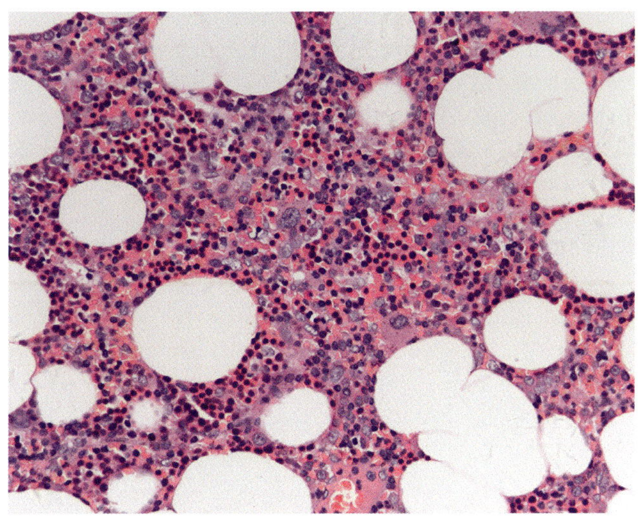

Fig. 6.77 Myelolipoma. Microscopic observation showed that the tumor was mainly composed of mature fat cells and hematopoietic cells

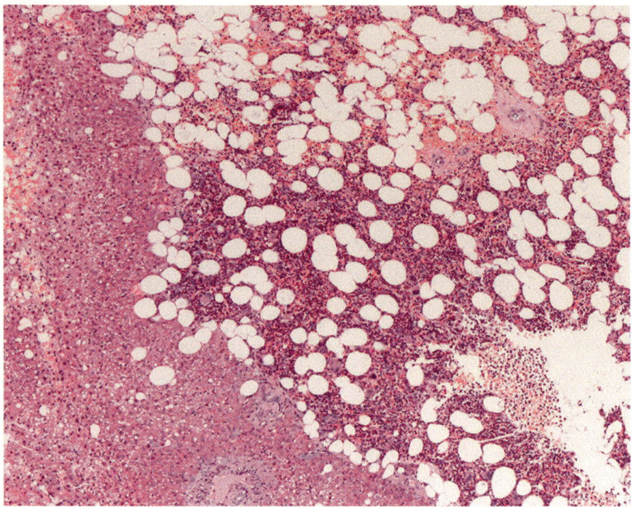

Fig. 6.78 Myelolipoma. With no capsule in the surrounding area, and tumor tissue forming an "infiltration border"

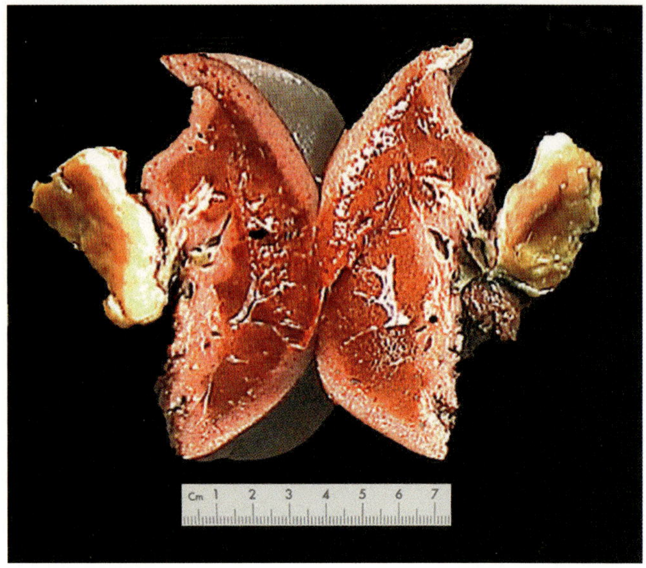

Fig. 6.79 Neurilemmoma. With a complete capsule and the section is *pale yellow*, crisp in nature

6.5 Neurological and Endocrinic Tumors

Wen-Ming Cong, Yu-Yao Zhu, and Yu-Yao Zhu
Department of Pathology, Eastern Hepatobiliary Surgery Hospital, Second Military Medical University, Shanghai, China

6.5.1 Neurilemmoma/Schwannoma

6.5.1.1 Pathogenesis and Mechanism

Neurilemmoma is a benign tumor derived from the nerve sheath cells (Schwann cells), also known as schwannoma or perineural fibroblastomas. In 1920, Antoni divided the tumor into cell rich zone (Antoni A type) and loose myxoid zone (Antoni B type). The patients with neurofibromatosis type I account for 20–50%, and neurilemmoma has been suggested to be a subtype of gastrointestinal stromal tumors, but inconsistency exists in immunohistochemical staining results for CD117. Neurilemmoma is mostly found in the head, neck, upper and lower limbs, and other parts of the body surface, and mediastinum is the major location in vivo, while abdominal cavity is less involved. Pereira et al. first reported hepatic neurilemmoma in 1978, and more than 20 cases have been reported in the literature by December 2013 [134, 135]. Hepatic neurilemmoma originates from various sympathetic nerve and parasympathetic nerve branches distributed in the connective tissue of the hepatic lobules or along the portal vein branches.

6.5.1.2 Clinical Features

Hepatic neurilemmoma is more common in elderly female patients, and the male to female ratio is 1: 4.5 with a mean age of 54.6 (35–70) years old. The main clinical manifestations include abdominal pain or back pain, and the course of the disease can be as long as 20 years due to slow growth of the tumor. Increased serum alkaline phosphatase and gamma GT can be detected, while AFP and CEA are normal. And elevation of serum collagenase type IV level was the important marker for peripheral neurilemmoma. B-ultrasound and CT images display hepatic nodular masses, and huge cystic occupying lesions with multiple calcification foci can be easily mistaken as parasitic cysts of the liver. Kim et al. [136] reported a case of hepatic neurilemmoma with positive finding on FDG-PE imaging, which is difficult to distinguish the nature of the tumor.

6.5.1.3 Gross Features

The tumors were more commonly located in the left lobe of the liver, often huge in size with an average diameter of 13 (2.3–24) cm and can be multinodular. The lesions appear in long fusiform, nodular, or lobulated shapes with a complete capsule, and the section is gray-white or pale yellow in color and crisp in nature, and interwoven structure can sometimes be observed (Fig. 6.79). Hemorrhage, necrosis, or cystic change can be found in cases with large lesions.

6.5.1.4 Microscopic Features

Hepatic neurilemmoma owns the mass morphology with neurilemmomas in other parts of the body, mainly consisting of Antoni A zone (bundle or compact type) and Antoni B zone (reticular type) in different proportions.

Antoni A zone contains abundant cells, fusiform or oval in shape with ambiguous cellar boundaries, pale staining cytoplasm, loosely arranged, and finely granular chromatin,

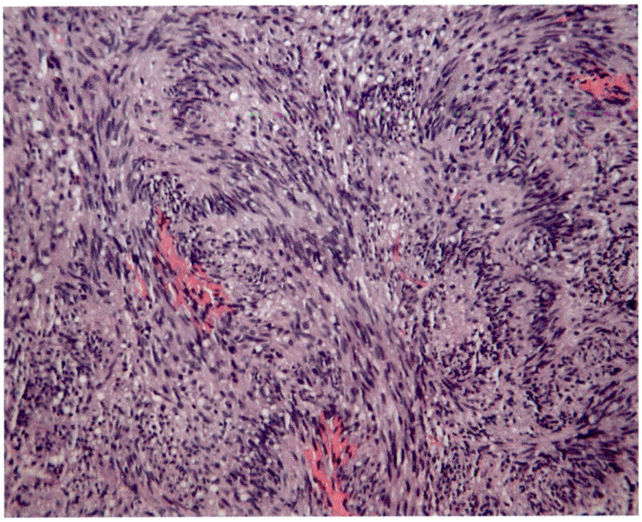

Fig. 6.80 Neurilemmoma. Antoni A zone: the tumor cells are arranged in a palisade shape, formed "Verocay bodies"

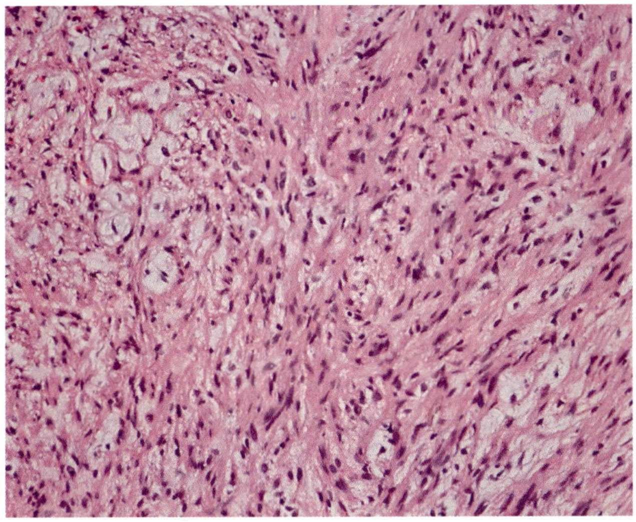

Fig. 6.81 Neurilemmoma. Antoni B zone: the tumor cells are loosely arranged and form a network

and visible slender fiber bundles can sometimes be seen at both ends of the nucleus, with no nuclear atypia, small or unclear nucleolus, and little karyokinesis. Nuclei of the tumor cells are arranged in a spiral or parallel palisade shape, between which is the slender homogeneous nuclear-free zone formed by cytoplasmic processes, and this is characteristic of Verocay bodies (Fig. 6.80).

Antoni B zone contains loosely arranged stellate tumor cells, and the cytoplasmic processes are connected to each other to form a network with grids expanded to be a small sac containing transparent matrix. There are three forms of the tumor cells, namely, lymphocyte-like cells, spindle cells, and stellate cells, the former of which are the most common type of cells with naked nucleus similar to lymphocyte. Antoni B zone contains numerous small thin-walled blood vessels, and piles of foam and yellow tumor cells are sometimes observed.

Neurilemmomas can be divided into several subtypes. The tumor with abundant cells and majorly composed by Antoni A zones is called cell-type neurilemmoma. The tumor mainly consisting of Antoni B zones and myxoid stroma is called myxoid neurilemmoma. And if the tumor contains significant melanin and positive HMB45, it is called melanin-type neurilemmoma, and if it is rich in small thin-walled blood vessels, the tumor is called angiomatous neurilemmoma, while for the tumor with cytoplasm containing eosinophilic granules, positive PAS, and anti-diastase digestion, it is called granulosa cell-type neurilemmoma (Fig. 6.81).

6.5.1.5 Immunohistochemistry

The tumors are NSE, S-100 (Fig. 6.82), CD57, glial fiber acidic protein (GFAP), and vimentin positive and SMA, desmin, and CK negative, with Ki-67 index < 5%.

6.5.1.6 Differential Diagnosis

1. Malignant neurilemmoma. Neurilemmoma with abundant cells should be identified from a malignant neurilemmoma. The former has a clear boundary even in the absence of a capsule, with no or mild atypia, and karyokinesis is rarely seen. The latter is often large in volume with an incomplete capsule, abundant cells, and obvious atypia, losing typical structures of Antoni A and B zoned, lack of Verocay bodies, and significant karyokinesis (> 5/10HPF), and tumor cells are distributed surrounding blood vessels forming a peripheral vascular sheath.
2. Neurofibroma and neurofibromatosis. There are no Verocay bodies, nuclei arranged in palisade shape or glass-like thickness of vascular wall, and neurofibromatosis also has corresponding genetic characteristics.
3. Leiomyoma. The tumor cells were arranged in a wave shape, with palisading arranged nuclei in some cases, abundant and eosinophilic cytoplasm, and visible myofilaments, and the nuclei are larger than those of the neurilemmoma cells, with both nuclear blunt ends, and no Antoni A and B zones. VG staining shows yellow green, rather than orange. And immunohistochemistry examination shows negative S-100 and positive actin and SMA.
4. Gastrointestinal stromal tumors. They are S-100 positive, as well as CD117 and CD34 positive, which can be distinguished from neurilemmomas. Moreover, it should be differentiated from fibrosarcoma and leiomyosarcoma.

6.5.1.7 Treatment and Prognosis

Surgical resection is a proper treatment for neurilemmoma with a good prognosis, and occasionally postoperative recurrence is related to incomplete resection of the tumor. And about 2–3% of the neurofibromatosis will evolve into malignant neurilemmomas.

6.5.2 Neurofibroma

6.5.2.1 Pathogenesis and Mechanism

Neurofibroma is a local or solitary benign tumor originating from neurilemma cells, consisting of proliferated Schwann cells and fibroblasts, mainly found in the skin, neck, mediastinum, etc. and related to type I neurofibromatosis (NF1). Hepatic neurofibroma is extremely rare, and only two cases have been reported in the English literature. Five cases have been diagnosed in the Department of Pathology, Eastern Hepatobiliary Surgery Hospital, of Second Military Medical University.

6.5.2.2 Clinical Features

All the five cases of hepatic neurofibroma, diagnosed in the Department of Pathology, Eastern Hepatobiliary Surgery Hospital, of Second Military Medical University, were female patients (Table 6.7), with an average age of 53.5 (3.5–84) years old. The tumor growth is slow, and the patients have no symptoms or only general gastrointestinal, local compression symptoms or radioactive pain. Elevated levels of serum alkaline phosphatase and γ-GT and normal AFP and CEA can be found. B-ultrasound and CT scan show intrahepatic solid lesions.

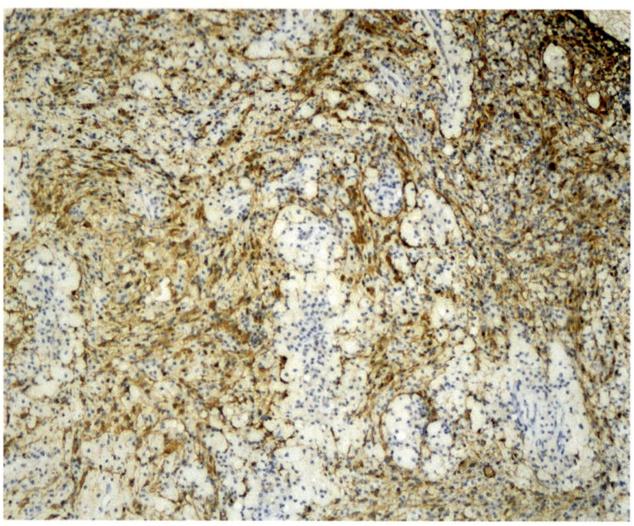

Fig. 6.82 Neurilemmoma. S-100 positive

6.5.2.3 Gross Features

The tumors were mainly located in the left lobe of the liver, and the average diameter of the tumors was 6.2 (4–13.5) cm. The gross morphology of neurofibromas varies greatly in different cases (Fig. 6.83), with no capsule or incomplete capsules and soft or hard and mildly flexible in texture. The section appears gray or grayish yellow, moist, and semitranslucent with luster and bundle or spiral structures (Fig. 6.84). The tumors are often solid with no obvious hemorrhage, or necrosis, and little cystic degeneration can be found.

6.5.2.4 Microscopic Features

Neurofibromas are composed by a proliferation mixture of all components of peripheral nerve, including neurilemma cells, axons, perineurium cells, and fibroblasts, and neurilemma cells are the major cellular component. The tumors are characterized by nerve fibers scattered within the tumor. And the tumor cells and nuclei were long wave shaped, with both tip ends of the nuclei and rare mitosis (Fig. 6.85). There is no Antoni A or Antoni B zone and the interstitial tissue is rich in collagen fibers with mucoid degeneration. The characteristics of neurofibromas developing into malignant neurilemmoma include increased cell density, polymorphism, nuclear mitosis, and vascular sheath formed by tumor cells.

6.5.2.5 Immunohistochemistry

S-100 and vimentin staining are positive, while CD34 and CD117 are negative.

6.5.2.6 Differential Diagnosis

The pathological diagnosis of neurofibromatosis is generally of no difficulties, and it should be differentiated from neurilemmoma which contains Antoni A and Antoni B zones.

6.5.2.7 Treatment and Prognosis

Recurrence after surgical resection of the tumor is rare; however, malignancy (malignant change rate of 3–13%) or involvement of other organ has been found; thus, the patients after surgical resection should be closely followed up.

Table 6.7 General features of five hepatic neurofibroma cases

Case	Gender	Age (years)	Location in the liver	Capsule	Tumor diameter (cm)	S-100 staining
1	Female	56	Left lobe	None	8	Positive
2	Female	3.5	Left lobe	None	12	Positive
3	Female	61	Left lobe	None	13.5	Positive
4	Female	63	Portal	None	3.5	Positive
5	Female	84	Portal	None	4	Positive

6.5.3 Plexiform Neurofibroma

6.5.3.1 Pathogenesis and Mechanism

Plexiform neurofibroma is characterized by masses consisting of nerve axons, nerve sheath cells, and fibroblasts in collagen or myxoid stroma, which mainly occurred in regions rich in innervation, and hepatic plexiform neurofibroma is rare. Zacharia et al. [137] reported that hepatic plexiform neurofibromas account for about 2.3% of the total number of abdominal and pelvic plexiform neurofibromas. And less than 20 cases have been reported in the literature. Hepatic plexiform neurofibromas are also common in NF1 patients. And plexiform neurofibromatosis is an autosomal dominant genetic disease with several cases of hepatic plexiform neurofibromatosis reported.

6.5.3.2 Clinical Features

Hepatic plexiform neurofibromas are common in adults and rare in children. The patients usually manifest no symptoms or only general gastrointestinal symptoms, local compression symptoms, or radioactive pain, and the severity of these symptoms varies depending on the location and size of the tumor. Some cases involving the hepatic hilus, small intestine, and biliary obstruction have been reported. The liver function in the patients is generally normal. MRI image characteristics are basically identical to the same tumors in other parts, and it is showed that all tumors are distributed along the intrahepatic portal tracts, sometimes involving the pancreas and gall bladder [138, 139]. Hepatic plexiform neurofibromas develop slowly, and stable condition of the tumor has been observed during years of follow-up.

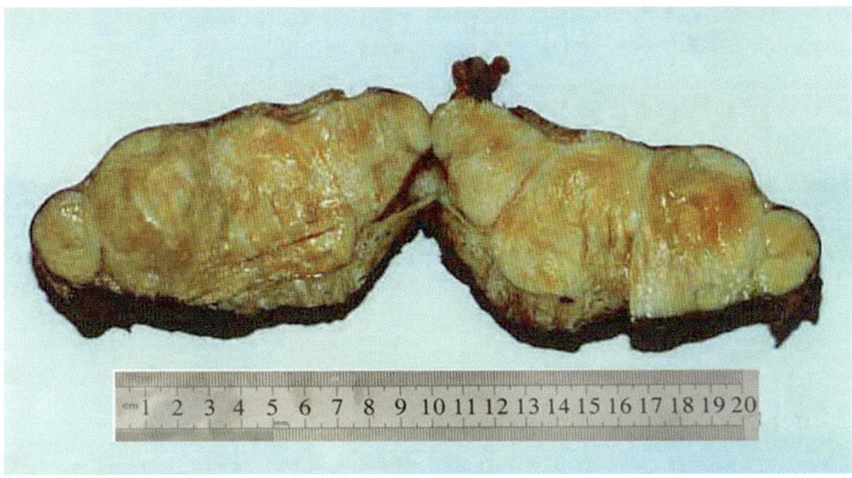

Fig. 6.83 Neurofibroma. The section appears *grayish yellow*, hard in texture

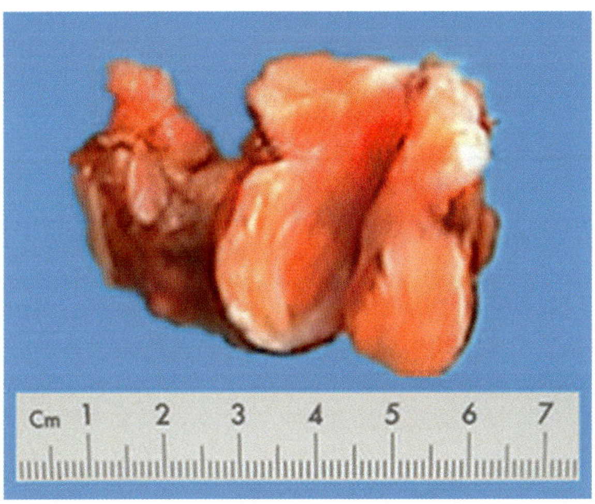

Fig. 6.84 Neurofibroma. The section appears *grayish white*, hard in texture

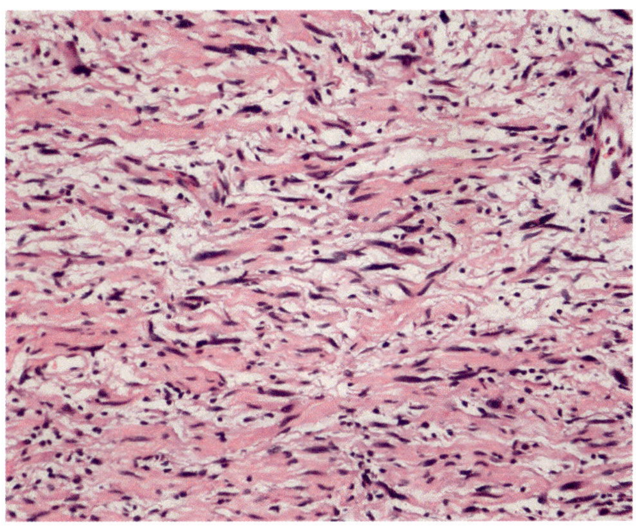

Fig. 6.85 Neurofibroma. The tumor cells and nuclei were long wave shaped, with both tip ends of the nuclei

6.5.3.3 Gross Features

Hepatic neoplasms can be huge with extensive involvement of the liver. The tumors are irregularly cylindrical, wormlike cords, spindle shaped, or spherically enlarged, often forming multiple nodules or beads (i.e., “plexiform”). Sometimes a tumor grows into a huge mass. The section of the tumor is often grayish white, soft in texture with elasticity, and a jelly part can be observed in some region of the tumor, while cystic change is rarely seen.

6.5.3.4 Microscopic Features

The lesions are characterized by a mixture of plexiform structure, peripheral proliferated collagen fibers, and stroma with mucoid degeneration, which is formed by all components of peripheral nerves, including axons, neurilemma cells, fibroblasts, and perineurium cells, and neurilemma cells are the main components, which are of spindle shape and loosely arranged, with light-stained cytoplasm, unclear cellular boundaries, long or wave-shaped nuclei with both tip ends, and dark nuclear chromatin. Generally, tumors which are > 5 cm in diameter, with infiltration into the surrounding liver tissue, tumor necrosis, calcification, and disappearance of target signs which is often central low signals in the tumor on MRI T_2-weighted images, suggest potential malignancy [140].

6.5.3.5 Immunohistochemistry

S-100 staining shows neurilemma cells, and EMA staining can display the perineurium cells, while NSE and NFP (neurofilament) staining shows the axons.

6.5.3.6 Differential Diagnosis

The pathological diagnosis is not difficult, but we should pay attention to the identification whether it is one of the concomitant lesions of the visceral neurofibromatosis.

Table 6.8 Features of NF1 and NF2

Features	NF1	NF2
Genetic features	Dominant heredity	Dominant heredity
Gene location	17q11.2	22q12.2
Gene property	Suppressor	Suppressor
Gene length	350 kb	110 kb
Coding protein	Neurofibromin	Schwannomin
Incidence at birth	1:2500–3300	1:5000
Incidence in population	1:33,000–40,000	1:210,000
Percentage of neurofibromatosis	96–97%	3–4%
Family history	None in 30–50%	None in 50%
Common tumor	Plexiform neurofibroma	Bilateral acoustic neuroma
Common sites	Bone, skin, soft tissue	Central nervous system

6.5.3.7 Treatment and Prognosis

The lifetime risk of malignancy for plexiform neurofibromas to develop into malignant peripheral neurilemmomas (malignant peripheral nerve sheath tumors (MPNSTs)) is 7–13%, and surgical resection is the optimal choice. Robertson et al. reported that treatment with imatinib mesylate facilitates the reduction of the size of plexiform neurofibroma [141].

6.5.4 Neurofibromatosis

6.5.4.1 Pathogenesis and Mechanism

Neurofibromatosis is an autosomal dominant genetic disease with onset of the disease in every generation of the family. According to the different pathogenic genes, it is divided into type I (NF1) and type II (NF2). NF1 was first described by Von Recklinghausen in 1882, characterized by peripheral neurofibroma, also known as Von Recklinghausen disease (VRD). NF2 was characterized by multiple tumors of the central nervous system, such as bilateral acoustic neuroma, spinal cord astrocytomas, meningiomas, retinal hamartoma, and ependymoma. The similarities and differences between NF1 and NF2 are summarized in Table 6.8. In addition, there are NF3–NF7 subtypes. The pathogenesis of NF1 is associated with multiple gene variants including NF1 gene, and 3–18% of the NF1 patients have the risk of other malignant tumors, including plexiform neurofibroma, glioma, pheochromocytoma, malignant schwannoma, carcinoid tumors, rhabdomyosarcoma, osteosarcoma, Wilms' tumor, and medulloblastoma. More than ten cases of neurofibromatosis with hepatic involvement have been reported so far, among which are cases of NF1 patients with hepatoblastoma [142], hepatic plexiform neurofibromas, liver plexiform neurofibroma and hepatic angiosarcoma [143], malignant hepatic neurilemmoma complicated with hepatic angiosarcoma [144], hepatic neurofibroma [145], as well as NF2 patients with hepatic angiomyolipoma [146]. Furthermore, one case of NF1 in a 44-year-old patient after liver transplantation treated with immunosuppressant has also been reported [147].

6.5.4.2 Clinical Features

The patients with hepatic neurofibromatosis are often young people, including children aged 4–17. The American National Institutes of Health (NIH) proposed the diagnostic standards for NF1 in 1988 which is still in use till now, including:

1. Prepuberty, the number of cafe-au-lait spots ≥ 6 with the maximum diameter ≥ 5 mm; postpuberty, the number of cafe-au-lait spots ≥ 6 with the maximum diameter ≥15 mm

2. The number of neurofibroma ≥2 or one plexiform neurofibroma
3. Visible nevoid lentigo in the armpit or groin area
4. Optic glioma
5. More than two iris pigment hamartoma (Lisch nodules)
6. Defined damage to the bone, such as sphenoid dysplasia or cortical thinning of long bones, with or without pseudoarthrosis
7. The first-degree relatives of NF1

Patients with two or more than two items of the above criteria can be diagnosed as NF1, and for those who do not meet the criteria but are highly suspected of NF1, genetic analysis could be considered.

6.5.4.3 Pathological Diagnosis

According to the corresponding histological features of hepatic tumors, the diagnosis can be made. And genetic testing can also provide an important evidence for the diagnosis. Mutations of NF1 gene located around the center of 17q11.2 are an important cause of NF1; therefore, PCR detection for microsatellite heterozygosity deletion near the related genes is useful, such as heterozygous deletions of microsatellites D22S929 and D22S1169 in NF2 patients, suggesting NF2 gene deletion in the tumor [148].

6.5.4.4 Differential Diagnosis

Patients with NF1 are the most common, and the differential diagnosis of tumors with no genetic factors according to the diagnostic criteria of NF1 should be paid much attention to.

6.5.4.5 Treatment and Prognosis

Surgery is the major treatment. And gene therapy is the most promising and the most important technique in the future. For instance, it has been discussed to introduce the normal NF1 gene into the diseased cells, so that it encodes normal fibrin to treat NF1 [149].

6.5.5 Paraganglioma

Wen-Ming Cong and Yu-Yao Zhu
Department of Pathology, Eastern Hepatobiliary Surgery Hospital, Second Military Medical University, Shanghai, China

6.5.5.1 Pathogenesis and Mechanism

Paraganglioma is a kind of neoplasm, derived from the sympathetic-adrenal neuroendocrine system and originated from the embryonic neural crest cells, usually referring to tumors of sympathetic and parasympathetic ganglion at sites except adrenal glands, and those in adrenal medulla are specifically known as pheochromocytoma. About 30% of patients with pheochromocytoma or paraganglioma have familial predisposition, and the pathogenesis involves mutations of VHL, MEN1, RET, and NF1. Hepatic paraganglioma is rare, and 16 cases have been reported so far [150].

6.5.5.2 Clinical Features

Among the16 cases of hepatic paraganglioma reported in the literature, the male to female ratio is 1:1.3, and the average age of the patients was 43 (ranged 14–71) years old. Hepatic paraganglioma is often nonfunctional due to the metabolism of catecholamine in liver cells; therefore, it generally manifests no clinical symptoms such as increased peripheral blood and urinary catecholamine concentrations, hypertension, heart palpitations, dizziness, and metabolic disorders. CT images display round or oval soft tissue masses in the liver, and tumors are lobulated, heterogeneous in density, clearly bounded, and irregularly hypodense, and marked enhancement in non-cystic parts can be found in cases with cystic change. High positive rate has been reported in radiation scanning with ^{131}I metaiodobenzylguanidine, but cases of false-negative results are found in a few cases.

6.5.5.3 Gross Features

Of the reported 16 cases of hepatic paraganglioma, 14 cases concerned intrahepatic solitary tumors, 2 cases exhibited multiple masses, and most of the lesions were located in the right lobe of the liver. The tumors are often large in volume with an average diameter of 8.2 (1.2–18) cm, round or lobulated in shape, and the sections are grayish white or brown in color, solid in texture, and hard and flexible, and brown-black hemorrhage and cystic cavities can be found inside the tumors. Koh et al. [151] reported one case of huge hepatic paraganglioma, 12 cm × 18 cm × 18 cm in size, which was treated by surgical resection.

6.5.5.4 Microscopic Features

The histological features of hepatic paraganglioma are similar to those of the same kind of tumor in other parts, including large amounts of capillaries which separate the tumor to form nests, acinar, or pseudorosette shapes. The cell nests are wrapped by flat supporting cells and surrounded by rich blood sinus, forming organ-like structures. The main cellular components are chief cells and supporting cells, and the former are polygonal, round, or oval shaped, densely arranged with abundant cytoplasm, rich in eosinophilic and basophilic or amphophilic particles of varying sizes (Figs. 6.86 and 6.87). And eosinophilic hyaline bodies can sometimes be found in the cytoplasm, which are positive for PAS staining after diastase digestion. The nuclei of the tumor cells are round or oval, with obvious nucleolus and intranuclear pseudoinclusion-like structures due to invagination of the cytoplasm. Cells in parts of the tumor are with atypia, abnormal nuclei, and less nuclear division. The supporting cells

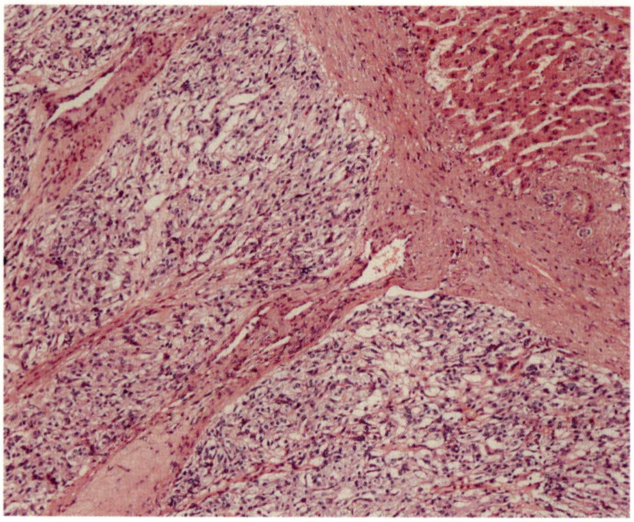

Fig. 6.86 Paraganglioma. The tumor arranged in a nest or interlaced shape; the tumor cells are polygonal shaped, with abundant cytoplasm

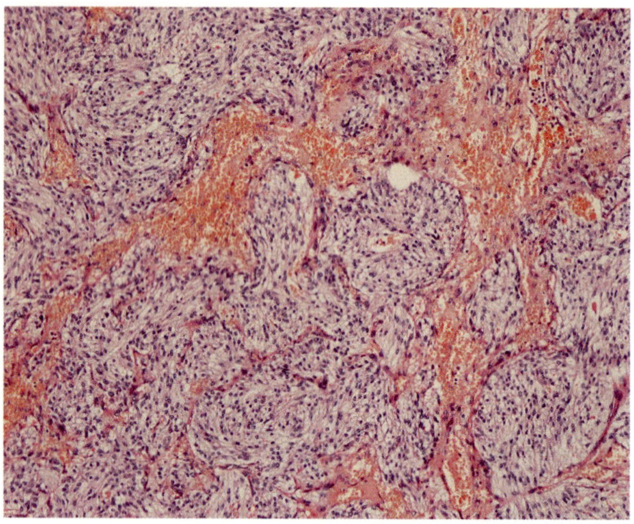

Fig. 6.87 Paraganglioma// pheochromocytoma?? The tumor arranged in a nest or interlaced shape; the tumor cells are spindle shaped, with abundant vessels

are spindle and distributed surrounding the tumor cell nests or interspersed between the chief cells. And no invasion of the tumor into the surrounding liver tissue has been found.

6.5.5.5 Immunohistochemistry

The chief cells of the ganglioma are positive for NSE, CgA (Fig. 6.88), Syn, and GFAP, and the supporting cells are positive for S-100, while both cells are negative for CD10, nestin, Bcl-2, SMA, EMA, etc.

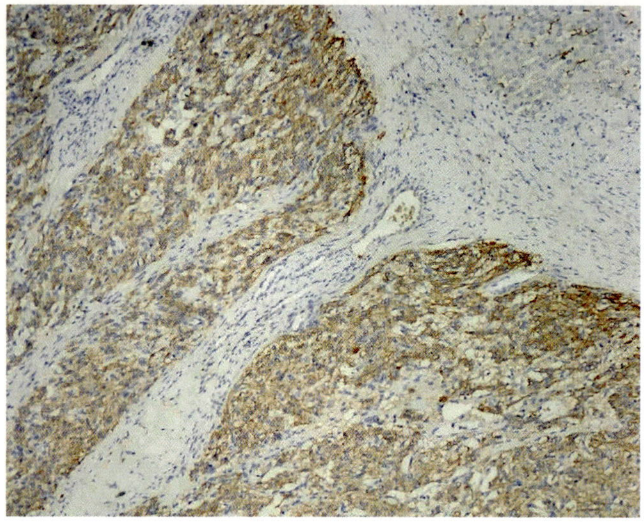

Fig. 6.88 Paraganglioma. CgA positive

6.5.5.6 Differential Diagnosis

1. Metastatic paraganglioma. The diagnosis of primary hepatic pheochromocytoma should first rule out metastasis of adrenal pheochromocytoma, with the bone and liver as the most common sites for metastasis. Three cases of hepatic metastatic paraganglioma have been diagnosed in the Department of Pathology, Eastern Hepatobiliary Surgery Hospital, Second Military Medical University, which were wrapped by a thick fibrous capsule.
2. Malignant paraganglioma. The identification of benign and malignant nature of a paraganglioma is of certain difficulties, and about 10% of all the cases were malignant. The histological findings may be inconsistent with the biologic behaviors. Of the reported 16 cases both at home and abroad, 2 cases with multiple hepatic masses were diagnosed as malignant lesions. Generally, when the tumor is larger than 6 cm in diameter, breaks through the capsule, and invades the adjacent liver tissue, with vascular infiltration, formation of tumor thrombus, abnormal increase of pathologic mitosis, metastasis, and diagnosis of malignant paraganglioma can be made.

6.5.5.7 Treatment and Prognosis

Surgical resection is the preferred treatment for paraganglioma. Due to the lower incidence, there are fewer reports of the tumor. The biological characteristics of this disease are not clear, and it has been reported that paraganglioma in the pancreas was a tumor with potential function and malignancy; thus, close follow-up should be carried out for a long term after surgery [152]. According to the reports on cases with no recurrence or metastasis during the 3-year follow-up after surgical resection, hepatic ganglioma treated with surgical removal is of good prognosis.

6.5.6 Adrenal Rest Tumor

6.5.6.1 Pathogenesis and Mechanism

Adrenal rest tumor was first reported by Hyams in 1960, and nine cases have been reported so far in the literature. The tumor is composed of adrenocortical cells, and its pathogenesis may involve ectopic location of the primordium or the whole organ of the right adrenal gland inside the hepatic capsule during embryonic development.

6.5.6.2 Clinical Features

Hepatic residual adrenal tumors can be both nonfunctional or functional, with the male to female ratio of 1:1, and the onset age in patients ranges 1–62 years old. Nonfunctional ones are hepatic pseudo-residual adrenal tumors, most without clinical symptoms, while patients with functional residual adrenal tumors manifest endocrine disorders such as Cushing syndrome or virilization or elevated serum levels of steroid hormones in some cases. Angiography shows the tumors in the liver parenchyma which are homogeneous in texture and rich in blood vessels. B-ultrasound examination shows round, clearly bounded, heterogeneous solid masses. And CT images display hypervascular densities of fat or soft tissue masses [153].

6.5.6.3 Gross Features

The tumors are mainly located in the hepatic capsule of the right lobe, which is associated with the blood supply of the tumor by hepatic artery. The tumors are 0.7–2.5 cm in diameter, and the cross sections are gray or yellowish gray, with or without calcification and cystic degeneration, and tumor often oppresses the adjacent liver tissue resulting in the formation of a thin pseudofibrous capsule.

6.5.6.4 Microscopic Features

The tumor exhibits expansive growth resulting in oppression on the adjacent liver tissue and the formation of thin pseudofibrous capsules. The tumor cells, resembling the pale cells in the adrenal cortex, are polygonal containing eosinophilic particles in the cytoplasm, oval nucleus, and no nucleolus and are arranged in wide trabecula or acinar shape, separated by slender fibrovascular septa. Some cells in certain regions are pleomorphic with transparent cytoplasm. Visible adrenal tissue can be sometimes found at the margins of the liver tissues. Tumors with huge sizes and obvious atypia of the tumor cells may be malignant. The tumor cells are positive in Sudan III staining (frozen section).

6.5.6.5 Immunohistochemistry

Steroid hormone contained in the tumor tissue is a key evidence for the diagnosis of the tumor. And the tumor cells are stained positive for adrenal 4-binding protein (Ad4BP) and CgA, but negative for EMA, S-100, CK, and vimentin.

6.5.6.6 Differential Diagnosis

1. Hepatic adenoma. Cholestasis and Mallory bodies can be found, and the tumors often contain small thin-walled veins or arteries with dilated lumen in diffuse distribution. PAS staining is positive in the tumor cells, while adrenal rest tumor shows negative result in PAS staining.
2. Metastatic adrenocortical carcinoma. The key point is to determine completeness and existence of tumor in the right adrenal gland.
3. Metastasis of renal cell carcinoma. Metastatic tumors in the liver of renal cell carcinoma are multiple nodular lesions, with transparent or eosinophilic cytoplasm of the tumor cells, positive staining for glycogen CD10. While adrenal rest tumor is often a solitary nodule and its glycogen staining and expression test of CD10 are both negative.
4. Hepatocellular carcinoma. HCC has a background of hepatitis or cirrhosis, and the cancer cells contain bile in the cytoplasm, with obvious nuclear atypia, and positive pCEA and Hep Par 1 result in immunohistochemistry.
5. Metastatic melanoma. The tumor cells contain melanin granules and are positive for HMB45 staining.

6.5.6.7 Treatment and Prognosis

Recurrence of tumors treated by surgical resection is rarely seen. And effective ketoconazole treatment for hepatic adrenal rest tumor has been reported.

6.5.7 Pancreatic Rest Tumor

Ectopic pancreatic tissue is more common in the stomach (27.5%), duodenum (25.5%), and jejunum (15.9%), while intrahepatic pancreatic rest tumor or heterotopic pancreas is extremely rare, with less than ten reported cases. Early in 1909, Heinrich et al. classified the tumor into three types according to the histological characteristics of ectopic pancreatic tissues. Type I contains acini, ducts, and endocrine islets, similar to normal pancreatic tissue; type II contains a large number of acini and small amount of ducts, with no islets; and type III contains several ducts, a small amount of acini and no islet.

The major clinical and pathological significance of ectopic pancreas lies in two aspects. One is repeated reports of canceration of the heterotopic pancreas, and the other is the differential diagnosis from other tumors. Yan et al. [154] first reported a 45-year-old woman with a 3.0 cm×2.0 cm×2.0 cm lesion near the portal area of the left lobe in the liver, which was surgically excised, and microscopic observation showed acinar cells containing abundant eosinophilic granules, centroacinar cells, and pancreatic ducts in the pancreatic tissue. The adenocarcinoma derived from ectopic pancreatic tissue and grew outward resulting in invasion of nerve tissue, and the pathological diagnosis was moderately differentiated adenocarcinoma originating from hepatic heterotopic pancreas. Guillou et al. [155] proposed three criteria for the diagnosis of adenocarcinoma originating from ectopic pancreatic tissue, including: ① the tumors should be located within or around the ectopic pancreatic tissue; ② there is a transition between the pancreatic tissue and cancer tissue; ③ the nontumor pancreatic tissue should contain acini, epithelium, and ducts.

6.5.8 Gastrinoma

Wen-Ming Cong and Qian Zhao
Department of Pathology, Eastern Hepatobiliary Surgery Hospital, Second Military Medical University,
Shanghai, China

6.5.8.1 Pathogenesis and Mechanism

Gastrinoma is a neuroendocrine tumor of the gastrointestinal tract and the pancreas, derived from G cells distributed in mucous membrane of the gastric antrum, duodenum, and proximal jejunum and characterized by the secretion of gastrin. Around 20–30% of the gastrinomas belong to multiple endocrine neoplasia type 1 (MEN1), and it is an autosomal dominant syndrome involving multiple endocrine organs. Related cancer genes for the pathogenesis of gastrinoma include c-Myc and HER2/neu (ElbB-2), and tumor suppressor genes include MEN1 and P16 (INK4a). Sporadic gastrinomas (75–90%) were often solitary, while MEN1-type gastrinomas (10–25%) are often multiple lesions and can be complicated by lesions in the parathyroid glands, pituitary, islet, and adrenal cortex. Gastrinomas located in "gastrinoma triangle" (below the junction of the cystic duct and common bile duct, above the junction of the descending and cross parts of the duodenum, and out of the junction of the neck and body of the pancreas) are the most common, accounting for up to 80–90%, among which the pancreas (21–65%) and duodenum (6–32%) are more common sites for gastrinomas than other locations, such as lymph nodes, stomach, mesentery, liver, ovary, kidney, and heart. So far, less than 30 cases of primary hepatic gastrinoma have been reported in the literature, and the current suggestion of the potential origin for hepatic gastrinomas concerns the uptake of amine precursor in the biliary tree and APUD cells [157–159].

6.5.8.2 Clinical Features

It is reported that hepatic gastrinoma occurs mainly in children and the elderly (28–77 years old), involving more men than women. Most of the patients manifest Zollinger-Ellison syndrome (ZES), including refractory ulcers, watery diarrhea, stomach burning sensation, and esophageal reflux. Fasting serum gastrin levels are more than 1000 pg/ml, and ^{123}I-octreotide somatostatin receptor scintigraphy (SRS) demonstrating high expression of somatostatin in the tumor is of diagnostic value. And gastrin stimulation test is helpful in tumor location. CT images show intrahepatic masses with clear boundaries, a number of septa, and no enhancement in enhanced scan. Ogawa et al. [160] suggested that selective arterial calcium infusion (SACI) in insulin stimulation test helps to exclude gastrinomas in the "gastrinoma triangle." Ga-68-DOTATOC PET-CT examination is beneficial to exclude gastrinomas out of the "gastrinoma triangle" and metastasis.

6.5.8.3 Gross Features

According to the literature, hepatic gastrinoma is often a small solitary nodule, but multiple lesions can also be found, with the diameter of 1–5 cm and a clear boundary, with or without a capsule, and the tumor section was pink-white.

6.5.8.4 Microscopic Features

Consistent with the histological morphology of gastrinomas in other locations, hepatic gastrinoma is often arranged in the shape of a nest, cord, or acinar structure. The tumor cells are often small or medium in size, round, oval, polygonal, cuboidal, or columnar, consistent in morphology and size, without obvious atypia, and visible mitosis is rare. Ki-67 labeling index is not high, and abundant blood vessels can be found in the interstitial tissue. Whether the tumor is benign or malignant is difficult to determine based on the histological examination, and the basic evidences for a malignant tumor include invasive growth into the surrounding tissue and metastasis into lymph nodes and other organs.

6.5.8.5 Immunohistochemistry

The tumor is positive for gastrin staining, and the tumor cells may also express a variety of hormones, including glucagon, vasoactive intestinal peptide (VIP), somatostatin and its receptors, insulin, CgA, Syn, and NSE.

6.5.8.6 Differential Diagnosis

The liver is the most common metastatic site for gastrinomas, so the first step for differential diagnosis is to exclude hepatic metastasis of gastrinomas from the pancreas and other parts.

6.5.8.7 Treatment and Prognosis

Gastrinomas with malignancy and metastasis account for 60–90% of all the gastrinomas. Based on the reports in the literature, surgery is the preferred treatment method for hepatic gastrinomas. Naoe et al. [156] reported one case of a 77-year-old woman with persistent diarrhea for 8 months, weight loss, and serum gastrin levels >4000 pg/ml, and CT showed two low-attenuation rounded nodules in the right lobe of the liver, 1.6 cm and 1.9 cm in diameter, respectively. The tumors were treated by resection, and immunohistochemistry was positive for gastrin and Ki-67 index >20%. Cranial MRI and thyroid ultrasound examinations suggested no abnormalities. FDG PET showed no extrahepatic lesions, excluding MEN1. And the pathological diagnosis was primary hepatic gastrinoma. Postoperative follow-up of 12 months revealed the disappearance of Zollinger-Ellison syndrome and decrease of serum gastrin levels to normal, indicating that the surgery cured the patient.

6.5.9 Vasoactive Intestinal Polypeptide-Secreting Tumor

Wen-Ming Cong and Qian Zhao
Department of Pathology, Eastern Hepatobiliary Surgery Hospital, Second Military Medical University,
Shanghai, China

Vasoactive intestinal polypeptide-secreting tumor (VIP tumor) is a rare neuroendocrine tumor, which often derives from D1 cells in the pancreatic islets, and more than 60% of the VIP tumors are malignant. VIP tumors outside the pancreas are generally neurogenic. Since the first case of primary hepatic VIP tumor reported by Ayub et al. [161] in 1993, only five cases have been found in the literature. The patients are often middle-aged men, aged 35–41 years old, with elevated serum levels of VIP due to secretion of large amounts of VIP, by D1 cells, resulting in periodic intractable watery diarrhea, hypokalemia caused by massive discharge of potassium via the intestinal tract, and lack of gastric acid due to inhibition by VIP. All of the above manifestations are called Verner-Morrison syndrome.

Primary hepatic VIP tumor is generally located in the right lobe of the liver, large in size with a maximum diameter of 10 cm. Microscopic observation shows well-differentiated tumor in nest or acinar-like structures, similar to the morphology of islet cell tumor. Immunohistochemistry demonstrates positive results for vasoactive intestinal peptide (VIP), CgA, Syn, and NSE and negative for gastrin. VIP tumors are of high malignancy, and more than 70% of the patients are found to have metastasis at the time of diagnosis, so exclusion of metastatic tumor in the liver derived from VIP tumors of pancreas or digestive tract. Dohmen et al. reported one case of a 33-year-old male patient with primary VIP tumor in the pancreatic tail, which was small in volume; however, two large metastatic nodules were found in the liver. It should also be differentiated from primary hepatic neuroendocrine tumors. Surgical resection is the first choice for the treatment and can be combined with radiofrequency and somatostatin therapies. After the tumor is excised, the clinical symptoms will be improved or completely disappear, and serum VIP levels will decrease to normal. Hachicha et al. [162] reported one case of primary hepatic VIP tumor which was treated with surgical resection, and no abnormality was found during the 42-month follow-up.

6.5.10 Somatostatinoma

Wen-Ming Cong and Yu-Yao Zhu
Department of Pathology, Eastern Hepatobiliary Surgery Hospital, Second Military Medical University,
Shanghai, China

Somatostatinoma is often found in the pancreas and small intestine, and over 200 cases have been reported globally. Primary hepatic somatostatinoma is rare, with only two cases found in the literature, and its origin is not clear. However, it is found that the cells containing somatostatin exist in the branches of the biliary tree, suggesting these endocrine cells may be the origin for hepatic somatostatinoma. Patients with somatostatinomas in the pancreas or duodenum often manifest "inhibition syndrome," including diabetes, diarrhea, abdominal pain, and cholelithiasis, due to the release of a large number of somatostatin. And laboratory examination showing elevated levels of serum somatostatin and calcitonin is helpful for the diagnosis [163].

Among the two reports on hepatic somatostatinoma, one case concerned a 56-year-old male patient with NF1 and multiple small lesions in the liver, which were confirmed as hepatic somatostatinomas via liver biopsy [164]. The other one concerned a 48-year-old woman with a huge abdominal mass as the first clinical manifestation, which was 20 cm×20 cm×10 cm in size and surgically excised, but recurrence occurred 5 years later and a hepatic mass of 11 cm×10 cm×10 cm was excised [165]. On gross appearance, the tumor is round with a thin capsule, and its section is grayish yellow, with no bleeding or necrosis, and the boundary is clear. Microscopic observation shows cuboidal tumor cells of medium sizes, with abundant and red-stained cytoplasm containing fine granules, round or oval nuclei, clear nucleolus, with mild atypia and mitosis. Tumor tissues are in trabecular, nest, banded, or glandular arrangement, surrounded by fibrovascular stroma. Most of the tumor cells are positive stained for somatostatin (SS), NSE, Syn, and CgA and negative for VIP, insulin, and gastrin (GAS) in immunohistochemistry.

The liver is the most common organ for metastasis of somatostatinoma, and metastatic hepatic somatostatinoma should be first excluded at the time of diagnosis. It is a high differentiated tumor with slow growth and low degree of malignancy, and the natural course can be several years. However, the discovery of hepatic somatostatinoma is usually complicated with metastasis, and invasion and metastasis into the surrounding liver tissue and blood vessels indicate malignancy. The treatment for extrahepatic somatostatinomas can be divided into two methods. For cases with no liver metastasis, radical resection of the primary lesions and dissection of lymph nodes are recommended. While surgical resection can also be applied in cases with liver metastasis [166], for unresectable lesions, liver transplantation is a proper choice which can improve the postoperative survival rates at 5 years and 10 years. For patients with somatostatinoma and expression of somatostatin receptors, injection of octreotide can help decrease the plasma somatostatin level and further improve symptoms such as diabetes and diarrhea [167].

6.6 Other Benign Tumors in the Liver

6.6.1 Teratoma

6.6.1.1 Pathogenesis and Mechanism

Teratoma is a tumor associated with abnormal embryonic tissue growth and development, originating from pluripotent germ cells, with the potential to differentiate into all three germinal layers to produce a variety of tissues and organs. The predilection sites for teratoma are distributed along the center line of the body, namely, the embryonic notochord line, including the ovary, testis, anterior mediastinum, retroperitoneal region, presacral space, and tail and pineal gland, sequenced by frequency. Teratomas can be divided into benign (mature) and malignant (immature) teratoma according to the degree of differentiation. To date, more than 30 cases of hepatic teratoma have been reported, which may derive from ectopic primordial germ cells, developed from residual primordial germ cells in the liver during the early development of embryos (blastocysts or morula) [168–171]. Three cases of hepatic teratoma have been diagnosed in the Department of Pathology, Eastern Hepatobiliary Surgery Hospital, of Second Military Medical University.

6.6.1.2 Clinical Features

Patients are often female infants younger than 1 year old, among whom 25% of them are diagnosed at birth. The patients of the three cases of hepatic teratoma diagnosed in the Department of Pathology, Eastern Hepatobiliary Surgery Hospital, of Second Military Medical University, were a 7-and-a-half-month female infant, a 32-year-old woman, and a 65-year-old man. Hepatic teratoma is often a benign tumor with no specific clinical manifestations, and the main symptoms include right upper abdominal pain, nausea, and vomiting due to tumor compression on the adjacent organs. And some patients go to hospital because of accidental discovery of abdominal mass with normal serum AFP. Imaging shows cystic lesions in the liver, which should be differentiated from liver abscess and liver parasitic cyst. CT shows cystic fat dilution in the liver with teeth and calcification. Cases of simple teratoma or mature teratoma have normal serum AFP and β-HCG levels, which are often significantly increased in cases of malignant teratoma or immature teratoma, and AFP can be used as a biomarker in distinguishing benign and malignant teratomas. The serum level of CA19–9 > 570 U/ml in one case in our hospital was significantly decreased after tumor resection.

6.6.1.3 Gross Features

The three cases of hepatic teratoma diagnosed in our hospital varied in the structure and morphology. These tumors were 13–25 cm in diameter, cystic or cystic-solid, with an uneven surface, soft or hard in texture, and solitary or multiple. Some lesions could grow into a huge mass, even occupying half of the liver. Structures such as cysts, bone, cartilage, hair, and teeth can be observed on the sections (Figs. 6.89 and 6.90), and cystic teratoma contains fetal fatlike or jelly-like liquid in the sac.

6.6.1.4 Microscopic Features

Teratoma is composed of three layers of mesodermal tissues. Ectodermal tissues include the skin, hair, sebaceous glands,

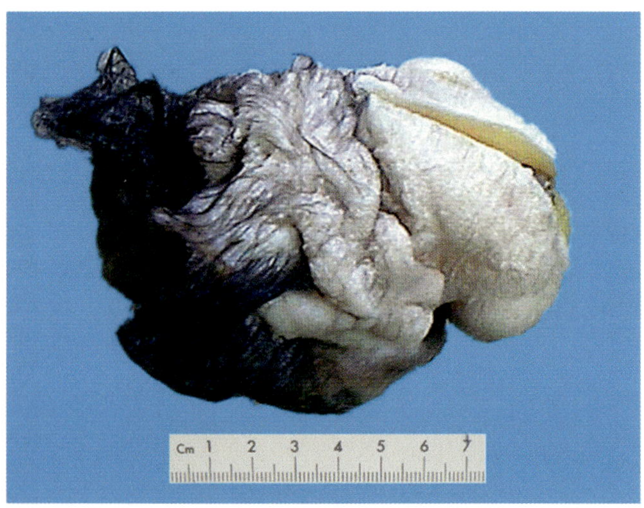

Fig. 6.89 Teratoma. An uneven surface, soft or hard in texture; hair can be observed on the sections

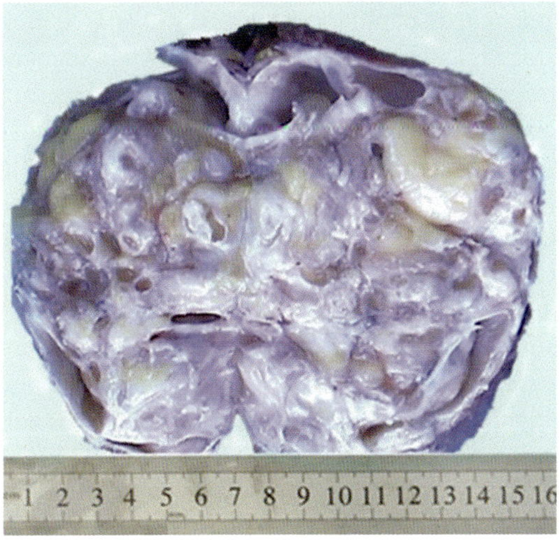

Fig. 6.90 Teratoma. Cystic-solid tumor, *yellow* and *white*

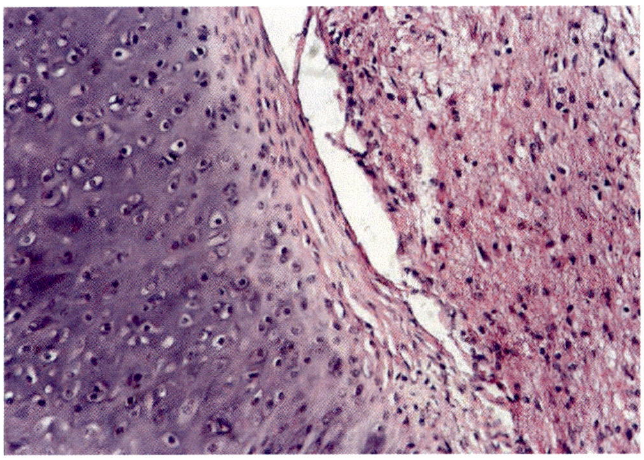

Fig. 6.91 Teratoma. Mature cartilage (*left*) and nerve tissue (*right*)

sweat glands, and nerve tissue (Fig. 6.91); the mesoderm contains bone, cartilage, bone marrow, skeletal muscle, lymph tissue, and connective tissue; and endodermal tissues contain the epithelium of the digestive tract (Fig. 6.92), fallopian tube, thyroid tissue, and respiratory epithelium. And extramedullary hematopoiesis in the liver can be found in some cases. Hepatic teratoma can also be complicated by yolk sac tumor and hepatocellular carcinoma.

6.6.1.5 Differential Diagnosis

1. Malignant teratoma. It is also known as immature teratoma. And when teratomas contain yolk sac carcinoma, embryonal carcinoma, or choriocarcinoma, the level of serum alpha-fetoprotein and chorionic gonadotropin will increase, which can be used as biomarkers for malignant teratoma.

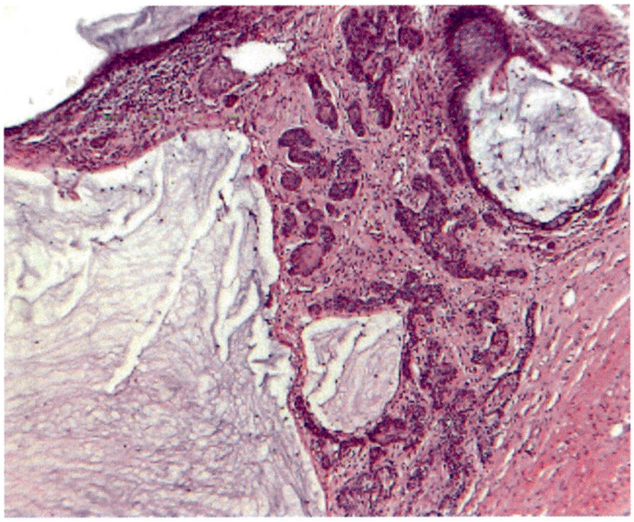

Fig. 6.92 Teratoma. Secreting epithelium of the digestive tract

2. Metastatic teratoma. The first step in diagnosis of primary hepatic teratoma is to exclude metastatic teratoma derived from predilection sites such as the ovary and testis.
3. Mesenchymal hamartoma of the liver. It is mainly myxoid matrix containing stellate and spindle primitive mesenchymal cells, thick-walled blood vessels, proliferated bile ducts, and liver cell clusters, the component of which are simple.

6.6.1.6 Treatment and Prognosis

Surgery is the first choice for the treatment of teratoma, and once the diagnosis is made, early surgical resection should be conducted and the prognosis is good. Follow-up and regular detection of AFP and β-HCG are recommended after the surgery.

6.6.2 Mesothelioma

6.6.2.1 Pathogenesis and Mechanism

Miller first reported mesothelioma in 1908, which occurs mainly in locations with mesepithelium covering, such as the pleura, peritoneum, and pericardium. The relation between the occurrence of some pleural and peritoneal mesotheliomas and inhalation of asbestos dusts has been defined. And patients with long-term use of immunosuppressants after organ transplantation have been found to develop peritoneal mesothelioma. Primary hepatic benign mesothelioma is rare, and Rout et al. [172] reported one case of hepatic mesothelioma in 1999, and Flemming et al. [173] reported one case of a 51-year-old woman with a 8 cm×6.5 cm×6 cm cystic mass in the left lobe of the liver, which was pathologically confirmed as a cystic mesothelioma after resection. Wang Jinbo et al. [174] reported one case of a 24-year-old male patient with surgically resected hepatic fibrous mesothelioma located in the right lobe underneath the hepatic capsule, and the tumor was 7 cm×6 cm×6 cm in size, gray or grayish yellow on the section, with swirling texture and greasy feeling. Hepatic mesothelioma may be derived from the mesothelial cells in the inner layer of the Glisson capsule.

6.6.2.2 Clinical Features

The majority of the patients are females aged 22–83 years old, and the major clinical manifestations include discomfort or pain in the liver zone, hypoglycemia-related symptoms, and elevation in serum CA19-9 levels. The X-ray or CT images show homogeneous densities in the liver which can be solitary, multinodular, or lobulated with clear boundaries. And qualitative examination depends on postsurgical pathological investigation.

6.6.2.3 Gross Features

The tumors are round and nodular with clear boundaries and complete capsules, and parts of the lesions are lobulated. The sections are gray or grayish yellow. The tumor is often large in size, even up to 15 cm × 9 cm × 8 cm and weighing up to 3800 g, moderate to hard in texture, and giant tumors may be complicated by mucinous degeneration, cystic degeneration, punctate hemorrhage, and necrosis. Multicystic mesothelioma contains sac cavities or cystic structures.

6.6.2.4 Microscopic Features

Benign mesothelioma can be divided into the following histological types:

1. Fibrous mesothelioma. The tumor tissue is mainly constituted by fibroblasts and epithelial spindle cells, with no nuclear atypia, covered by an intact layer of mesothelial cells, and parenchymal components of the liver can be bundled into the tumor. Immunohistochemistry shows positive CK, EMA, and vimentin and negative CD117 and CD34, while positive actin can be observed in a few tumors. The tumor tends to be recurrent with rare malignant transformation.
2. Epithelial mesothelioma. The tumor is papillary or tubular, lined with a single layer of cuboidal or low columnar cells with consistency in size, no obvious atypia, and rare mitosis. The tumor cells are positive for CK, CK7, CA-125, calretinin, D2–40, thrombomodulin, WT-1, and mesothelin (a kind of anti mesothelial cell antibody). And well-differentiated papillary mesothelioma is a tumor with weak malignancy.
3. Multicystic mesothelioma. It is known as a benign or indolent tumor, consisting of cystic cavities in varying sizes and round or irregular shapes. The cystic walls are lined with a single layer of well-differentiated flat or cuboidal epithelioid cells which protrude into the lumen in hobnail or papillary shapes. Positive CK, EMA and HBME-1, and negative F-VII are shown in immunohistochemistry tests. Recurrence has been observed in some cases with no metastasis, and a second resection can be conducted due to the malignant potential of the tumor.
4. Differentiated papillary mesothelioma. The tumor consists of diffuse papillary hyperplasia which appears as thick branched tubular papilla with fibrous tissue and blood vessel in the center. It is a borderline tumor with a benign course, while recurrence may be found several years after resection in a few cases, and development for malignant mesothelioma and distant metastasis will occur in individual cases.

6.6.2.5 Differential Diagnosis

Benign mesothelioma is rare, and malignant epithelial mesothelioma contains obvious hemorrhage and necrosis foci with abundant tumor cells in diffuse distribution and marked nuclear atypia with mitosis figures > 5/10HPF. It tends to metastasize to lymph nodes, and the tumor cells are negatively stained for desmin and positive in p53 and Ki-67 staining. In addition, it should be differentiated from other cystic tumors in the liver, such as parasitic cysts, biliary cystadenoma, or cystadenocarcinoma.

6.6.2.6 Treatment and Prognosis

Surgical resection is the first choice for the treatment of benign mesothelioma with a good prognosis when complete resection has been demonstrated.

6.6.3 Myxoma

Myxoma is a benign mesenchymal tumor characterized by myxoid matrix which is rich in acid mucopolysaccharides and glycoproteins, generally with no progression. Myxoma is often discovered in the myocardium, bone, skin, and urogenital system, while hepatic myxoma is rare. One case of hepatic myxoma has been diagnosed in the Department of Pathology, Eastern Hepatobiliary Surgery Hospital, Second Military Medical University, and the patient was a 19-year-old male who complained of a gradually increased mass in the right upper abdomen for 2 years, and his main symptoms included an upper abdominal mass, abdominal distension, and abdominal pain. He was generally in a good condition, with no history of hepatitis, and his serum AFP detection was negative, and the liver function was normal. A lobulated tumor in the right lobe of the liver was surgically excised, and it was 15 cm×12 cm×6.5 cm in size. Zhang Jianping et al. [175] reported one case of hepatic myxoma which was 19 cm×13 cm in size, and the section was gray and hard with no obvious hemorrhage or necrosis, with an intact capsule and no cirrhosis in the surrounding liver tissue (Fig. 6.93).

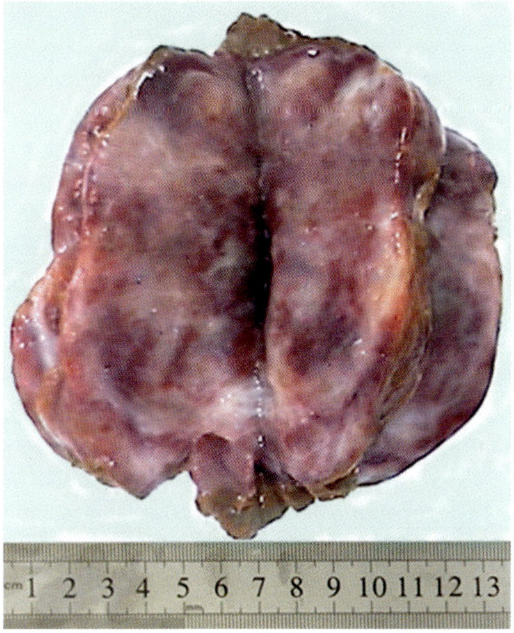

Fig. 6.93 Myxoma. The section was *gray* and *white*, lobulated, and hard in texture

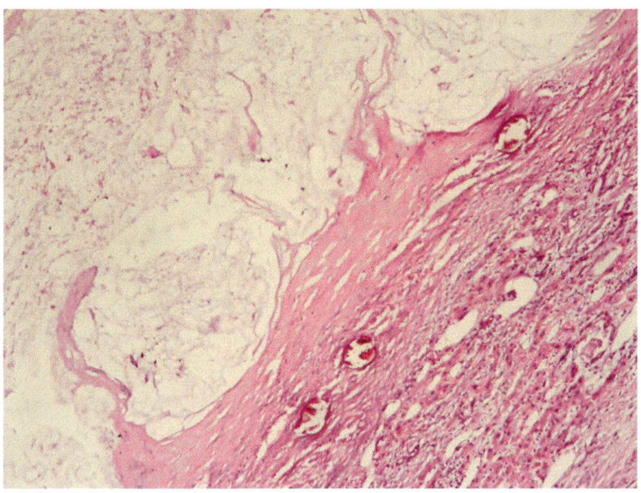

Fig. 6.94 Myxoma. Tumor tissue contained large amounts of mucus, with clear boundary and schistosome eggs in the capsule

Under the microscope, tumor tissue contained large amounts of mucus (Fig. 6.94) with varying numbers of fusiform and star-shaped mucous cells. The round or spindle nuclei of the tumor cells contain dense and dark-stained chromatin, no visible nucleolus, with no obvious atypia. The spindle-shaped tumor cells were positive for vimentin and SMA staining, and the abundant myxoid stroma was positive in Alcian blue staining. The adjacent liver tissue was compressed by the expansion of the tumor resulting in atrophy, but no invasive growth was observed.

The diagnosis of hepatic myxoma is generally of no difficulties; however, attention should be paid to differential diagnosis from other tumors with local mucinous degeneration. For an instance, mesenchymal hamartoma of the liver can have mucinous degeneration, but the mucus contains bile ducts and liver tissue, while myxoma contains homogeneous mucus mostly with single component. Hepatic myxoma is a benign mesenchymal tumor, which can be treated by surgical resection with a good prognosis.

6.6.4 Chondroma

Wen-Ming Cong and Qian Zhao
Department of Pathology, Eastern Hepatobiliary Surgery Hospital, Second Military Medical University,
Shanghai, China

Only one case of chondroma has been found in the current literature, which was reported by Fried in 1992. The patient was a 44-year-old female manifesting dull pain and oppression symptoms in the liver zone. She was followed up by CT imaging for 6 years, after when a surgical resection was conducted for the tumor which increased significantly in volume. Pathological examination showed that hepatic tumor was 19 cm×15 cm×9.5 cm in size with a clear boundary and was a huge oval nodular mass with an envelope and tender in texture similar to a rubber. The cross section was yellow and myxoid, or gray hyaline and cartilage-like, with calcification or ossification, and a jelly area of cystic degeneration was found in the center which was 6 cm×4.5 cm in size. Microscopic observation showed that it contained lobulated well-differentiated hyaline cartilage, fibrous cartilage, or myxoid cartilage, with mature hyaline cartilage as the majority. The cartilage was separated into lobules by fibrous tissue, and tumor cells were without atypia or obvious mitotic figures. And it was difficult to find hypertrophic or binucleate cells. Tumors with peripheral foci of fibrosis surrounding the lobules are called fibrochondroma, and those with obvious calcification and ossification are called osteochondroma, while tumors with abundant myxoid interstitial tissue in the center or the peripheral regions of the cartilage lobules are known as myxoid chondroma. The tumors were separated from the hepatic parenchyma by fibrous tissue, and infiltration of chronic inflammatory cells in surrounding liver tissues with formation of focal lymphoid follicles could be observed. Immunohistochemistry: cartilaginous cells were positive for vimentin and S-100 and negative for CK and SMA. Analysis via flow cytometry showed no heteroploid tumor cells.

6.6.5 Langerhans Cell Histiocytosis

Wen-Ming Cong and Xin-Yuan Lu
Department of Pathology, Eastern Hepatobiliary Surgery Hospital, Second Military Medical University, Shanghai, China

6.6.5.1 Pathogenesis and Mechanism

Langerhans cell histiocytosis (LCH) is caused by hyperplasia of histiocytes and dendritic cells in the mononuclear phagocytic system, and Langerhans cells (LCs) are equivalent to normal dendritic cells. The pathogenesis of LHC is unknown. Yousem et al. (2001) conducted human androgen receptor assay (HUMARA) of chromosome X polymorphism in CD1a-positive LCH cells by microdissection in women, finding that mono-organ (lung) LCH is non-clonal or polyclonal, while systemic LCH is monoclonal with potential tumorous properties. Recently, Badalian-Very et al. [176] discovered BRAF V600E mutations in LCH tissues, while mutations of TP53 and MET have also been found in individual cases, suggesting that LCH is a tumorous lesions and may be sensitive to inhibitors of the RAF pathway.

LCH can be either diffuse lesions involving multiple systems and organs or focal lesions involving a single system. And LCH accumulation and infiltration can be found to form masses in almost all organs of the body, and the predilection sites include the bone, skin, lymph nodes, and bone marrow, followed by the spleen, lung, endocrine organs, and gastrointestinal tract. The liver is often less involved and can be the only affected organ or as part of multiorgan diseases. LCH subtypes include three kinds of lesions:

1. Solitary or multiple bone destruction LCH (eosinophilic granuloma), confined to bone destruction
2. Local disseminated LCH with bone destruction and ectosteal soft tissue invasion (Hand-Schuller-Christian disease), the triad signs of which include skull defects, diabetes insipidus (pituitary involvement), and exophthalmos
3. Diffuse disseminated LCH involving multiple systems and organs (liver, spleen, lung, and bone marrow) (Letterer-Siwe disease)
4. Congenital self-healing reticulohistiocytosis (Hashimoto-Pritzker disease), the children patients of the disease are with skin damage as early as at birth [177, 178]

Diffuse disseminated LCH mainly involves infants and young children, and the incidence of cases with liver involvement was 40–60%, while cases of adult hepatic solitary LCH have been occasionally reported. Thus, LCH can be divided into single system with single lesion type, single system with multifocal type, and multisystem with multifocal type. The latter is further divided into low-risk group (involvement of multiple organs and systems except the hematopoietic system, liver, spleen, and lung) and high-risk group (involvement of multiple organs and systems including hematopoietic system, liver, spleen, and lung). The mechanism of the damage caused by hepatic LCH is associated with the invasion and destruction of bile ducts by LC, leading to damage and disappearance of bile ducts and further peribiliary fibrosis, inducing secondary sclerosing cholangitis changes, during which the chronic injury eventually evolved into biliary cirrhosis.

6.6.5.2 Clinical Features

Hepatic LCH is a visceral LCH, and the patients are predominantly infants and young children, affecting few adults and the elderly rarely. Shi et al. [179] reported 13 cases of diffuse LCH involving the liver and other organs and tissues, including seven males and six females, aged 13–52 months with an average of 28.9 months old. Kaplan et al. [184] reported one group of nine hepatic LCH cases, with a male to female ratio of 1:2 and a median age of 18 months old (ranged 7 days to 62 years old), among which five cases were solitary hepatic LCH and the remaining four cases were accompanied with involvement of the lymph nodes, skin, lung, thymus, spleen, pancreas, bone, and heart. Mulitifocal (multiple) LCH is more common in children, while monofocal (solitary) LCH can occur at any age. Adult patients with LCH can also be complicated by diseases, such as breast cancer, lymphoma, or leukemia. The clinical symptoms mainly relate to the number of organs involved, and the most common manifestations in pediatric patients are multisystem LCH, fever, and poor growth. Patients of hepatic LCH have normal extrahepatic bile ducts, and their intrahepatic bile ducts show segmental dilatation with stones, similar to the characteristics of sclerosing cholangitis. The patients usually manifest as chronic cholestasis, portal hypertension, ascites, hepatosplenomegaly, and abnormal liver function, including elevated serum alkaline phosphatase and γ-glutamyl transpeptidase in most cases. Braier et al. [180] reported 182 cases of children with LCH, including 36 cases with liver damage, among which 12 patients had cholestasis. Imaging examination primarily shows multiple liver nodular and beaded lesions distributed along the portal vein system with cholangitis. In 2009, the International Association of Tissue and Cells divided LCH into two groups: ① low risk group, patients older than 2 years without damage on the liver, lung, and bone, and ② high risk groups, with damage on multiple organs including the liver, lung, and bone.

6.6.5.3 Gross Features

The lesions are multiple nodular or intranodular cystic, ranging in diameter from 2 mm microgranulomas to 10 cm solid masses, brown yellow, tenacious, with clear boundaries.

6.6.5.4 Microscopic Features

Histologically, LCH can be divided into four stages: proliferation, granuloma, xanthoma, and fibrosis, mainly in the following three kinds of pathological presentations:

1. Formation of LC foci. Small granulomas or tumorlike lesions are of diagnostic value. Typical LCs are 10–12 μm in diameter, rich in eosinophilic cytoplasm with phagocytosis, and the nuclei are often oval, lobulated, and horseshoe shaped or twisted with obvious nuclear grooves, fine granular chromatin, and visible nucleolus. In most cases, the LCs are surrounded by varying amounts of eosinophilic granulocytes, lymphocytes, neutrophils, plasma cells, and non-LC multinucleated giant cells, which can be mingled with fibroblasts and hematopoietic cells.
2. LC infiltration into bile duct walls. LCs mainly invade the basement membrane of bile ducts, with infiltration of inflammatory cells, resulting in stripping of biliary epithelial cells from the basement membrane. Clinically, this can lead to chronic cholestasis, similar to the performance of primary sclerosing cholangitis. Residual small bile ducts can be observed in the LC clusters, or they are completely replaced by LC, and only the basement membrane of the bile duct can be seen, which is also considered to be the characteristic lesions of hepatic LCH. And a large number of LCs and infiltration of inflammatory cells can also be discovered in the lumen of large bile ducts, resulting in dilatation of the bile ducts.
3. Peribiliary fibrosis. It is observed in most cases. On the basis of second pathological lesions, the large bile ducts are surrounded by a large amount of fibrous tissue with dilatation of the bile ducts, presenting the changes of secondary sclerosing cholangitis, which is the main reason for jaundice. Other secondary changes include hyperplasia of small bile ducts and fibrous tissue in the portal district, expansion of periportal area, an "onion skin" appearance around the bile ducts, cholestasis in liver cells, and formation of fat nodules around the portal veins in the liver parenchyma.

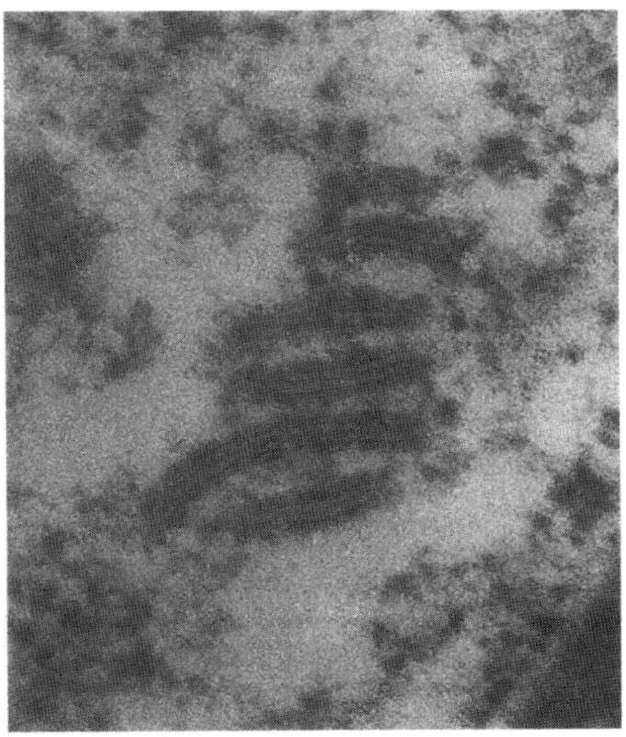

Fig. 6.95 Hepatic Langerhans cell histiocytosis. Birbeck bodies in the cytoplasm (From Kaplan[182])

In 1987, the International Association of Tissue and Cells classified LCH into three grades:

Grade I: according to findings, the clinical and laboratory tests, X-ray changes of organs including bone and lung, and abnormal LCs on histological sections, a preliminary diagnosis can be made.
Grade II: immunohistochemical staining shows S-100 positive in LC.
Grade III: visible Birbeck bodies or positive CD1a immunohistochemistry staining under electron microscope.

6.6.5.5 Immunohistochemistry

Positive CD1a (OKT-6) and langerin (CD207) are of the greatest diagnostic significance (Fig. 6.95). In addition, positive vimentin, CD11, S-100, and CD14, negative lymphocyte markers, and partial positive CD68 and lysozyme suggest the histiocyte origin of LC rather than lymphocyte lines.

6.6.5.6 Electron Microscopic Observation

Poor development of LC can be found, and Birbeck bodies in the cytoplasm are of diagnostic value with specificity [182] (Fig. 6.95).

6.6.5.7 Differential Diagnosis

The basis pathological change of LCH is sclerosing cholangitis, while LC is not visible in all cases, which makes it difficult to differentiate from primary sclerosing cholangitis; however, the latter is rare in children. Thus, the correct diagnosis of LC can be made if phenomenon in the portal area of a child's liver is discovered, including accumulation of histiocytes accompanied by infiltration of inflammatory cell, damage on bile ducts, the absence of small bile ducts, sclerosing cholangitis, cholestasis, confirmation of LC by immunohistochemical staining of S-100 and CD-1a, or visible LC in extrahepatic lesions. Moreover, IDC tumor is a progressive malignant tumor, which has long processed cytoplasm, decreased expression of CD-1a, and fewer Birbeck granules [181].

6.6.5.8 Treatment and Prognosis

LCH with hepatic involvement usually suggests a poor prognosis. However, the prognosis of patients varies greatly according to different ages, numbers, and severity of organs that are involved. LCH patients under 2 years old or over 65 years old with multiple organ involvement have a poorer prognosis. Generally, hepatic LCH is with a good prognosis, and the median follow-up period reaches 10 years and 6 months long. Yagita et al. (2001) reported a case of a 58-year-old patient who had hepatic and splenic LCH, including multiple lesions in the liver and a mass of 6 cm in diameter in the spleen. Excochleation of part of the hepatic lesions and splenectomy were conducted as well as CHOP chemotherapy, after which the volumes of the remaining hepatic lesions reduced, and the patients survived well 4 years later without recurrence, suggesting the benign nature of the LCH. Effective chemotherapy facilitates the reduction of the number and size of LCH lesions and long-term survival for the patients. For LCH patients with progressive sclerosing cholangitis, liver transplantation is an effective choice [183]. Hepatic LCH can be complicated by hepatocellular carcinoma in a few cases.

6.6.6 Spongiotic Pericytoma

Wen-Ming Cong and Yu-Yao Zhu
Department of Pathology, Eastern Hepatobiliary Surgery Hospital, Second Military Medical University, Shanghai, China

In 2005, Kaiserling et al. [185] reported a case of a 35-year-old woman with a history of several years' oral contraceptive, who received a surgical resection of a 6 cm×5 cm×3 cm spongiotic pericytoma. The cross section of the tumor was brownish red, with gray-white fibrous septa and a clear boundary with the surrounding tissue. Under the microscope, the spindle-shaped tumor cells were rich in translucent cytoplasm, with a vascular fibrous septa in the center, arranged in nests, in diffuse nodular distribution. Liver plates, hepatic lobule, and hepatic sinusoid remain in the tumor with no envelope. The immunohistochemical staining shows that the tumor cells express VI, CD34, CD105 (endoglin), CD99 (Mic1), CD56, and SMA, and the stroma cells around the tumor express collagens I, III, and V and fibronectin, while Syn and sGFAP are negative, and a small amount of CD105 (endoglin)-positive staining cells are found in the adjacent hepatic sinusoid, which are fibroblast-like but contain fat droplets under electron microscope. Kaiserling et al. suggested that the tumor was similar to cell tumor discovered in animal experiments, which expressed CD34 along with the hepatic sinusoidal endothelium, suggesting that the tumor derived from the lining cells of the hepatic sinusoid.

This is the only case report on human hepatic spongiotic pericytoma, and previous reports were on similar lesions in mice, rats, and fish induced by carcinogenic drugs on the liver [187, 188]. Karbe et al. [186] and Bannasch et al. [189] supported that astrocytoma is an independent tumor and that the tumor is the result of carcinogenic agents. However, Kerlin et al. [190] suggested that astrocytoma is not a true tumor. Though whether the tumor is benign or malignant has not been determined, it may have a good prognosis based on the evidence of low proliferation activity of the tumor cells and no recurrence or metastasis during the 12-month follow-up.

References

1. Rebouissou S, Bioulac-Sage P, Zucman-Rossi J. Molecular pathogenesis of focal nodular hyperplasia and hepatocellular adenoma. J Hepatol. 2008;48(1):163–70.
2. Van Aalten SM, Terkivatan T, De Man RA, et al. Diagnosis and treatment of hepatocellular adenoma in the Netherlands: similarities and differences. Dig Surg. 2010;27(1):61–7.
3. Socas L, Zumbado M, Perez-Luzardo O, et al. Hepatocellular adenomas associated with anabolic androgenic steroid abuse in bodybuilders: a report of two cases and a review of the literature. Br J Sports Med. 2005;39(5):e27.
4. Labrune P, Trioche P, Duvaltier I, et al. Hepatocellular adenomas in glycogen storage disease type I and III: a series of 43 patients and review of the literature. J Pediatr Gastroenterol Nutr. 1997;24(3):276–9.
5. Jeannot E, Mellottee L, Bioulac-Sage P, et al. Spectrum of HNF1A somatic mutations in hepatocellular adenoma differs from that in patients with MODY3 and suggests genotoxic damage. Diabetes. 2010;59(7):1836–44.
6. Bioulac-Sage P, Taouji S, Possenti L, et al. Hepatocellular adenoma subtypes: the impact of overweight and obesity. Liver Int. 2012;32(8):1217–21.
7. Chang CY, Hernandez-Prera JC, Roayaie S, et al. Changing epidemiology of hepatocellular adenoma in the United States: review of the literature. Int J Hepatol. 2013;2013:604860.
8. Liu HP, Cong WM. Hepatocellular adenoma: new understandings of molecular pathology and novel model of clinical diagnosis and therapy. Chin J Clin Hepatol. 2013;29(11):801–4.
9. Bioulac-Sage P, Laumonier H, Couchy G, et al. Hepatocellular adenoma management and phenotypic classification: the Bordeaux experience. Hepatology. 2009;50(2):481–9.
10. Grazioli L, Bondioni MP, Haradome H, et al. Hepatocellular adenoma and focal nodular hyperplasia: value of gadoxetic acid-enhanced MR imaging in differential diagnosis. Radiology. 2012;262(2):520–9.
11. Bioulac-Sage P, Rebouissou S, Thomas C, et al. Hepatocellular adenoma subtype classification using molecular markers and immunohistochemistry. Hepatology. 2007;46(3):740–8.
12. Zhang LH, Xu JJ. Molecular subtypes and clinical significance of Hepatocellular adenoma. Chin J Pathol. 2014;43(6):428–30.
13. Rebouissou S, Amessou M, Couchy G, et al. Frequent in-frame somatic deletions activate gp130 in inflammatory hepatocellular tumours. Nature. 2009;457(7226):200–4.
14. Bioulac-Sage P, Balabaud C, Zucman-Rossi J. Subtype classification of hepatocellular adenoma. Dig Surg. 2010;27(1):39–45.
15. Pan J, Cong WM. Analysis on loss of heterozygosity of four tumor suppressor genes in hepatocellular adenoma. Chin J Clin Exp Pathol. 2003;19(5):481–3.

16. Fu HH, JIN GZ, Liu HP, et al. Analysis of microsatellite instability in hepatocellular adenoma cases with overweight and obesity. Chin J Cancer Prev Treat. 2013;20(20):1557–60.
17. Chen LL, JI Y, Xu JF, et al. Focal nodular hyperplasia of liver: a clinicopathologic study of 238 patients. Chin J Pathol. 2011, 40(1): 17–22.
18. Tanaka J, Baba N, Arii S, et al. Typical fibrolamellar hepatocellular carcinoma in Japanese patients: report of two cases. Surg Today. 1994;24(5):459–63.
19. Nault JC, Bioulac-Sage P, Zucman-Rossi J. Hepatocellular benign tumors-from molecular classification to personalized clinical care. Gastroenterology. 2013;144(5):888–902.
20. Flejou JF, Barge J, Menu Y, et al. Liver adenomatosis. An entity distinct from liver adenoma? Gastroenterology. 1985;89(5):1132–8.
21. De Kock I, Mortele KJ, Smet B, et al. Hepatic adenomatosis: MR imaging features. JBR-BTR. 2014;97(2):105–8.
22. Liu LG, Wu F, Wu JX, et al. Hepatocellular adenoma and liver adenomatosis: a report of 11 patients. Chin J Hepatobiliary Surg. 2012;18(3):166–8.
23. Greaves WO, Bhattacharya B. Hepatic adenomatosis. Arch Pathol Lab Med. 2008;132(12):1951–5.
24. Asran MK, Loyer EM, Kaur H, et al. Case 177: congenital absence of the portal vein with hepatic adenomatosis. Radiology. 2012;262(1):364–7.
25. Babaoglu K, Binnetoglu FK, Aydogan A, et al. Hepatic adenomatosis in a 7-year-old child treated earlier with a Fontan procedure. Pediatr Cardiol. 2010;31(6):861–4.
26. Iwen KA, Klein J, Hubold C, et al. Maturity-onset diabetes of the young and hepatic adenomatosis - characterisation of a new mutation. Exp Clin Endocrinol Diabetes. 2013;121(6):368–71.
27. Shen WF, Yang JM. Diagnosis and treatment of hepatic adenoma and liver adenomatosis. Chin J Hepatobiliary Surg. 2007;13(9):646–8.
28. An C, Park S, Choi YJ. Diffusion-weighted MRI in intrahepatic bile duct adenoma arising from the cirrhotic liver. Korean J Radiol. 2013;14(5):769–75.
29. Koga F, Tanaka H, Takamatsu S, et al. A case of very large intrahepatic bile duct adenoma followed for 7 years. World J Clin Oncol. 2012;3(4):63–6.
30. Wu WW, Gu M, Lu D. Cytopathologic, histopathologic, and immunohistochemical features of intrahepatic clear cell bile duct adenoma: a case report and review of the literature. Case Rep Pathol. 2014;2014:874826.
31. Johannesen EJ, Wu Z, Holly JS. Bile duct adenoma with oncocytic features. Case Rep Pathol. 2014;2014:282010.
32. Albores-Saavedra J, Hoang MP, Murakata LA, et al. Atypical bile duct adenoma, clear cell type: a previously undescribed tumor of the liver. Am J Surg Pathol. 2001;25(7):956–60.
33. Arena V, Arena E, Stigliano E, et al. Bile duct adenoma with oncocytic features. Histopathology. 2006;49(3):318–20.
34. Hastir D, Verset L, Demetter P. Intrahepatic bile duct adenoma with oncocytic features. Liver Int. 2013;33(2):273.
35. Bhathal PS, Hughes NR, Goodman ZD. The so-called bile duct adenoma is a peribiliary gland hamartoma. Am J Surg Pathol. 1996;20(7):858–64.
36. Sasaki M, Matsubara T, Kakuda Y, et al. Immunostaining for polycomb group protein EZH2 and senescent marker p16INK4a may be useful to differentiate cholangiolocellular carcinoma from ductular reaction and bile duct adenoma. Am J Surg Pathol. 2014;38(3):364–9.
37. Komuta M, Spee B, Vander Borght S, et al. Clinicopathological study on cholangiolocellular carcinoma suggesting hepatic progenitor cell origin. Hepatology. 2008;47(5):1544–56.
38. Nishihara Y, Aishima S, Hayashi A, et al. CD10+ fibroblasts are more involved in the progression of hilar/extrahepatic cholangiocarcinoma than of peripheral intrahepatic cholangiocarcinoma. Histopathology. 2009;55(4):423–31.
39. Tretiakova M, Antic T, Westerhoff M, et al. Diagnostic utility of CD10 in benign and malignant extrahepatic bile duct lesions. Am J Surg Pathol. 2012;36(1):101 8.
40. Haas S, Gutgemann I, Wolff M, et al. Intrahepatic clear cell cholangiocarcinoma: immunohistochemical aspects in a very rare type of cholangiocarcinoma. Am J Surg Pathol. 2007;31(6):902–6.
41. Toriyama E, Nanashima A, Hayashi H, et al. A case of intrahepatic clear cell cholangiocarcinoma. World J Gastroenterol. 2010;16(20):2571–6.
42. Nakanuma Y, Tsutsui A, Ren XS, et al. What are the precursor and early lesions of peripheral intrahepatic cholangiocarcinoma? Int J Hepatol. 2014;2014:805973.
43. Rafiq E, Alaradi O, Bawany M, et al. A combination of snare polypectomy and apc therapy for prolapsing common bile duct adenoma. J Interv Gastroenterol. 2012;2(4):193–5.
44. Munshi AG, Hassan MA. Common bile duct adenoma: case report and brief review of literature. Surg Laparosc Endosc Percutan Tech. 2010;20(6):e193–4.
45. Soares KC, Arnaoutakis DJ, Kamel I, et al. Cystic neoplasms of the liver: biliary cystadenoma and cystadenocarcinoma. J Am Coll Surg. 2014;218(1):119–28.
46. Yang ZZ, Li Y, Liu J, et al. Giant biliary cystadenoma complicated with polycystic liver: a case report. World J Gastroenterol. 2013;19(37):6310–4.
47. Abhishek S, Jino T, Sarin GZ, et al. An uncommon cause of ascites: spontaneous rupture of biliary cystadenoma. Australas Med J. 2014;7(1):6–10.
48. Yu YQ, Lou BH, Yan HC, et al. Intrahepatic biliary cystadenoma presenting with pleural effusion. Chin Med J. 2012;125(7):1355–7.
49. Sang X, Sun Y, Mao Y, et al. Hepatobiliary cystadenomas and cystadenocarcinomas: a report of 33 cases. Liver Int. 2011;31(9):1337–44.
50. Wang C, Miao R, Liu H, et al. Intrahepatic biliary cystadenoma and cystadenocarcinoma: an experience of 30 cases. Dig Liver Dis. 2012;44(5):426–31.
51. Rayapudi K, Schmitt T, Olyaee M. Filling defect on ERCP: Biliary Cystadenoma, a Rare Tumor. Case Rep Gastroenterol. 2013;7(1):7–13.
52. Zen Y, Pedica F, Patcha VR, et al. Mucinous cystic neoplasms of the liver: a clinicopathological study and comparison with intraductal papillary neoplasms of the bile duct. Mod Pathol. 2011;24(8):1079–89.
53. Abdul-Al HM, Makhlouf HR, Goodman ZD. Expression of estrogen and progesterone receptors and inhibin-alpha in hepatobiliary cystadenoma: an immunohistochemical study. Virchows Arch. 2007;450(6):691–7.
54. Daniels JA, Coad JE, Payne WD, et al. Biliary cystadenomas: hormone receptor expression and clinical management. Dig Dis Sci. 2006;51(3):623–8.
55. Ahanatha Pillai S, Velayutham V, Perumal S, et al. Biliary cystadenomas: a case for complete resection. HPB Surg. 2012;2012:501705.
56. Kazama S, Hiramatsu T, Kuriyama S, et al. Giant intrahepatic biliary cystadenoma in a male: a case report, immunohistopathological analysis, and review of the literature. Dig Dis Sci. 2005;50(7):1384–9.
57. Ratti F, Ferla F, Paganelli M, et al. Biliary cystadenoma: short- and long-term outcome after radical hepatic resection. Updat Surg. 2012;64(1):13–8.
58. Diaz De Liano A, Olivera E, Artieda C, et al. Intrahepatic mucinous biliary cystadenoma. Clin Transl Oncol. 2007;9(10):678–80.

59. Delis SG, Touloumis Z, Bakoyiannis A, et al. Intrahepatic biliary cystadenoma: a need for radical resection. Eur J Gastroenterol Hepatol. 2008;20(1):10–4.
60. Meng XF, Li J, Zhang WZ, et al. Intrahepatic biliary cystadenoma: experience with 10 consecutive cases at a single center. J South Med Univ. 2011;31(10):1733–6.
61. Sun ZP, Peng C, Jiang B, et al. Intrahepatic biliary cystadenoma: diagnosis and Treatment experience of 15 cases. J Clin Res. 2013;30(5):1030–2.
62. Shen H. Diagnoses and treatments of 11 cases of intrahepatic Bile Duct Cystadenoma. Zhejiang Pract Med. 2012;17(3):196–8.
63. Romagnoli R, Patrono D, Paraluppi G, et al. Liver transplantation for symptomatic centrohepatic biliary cystadenoma. Clin Res Hepatol Gastroenterol. 2011;35(5):408–13.
64. Yeh TS, Tseng JH, Chen TC, et al. Characterization of intrahepatic cholangiocarcinoma of the intraductal growth-type and its precursor lesions. Hepatology. 2005;42(3):657–64.
65. Lee SS, Kim MH, Lee SK, et al. Clinicopathologic review of 58 patients with biliary papillomatosis. Cancer. 2004;100(4):783–93.
66. Zhang XF, Qiu FB, He JC, et al. Clinical epidemiology of biliary papillomatosis in China during the past 32 years(1979~2011). Chin J Curr Adv Gen Surg. 2012;15(6):455–8.
67. Nakanuma Y, Sato Y, Ojima H, et al. Clinicopathological characterization of so-called "cholangiocarcinoma with intraductal papillary growth" with respect to "intraductal papillary neoplasm of bile duct (IPNB)". Int J Clin Exp Pathol. 2014;7(6):3112–22.
68. White AD, Young AL, Verbeke C, et al. Biliary papillomatosis in three Caucasian patients in a Western centre. Eur J Surg Oncol. 2012;38(2):181–4.
69. Sasaki M, Matsubara T, Yoneda N, et al. Overexpression of enhancer of zeste homolog 2 and MUC1 may be related to malignant behaviour in intraductal papillary neoplasm of the bile duct. Histopathology. 2013;62(3):446–57.
70. Murakami S, Ajiki T, Hori Y, et al. Establishment of a novel cell line from intraductal papillary neoplasm of the bile duct. Anticancer Res. 2014;34(5):2203–9.
71. Rocha FG, Lee H, Katabi N, et al. Intraductal papillary neoplasm of the bile duct: a biliary equivalent to intraductal papillary mucinous neoplasm of the pancreas? Hepatology. 2012;56(4):1352–60.
72. Kim KM, Lee JK, Shin JU, et al. Clinicopathologic features of intraductal papillary neoplasm of the bile duct according to histologic subtype. Am J Gastroenterol. 2012;107(1):118–25.
73. Tsui WM, Loo KT, Chow LT, et al. Biliary adenofibroma. A heretofore unrecognized benign biliary tumor of the liver. Am J Surg Pathol. 1993;17(2):186–92.
74. Parada LA, Bardi G, Hallen M, et al. Monosomy 22 in a case of biliary adenofibroma. Cancer Genet Cytogenet. 1997;93(2):183–4.
75. Akin O, Coskun M. Biliary adenofibroma with malignant transformation and pulmonary metastases: CT findings. AJR Am J Roentgenol. 2002;179(1):280–1.
76. Varnholt H, Vauthey JN, Dal Cin P, et al. Biliary adenofibroma: a rare neoplasm of bile duct origin with an indolent behavior. Am J Surg Pathol. 2003;27(5):693–8.
77. Xu L, Wang FS, Chen L, et al. Biliary adenofibroma of the liver: report of a case. Chin J Gen Surg. 2009;11:925–925.
78. Gurrera A, Alaggio R, Leone G, et al. Biliary adenofibroma of the liver: report of a case and review of the literature. Pathol Res Int, 2010, 504584.
79. Fu XH, Chun KJ, Lu CD, et al. Hepatic cavernous hemangioma: an analysis of 172 cases. Chin J Pract Surg. 2009;9:756–8.
80. Mazereeuw-Hautier J, Hoeger PH, Benlahrech S, et al. Efficacy of propranolol in hepatic infantile hemangiomas with diffuse neonatal hemangiomatosis. J Pediatr. 2010;157(2):340–2.
81. Mo JQ, Dimashkieh HH, Bove KE. GLUT1 endothelial reactivity distinguishes hepatic infantile hemangioma from congenital hepatic vascular malformation with associated capillary proliferation. Hum Pathol. 2004;35(2):200–9.
82. Zhou W, Li A, Pan Z, et al. Selective hepatic vascular exclusion and Pringle maneuver: a comparative study in liver resection. Eur J Surg Oncol. 2008;34(1):49–54.
83. Mcgrath FP, Gibney RG, Morris DC, et al. Case report: multiple hepatic and pulmonary haemangioblastomas--a new manifestation of von Hippel-Lindau disease. Clin Radiol. 1992;45(1):37–9.
84. Hayasaka K, Tanaka Y, Satoh T, et al. Hepatic hemangioblastoma: an unusual presentation of von Hippel-Lindau disease. J Comput Assist Tomogr. 1999;23(4):565–6.
85. Rojiani AM, Owen DA, Berry K, et al. Hepatic hemangioblastoma. An unusual presentation in a patient with von Hippel-Lindau disease. Am J Surg Pathol. 1991;15(1):81–6.
86. Rapini N, Lidano R, Pietrosanti S, et al. De novo 13q13.3-21.31 deletion involving RB1 gene in a patient with hemangioendothelioma of the liver. Ital J Pediatr. 2014;40:5.
87. Riley MR, Garcia MG, Cox KL, et al. Hepatic infantile hemangioendothelioma with unusual manifestations. J Pediatr Gastroenterol Nutr. 2006;42(1):109–13.
88. Sondhi V, Kurkure PA, Vora T, et al. Successful management of multi-focal hepatic infantile hemangioendothelioma using TACE/surgery followed by maintenance metronomic therapy. BMJ Case Rep. 2012;2012:1–4.
89. Kochin IN, Miloh TA, Arnon R, et al. Benign liver masses and lesions in children: 53 cases over 12 years. Isr Med Assoc J. 2011;13(9):542–7.
90. Choi WJ, Jeong WK, Kim Y, et al. MR imaging of hepatic lymphangioma. Korean J Hepatol. 2012;18(1):101–4.
91. Ra SH, Bradley RF, Fishbein MC, et al. Recurrent hepatic lymphangiomatosis after orthotopic liver transplantation. Liver Transpl. 2007;13(11):1593–7.
92. Zhang YZ, Ye YS, Tian L, et al. Rare case of a solitary huge hepatic cystic lymphangioma. World J Clin Cases. 2013;1(4):152–4.
93. Datz C, Graziadei IW, Dietze O, et al. Massive progression of diffuse hepatic lymphangiomatosis after liver resection and rapid deterioration after liver transplantation. Am J Gastroenterol. 2001;96(4):1278–81.
94. Liu XW, Sun B, Guo TG. CT, MRI diagnosis of hepatic leiomyoma. Chin J Lab Diagn. 2011;5(15):2.
95. Liu Q, Liu J, Chen W, et al. Primary solitary fibrous tumors of liver: a case report and literature review. Diagn Pathol. 2013;8:195.
96. Fisher C. Atlas of soft tissue tumor pathology. New York/Heidelberg/Dordrecht/London: Springer; 2013.
97. Theise ND, Park YN, Curado MP, et al. Tumours of the liver and intrahepatic bile ducts. In: Bosman FT, Carneiro F, Hruban RH, et al., editors. WHO classification of tumours of the digestive system. Geneva: WHO Press; 2010. p. 195–261.
98. Beyer L, Delpero JR, Chetaille B, et al. Solitary fibrous tumor in the round ligament of the liver: a fortunate intraoperative discovery. Case Rep Oncol. 2012;5(1):187–94.
99. Yilmaz S, Kirimlioglu V, Ertas E, et al. Giant solitary fibrous tumor of the liver with metastasis to the skeletal system successfully treated with trisegmentectomy. Dig Dis Sci. 2000;45(1):168–74.
100. Wang H, Shen D, Hou Y. Malignant solitary tumor in a child: a case report and review of the literature. J Pediatr Surg. 2011;46(3):e5–9.
101. Munoz E, Prat A, Adamo B, et al. A rare case of malignant solitary fibrous tumor of the spinal cord. Spine (Phila Pa 1976). 2008;33(12):e397–9.

102. Sasaki H, Kurihara T, Katsuoka Y, et al. Distant metastasis from benign solitary fibrous tumor of the kidney. Case Rep Nephrol Urol. 2013;3(1):1–8.
103. Cong WM, Wu MC, Chen H, et al. Hepatic angiomyolipoma: a case report. Chin J Surg. 1992,30(10).618.
104. Ren N, Qin LX, Tang ZY, et al. Diagnosis and treatment of hepatic angiomyolipoma in 26 cases. World J Gastroenterol. 2003;9(8):1856–8.
105. Ji Y, Zhu X, Xu J, et al. Hepatic angiomyolipoma: a clinicopathologic study of 10 cases. Chin Med J. 2001;114(3):280–5.
106. You J, Xu W, Zhu JH. The diagnostic imaging and interventional therapy of hepatic angiomyolipoma associated with tuberous sclerosis. J Interven Radiology. 2001;10(6):333–5.
107. Wang JR, Qiu FB, Li ZC, et al. The epidemiological characteristics, diagnosis and treatment of hepatic angiomyolipoma(HAML) in China in the past 23 years. J Hepatopancreatobiliary Surg. 2012;24(3):183–7.
108. Wang JR, Qiu FB. Diagnosis and treatment of Hepatic Angiomyolipoma. Med Recapitulate. 2011;17(12):1826–8.
109. Zhu L, Hao YZ, Huang SL, et al. Ultrasonographic diagnosis of hepatic angiomyolipoma. Chin J Clin Oncol Rehabil. 2004;11(3):244–6.
110. Li SL, Qian JZ, Xu HM. Analysis of the imaging and clinicopathological features of hepatic angiomyolipoma. Chin J Gen Surg. 2011;20(7):696–9.
111. Yang B, Chen WH, Li QY, et al. Hepatic angiomyolipoma: dynamic computed tomography features and clinical correlation. World J Gastroenterol. 2009;15(27):3417–20.
112. Jeon TY, Kim SH, Lim HK, et al. Assessment of triple-phase CT findings for the differentiation of fat-deficient hepatic angiomyolipoma from hepatocellular carcinoma in non-cirrhotic liver. Eur J Radiol. 2010;73(3):601–6.
113. Zhang LP, Tang BH, Li LC, et al. CT features of epithelioid angiomyolipoma in liver: report of 2 cases and literature review. J Clin Radiology. 2012;31(12):1805–7.
114. Balci NC, Akinci A, Akun E, et al. Hepatic angiomyolipoma: demonstration by out of phase MRI. Clin Imaging. 2002;26(6):418–20.
115. Ji Y, Zhu XZ. Hepatic angiomyolipoma-a clinicopathologic study. Chin J Clin Exp Pathol. 2000;16(3):192–5.
116. Li M, Liu JS, Xu GR, et al. Clinicopathological Analysis for Hepatic Angioleiomyolipoma: a Report of Two Cases and Review of Literature. Chin J Clin Exp Pathol. 2012;28(9):1049–51.
117. Ji XL, Ji Y, Zhong DR, et al. Hepatic angiomyolipoma: a clinicopathological study of 21 cases. Chin J Diagn Pathol. 2001;8(5):267–9.
118. Tsui WM, Colombari R, Portmann BC, et al. Hepatic angiomyolipoma: a clinicopathologic study of 30 cases and delineation of unusual morphologic variants. Am J Surg Pathol. 1999;23(1):34–48.
119. Zhou Y, Chen F, Jiang W, et al. Hepatic epithelioid angiomyolipoma with an unusual pathologic appearance: expanding the morphologic spectrum. Int J Clin Exp Pathol. 2014;7(9):6364–9.
120. Nonomura A, Enomoto Y, Takeda M, et al. Angiomyolipoma of the liver: a reappraisal of morphological features and delineation of new characteristic histological features from the clinicopathological findings of 55 tumours in 47 patients. Histopathology. 2012;61(5):863–80.
121. Rao Q, Cheng L, Xia QY, et al. Cathepsin K expression in a wide spectrum of perivascular epithelioid cell neoplasms (PEComas): a clinicopathological study emphasizing extrarenal PEComas. Histopathology. 2013;62(4):642–50.
122. Makhlouf HR, Ishak KG, Shekar R, et al. Melanoma markers in angiomyolipoma of the liver and kidney: a comparative study. Arch Pathol Lab Med. 2002;126(1):49–55.
123. Lenci I, Angelico M, Tisone G, et al. Massive hepatic angiomyolipoma in a young woman with tuberous sclerosis complex: significant clinical improvement during tamoxifen treatment. J Hepatol. 2008;48(6):1026–9.
124. Gennatas C, Michalaki V, Kairi PV, et al. Successful treatment with the mTOR inhibitor everolimus in a patient with perivascular epithelioid cell tumor. World J Surg Oncol. 2012;10:181.
125. Higa F, Uchihara T, Haranaga S, et al. Malignant epithelioid angiomyolipoma in the kidney and liver of a patient with pulmonary lymphangioleiomyomatosis: lack of response to sirolimus. Intern Med. 2009;48(20):1821–5.
126. Deng YF, Lin Q, Zhang SH, et al. Malignant angiomyolipoma in the liver: a case report with pathological and molecular analysis. Pathol Res Pract. 2008;204(12):911–8.
127. Folpe AL, Mentzel T, Lehr HA, et al. Perivascular epithelioid cell neoplasms of soft tissue and gynecologic origin: a clinicopathologic study of 26 cases and review of the literature. Am J Surg Pathol. 2005;29(12):1558–75.
128. Brimo F, Robinson B, Guo C, et al. Renal epithelioid angiomyolipoma with atypia: a series of 40 cases with emphasis on clinicopathologic prognostic indicators of malignancy. Am J Surg Pathol. 2010;34(5):715–22.
129. Martin-Benitez G, Marti-Bonmati L, Barber C, et al. Hepatic lipomas and steatosis: an association beyond chance. Eur J Radiol. 2012;81(4):e491–4.
130. Moreno Gonzalez E, Seoane Gonzalez JB, Bercedo Martinez J, et al. Hepatic myelolipoma: new case and review of the literature. Hepato-Gastroenterology. 1991;38(1):60–3.
131. Allison KH, Mann GN, Norwood TH, et al. An unusual case of multiple giant myelolipomas: clinical and pathogenetic implications. Endocr Pathol. 2003;14(1):93–100.
132. Radhi J. Hepatic myelolipoma. J Gastrointestin Liver Dis. 2010;19(1):106–7.
133. Chen XX, Jiang XW, Huang W. Hepatic myelolipoma: a case report. Chin J Intern Med. 2010; 49(3):262–262.
134. Hayashi M, Takeshita A, Yamamoto K, et al. Primary hepatic benign schwannoma. World J Gastrointest Surg. 2012;4(3):73–8.
135. Kapoor S, Tevatia MS, Dattagupta S, et al. Primary hepatic nerve sheath tumor. Liver Int. 2005;25(2):458–9.
136. Kim YC, Park MS. Primary hepatic schwannoma mimicking malignancy on fluorine-18 2-fluoro-2-deoxy-D-glucose positron emission tomography-computed tomography. Hepatology. 2010;51(3):1080–1.
137. Zacharia TT, Jaramillo D, Poussaint TY, et al. MR imaging of abdominopelvic involvement in neurofibromatosis type 1: a review of 43 patients. Pediatr Radiol. 2005;35(3):317–22.
138. Malagari K, Drakopoulos S, Brountzos E, et al. Plexiform neurofibroma of the liver: findings on mr imaging, angiography, and CT portography. AJR Am J Roentgenol. 2001;176(2):493–5.
139. Delgado J, Jaramillo D, Ho-Fung V, et al. MRI features of plexiform neurofibromas involving the liver and pancreas in children with neurofibromatosis type 1. Clin Radiol. 2014;69(6):e280–4.
140. Imbert JP, Pilleul F, Valette PJ. Value of MRI in hepatic plexiform neurofibromatosis. Case report. Gastroenterol Clin Biol. 2002;26(8–9):791–3.
141. Robertson KA, Nalepa G, Yang FC, et al. Imatinib mesylate for plexiform neurofibromas in patients with neurofibromatosis type 1: a phase 2 trial. Lancet Oncol. 2012;13(12):1218–24.
142. Ucar C, Caliskan U, Toy H, et al. Hepatoblastoma in a child with neurofibromatosis type I. Pediatr Blood Cancer. 2007;49(3):357–9.
143. Andreu V, Elizalde I, Mallafre C, et al. Plexiform neurofibromatosis and angiosarcoma of the liver in von Recklinghausen disease. Am J Gastroenterol. 1997;92(7):1229–30.

144. Lederman SM, Martin EC, Laffey KT, et al. Hepatic neurofibromatosis, malignant schwannoma, and angiosarcoma in von Recklinghausen's disease. Gastroenterology. 1987;92(1):234–9.
145. Kakitsubata Y, Kakitsubata S, Sonoda T, et al. Neurofibromatosis type 1 involving the liver: ultrasound and CT manifestations. Pediatr Radiol. 1994;24(1):66–7.
146. Levi Sandri GB, Ettorre GM, Vennarecci G. Hepatic angiomyolipoma and neurofibromatosis type 2: a novel association. Liver Int. 2014;34(9):1445.
147. Miller MB, Tonsgard JH, Soltani K. Late-onset neurofibromatosis in a liver transplant recipient. Int J Dermatol. 2000;39(5):376–9.
148. Yohay KH. The genetic and molecular pathogenesis of NF1 and NF2. Semin Pediatr Neurol. 2006;13(1):21–6.
149. Maruta H. Effective neurofibromatosis therapeutics blocking the oncogenic kinase PAK1. Drug Discov Ther. 2011;5(6):266–78.
150. Roman SA, Sosa JA. Functional paragangliomas presenting as primary liver tumors. South Med J. 2007;100(2):195–6.
151. Koh PS, Koong JK, Westerhout CJ, et al. Education and imaging. Hepatobiliary and pancreatic: A huge liver paraganglioma. J Gastroenterol Hepatol. 2013;28(7):1075.
152. Zhang L, Liao Q, Hu Y, et al. Paraganglioma of the pancreas: a potentially functional and malignant tumor. World J Surg Oncol. 2014;12(1):218.
153. Baba Y, Beppu T, Imai K, et al. A case of adrenal rest tumor of the liver: radiological imaging and immunohistochemical study of steroidogenic enzymes. Hepatol Res. 2008;38(11):1154–8.
154. Yan ML, Wang YD, Tian YF, et al. Adenocarcinoma arising from intrahepatic heterotopic pancreas: a case report and literature review. World J Gastroenterol. 2012;18(22):2881–4.
155. Guillou L, Nordback P, Gerber C, et al. Ductal adenocarcinoma arising in a heterotopic pancreas situated in a hiatal hernia. Arch Pathol Lab Med. 1994;118(5):568–71.
156. Naoe H, Iwasaki H, Kawasaki T, et al. Primary hepatic gastrinoma as an unusual manifestation of zollinger-ellison syndrome. Case Rep Gastroenterol. 2012;6(3):590–5.
157. Moriura S, Ikeda S, Hirai M, et al. Hepatic gastrinoma. Cancer. 1993;72(5):1547–50.
158. Diaz R, Aparicio J, Pous S, et al. Primary hepatic gastrinoma. Dig Dis Sci. 2003;48(8):1665–7.
159. Tsalis K, Vrakas G, Vradelis S, et al. Primary hepatic gastrinoma: report of a case and review of literature. World J Gastrointest Pathophysiol. 2011;2(2):26–30.
160. Ogawa S, Wada M, Fukushima M, et al. Case of primary hepatic gastrinoma: diagnostic usefulness of the selective arterial calcium injection test. Hepatol Res. 2014;45(7):823–6.
161. Ayub A, Zafar M, Abdulkareem A, et al. Primary hepatic vipoma. Am J Gastroenterol. 1993;88(6):958–61.
162. Hachicha I, Zayene A, Mnif Hachicha L, et al. Primary hepatic vipoma. Gastroenterol Clin Biol. 2003;27(5):551–4.
163. Ohwada S, Joshita T, Ishihara T, et al. Primary liver somatostatinoma. J Gastroenterol Hepatol. 2003;18(10):1218–9.
164. Morisawa Y, Tanaka A, Yamamoto T, et al. Primary hepatic somatostatinoma developed in a patient with von Recklinghausen's disease. J Gastroenterol. 2006;41(4):389–91.
165. Do Cao C, Mekinian A, Ladsous M, et al. Hypercalcitonemia revealing a somatostatinoma. Ann Endocrinol (Paris). 2010;71(6):553–7.
166. Zhang ZY, Zhou GW, Shen C, et al. Liver transplantation revealing a case of metastatic pancreatic somatostatinoma. Chin J Surg. 2007;45(15):1075–6.
167. Rosenau J, Bahr MJ, Von Wasielewski R, et al. Ki67, E-cadherin, and p53 as prognostic indicators of long-term outcome after liver transplantation for metastatic neuroendocrine tumors. Transplantation. 2002;73(3):386–94.
168. Einarsson JI, Edwards CL, Zurawin RK. Immature ovarian teratoma in an adolescent: a case report and review of the literature. J Pediatr Adolesc Gynecol. 2004;17(3):187–9.
169. Karlo C, Leschka S, Dettmer M, et al. Hepatic teratoma and peritoneal gliomatosis: a case report. Cases J. 2009;2:9302.
170. Col C. Immature teratoma in both mediastinum and liver of a 21-Year-old female patient. Acta Med Austriaca. 2003;30(1):26–8.
171. Certo M, Franca M, Gomes M, et al. Liver teratoma. Acta Gastroenterol Belg. 2008;71(2):275–9.
172. Rout P, Rameshkumar K, Srikrishna NV. Hepatic mesothelioma. Indian J Gastroenterol. 1999;18(4):176–7.
173. Flemming P, Becker T, Klempnauer J, et al. Benign cystic mesothelioma of the liver. Am J Surg Pathol. 2002;26(11):1523–7.
174. Wang JB, Cao BK. One case of hepatic fibrous mesothelioma. Chin J Gen Surg. 2004;19(12):715–715.
175. Zhang JP, Ni JL. One case of large hepatic myxoma. Chin J Hepatobiliary Surg. 2007;9(13):610–1.
176. Badalian-Very G, Vergilio JA, Degar BA, et al. Recurrent BRAF mutations in Langerhans cell histiocytosis. Blood. 2010;116(11):1919–23.
177. Wu ZS, Li DH, Kong LB, et al. One case of liver Langerhans cell histiocytosis. Chin J Hepatobiliary Surg. 2012;18(2):138–138.
178. Hu X, Dong A, Lv S, et al. F-18 FDG PET/CT imaging of solitary liver Langerhans cell histiocytosis: preliminary findings. Ann Nucl Med, 2012, 2012.
179. Shi Y, Qiao Z, Xia C, et al. Hepatic involvement of Langerhans cell histiocytosis in children–imaging findings of computed tomography, magnetic resonance imaging and magnetic resonance cholangiopancreatography. Pediatr Radiol. 2014;44(6):713–8.
180. Braier J, Ciocca M, Latella A, et al. Cholestasis, sclerosing cholangitis, and liver transplantation in Langerhans cell Histiocytosis. Med Pediatr Oncol. 2002;38(3):178–82.
181. Ma J, Jiang Y, Chen X, et al. Langerhans cell histiocytosis misdiagnosed as liver cancer and pituitary tumor in an adult: a case report and brief review of the literature. Oncol Lett. 2014;7(5):1602–4.
182. Valladeau J, Ravel O, Dezutter-Dambuyant C, et al. Langerin, a novel C-type lectin specific to Langerhans cells, is an endocytic receptor that induces the formation of Birbeck granules. Immunity. 2000;12(1):71–81.
183. Lee RJ, Leung C, Lim EJ, et al. Liver transplantation in an adult with sclerosing cholangitis due to multisystem Langerhans cell histiocytosis. Am J Transplant. 2011;11(8):1755–6.
184. Kaplan KJ, Goodman ZD, Ishak KG. Liver involvement in Langerhans' cell histiocytosis: a study of nine cases. Mod Pathol. 1999;12(4):370–8.
185. Kaiserling E, Muller H. Neoplasm of hepatic stellate cells (spongiotic pericytoma): a new tumor entity in human liver. Pathol Res Pract. 2005;201(11):733–43.
186. Karbe E, Kerlin RL. Cystic degeneration/Spongiosis hepatis in rats. Toxicol Pathol. 2002;30(2):216–27.
187. Couch JA. Spongiosis hepatis: chemical induction, pathogenesis, and possible neoplastic fate in a teleost fish model. Toxicol Pathol. 1991;19(3):237–50.
188. Stroebel P, Mayer F, Zerban H, et al. Spongiotic pericytoma: a benign neoplasm deriving from the perisinusoidal (Ito) cells in rat liver. Am J Pathol. 1995;146(4):903–13.
189. Bannasch P. Comments on R. Karbe and R. L. Kerlin (2002). Cystic degeneration/spongiosis hepatis (Toxicol Pathol 30 (2), 216–227). Toxicol Pathol, 2003, 31(5): 566–570.
190. Kerlin RL, Karbe E. Response to comments on E. Karbe and R. L. Kerlin (2002). Cystic degeneration/spongiosis hepatis (Toxicol Pathol 30(2): 216–227). Toxicol Pathol, 2004; 32(2): 271.

Malignant Tumors of the Liver and Intrahepatic Bile Ducts

7

Wen-Ming Cong, Hui Dong, Yu-Yao Zhu, and Zhen Zhu

7.1 Malignant Hepatocellular Tumors

Wen-Ming Cong
Department of Pathology, Eastern Hepatobiliary Surgery Hospital, Second Military Medical University, Shanghai, China

7.1.1 Hepatocellular Carcinoma

7.1.1.1 Epidemiology

It has been estimated that there are about 748,3000 cases of newly diagnosed liver cancer worldwide with a mortality of 695,900 cases each year. More than 80% of hepatocellular carcinoma (HCC) is discovered in sub-Saharan Africa or Asia, while the Western countries have a lower incidence. For example, the annual incidence rate of HCC in the United States is (1.5–4.9)/100,000 people. And according to the prediction by American Cancer Society, the new cases of liver cancer would reach 28,720, with 20,550 deaths in 2013, but it did not belong to the top ten malignant tumors with high incidence. In our country, the annual incidence of liver cancer was 25.7/100,000, and the mortality rate was 23.7/100,000, ranking the third and second the incidence and mortality of malignant tumor, respectively. Among 40,656 cases of hepatobiliary tumor diagnosed in the Department of Pathology, Eastern Hepatobiliary Surgery Hospital (EHBH),the Second Military Medical University during the past 30 years, malignant hepatic tumors account for 80% of all the cases, and the top two are HCC (86%) and intrahepatic cholangiocarcinoma (ICC, 8%). The number of surgical cases of both cancers is still increasing (Fig. 7.1), suggesting the high incidence of liver cancers in our country [1–3].

7.1.1.2 Histological Classification

The World Health Organization (WHO) formulated the *Histological Classification of Hepatic and Intrahepatobiliary Tumors* (2010 edition) involving about 30 kinds of nodular space-occupying lesions [4]; however, the actual histological classification of hepatobiliary tumors is much more complex than the traditional understanding. We put forward "three types" based on the comprehensive data found in the domestic and foreign pathological studies on pathology of hepatic tumors, including tumor-like lesions (6%), benign tumors (11.1%), and malignant tumors (82.9%) (Fig. 7.2), and "six subtypes" including hepatocellular tumors; bile duct epithelial tumors; vascular, lymphoid, and hematopoietic tumors; muscle, fibrous, and adipocytic tumors; neuroendocrine tumors; and miscellaneous tumors, all of which were accounted for more than 100 kinds of pathological types of hepatobiliary tumors [5]. For a period of 30 years from January 1982 to December 2011, a total of more than 40,000 cases of large series of surgically resected hepatobiliary tumors were pathologically diagnosed in the Department of Pathology of EHBH, Second Military Medical University, which provides necessary evidences on histological classification in diagnosis, differential diagnosis, and treatment for pathologists and surgeons on the basis of a comprehensive knowledge of heaptobiliary tumor spectrum. Pathology on various kinds of hepatobiliary tumors needs to be further studied covering pathogenesis, pathodiagnostic criteria, and biological behaviors. Furthermore, hepatobiliary surgeons need to understand the pathological features of hepatobiliary tumors and put emphasis on the individual strategy of diagnosis, treatment, and prognosis evaluation according to the pathobiological characteristics of the tumors, thus constantly improving treatment levels in hepatobiliary surgery.

7.1.1.3 Pathogenesis and Mechanism

Currently, it is suggested that HCC relates to the following pathogenic factors:

W.-M. Cong (✉) • H. Dong • Y.-Y. Zhu • Z. Zhu
Department of Pathology, Eastern Hepatobiliary Surgery Hospital, Second Military Medical University, Shanghai, China
e-mail: wmcong@smmu.edu.cn

W.-M. Cong (ed.), *Surgical Pathology of Hepatobiliary Tumors*, DOI 10.1007/978-981-10-3536-4_7

Fig. 7.1 The proportion of surgical resected HCC/ICC in the EHBH over the 30 years

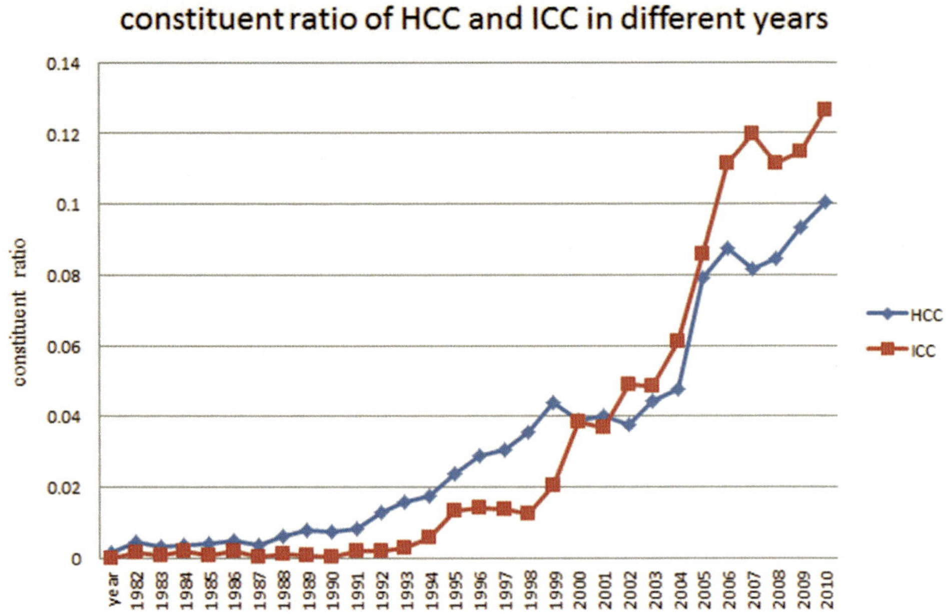

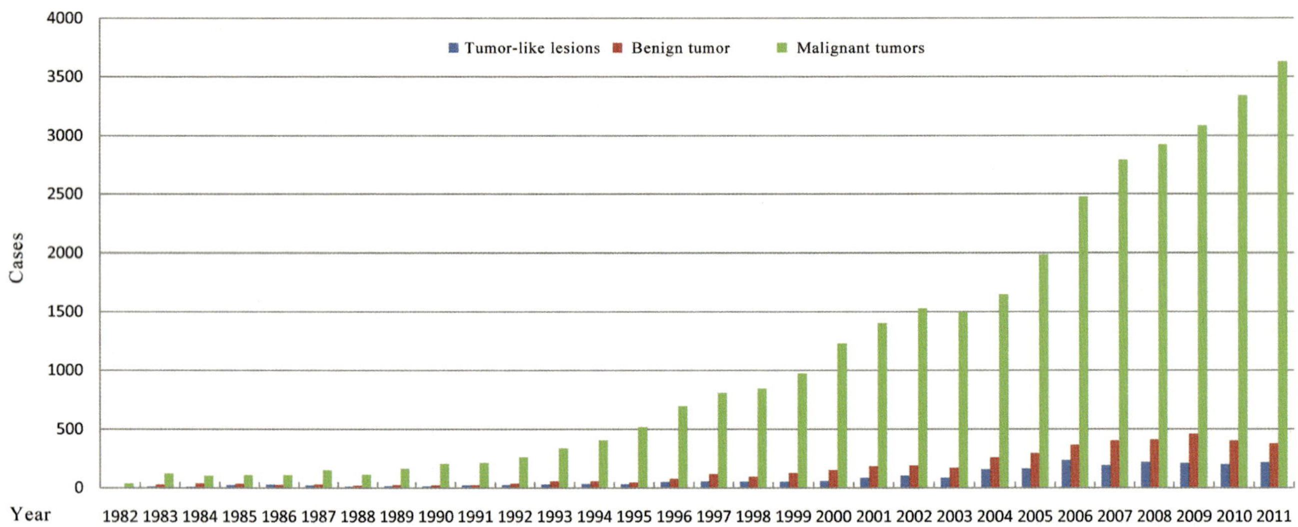

Fig. 7.2 Surgical resection of hepatobiliary tumors during the 30-year period in the EHBH

(1) Infection of hepatitis viruses

1. Infection of hepatitis B virus (HBV). According to the estimation by WHO, about two billion out of six billion of the world's populations have infected with HBV, and 300 million people suffer from chronic HBV infection. In China, HCC with HBV infection is the most common epidemiological manifestations, and HBV infection is the main cause for 75–95% of HCC cases. Generally, patients with positive serum HBsAg for more than 6 months are known to have chronic HBV infection, and the risk of developing HCC in chronic HBV carriers is 200 times higher than that in non-HBV carriers. According to the national epidemiological survey on serum in 1992, HBV infection rate was about 60% in the population, with 700–800 million people infected with HBV, and the number of HBV carriers was about 120 million. However, the national epidemiological survey on serum epidemiology carried out by the Ministry of Health of China in 2006 demonstrated that HBsAg carrying rate in Chinese population was 7.18% and the carrying rate of HBsAg in children under 4 years old was lower than 1%. From the perspective of HBsAg carrying rate and HBV prevalence rate, the number of children infected with HBV in China had reduced by nearly 80 million people since 1992, with a reduction of nearly 19 million children carriers of HBsAg, and the national inoculation rate of hepatitis B vaccine had been raised

from 39.95% in 1995 to 94.2% in 2005 according to the related investigations in China. And by 2010, both the incidence of hepatitis B and the rate of hepatitis B surface antigen carrying have decreased significantly, which is of great significance for the primary prevention of liver cancers and reduction in the incidence.

Based on the statistics of HCC patients who received surgical resection during the past 30-year period in the EHBH, the infection rate of HBV (either serum or immunohistochemical HBsAg positive) in these HCC patients was 85.86%. Due to the large population infected with HBV, the carrying rate of hepatitis B surface antigen in people aged from 15 to 59 years old was 8.57%. And according to the data released by Chinese Society of Hepatology, Chinese Medical Association, among about 93 million people with chronic HBV infection in China, there were 20 million patients, and the number of HBV infections would continue to increase in the future. Furthermore, 15–25% of people with chronic HBV infection develop into hepatic cirrhosis or liver cancer, which is the major cause responsible for the high incidence of HCC in China currently; thus, prevention and treatment of liver cancers are long and arduous tasks.

Researchers showed that the insertion of HBV-DNA gene into adjacent regions of the cancer gene or suppressor genes in the liver cells would cis-change the function of the gene resulting in disruption of related protein-encoding sequence. The integration of HBx gene into the host genome is the most crucial event, which can be found in genes of any length, and in 96% of the HCC specimens, all X genes are found to insert into the host cell DNA in the truncated form, suggesting trans-carcinogenic effects of the truncated X protein, such as exertion of the trans-transcription activity by the interaction between protein and protein. X protein encoded by HBx gene is a multifunctional regulatory protein and plays a key regulatory role in viral infection, replication, pathogenic, and carcinogenic processes. HBV integration results in a series of molecular variations, such as insertion mutation into the host genome, upregulated transcription driven by virus promoter, human-virus transcriptional fusion, variation of DNA copy number and induction of genomic instability, including activation of oncogenes (such as C-myc, KRAS, C-fos, IGF- II, IGF-IR) via trans-activation mechanism, inactivation of tumor suppressor genes (such as p53, RB, Bcl-2, DNA mismatch repair genes), regulation of epigenetic proteins via mediation of DNA methylation, or regulation of cell apoptosis, DNA damage and repair, cell cycle, and miRNA functions through transcriptional activation of various signal transduction pathways to promote the abnormal proliferation of liver cells leading to the formation of HCC, which is HBV-DNA integrated-type HCC. Recent studies demonstrated HBx can induce epithelium-mesenchymal transformation (EMT) via PI3K/AKT/GSK3β/Snail signaling pathway, promote the invasion and metastasis of HBV-HCC via formation of HBx-YAP conjugates [6, 7], or exert target inhibition of the function of tumor suppressor genes by regulating miRNA.

2. Infection of hepatitis C virus (HCV). The global population of HCV infection reaches about 170 million, and there are about 35,000 new cases emerging each year. The Japanese HCV-related HCC account for 80–90% of all the cases. And the national serum epidemiological survey of China for virus hepatitis in 2006 showed that the prevalence rate of anti-HCV was 0.43% in Chinese population aged 1–59 years old, indicating that China was a low HCV endemic area in the global scope; however, the infection rate in China is increasing. It has been evaluated that the number of cumulative HCV infection in China exceeded 43 million. The serum anti-HCV positive rate in Chinese HCC patients is 6–32%, and the statistics of patients with HCC treated in the EHBH during the period of 30 years showed that HCV infection rate was 9.76%.

HCV is a single-stranded RNA virus encoding a single polyprotein precursor of about 3000 amino acids, generating more than ten proteins, among which NS5A protein, a transcription factor for cell growth, plays a key role in the canceration of liver cells through interaction with other proteins, such as participation in HCV protein mutation and replication of RNA, regulation of the expression of multiple genes in the host cells, stimulation of cell proliferation, inhibition of apoptosis, and reducing the curative effects of interferon [8]. Wurmbach et al. (2007) studied the signal pathways involving multiple stages in the development of HCV-related HCC and found dysregulation of several pathways, including Notch- and Toll-like receptor in the precancerous stage of hepatic cirrhosis, and several components of JAK/STAT pathway in the early stage of carcinogenesis, upregulation of expression of genes participating in DNA replication, and repair and cell cycle in late stage of carcinogenesis [9]. Because of no discovery of reverse transcriptase in the liver cells, HCV cannot integrate into the host genome but produce severe cytotoxic damage on the infected liver cells and modification of the host's immune system through indirect interaction similar to oncogene proteins. In order to evade the host immune surveillance, HCV can constantly mutate to form variant strains after infection of host cells, resulting in constant degeneration necrosis, repeated regeneration, and proliferation of the host cells and finally causing chronic hepatic injury [10].

Generally, about 20% of the chronic HCV hepatitis will develop into hepatic cirrhosis, including 1–4% of the cases evolving into HCC. Therefore, the development from infection of HBV or HCV to HCC generally includes a stage ofchronic hepatitis and cirrhosis. Compared with HBV hepatitis, the period for chronic hepatitis HCV to develop into hepatic cirrhosis may be shorter. According to statistics of 26,330 cases of surgically excised HCC diagnosed in the Department of Pathology of EHBH, patients with cirrhosis accounted for 73% of all the cases. From the temporal perspective, the proportion of HCC cases with hepatic cirrhosis reached 95–100% before 2000, while it was 50–95% for HCC cases diagnosed after 2001, suggesting a potential increase in the number of non-cirrhotic HCC, and the pathological significance of this type of HCC needs further studies. For patients of chronic hepatitis or cirrhosis with persistent positive serum HBV/HCV, regardless of clinical symptoms and signs, physical examinations should be carried out regularly, including the monitoring of HCC markers, such as serum AFP, and standardized antiviral treatment should be adopted.

(2) Environmental pollution

1. Food contamination aflatoxin (AFB1) is highly mutagenic, teratogenic, and carcinogenic and belongs to the first-degree carcinogens. High intake of AFB1 is associated with the pathogenesis of HCC in high-incidence area [11]. AFB1 can integrate with DNA in the liver cells to form AFB1-DNA adducts. The results of immunohistochemistry show that positive signals of AFB1-DNA adduct are located in the nuclei of the hepatocytes, the expression level of which is a biomarker reflecting the degree of AFB1 exposure. It can induce the transversion of arginine (AGG) to serine (AGT) on codon 249th of p53 gene in synergy with HBV, inducing gene mutation, or directly induce chromosome aberration. It has been shown that the exposure dose of AFB1 is 10–200 ng/kg in population in endemic areas of HCC, such as Southeast Asia, Africa, and Asia-Sahara area, while it is less than 3 ng/kg in the United States. Therefore, it is of importance to avoid intake of AFB1-contaminated food for the prevention of HCC.
2. Drinking water contamination. The pollution of drinking water by substances, such as ammonia nitrogen, nitrite nitrogen, blue-green algae toxin, and humic acid, is closely related to the pathogenesis of HCC, and microcystin has a synergistic effect on the induction of HCC with chemical substances, such as AFB1.
3. Environmental pollution. Chemical substances used in industries, such as vinyl chloride, phenol, arsenic, and aromatic amine compounds, have a strong induction effect on HCC.

(3) Obesity and diabetes

According to a recent survey, children aged 7–13 years of age with an excess body mass index (BMI) have a significantly higher risk of HCC in their adulthood. An American study showed that patients with BMI $\geq$ 35 kg/m^2 have a morality rate 4.5 times higher than that of the people with a normal BMI, and the relative risks of HCC in people with overweight and obesity are 117% and 189%, respectively. The risk of HCC developing in diabetic patients increases by three times compared to their nondiabetic counterparts [12]. The incidences of nonalcoholic fatty liver disease (NAFLD) in many countries have increased significantly, and it has become the second major liver disease after viral hepatitis. The cumulative incidence rate of HCC with NAFLD-related cirrhosis is 2.6%. And in the past 10 years, at least 300 cases of NAFLD with HCC have been reported in the literature, and defined risk factors for NAFLD include obesity, diabetes, hyperlipidemia, and insulin resistance. About 20% cases of NAFLD are complicated by fatty hepatitis, the latter of which is a risk factor for the development of cirrhosis and HCC. A German study showed that fatty hepatitis is an underlying cause in 24% of HCC patients, and average 55% of HCV patients in Western countries have NAFLD. In addition, there are also cases of HCC developed from non-cirrhosis NAFLD and nonfibrous fatty hepatitis.

(4) Genome variation

Mutations of cancer genes and/or inactivation of tumor suppressor genes (TSG) results in canceration of liver cells due to lack of regulation in signal transduction, cell cycle and growth, and proliferation by normal genes. The various molecular mechanisms and molecular types of HCC genomic variation are complex, and it has been found that human body has at least more than 1000 HCC-related genes with increasing discoveries of new HCC-related oncogenes, tumor suppressor genes, signal transduction pathways, and molecular targets. For example, He et al. (2011) conducted a genome-wide SNP microarray analysis on HCC tissues, screened out 1241 somatic copy number variation regions, and further identified 362 differentially expressed genes. They found that 60% of the HCC demonstrated lower expression >twofolds of TRIM35 gene which is a tumor suppressor and inhibits the proliferation of HCC cells. Higher expression (>twofolds) of HEY1 gene was found in 42.6% of the HCC, which is a cancer gene and promotes the proliferation of HCC cells [13]. Li et al. (2011) conducted a detection study on 18 thousand exons of coding genes using massively parallel sequencing technique, finding that 18.2% of HCV-HCC cases contain inactivating mutations of ARID2 gene, suggesting that it is a tumor suppressor gene for HCC [14]. A China-US joint research demonstrated a study using whole genome sequencing (WGS), and the results showed that β-catenin gene was the most common oncogene which mutate (15.9%) in HBV-HCC tissue, and TP53 gene was most susceptible to inactivation of anti-oncogenes (35.2%), while Wnt/beta-catenin pathway (62.5%) and JAK/STAT pathway (45.5%) were two signal pathways in which variations are the most frequently found for HCC [15].

Liu et al. (2014) investigated chromosomal DNA copy number changes in HCC by comparative genomic hybridization and detected the overexpression (>2-folds) of a new oncogene Maelstrom (MAEL) in 59.7% of the HCC cases. The experimental results showed that the MAEL is located on chromosome 1q24 and can activate Akt/ GSK-3β/Snail signaling pathway, inducing epithelial-mesenchymal transition (EMT) to promote the invasion and metastasis of HCC, and it also correlates with the recurrence and prognosis of these patients [16]. DLC-1 (deleted in liver cancer-1) gene is located on chromosome 8p21–22, encoding GTPase activator and can inhibit tumor metastasis. Deletion of DLC-1 gene has been found in 20% of HCC samples and 40% of HCC cell lines, and the growth of HCC cell strains transfected with DLC-1 was significantly inhibited, suggesting it is an inhibitory gene for HCC.

The biological characteristics of HCC are regulated by a complex cell signaling system, which are studied widely in aspects including the pathogenesis, growth, apoptosis, angiogenesis, invasion, metastasis, molecular therapeutic targets, and prognosis evaluation of HCC. And the representatives are tyrosine kinase pathway, Wnt/β-catenin pathway, P53 pathway, Notch pathway, NF-κB pathway, Hedgehog (Hh) pathway, Ras/Raf/MAPK pathway, VEGF pathway, JAK-STAT pathway, PI3K/Akt/mTOR pathway, HGF/c-Met pathway, and TGFβ1/Smads pathway, each of which is composed by diverse and complex key molecules. These pathways may be regulated by upstream miRNAs or target genes and exert the functions via the downstream target genes. Molecular analysis of molecules and function modes of HCC-related signal pathways is of clinical practice in aspects such as molecular typing, molecular diagnosis, and molecular-targeted therapy.

(5) Other factors

The association between alcoholic fatty liver disease (AFLD) and HCC has been recognized, and smoking can increase the risk of HCC development. And cases of HCC in patients with hereditary, congenital, allergic, or metabolic liver diseases, such as α1-antitrypsin protease deficiency, hereditary hemochromatosis, hereditary tyrosinemia, autoimmune hepatitis, primary biliary cirrhosis, have also been reported.

In a word, the genesis of HCC is a complex process involving multiple causes, mechanisms, steps, and genes. We briefly summarize the common causes of HCC, 16 key canceration mechanisms or research focus, and multistages during the pathological development (Fig. 7.3).

7.1.1.4 Clinical Features

According to the statistics of clinical data in 28,869 cases of surgically excised HCC cases in the Department of Pathology, Eastern Hepatobiliary Surgery Hospital, Second Military Medical University, the ratio of male to female was 6.72:1, and the average age of HCC patients in each year during the 30 years was stable at around the age of 50 years old, younger than the average age of ICC patients of 54.9 years old and older than the average age of patients with benign liver tumors of 44.9 years old. And 86% of the HCC patients had a history of HBV infection, while about 10% of the patients had a history of HCV infection. The serum AFP level increased with the growth of the tumor, and the positive rates of serum AFP were 69.6, 59.1, 57.6, and 68.2% in HCC

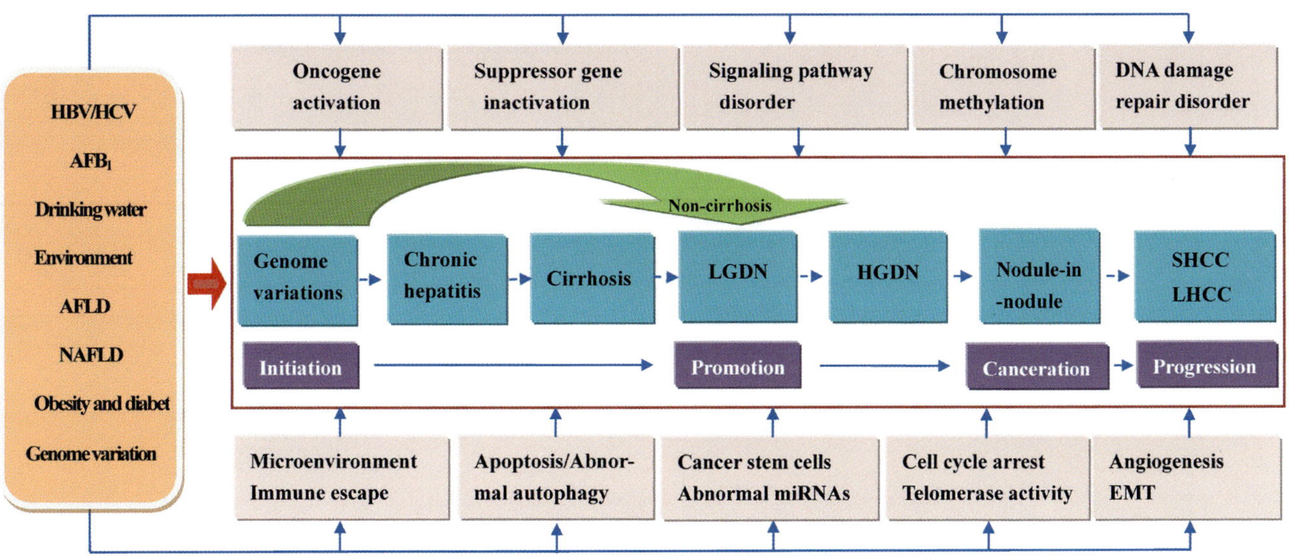

Fig. 7.3 Molecular mechanism of multistage carcinogenesis and progression of hepatocellular carcinoma

patients with tumors <1 cm, <2 cm, <3 cm, and >3 cm in diameter, respectively, with 20 μg/ml as the threshold, while the positive rates of serum AFP were 39.6, 25.7, 26.4, and 44.7% with 400 μg/ml as the threshold, showing that the serum AFP is still one of the serological markers for diagnosis of HCC, but negative serum AFP was found in more than 50% of these patients with HCC.

Most of HCC patients with tumor <3–5 cm in diameter are in early subclinical stage and may manifest no obvious clinical symptoms or signs, while the manifestations in HCC patients with tumors >3–5 cm in diameter include pain in hepatic zone, hepatosplenomegaly, general gastrointestinal symptoms (abdominal distention, diarrhea, decreased appetite), upper abdominal mass, fatigue, emaciation, persistent fever, jaundice, weight loss, abnormal liver function, and paraneoplastic syndrome.

According to clinical features, HCC can be divided into cirrhosis-type HCC characterized by hepatic cirrhosis, portal hypertension, and upper gastrointestinal hemorrhage; fever-type HCC with fever, increased white blood cells, and multiple concurrent infections, which is similar to liver abscess as the main characteristics; hepatitis-type HCC with progressive liver failure and hepatic encephalopathy (hepatic coma) in severe cases, similar to acute severe hepatitis; acute abdomen-type HCC with tumor rupture hemorrhage as the first symptom; cholestasis-type HCC manifested obstructive jaundice involving common bile duct; and metastasis-type HCC with metastasis of extrahepatic organs as the first clinical manifestation.

Type B ultrasonic (B-US) images display hypoechoic lesions in small HCC and hypoechoes or mixed echoes in large HCC, and the detection rate was 85–95% for lesions of 3–5 cm in diameter, while the sensitivity can reach 60–80% for lesions of 1 cm in diameter. Computer tomography (CT) images are more clear and stable with high resolution and show low densities for HCC lesions. Dynamic enhancement CT shows a curve of rapidly increased and then rapidly decreased densities of contrast agent in arterial phase, showing the characteristic "fast in fast out" performance. Magnetic resonance imaging (MRI) images of HCC is characterized by low signal on T_1-weighted images and high signal on T_2-weighted images, and MRI is especially sensitive for small lesions.

7.1.1.5 Gross Features

(1) Gross classification of HCC

Current gross classification of HCC mainly includes the following three models:

1. Eggel's classification: Suggested by Eggel (1901), the HCC can be divided into nodular type (<10 cm in diameter), massive type (>10 cm in diameter), and diffuse type (cancer nodules in varying sizes and diffuse distribution throughout the liver).
2. Chinese's classification: Formulated by Chinese Cooperation Group on Pathology of Liver Cancers in 1979 and included in *Standards of Diagnosis and Treatment for Malignant Tumors* promulgated by the Ministry of Health, the Chinese's classification divided HCC into five major types and six subtypes, namely:
   ① Diffuse type: small nodules in diffuse distribution in the liver.
   ② Giant block type: The tumor is >10 cm in diameter (Figs. 7.4 and 7.5).

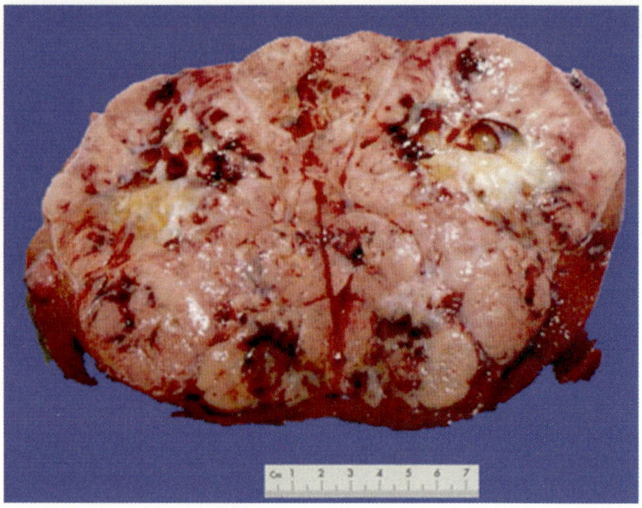

Fig. 7.4 HCC, giant block type, with liquefied necrosis and cystic changes

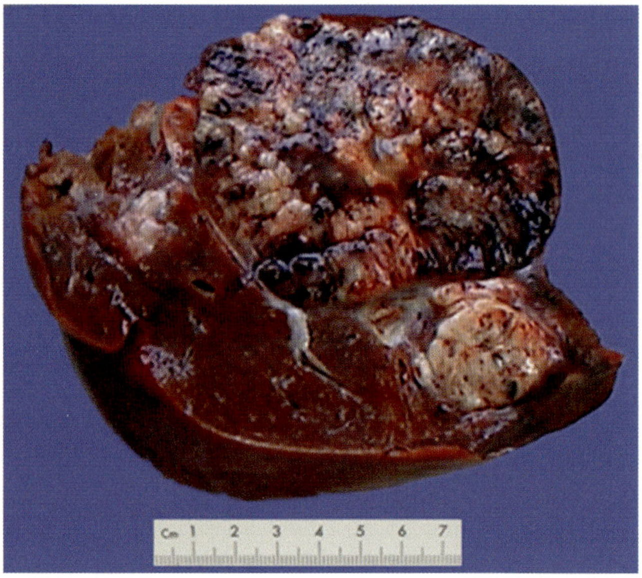

Fig. 7.5 HCC, giant block type, two nodules adjacent to the main tumor

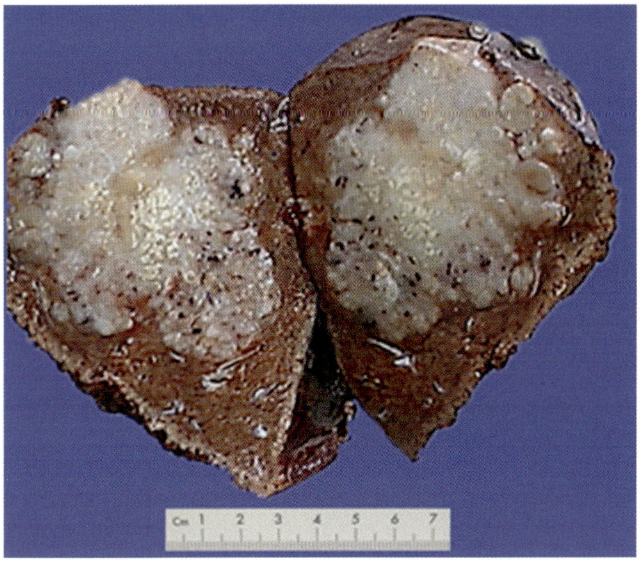

Fig. 7.6 HCC, block type, infiltrative growth without encapsulation

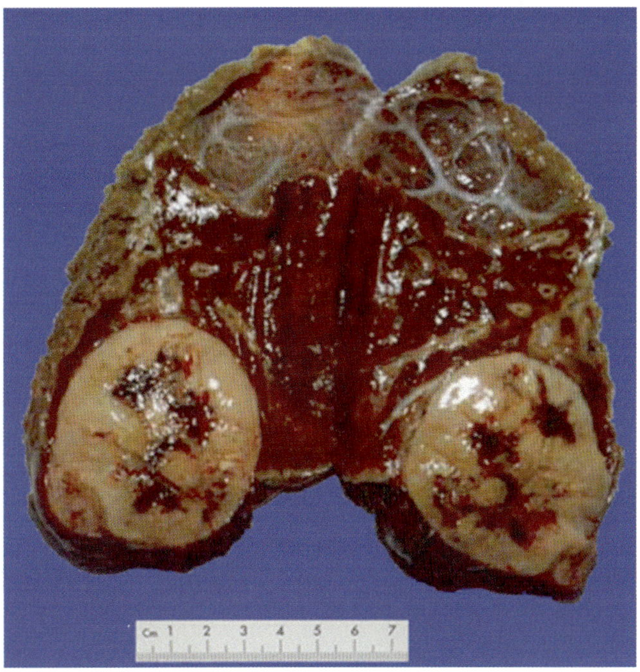

Fig. 7.7 HCC, solitary type, clear boundary with hepatic cyst

③ Block type: The tumor is 5–10 cm in diameter and can be divided into solitary (Fig. 7.6), confluent, and multiblock types according to the number and the morphology of the lesions.

④ Nodular type: The tumor is 3–5 cm in diameter and can be divided into solitary (Fig. 7.7), confluent (Fig. 7.8), and multinodular types (Fig. 7.9) according to the number and the morphology of the lesions.

⑤ Small HCC: Three nodules ≤3 cm in diameter (Fig. 7.10).

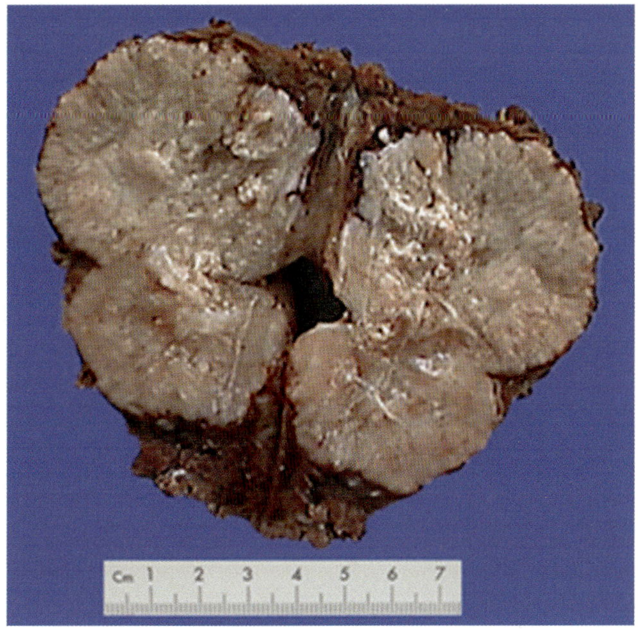

Fig. 7.8 HCC, confluent type, two fused tumor nodules in a gourd shape

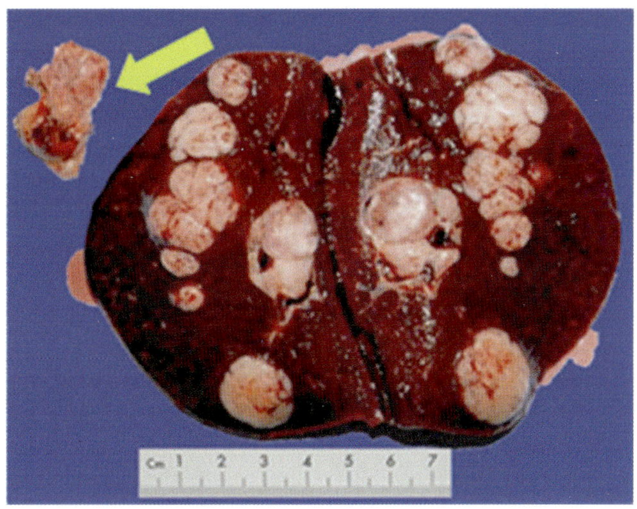

Fig. 7.9 HCC, multinodular type, multiple tumor nodules with portal vein tumor thrombus (*arrow*)

According to the statistics on the pathological data of 8580 cases of HCC with surgical resection in our hospital during 2009–2011, huge, massive, nodular, and small types of HCC accounted for 15.1, 30.2, 27.8, and 26.9%, respectively. Following the late 1970s when Chinese Cooperation Group on Pathology of Liver Cancers first proposed the pathological characteristics of small HCC ≤3 cm in diameter and classified it as an independent type, we suggested that ≤3 cm small HCC was a key transition of biological characteristics between benign and malignant tumors in the 1990s (refer to the chapter *Small Hepatocellular Carcinoma*). In

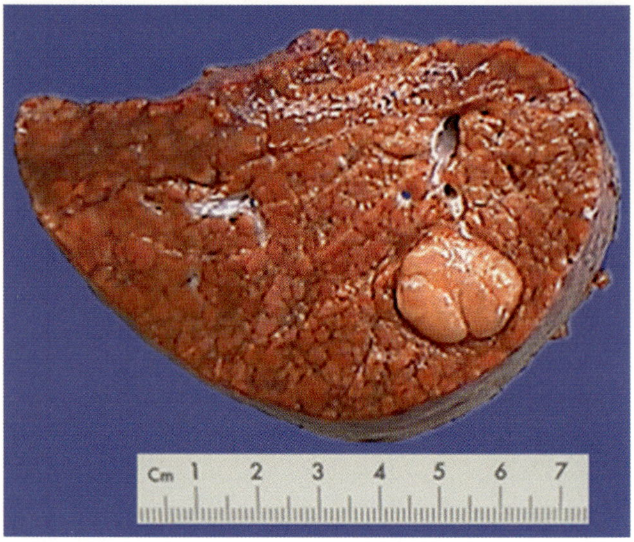

Fig. 7.10 Small HCC, with cirrhosis

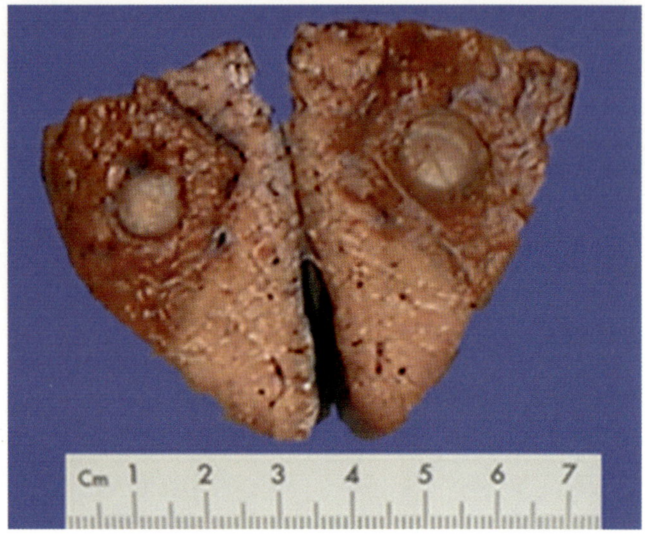

Fig. 7.11 Minute HCC, without cirrhosis

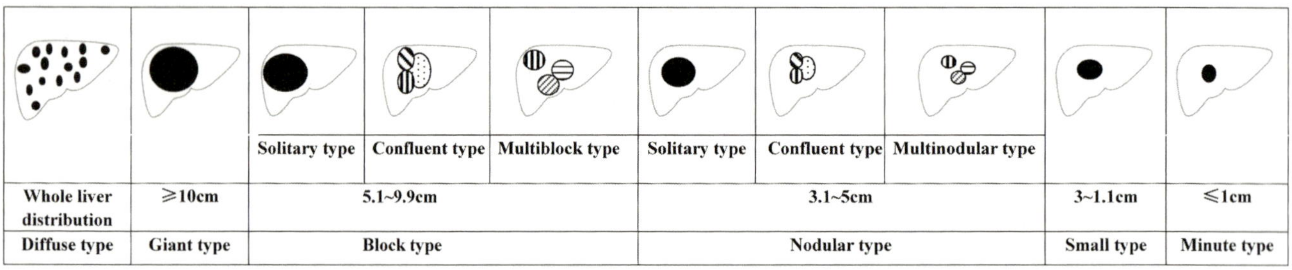

Fig. 7.12 Gross pathological classification of liver cancer in China

the *Practice guidelines for the pathological diagnosis of primary liver cancer: 2015 update* issued by the Chinese Pathological Group of Hepatobiliary Tumor and Liver Transplantation, a single tumor ≤1 cm in diameter is defined as minute HCC, and a single tumor with a diameter from >1 cm to ≤3 cm is defined as SHCC (Fig. 7.11). All the above viewpoints represent the basic understanding of gross typing of liver cancers in China at present (Fig. 7.12). In a word, HCC is currently in a lack of a unified international standard on the gross classification, but the major trend is to combine morphological, biological, and molecular characteristics affecting the clinical prognosis, and analysis of gene spectrum may lead to the suggestion of a new model of HCC molecular typing.

3. Kanai's classification: Nodular HCC was suggested to be divided into three types by Kanai et al. in 1987: type I, solitary nodule type; type II, solitary nodule type with extranodular growth; and type III, contiguous multinodular type [17]. The rate of tumor thrombus and intrahepatic metastasis is the highest in type II (71.4%) and the lowest in type I (7.7%), and the response to TAE is poor, and the prognosis is the worst in the type III.

4. Kojiro's classification: Proposed by Nakashima and Kojiro in 1987 and based on the gross classification of Okuda in 1984, Kojiro typing classified HCC into five major types and four subtypes:

   Infiltrative type (type I): Dissemination in the adjacent liver tissues.

   Expansive type (type II): The tumor grows expansively and compresses the surrounding tissue, with a clear border, including single nodular type and multiple nodular type.

   Mixed infiltrative and expansive type (type III): Single nodular mixed type and multinodular mixed type.

   Diffuse type (type IV).

   Special type (type V): such as exophytic HCC.

Exophytic HCC may be connected to the hepatic capsule by fibrous pedicles or directly adheres to the visceral or diaphragmatic surface of the hepatic capsule, and the outward growth of the main part of the tumor into extrahepatic regions can be found due to low resistance, compressing the surrounding organs, while the liver parenchyma is less involved, similar to abdominal massed clinically. One case of HCC in the caudate lobe of the liver was reported in China, with a

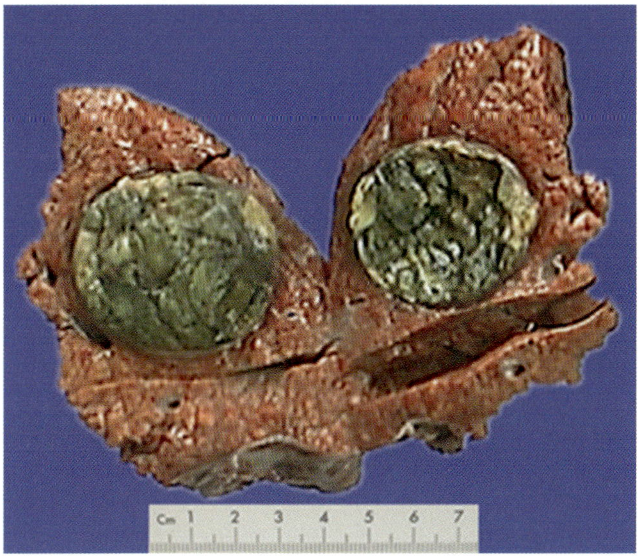

Fig. 7.13 HCC, block type, *green-colored* tumor by bile staining

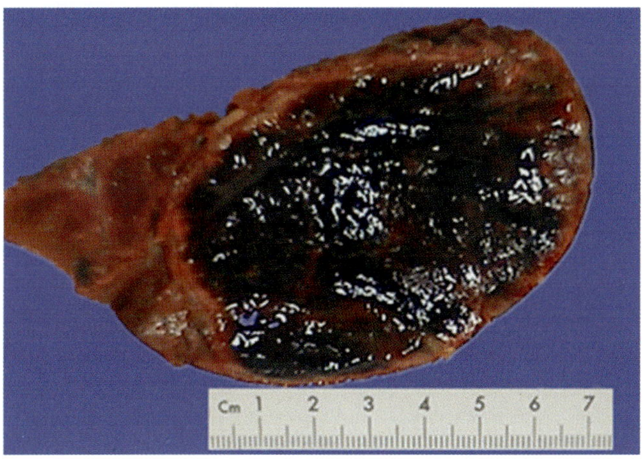

Fig. 7.14 HCC, block type, *dark brown* by severe hemorrhage

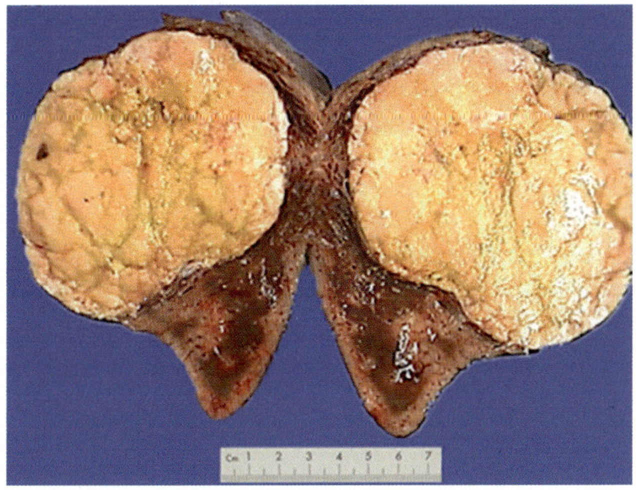

Fig. 7.15 HCC, block type, *pale yellow* by severe steatosis

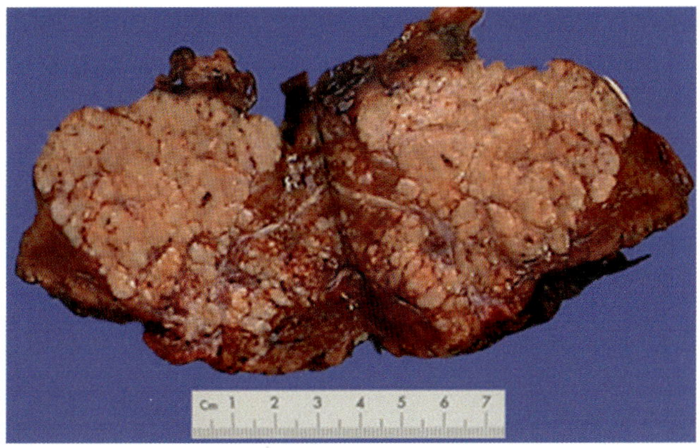

Fig. 7.16 HCC, block type, with a multifocal growth pattern

tumor of 21 cm in diameter protruding into the lessor omental bursa. Among the eight cases of huge exophytic HCC with surgical resection reported by Zhang HB of our hospital, the average diameter of the tumors was 18 cm, and all the patients had a history of HBV infection, of which seven cases concerned lesions on the visceral surface of the liver, seven cases with different degrees of invasion into the adjacent hepatic lobes, and patients in six cases demonstrated long-term survival.

(2) Characteristics of gross specimens

Morphological features of HCC include the tumor size, number, and the association with the surrounding liver tissue, such as capsular integrity, focal infiltration, cancer embolus in the vessels, satellite nodules, intrahepatic metastasis, and other biological behaviors, all of which are the main basis for pathological typing of HCC. The section of a HCC mass is often solid, gray white, and soft in texture, with hemorrhage and necrosis, or dark green in cases with cholestasis (Fig. 7.13), dark brown in cases with severe hemorrhage (Fig. 7.14), and pale yellow due to severe fatty degeneration (Fig. 7.15). Cystic degeneration can be observed in cases with severe liquefaction necrosis, and fibrous scars can be found in the lesions of sclerosing HCC. Special attention should be paid to the invasion of capsule and the boundary invasion (Fig. 7.16).

In addition, cirrhosis-like HCC (CL-HCC) was also reported in the literature, characterized by diffuse micronodular cirrhosis like microcarcinoma in the background of cirrhosis [18], with mild elevation in serum AFP level and difficulty in distinguishing it from liver cirrhosis nodules. Although it is similar to diffuse HCC, most CL-HCC nodules have a fibrous capsule and a clear boundary. Histologically, it is composed by moderate, well-differentiated HCC cells, often with visible pseudoglandular tubular structures, and 80% of the cases contain visible

Mallory bodies. These morphological features of CL-HCC suggest its polyclonal origin, and liver transplantation is a choice for the treatment during which cirrhosis lesions and tumor nodules in the liver can be removed.

(3) Sampling of gross specimen

With the deepening understanding on the biological characteristics and tumor microenvironment of HCC, and based on the clinical demand for prognosis evaluation and individualized treatment, more attention should be paid to the examination on invasion of the surrounding liver tissue (microvascular invasion and satellite lesions) and the lesions around the tumors (precancerous lesions). Therefore, the pathological sampling should focus on comprehensive evaluation of the condition of the tumor and the adjacent liver tissues, rather than tumor itself as previous experience, and the specification of sampling will directly affect the statistical accuracy and scientific significance of pathological parameters (number and distribution of microvascular invasion and satellite foci). According to our experience in operability of practical work in the Department of Pathology, the basic method of sampling for HCC is as follows. Make vertical sections in an interval of 0.5–1 cm, select a representative one, and harvest 7-point baseline sampling protocol, which stipulates that at least four tissue specimens should be sampled at the junction of the tumor and adjacent liver tissues (1:1 ratio) at the 12, 3, 6, and 9 o'clock reference positions, making sure that every sample contains both the tumor tissue and the peritumorous liver tissue for observation of the invasion of capsule, blood vessels, and the surrounding liver tissue. For the purposes of molecular pathological examination, at least one specimen should be sampled at the intratumoral zone. In addition, harvest of liver tissue within the distance of ≤1 cm (adjacent peritumoral liver tissues) and >1 cm (distant peritumoral liver tissues) (Fig. 7.17) is for observation of satellite foci, microvascular invasion, residual cancer cells, as well as the background of the liver tissue (inflammation, fibrosis, cirrhosis). Sampling in the cutting edge should be used to determine whether a positive cutting edge can be found.

Of course, the number and sites of the samples depend on the size, shape, and number of the lesions of the tumor. For ≤3 cm small HCC, the whole tumor with peritumorous tissue should harvested, and more samples should be harvested corresponding the increased amount of peritumorous liver tissue and number of tumor nodules. The size of each sample should be 1.5–2.0 cm × 1.0 cm × 0.2 cm, and the sampling sites should be marked, with picture of the samples taken for file keeping.

7.1.1.6 Microscopic Features

(1) Histological classification

The architectural patterns of HCC mainly include the following types:

1. Thin trabecular pattern: This is a common histological type of well-differentiated HCC. The cancer cells are arranged in 1~3 layers of cell-thick cords between which are micro-blood vessels lined with endothelial cells, similar to normal hepatic cords (Fig. 7.18), and should be carefully distinguished especially in cases with no capsule around the tumor and transition is found between it with the surrounding trabeculae hepaticae (Fig. 7.19). When a fibrous capsule is visible, increased blood sinus gaps are found between hepatic cellular cords, and well-differentiated HCC is located on the side with disorderly arrangement (Fig. 7.20). A diffuse-type distribution of capillarization (microvessel structure) shown in CD34

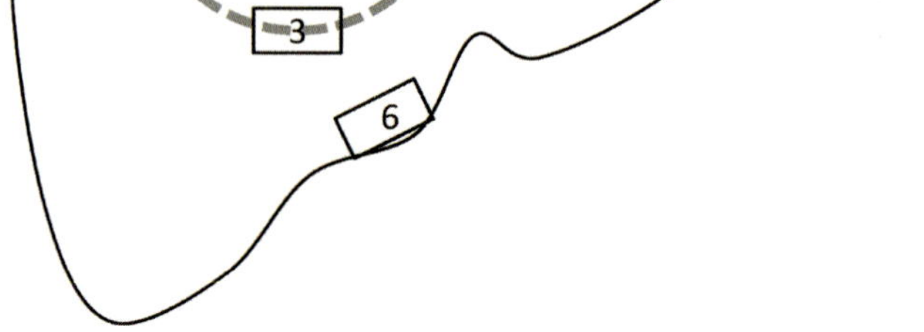

Fig. 7.17 Illustration of sampling HCC specimen

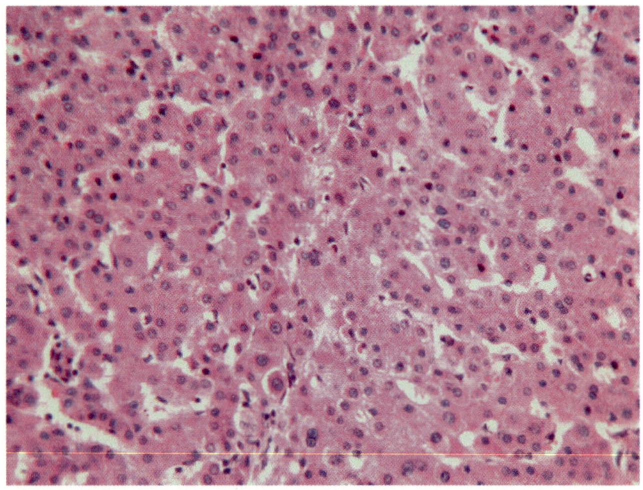

Fig. 7.18 HCC, thin trabecular pattern in 1–3 cells thick

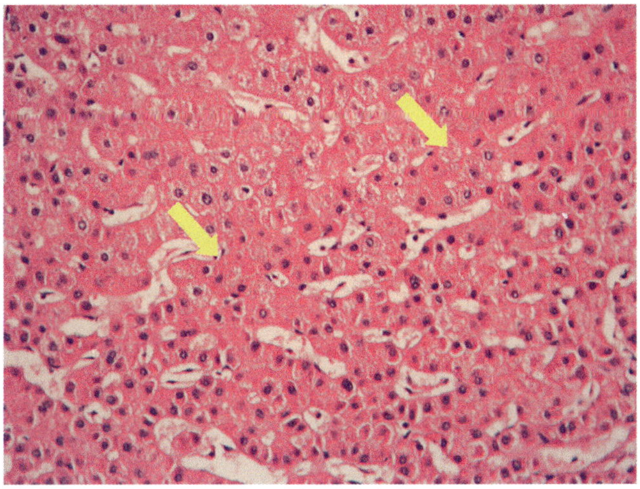

Fig. 7.19 HCC, transition between HCC thin trabecular plates and liver cell cords

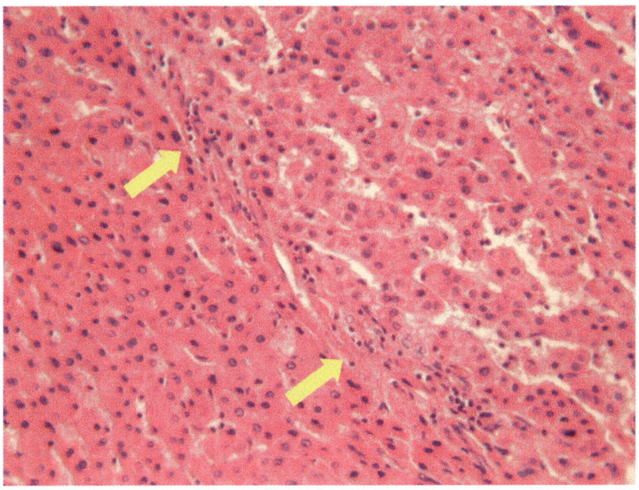

Fig. 7.20 HCC, thin fibrous capsule around tumor tissue

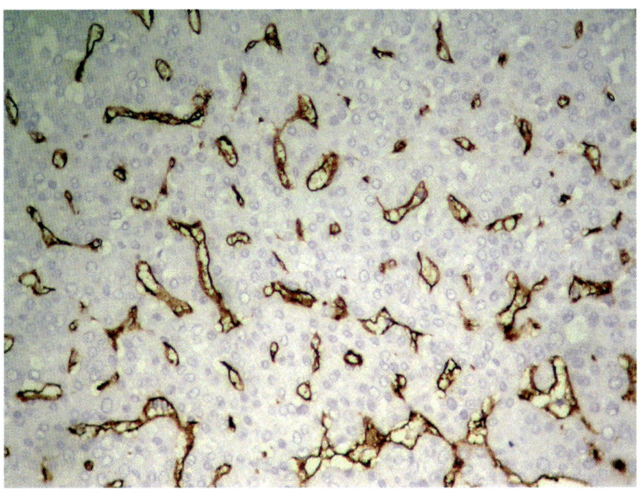

Fig. 7.21 HCC, thin trabecular pattern, CD34 immunohistochemical staining showing diffuse and uniform distribution of microvessels

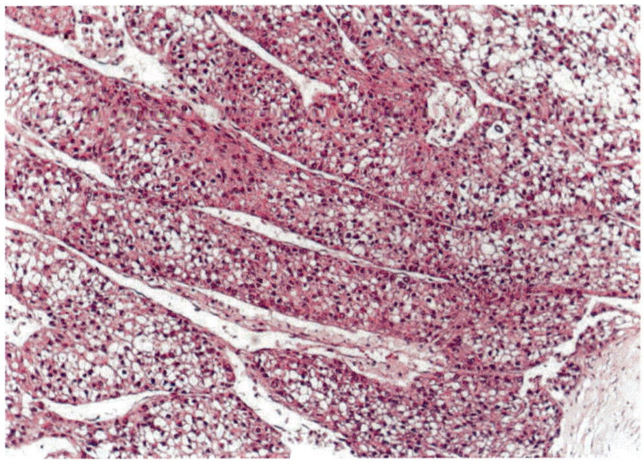

Fig. 7.22 HCC, thick trabecular pattern, HCC cells arranged as thick trabecular cords

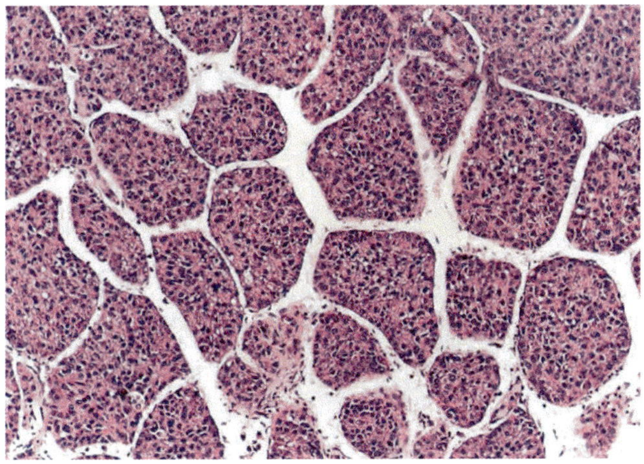

Fig. 7.23 HCC, thick trabecular pattern, ten cells or more thick

staining is helpful for diagnosis (Fig. 7.21). And high-differentiated HCC should be differentiated from focal nodular hyperplasia of the liver, hepatocellular adenoma, and high-grade dysplastic nodules.

2. Thick trabecular pattern: This is the most common histological type of moderately differentiated HCC. The cancer cells are arranged in a thick trabecular pattern with four to several layers of cells which have increased nuclear to cytoplasmic ratio, obvious nuclear atypia, and increased mitotic nuclear divisions (Figs. 7.22 and 7.23), and CD34 staining shows the thick cellular cords outlining the sinusoid-like blood spaces (Fig. 7.24).

3. Pseudoglandular pattern: It is also known as acinar type, which was considered to be formed by expansion of bile canalicular-like structures between the cancer cells, and the glandular tubes are lined with a single layer of cuboi-

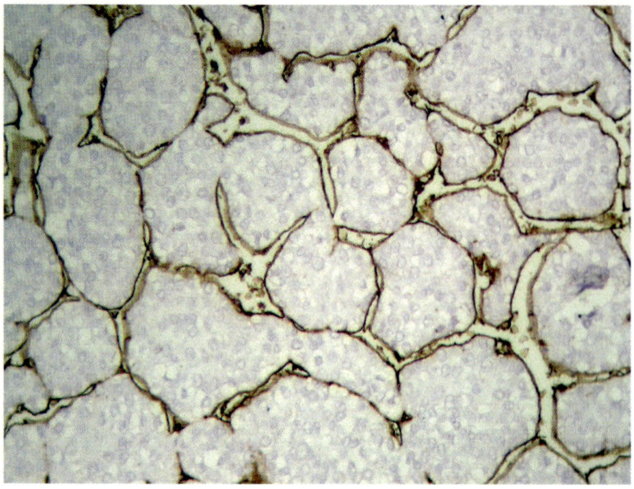

Fig. 7.24 HCC, CD34 immunohistochemical staining outlining thick trabecular cords

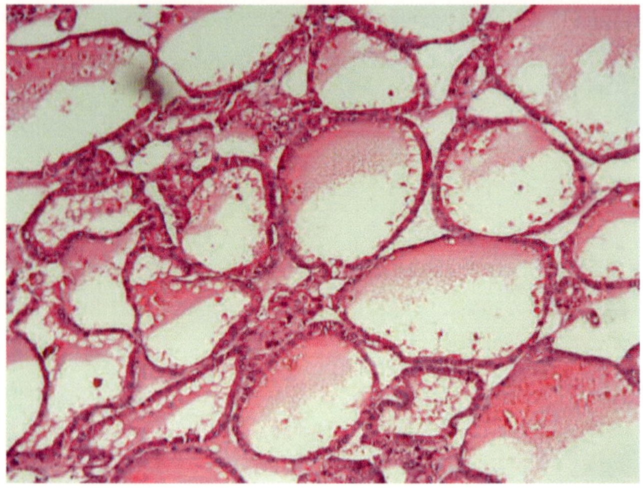

Fig. 7.26 HCC, pseudoglandular pattern, pseudoglands with cystic dilatation containing proteinaceous, similar to the thyroid follicles

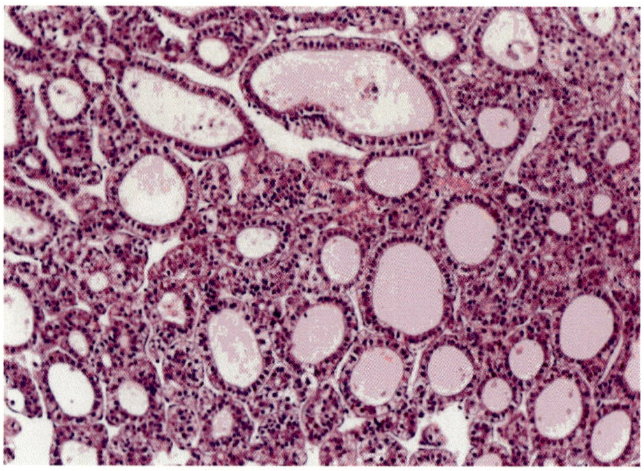

Fig. 7.25 HCC, pseudoglandular pattern, small cuboidal epithelioid HCC cells arranged in gland-like/tubular structures

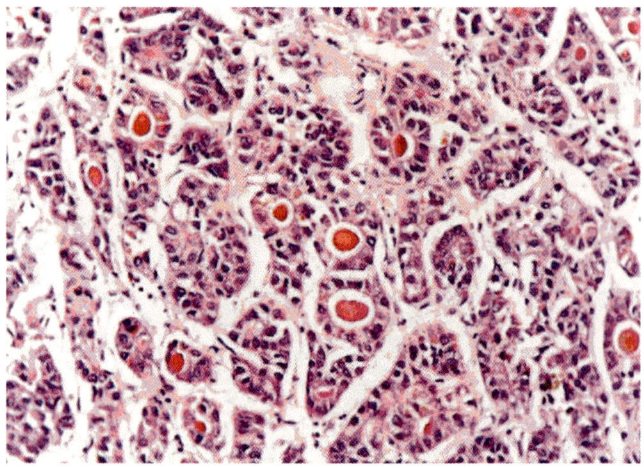

Fig. 7.27 HCC, pseudoglandular pattern with bile plugs

dal epithelioid HCC cells (Fig. 7.25), often containing light-stained proteinaceous material in the dilated lumen with absorptive vesicles in the surroundings, similar to thyroid follicle-like structures (Fig. 7.26). The acini may also contain bile (Fig. 7.27). And the paratumorous new foci can also be well-differentiated pseudoglandular-type HCC (Fig. 7.28).

Cases with diffuse pseudoglandular structures should be distinguished from intrahepatic cholangiocarcinoma and metastatic adenocarcinoma in the liver. These pseodoglandular tubes are positive for a hepatocellular marker Hep Par-1 (Fig. 7.29), and polyclonal carcinoembryonic antigen (CEA) and CD10 staining shows a characteristic canalicular staining pattern on the membrane of the pseudoglandular cells (Fig. 7.30), which suggest these are liver cells rather than real glandular epithelium. CK19 staining demonstrates generally negative results, and its positive results may suggest bile duct epithelial differentiation of the HCC cells (Fig. 7.31), and it belongs to a new subtype of HCC, so we named dual-phenotype HCC (see below). Pseudoglands do not contain myxoid components, and AB/PAS mucus staining is negative, and MUC-1 staining shows bile-like secretion (Fig. 7.32), also suggesting the lumen derives from specialized transformation of capillary bile ducts.

4. Compact pattern: It is also known as solid type. The cancer cells are arranged in flaky or solid patterns, with insignificant or slit-like hepatic sinusoid capillarization due to serious compression (Figs. 7.33, 7.34, and 7.35), suggesting active growth and poor differentiation of the tumor cells. And CD34 immunohistochemical staining shows

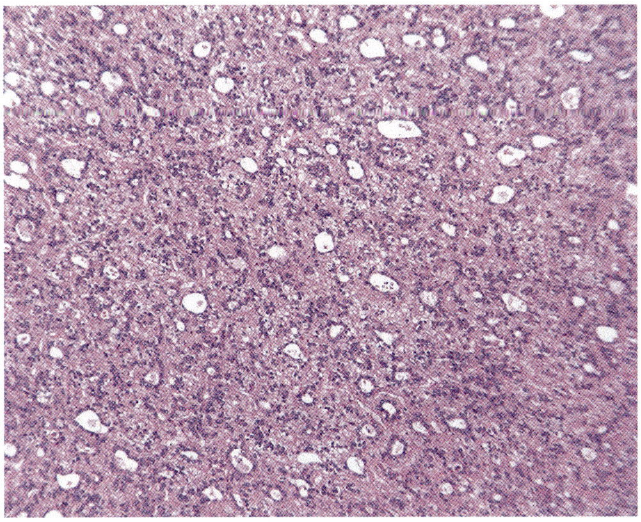

Fig. 7.28 HCC, pseudoglandular pattern, showing diffuse pseudoglandular structures

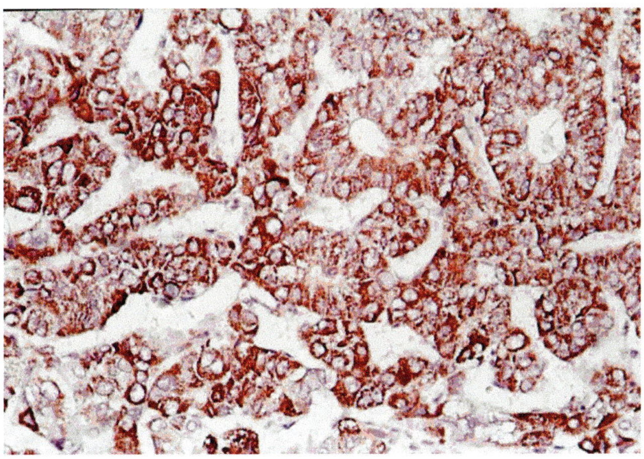

Fig. 7.29 HCC, pseudoglandular pattern, showing positive immunohistochemical staining of Hep Par-1

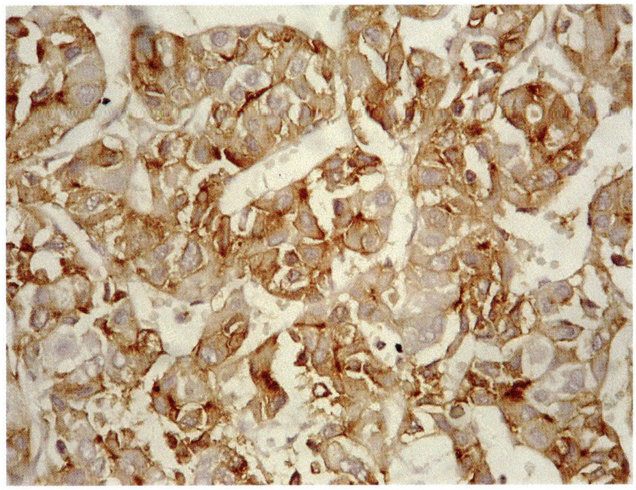

Fig. 7.30 HCC, pseudoglandular pattern, immunohistochemical staining ofCD10 showing canalicular membrane of HCC cells

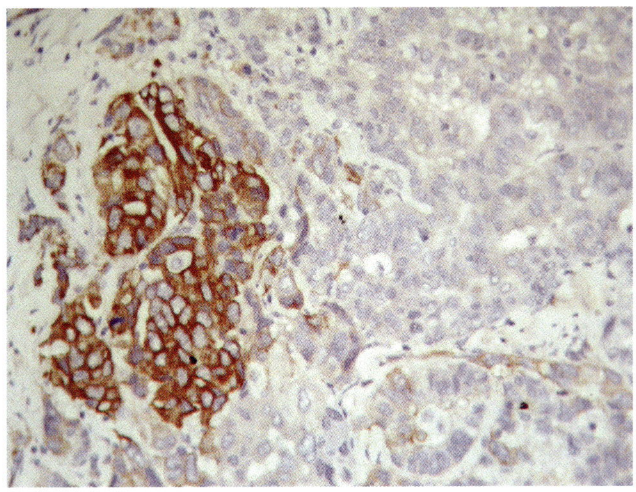

Fig. 7.31 HCC, pseudoglandular pattern, immunohistochemical staining showing some CK19-positive HCC cells

sparsely distributed microvessels, significantly different from densely arranged microvessels of trabecular-type HCC (Fig. 7.36).

5. Sclerosing (or scirrhous) pattern: Visible gray-white fibrous scars can be found on the section of the tumor (Figs. 7.37 and 7.38). Under the microscope, the tumor contains abundant collagen fibrous tissue and is divided by thick fibrous connective tissue into varying sizes of cell nests (Fig. 7.39), similar to the morphology of metastatic tumors or intrahepatic cholangiocarcinoma in some cases (Fig. 7.40). And hyaline degeneration can also be observed in some cancer cells. Positive Hep Par-1 staining (Fig. 7.41) is helpful in differential diagnosis. Sclerosing type of HCC indicates a strong local immune response in the body, which is also common as a histological reaction in cases treated with radiotherapy or chemotherapy.

6. Purpura pattern: The tumor is rich in highly dilated vessels containing abundant blood in the lumen, and the sections are often dark red, similar to that of the hemangioma (Fig. 7.42). Under a microscope, blood sinuses in the tumor tissue are highly expanded or similar to cavernous hemangioma-like structures (Figs. 7.43 and 7.44), with flat peripheral cancer cells due to compression. In addition, focal purpura-like vascular expansion can be observed in many HCC tissues.

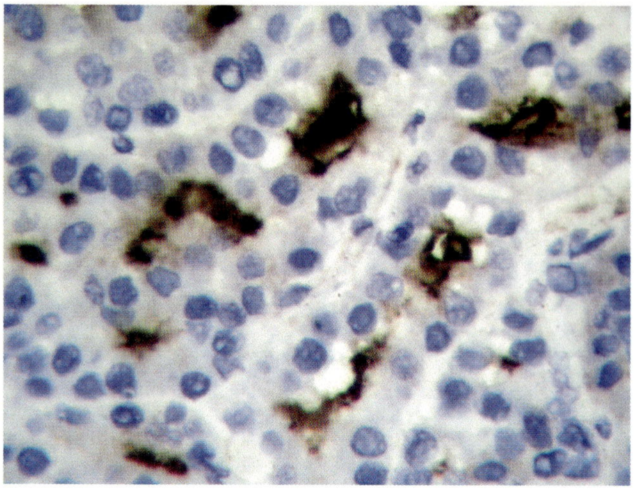

Fig. 7.32 HCC, pseudoglandular pattern, immunohistochemical staining showing MUC-1-positive glandular tubules

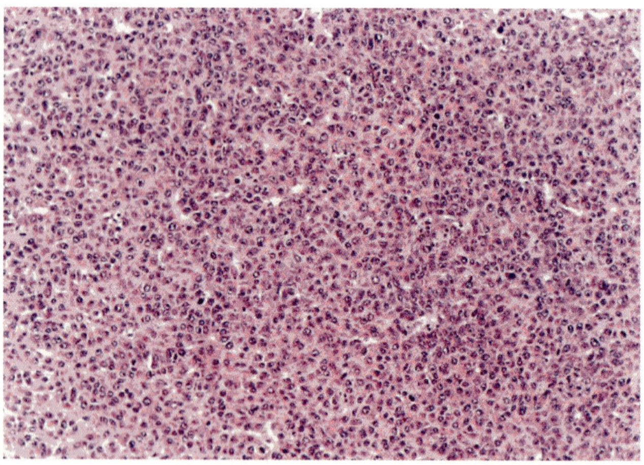

Fig. 7.33 HCC, compact pattern, closely arranged cells with no obvious hepatic sinusoids

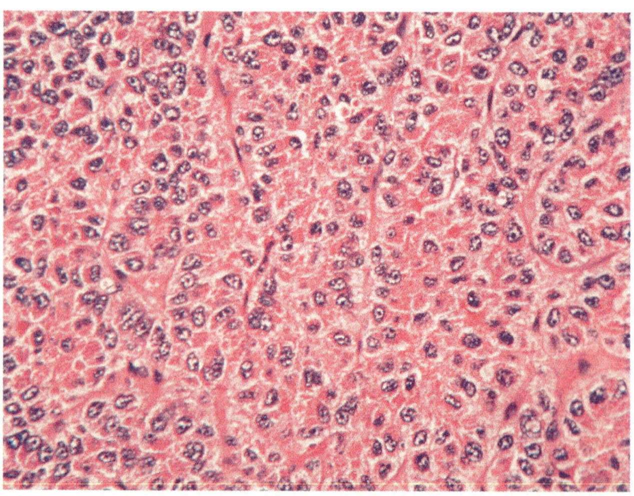

Fig. 7.34 HCC, compact pattern, HCC cells arranged in solid cord-like structures with no obvious hepatic sinusoids

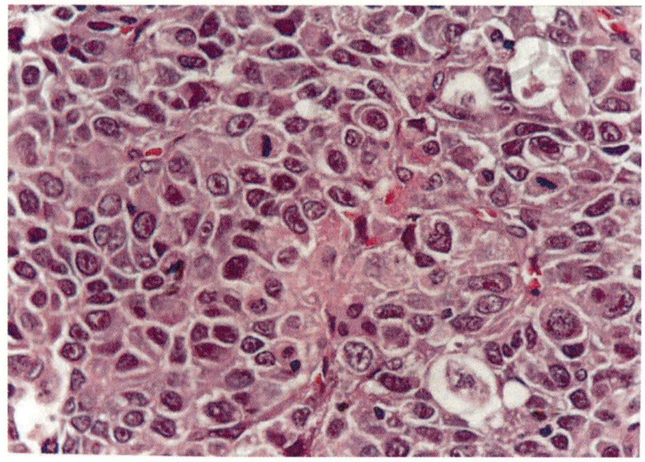

Fig. 7.35 HCC, compact pattern, showing a mosaic arrangement of tumor cells with frequent mitotic figures

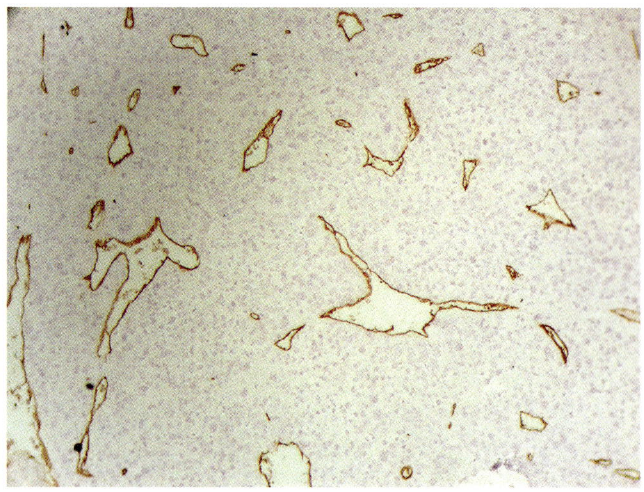

Fig. 7.36 HCC, compact pattern, CD34 staining showing sparse microvessels

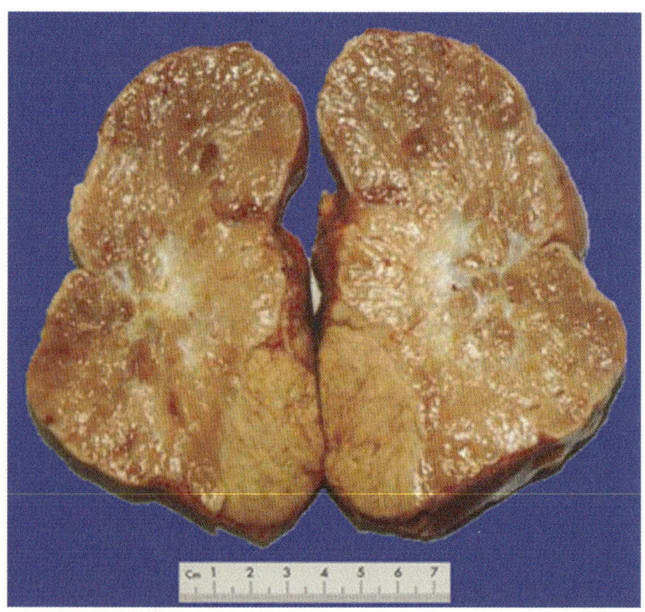

Fig. 7.37 HCC, sclerosing type, showing central fibrous scar

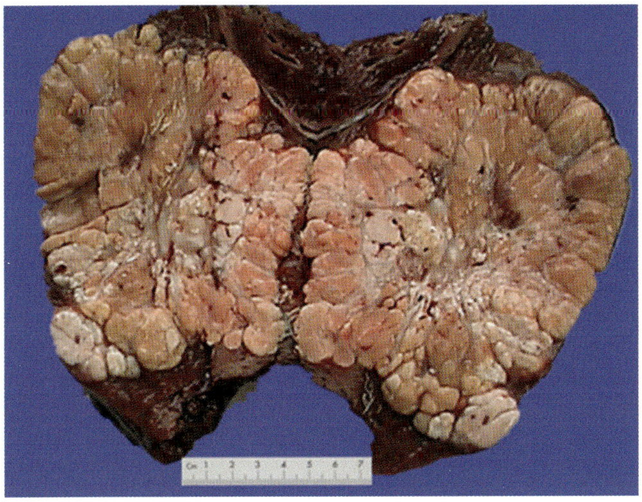

Fig. 7.38 HCC, sclerosing type, showing lobulated mass due to fibrous septa

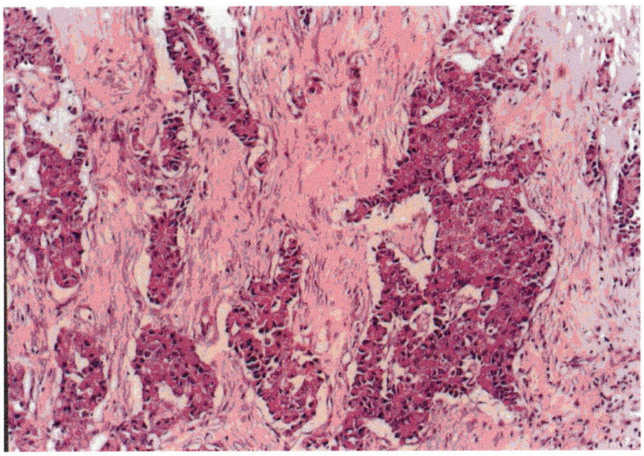

Fig. 7.39 HCC, sclerosing type, showing nested structures divided by fibrous septa

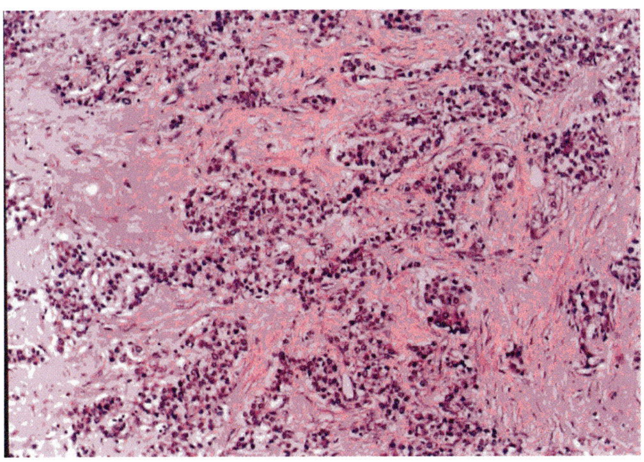

Fig. 7.40 HCC, sclerosing type, tumor cells arranged in solid nests with rich fibrous stroma

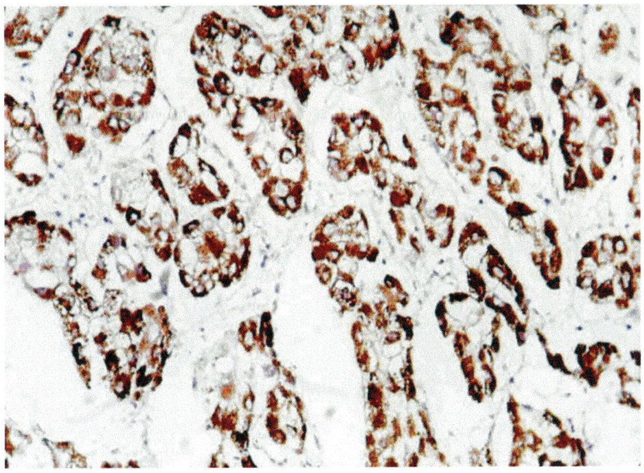

Fig. 7.41 HCC, sclerosing type, showing positive immunohistochemical staining of Hep Par-1

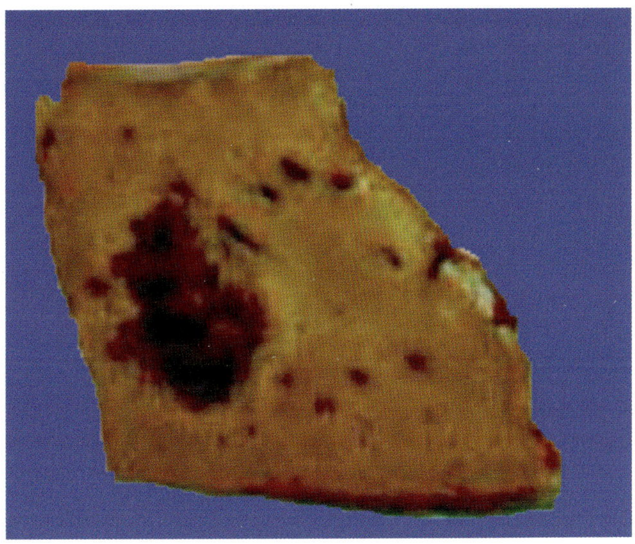

Fig. 7.42 HCC, purpura pattern, the cut surface looks like hemangioma

7. Rosette-like pattern: Little round groupings of HCC cells consist of a spoke-wheel or halo arrangement surrounding a central, acellular region. A minority of HCC tissue can be arranged in a rosette-like structure, with each rosettes surrounded by about more than 20 cells at an equal interval distance in peripheral regions of the rosettes, with or without significant central lumen. The cells are consistent in size with eosinophilic cytoplasm and unclear boundaries (Fig. 7.45a, b), and immunohistochemistry shows strongly positive Hep Par-1 (Fig. 7.46).

8. Private-like arrangement HCC cells contain sparse cytoplasm and vacuolation, with small remaining of pale-stained cytoplasm. The blue-stained nuclei of the cancer cells are arranged in a single layer near the sinusoidal sur-

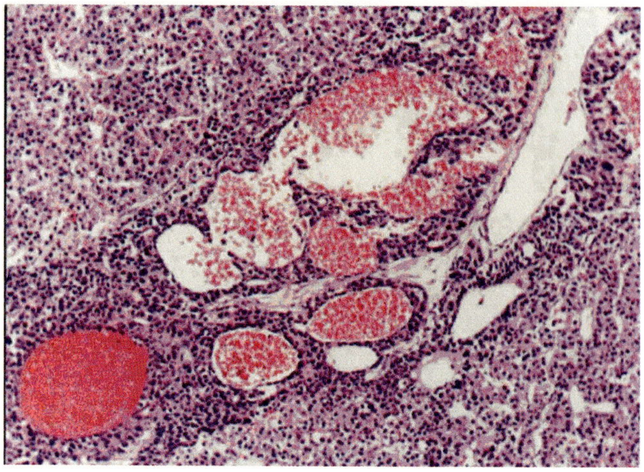

Fig. 7.43 HCC, purpura pattern, the tumor tissue contains dilated lacunae vasorum

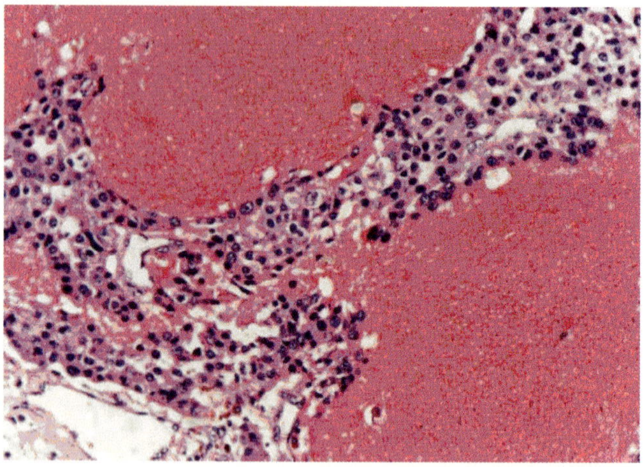

Fig. 7.44 HCC, purpura pattern, the dilated lacunae vasorum contains numerous erythrocytes

face of the trabecular structure which is like privates (Fig. 7.47), and CD34 staining shows increase of microvascular density (Fig. 7.48).

9. Spontaneous necrosis type: The diagnosis of HCC is based on the clinical history of viral hepatitis in patients, previous elevated serum AFP level, liver masses found in imaging examination, as well as other clinical indications. And in cases without any special treatment, after the levels of serum AFP decreased or become negative, complete coagulation necrosis is found in the tumors. In addition, about 100 cases of spontaneous regression of HCC have been reported in the literature, and the imaging results during the follow-up for HCC patients showed part or complete disappearance of liver masses or extrahepatic metastases. And I diagnosed one case in accordance to the criteria of spontaneous necrosis-type HCC, and it was treated with surgical resection, the lesion of which demonstrated severe hemorrhagic necrosis in gross appearance (Fig. 7.49), while repetitive sampling failed to find remaining cancer cells, but only the remaining trabecular contour left by tumor necrosis (Fig. 7.50). The patient recovered well with a good prognosis and no recurrence was found during the long-term postoperative follow-up. And theses HCC cases with spontaneous necrosis or spontaneous regression are likely to be related to the strong immune function of the patients.

Supplementary: Posttreatment Necrotic HCC

Minimally invasive surgical methods are widely applied in the treatment of HCC, including transcatheter arterial chemoembolization (TACE), radiofrequency ablation (RFA), percutaneous ethanol injection (PEI), microwave

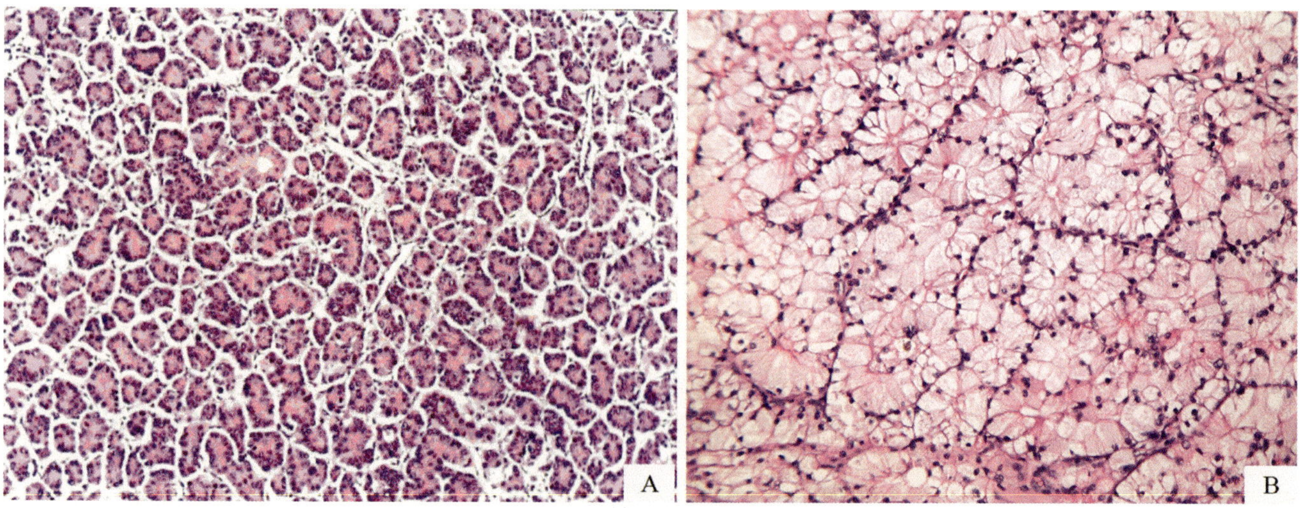

Fig. 7.45 (**a**) HCC, rosette-like pattern, tumor cells surrounding a central lumen that contains cytoplasmic extensions from the tumor cells, (**b**) HCC, rosette-like pattern, concentric arrangement of rosette-like hepatocytes with bright cytoplasm

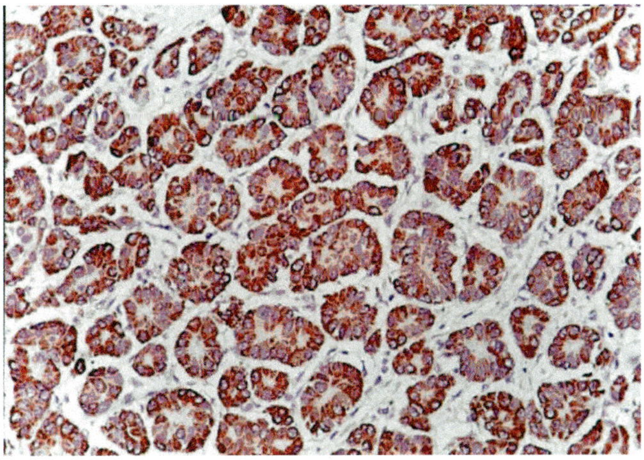

Fig. 7.46 HCC, rosette-like pattern, showing positive immunohistochemical staining of Hep Par-1

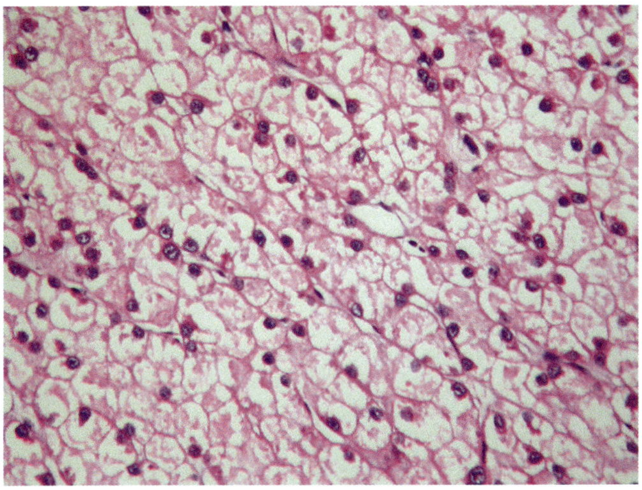

Fig. 7.47 HCC, private-like arrangement, cancer cells are arranged in a single layer along the trabecular cords

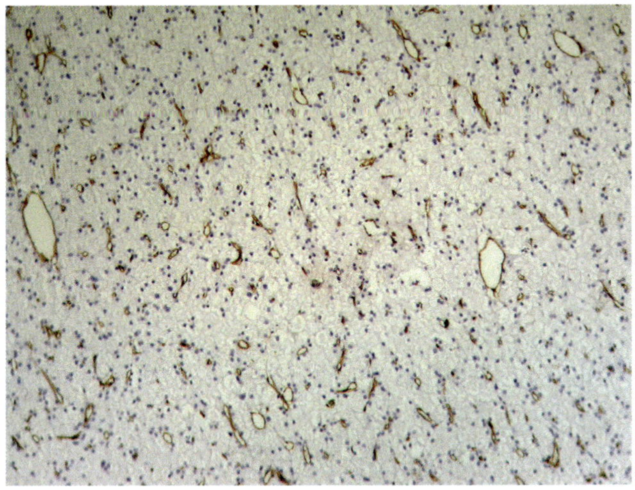

Fig. 7.48 HCC, private-like arrangement, CD34 staining showing diffuse microvessels

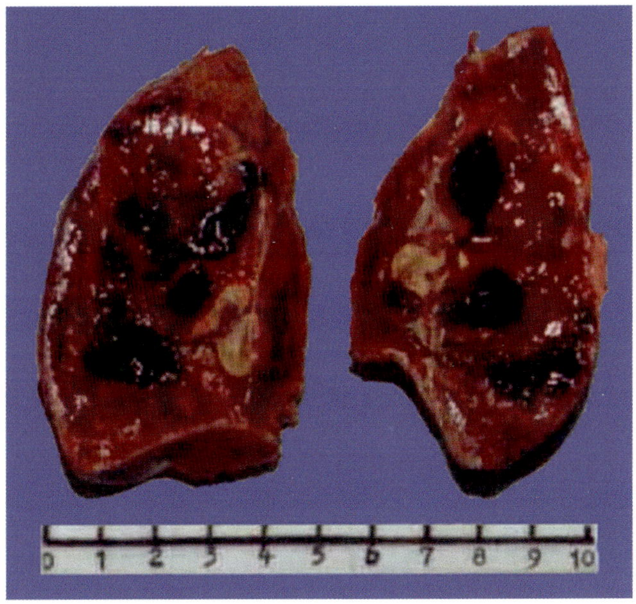

Fig. 7.49 HCC, spontaneous necrosis type, showing severe hemorrhage and necrosis

coagulation therapy (MCT), laser thermal ablation (LTA), and argon helium cryoablation surgery (AHCS), which can directly cause the coagulation necrosis of HCC cells and tissues. The main mechanism of minimally invasive treatment for hepatic tumors is physical or chemical destruction or ablation of cancer cells, so as to achieve the purpose of effective decrease of tumor load. However, the biggest difference between it and surgical resection is the tumor remaining in situ after interventional therapy; therefore, the efficacy of destruction or elimination of tumor cells is closely related to the effect of the interventional therapy which is affected by various important factors, such as tumor size, number, location, shape, growth pattern, biological characteristics, etc. Thus, in pathological examination, sampling in multiple parts and sites should be conducted as well as careful searching for tumor cells. The degree and scope of necrosis in the cancer tissue should also be described in pathological reports. Single-stranded DNA markers, lactate dehydrogenase staining, and Ki-67 labeling are all methods to determine the activity of degenerated and necrotic cancer cells. According to incomplete statistics, 102 cases of HCC treated by interventional therapy and subsequent surgical resection have been found in our hospital from September 2005 to November 2007, and pathological examinations displayed 78 cases (76.5%) of complete necrosis and cancer cell remaining in 24 cases (23.5%) (Figs. 7.51, 7.52, 7.53, and 7.54).

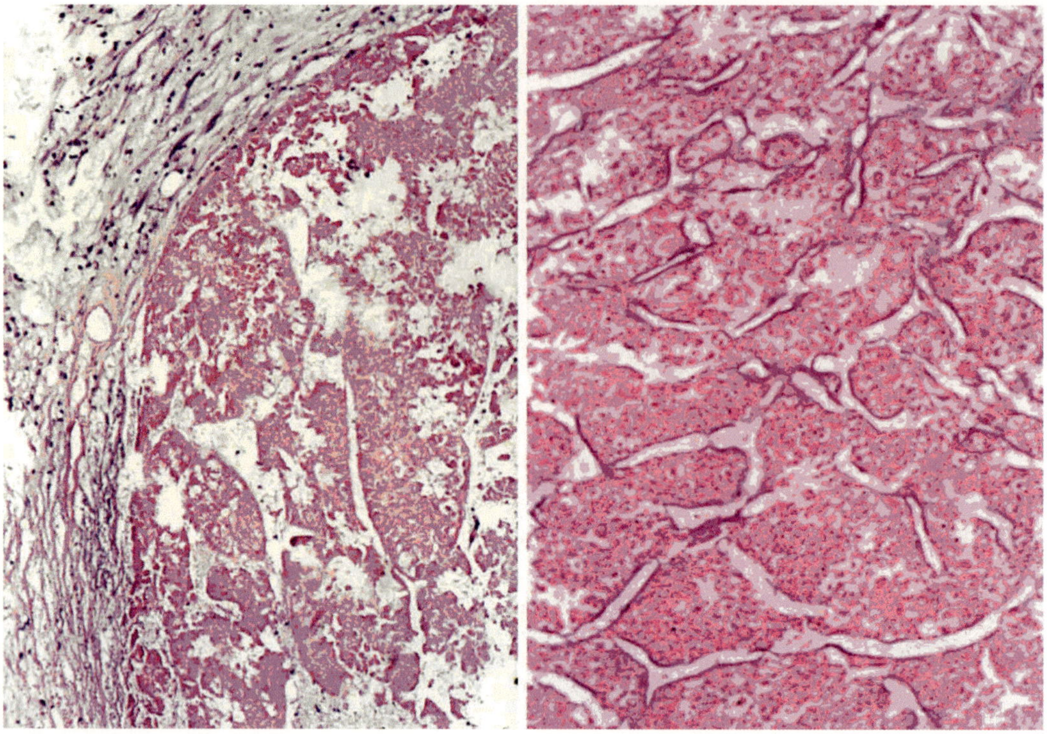

Fig. 7.50 HCC, spontaneous necrosis type, tumor tissue showed a complete coagulation necrosis, only remaining trabecular outline

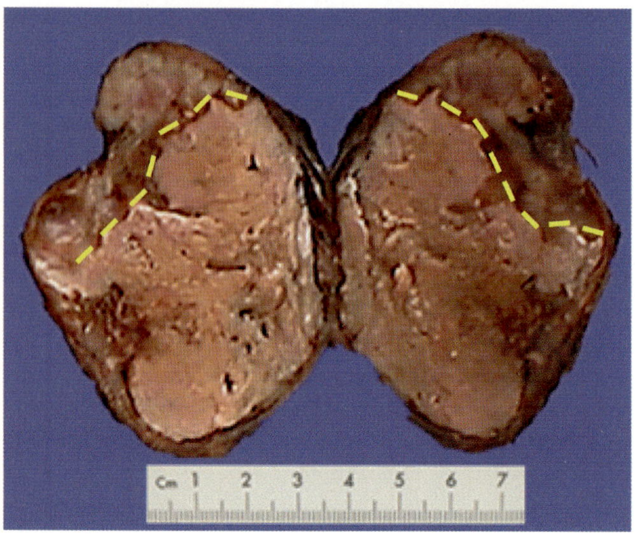

Fig. 7.51 Necrosis of HCC after TACE

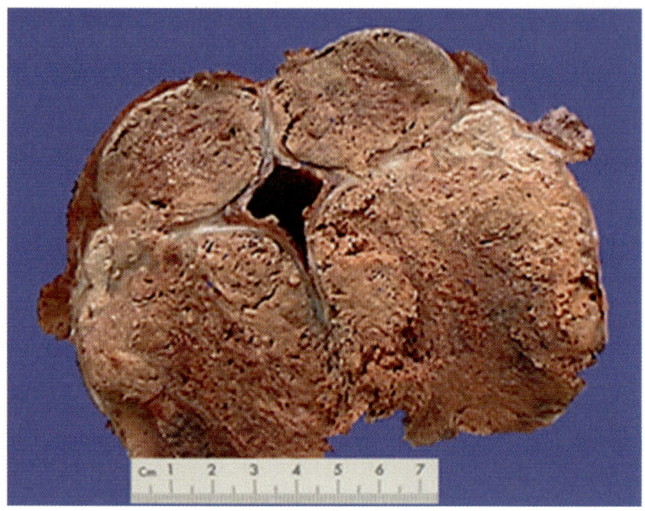

Fig. 7.52 Necrosis of HCC after TACE

(2) Cytological classification of HCC

HCC cells have a variety of morphological manifestations, even completely different from that of hepatocytes, mainly including the following types:

1. Liver cell type: This is the most common type, similar to that of normal hepatocytes, and the cancer cells were polygonal, with eosinophilic fine granular cytoplasm. The cell membrane contains specialized bile canalicular structure and bile plug, which is an important sign of hepatocyte differentiation. Poorly differentiated cancer cells are enlarged in volume significantly, with increased cytoplasmic basophilia, nuclear volume, and nucleus to cytoplasm ratio, and the nuclei are irregular shaped, darker stained with a variable number of mitotic figures.
2. Clear cell type: More than 50% of the cancer cells contain rich glycogens which are irregular and large vacuole-like

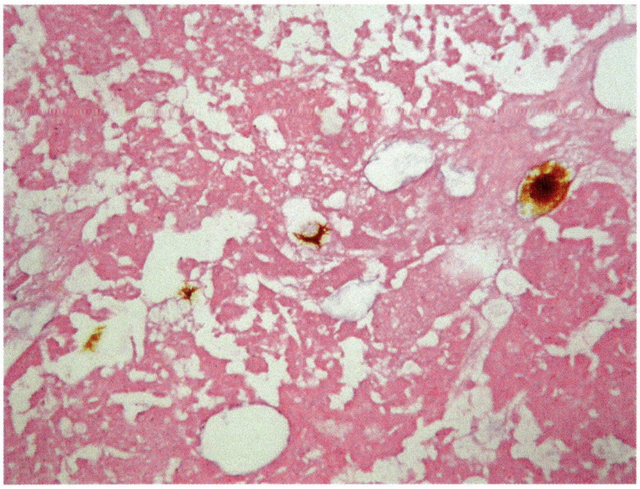

Fig. 7.53 Necrosis of HCC after TACE, no survival cancer cells under microscope

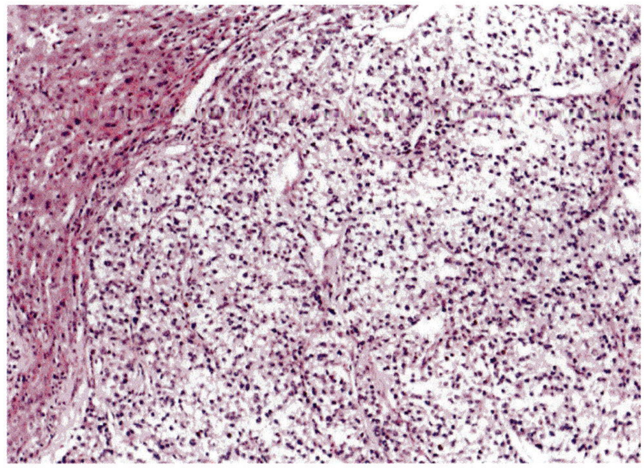

Fig. 7.55 HCC, clear cell type, showing vacuolated cytoplasm in clear cell

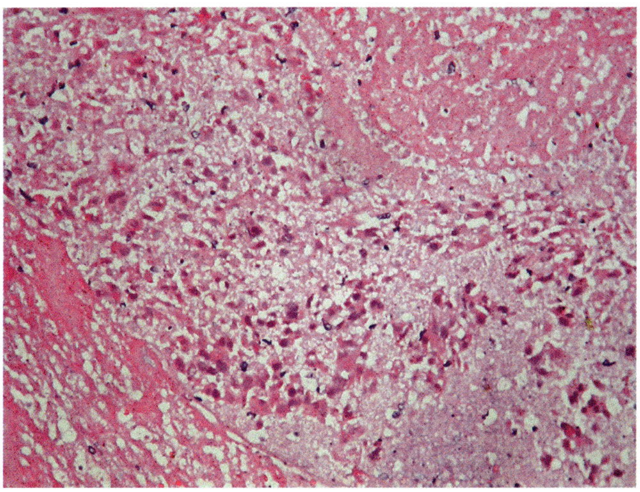

Fig. 7.54 Necrosis of HCC after TACE, a small amount of incompletely necrotic cancer cells under microscope

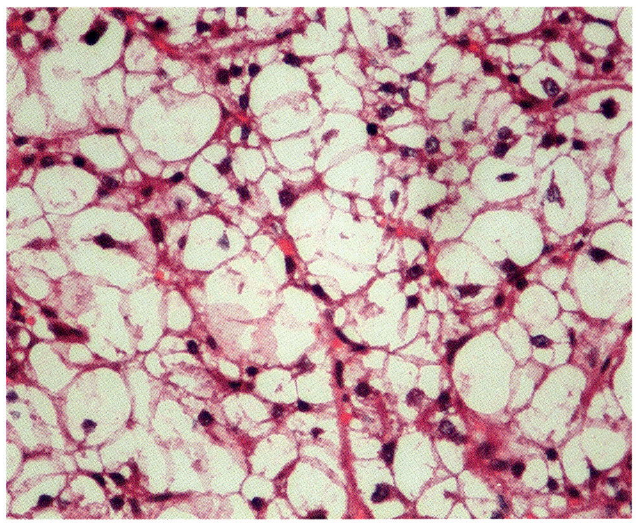

Fig. 7.56 HCC, clear cell type, the tumor cell cytoplasm showed hydropic-type vacuolar degeneration, like empty bubble

structures, resulting in transparent cytoplasm (Fig. 7.55), and nucleus can be found floating in the center of the cytoplasm (Fig. 7.56). The cancer cells are positive in PAS staining because of abundant glycogen content. In cases with transparent cells, as the majority of the tumor, it should be differentiated from metastatic clear cell carcinoma which originates in the kidney, while the latter is positive for EMA, Leu M-1, and broad-spectrum CK staining but negative for Hep Par-1, which is positively expressed in clear cell-type HCC (Fig. 7.57). Emile et al. (2001) studied tumor diameter, tumor number, and prognosis and conducted the detection of six microsatellite loci of the clear cell-type HCC; however, no obvious difference was found between liver cell-type HCC and clear cell-type HCC.

3. Fatty-rich type: Also known as fatty change, this type of HCC is formed by cancer cells with metabolism disorder of fat, characterized by circular lipid droplets with smooth surface and consistent size, occupying in the whole cytoplasm (macrovesicular steatosis), leading to nuclear deviation (Figs. 7.58 and 7.59). Occasionally, nucleated red cells can be found in the hepatic sinusoids, suggesting extramedullary hematopoiesis (3–5%). The fatty-rich type of HCC should be differentiated from angioleiomyolipoma and focal fatty change, and typical HCC samples should be harvested via multiple sampling to avoid misdiagnosis as benign lesions. Immunohistochemical staining shows positive results for GPC-3, Hep Par-1 (Fig. 7.60), CD34 (Fig. 7.61), and CK18 to facilitate the diagnosis.

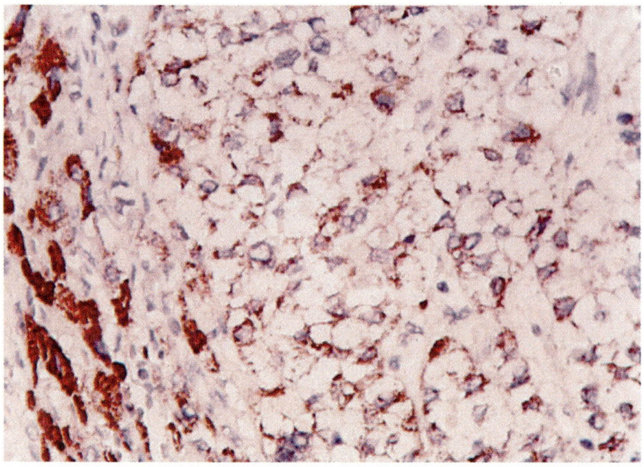

Fig. 7.57 HCC, clear cell type, showing positive immunohistochemical staining of Hep Par-1

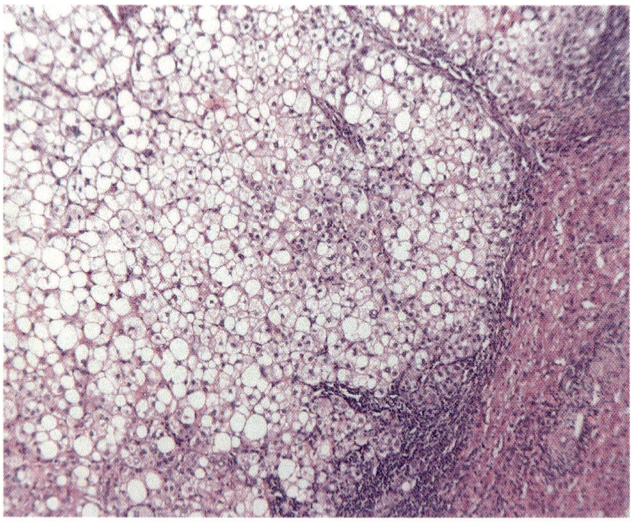

Fig. 7.58 HCC, fatty-rich type, showing diffuse fatty change in HCC cells

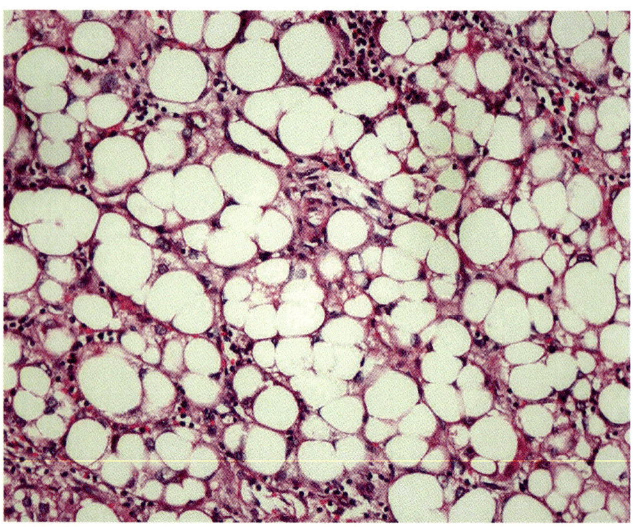

Fig. 7.59 HCC, fatty-rich type, showing hepatic macrovesicular steatosis

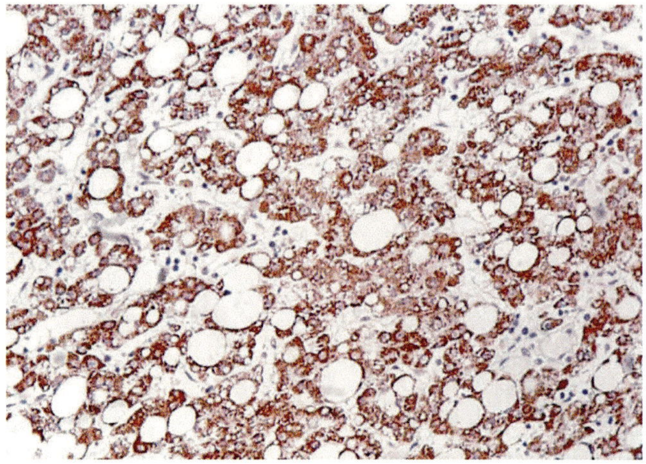

Fig. 7.60 HCC, fatty-rich type, showing positive immunohistochemical staining of Hep Par-1

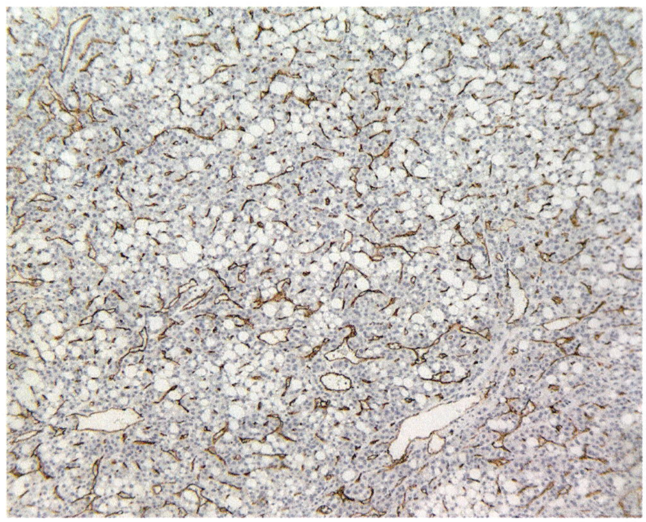

Fig. 7.61 HCC, fatty-rich type, CD34 staining showing diffuse microvessels

4. Spindle cell type: Also known as sarcomatoid type, it accounts for about 5% of HCC and is a special form of poorly differentiated HCC, of which approximately 46% of the patients are found with positive serum AFP. The tumor cells are spindle like with rod-shaped nucleus (Fig. 7.62) in fascicular or storiform arrangement (Figs. 7.63 and 7.64), similar to myogenic sarcoma, fibrosarcoma, or chondrosarcoma, with invasive growth on the boundary of the tumor, and are often concurrent with typical HCC; therefore, adequate samples should be harvested. Immunohistochemical staining shows that spindle cells express Hep Par-1 (Fig. 7.65), AFP, CK, EMA (Fig. 7.66), vimentin (Fig. 7.67), and S-100. Electron microscope demonstrates cancer cells with abundant rough endoplasmic reticulum, phagolysosomes, lipid droplets, and

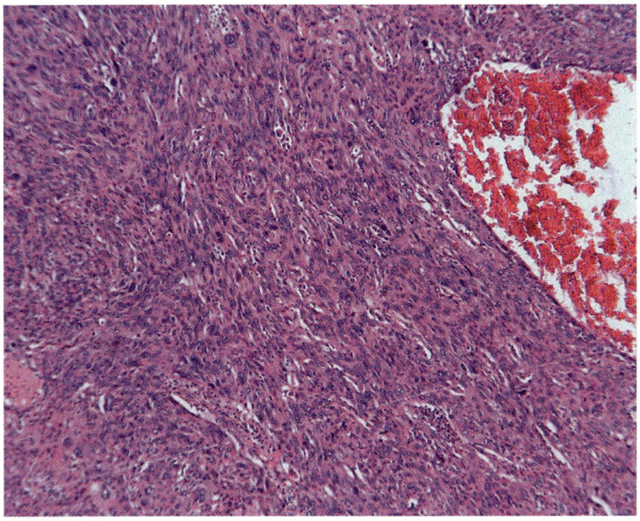

Fig. 7.62 HCC, spindle cell type, the tumors consisted of uniform long spindle cells

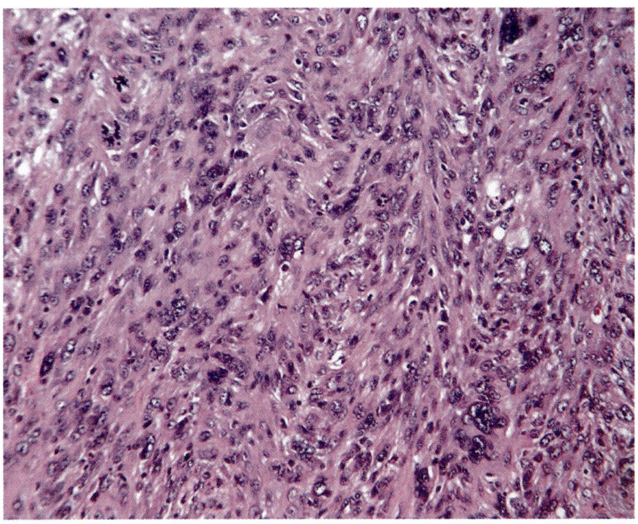

Fig. 7.63 HCC, spindle cell type, spindle tumor cells arranged in an interwoven pattern

microvillar projections, indicating that spindle cells derive from metaplasia or sarcomatoid change of HCC rather than real mesenchymal components. It can be diagnosed as sarcomatoid carcinoma but should be distinguished from carcinosarcoma, which is composed by both carcinoma and sarcoma elements. Spindle cell-type HCC has a poor prognosis with frequent invasion of portal vein and intrahepatic metastasis.

5. Foam cell-like type: According to our observations, the cells of this rare type of HCC are similar to the xanthoma cells, with cell volume one to two times greater than that of normal liver cells. Their cytoplasms are sparse and mesh filamentous, filled with microvesicles, and may also

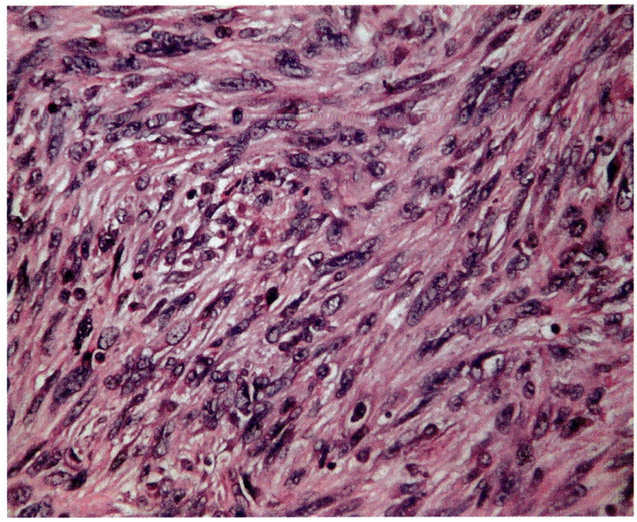

Fig. 7.64 HCC, spindle cell type, showing spindle tumor cells with rod-shaped nucleus

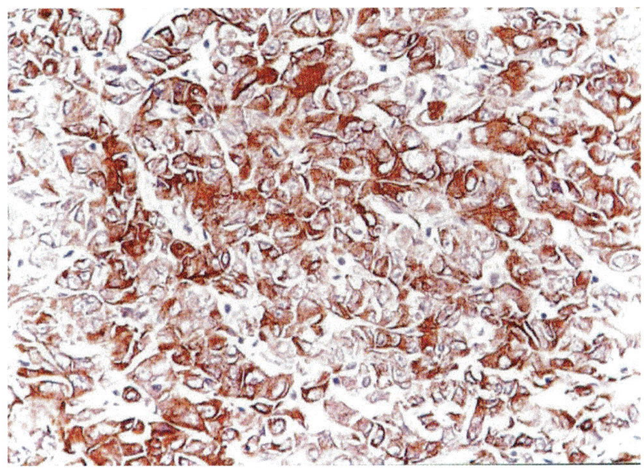

Fig. 7.65 HCC, spindle cell type, showing positive immunohistochemical staining of Hep Par-1

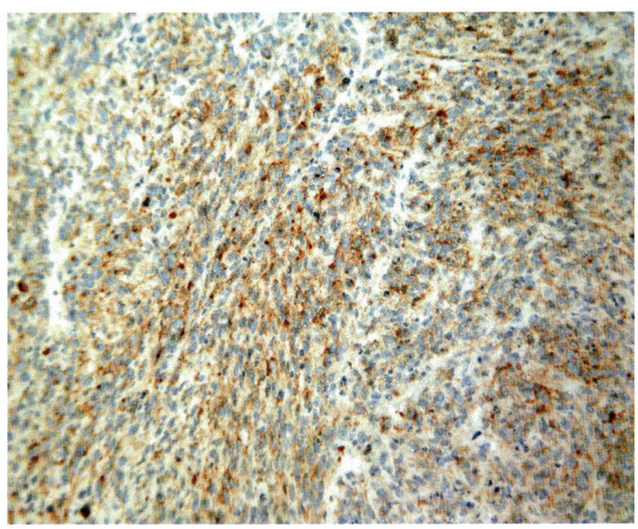

Fig. 7.66 HCC, spindle cell type, showing positive immunohistochemical staining of EMA

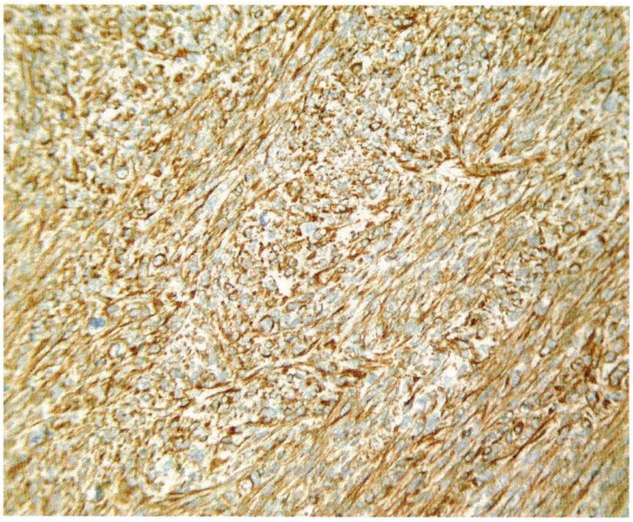

Fig. 7.67 HCC, spindle cell type, showing positive immunohistochemical staining of vimentin

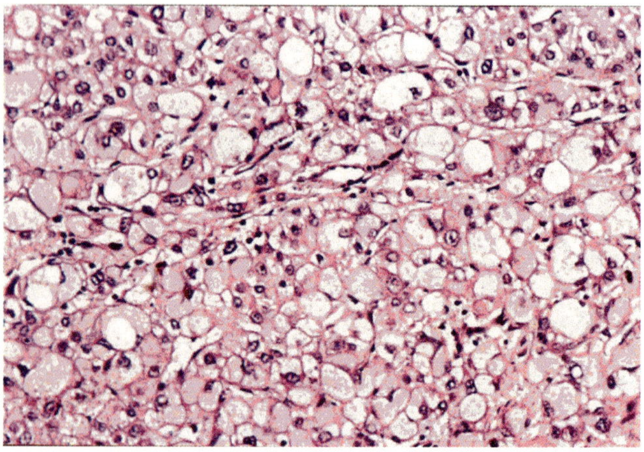

Fig. 7.68 HCC, foam cell-like HCC cells with a swollen vacuolated cytoplasm

contain tiny fat vacuoles. The nuclei are relatively small in size with no deviation (Figs. 7.68 and 7.69). The cancer cells lose the morphology of a liver cell, but the immunohistochemical staining shows positive Hep Par-1 (Fig. 7.70), which may be due to highly hydropic degeneration of the mitochondria in cancer cells, resulted in a more swelling and sparse cytoplasm than that in clear cell-type HCC.

6. Giant cell type: The cancer cells are pleomorphic in varying sizes and irregular shapes, with a large number of multiple or odd-shaped nuclei with megakaryocytes in horseshoe-shaped arrangement, and nuclear mitotic figures are commonly seen. The cells lack the morphology of liver cells (Fig. 7.71a–d), but immunohistochemical staining shows that they retain the hepatocytic phenotype.

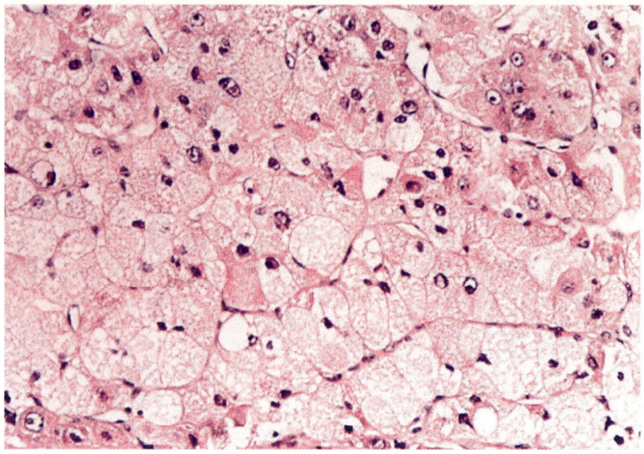

Fig. 7.69 HCC, foam cell-like type, the volume of foam cell-like HCC cells increased obviously

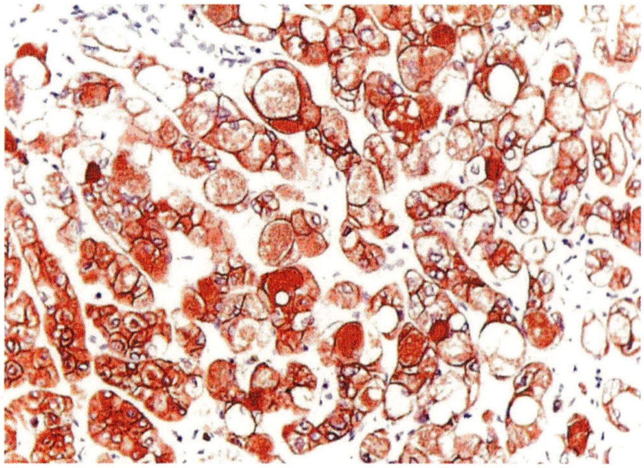

Fig. 7.70 HCC, foam cell-like type, showing positive immunohistochemical staining of Hep Par-1

In addition, osteoclast-like giant cells can be found in HCC tissues; thus, it is also known as osteoclast-like giant cell tumor of the liver, consisting of small mononuclear cells and osteoclast-like giant cells. The former are positive for AFP and CAM5.2, suggesting the origination from HCC, and it may be a metaplastic change of HCC, and the latter are strongly positive for CD68 and KP1, negative for AFP, CK, and P53, suggesting that it is a kind of reactive histiocyte.

(3) Grading of differentiation

Edmondson-Steiner grading is still widely used:

Grade I: The cancer cells are highly differentiated, with no obvious atypia, similar to normal liver cells, which are arranged in thin trabecules, similar to normal hepatic plates.

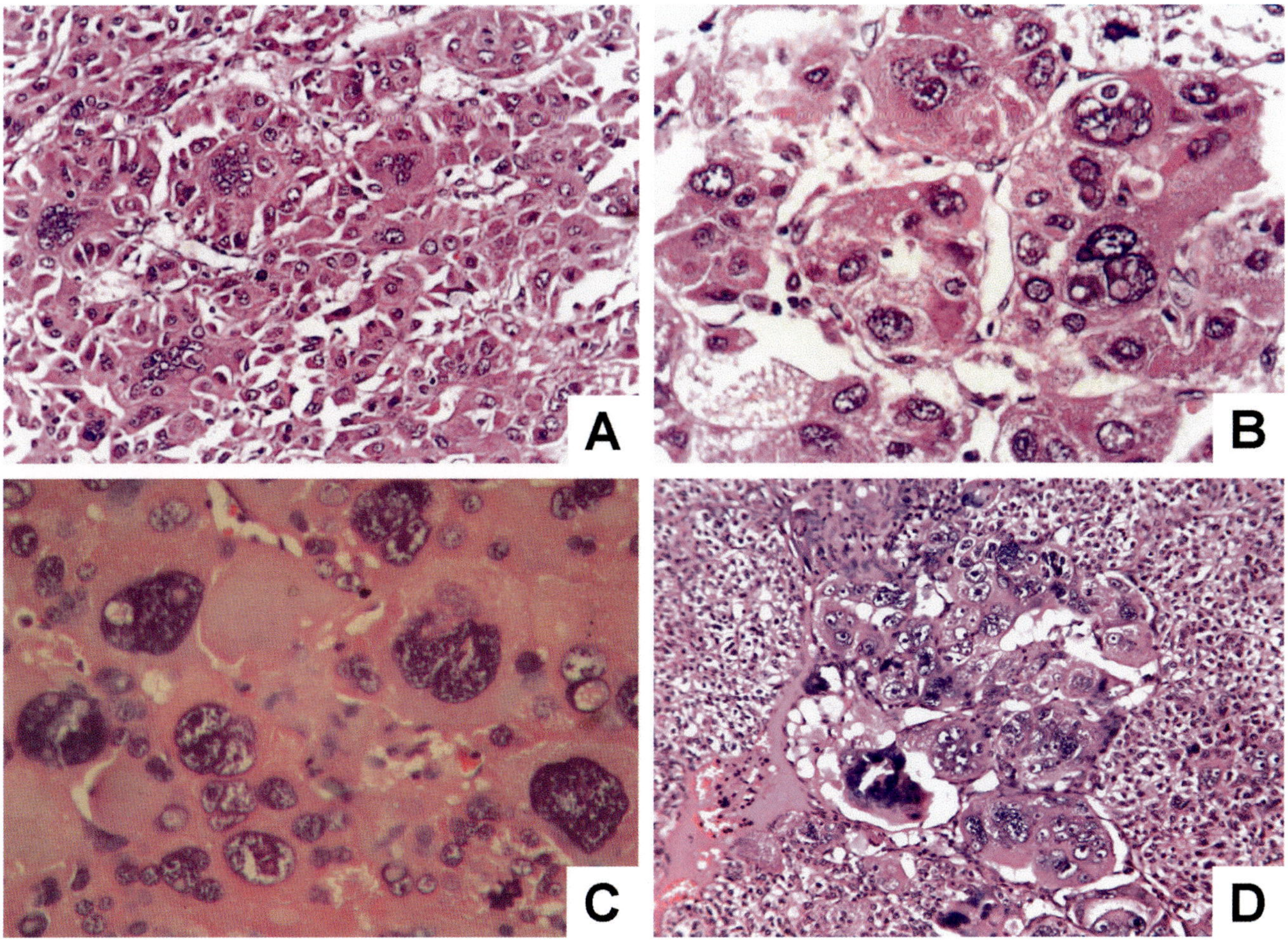

Fig. 7.71 HCC, giant cell type, showing multinucleated giant cells with odd-shaped nuclei

Grade II: The cancer cells are moderately differentiated with their morphology close to that of normal liver cells, arranged mainly in thin trabecules, but the karyoplasmic ratio is slightly increased, the nuclear staining darker, and the cytoplasm acidophilia increased. On the basis of trabecular structures, pseudoglandular structure may also be found.

Grade III: The differentiation of the cancer cells was poor, and the changes of nuclear volume, atypia, and mitotic figures were more obvious than that in Grade II; occasionally, a few tumor giant cells can be observed.

Grade IV: The cancer cells were undifferentiated or anaplastic, with extremely irregular shapes, or the tumor is an undifferentiated carcinoma. Tumor giant cells or tumor cells with odd-shaped nuclei are commonly seen, and highly pleomorphic carcinoma cells constitute the majority of them, with less cytoplasm, dark-stained nuclear chromatin, loose cell arrangement, and no significant trabecular structure.

In addition, a simple grading method recommended by WHO can also be adopted, with grades including well differentiation, moderate differentiation, poor differentiation, and undifferentiation. A potential relationship has been shown between clinical prognosis and differentiation of HCC; the grading of HCC can provide reference for the evaluation on the biological characteristics of HCC.

(4) Growth and infiltration

The diversification of HCC growth and invasion directly reflects the diversification of HCC biology behavior characteristics and is closely related to the prognosis of the patients, as well as an important reference for the designing of clinical individualized treatment mode. To sum up, HCC has at least the following eight patterns of growth and invasion:

1. Capsular invasion: It mainly contains two types. One is invasion inside the capsule, and the tumor has not invaded

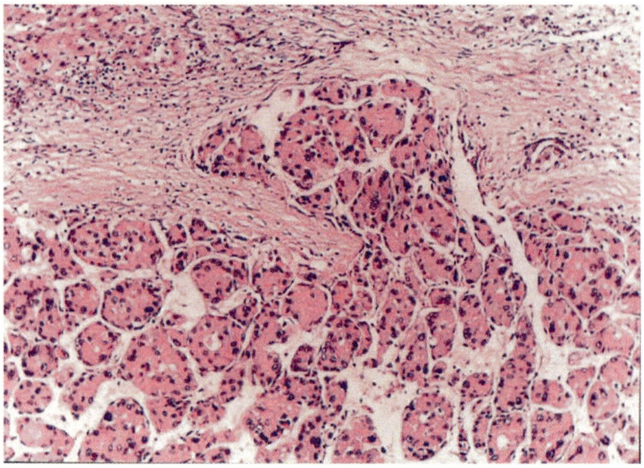

Fig. 7.72 HCC, tumor capsule vessel invasion

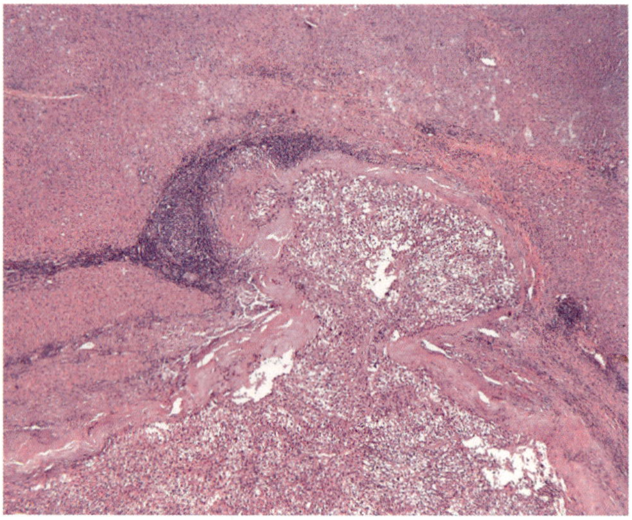

Fig. 7.73 HCC, tumor bursting into the capsule

the whole layers of the capsule and forms tumor thrombus in the capsule (Fig. 7.72). The other is a breakthrough of the capsule, forming satellite foci or tumor embolus outside the capsule. It is noted that the capsule is an important barrier against the dissemination of HCC, and the formation of a second capsule after the breakthrough of the first layer of the capsule is sometimes observed in HCC tissue (Fig. 7.73), as well as multiple layers of fibrous capsule formation (Fig. 7.74). Complete resection of the tumor can be achieved by expanding the resection area to a certain distance adjacent to the tumor capsule. HCC complicated by liver cirrhosis often has a capsule, while HCC cases without cirrhosis often contain no capsule with a potential of invasive growth into paracancerous liver tissue to form multifocal lesions due to lack of fibrous blockage.

2. Vascular invasion HCC can invade major hepatic vessels with observable tumor thrombus in them both grossly and

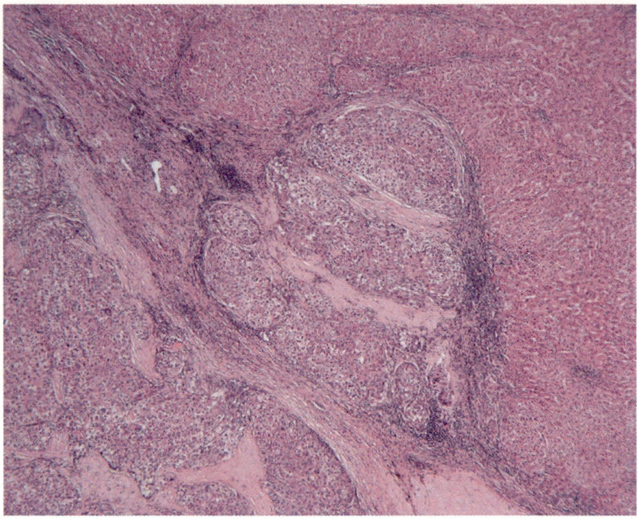

Fig. 7.74 HCC, showing repeated capsule invasion and repeated capsule enveloping

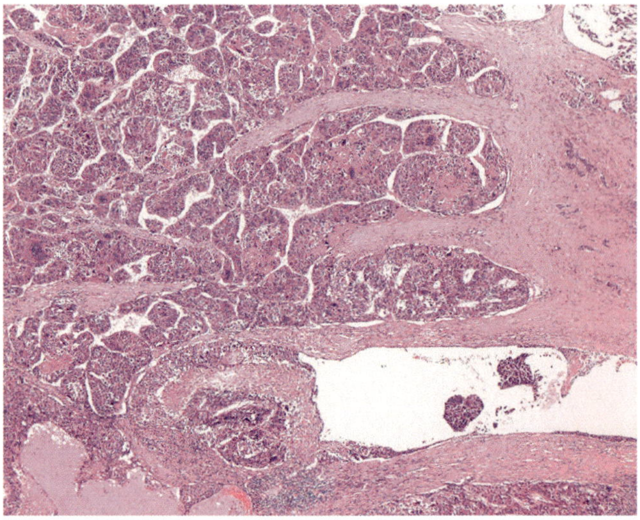

Fig. 7.75 HCC, tumor thrombus formation in tumor stroma

on images or presents microvascular invasion (MVI) or microvascular thrombus. At present, the definition, diagnostic criteria, and grading system of MVI have not reached a consensus. In view that HCC is rich in sinuses and lacks fibrous interstitial components, many scholars defined MVI as the microscopical observation of tumor thrombus inside the vessels lined with endothelial cells, mainly within the branches of the portal vein and tributaries of the hepatic vein or vessels of the tumor capsule. Occasionally, the liver cancer may invade the hepatic artery, bile duct, and lymphatic vessels, which should be reported independently because of their differences in clinical significance. As for trabecular patterns of HCC lined with sinusoidal endothelial cells, it is not a real MVI (Fig. 7.75). The MVI tends to adhere on endothelial cells or invades the vascular wall, resulting in interruption of

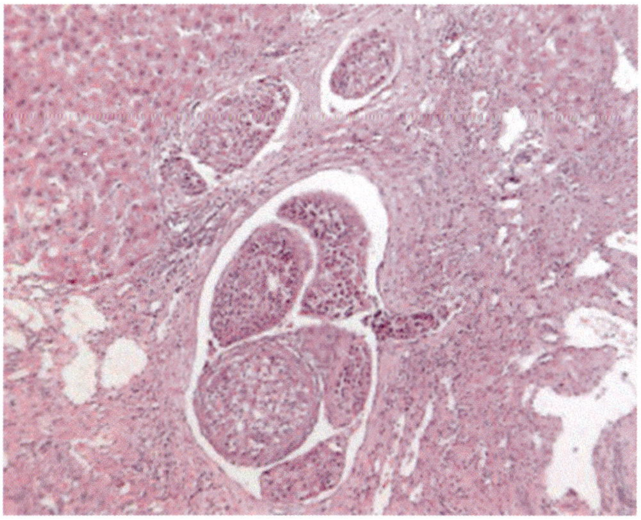

Fig. 7.76 HCC, tumor thrombus in the multilevel branch of the portal vein

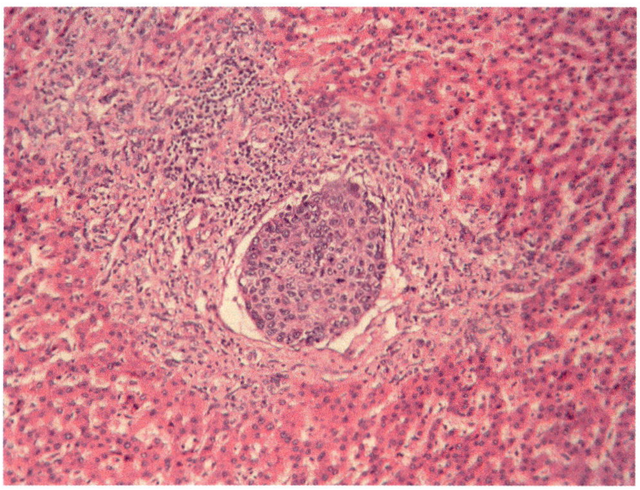

Fig. 7.77 HCC, microvascular thrombus in the portal interlobar vein

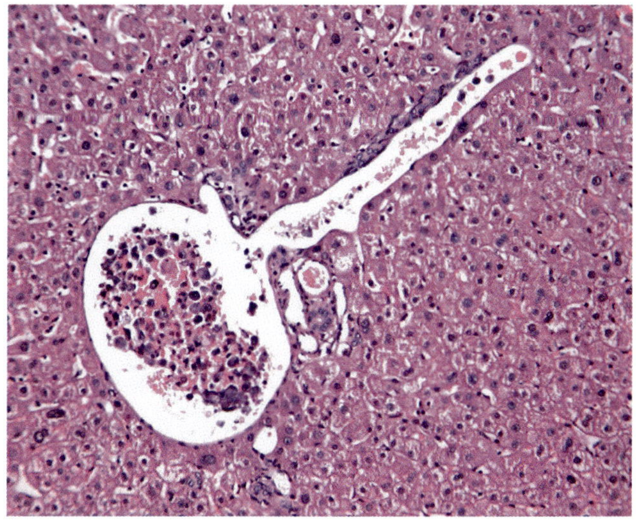

Fig. 7.78 HCC, showing intravascular floating tumor clusters in the branch of portal vein

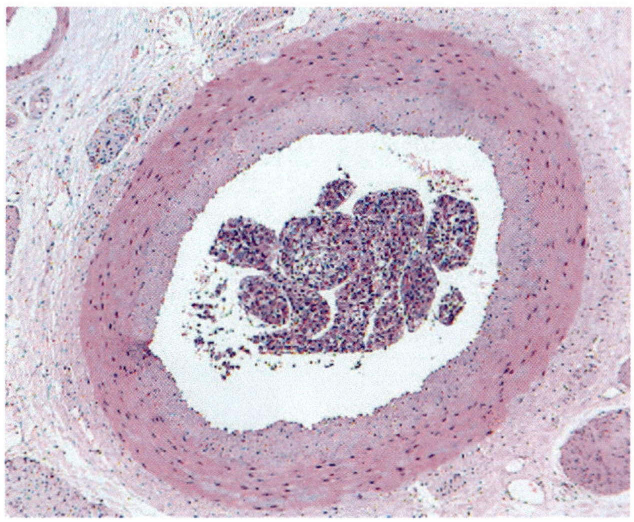

Fig. 7.79 HCC, tumor thrombi involving the branch of the hepatic artery

the vascular endothelium (Figs. 7.76, 7.77, and 7.78). Studies have shown that the cancer cells must enter the vessels lined by endothelial cells and they can escape from the host's immune attack and the coagulation cascade to survive and metastate. Other studies showed that >50 suspended carcinoma cells in the portal vein were markedly correlated to the prognosis (Fig. 7.79) [19]. The incidence of MVI increase with the increase of tumor size, which is a key pathological factor leading to high risk of recurrence and poor prognosis of HCC patients after surgical resection.

According to the literature, the incidence of MVI in HCC was 15–57%, which increases with the increase of HCC volume. MVI in the adjacent paracancerous liver tissue can be excised along with the primary tumor in operation, while those located in distant paracancerous liver tissue cannot be removed in whole easily. MVI occurs not only as late stage of HCC, and numerous and distant MVI can increase the risk of recurrence and metastasis of HCC. Most of the studies demonstrate that MVI is an indicator for highly invasive growth of HCC and is one of the independent pathological factors affecting the postoperative recurrence and long-term therapeutic efficacy of HCC, as well as the important pathological evidence for anti-recurrence treatment. Therefore, pathological examinations should include careful observation on the number, distance, vascular types, and distribution of MVI. In addition, lymphatic vessel invasion, metastasis along lymphatic vessels, or tumor thrombi in intrahepatic

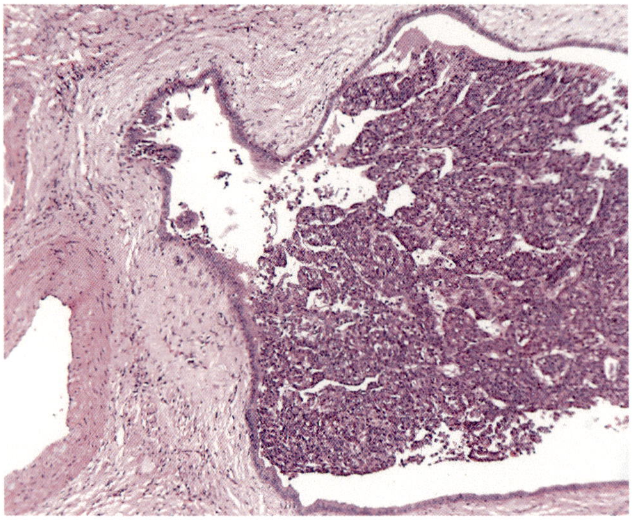

Fig. 7.80 HCC, tumor thrombi involving the branch of bile ducts

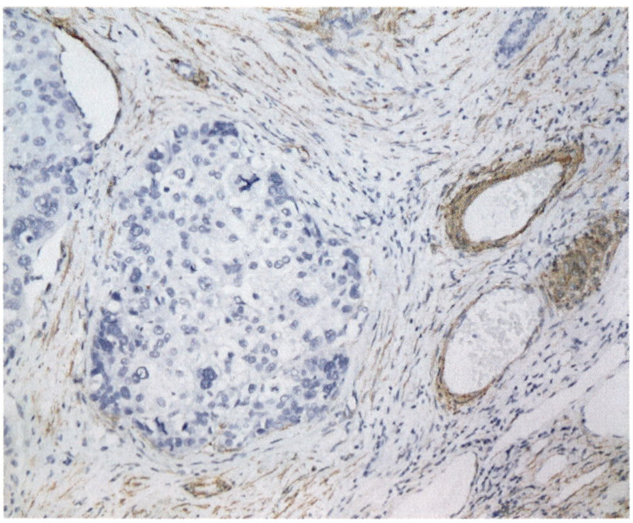

Fig. 7.81 HCC, showing negative immunohistochemical staining of SMA for carcinoma nests or satellites

bile ducts can be found in a few cases of HCC (Fig. 7.80). According to the *Practice guidelines for the pathological diagnosis of primary liver cancer: 2015 update* of China, risk grading of MVI should be done according to the quantity and distribution of MVI: M0, no visible MVI; M1 (low-risk group), ≤5 MVI in adjacent paracancerous liver tissue (≤1 cm); and M2 (high-risk group), > 5 MVI or MVI in distant paracencerous liver tissue (> 1 cm).

To avoid the misdiagnosis of fibrous tissue around the cancer cell nests as MVI, a selection of immunohistochemical staining is used. VEGF, CD31, CD34, SMA (Fig. 7.81), and h-caldesmon can label blood vascular endothelial cells and D2–40, podoplanin, and LYVE-1 can label lymphatic endothelial cells. Rodríguez-Perálvarez et al. (2013) pointed out that tumor thrombus within the vessels wrapped by a

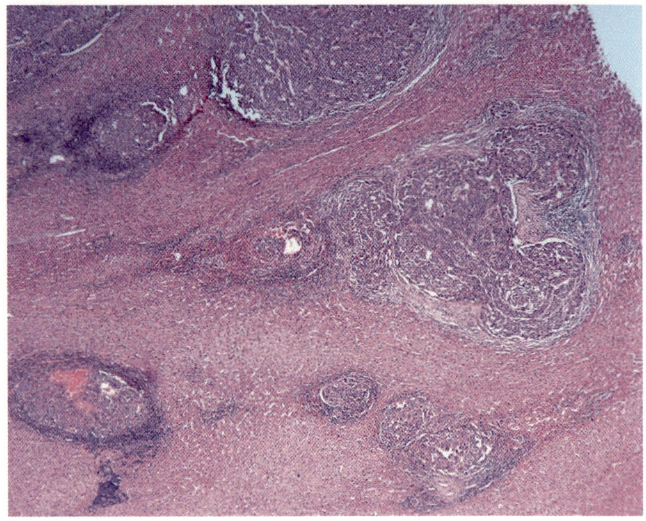

Fig. 7.82 HCC, showing multiple satellite nodules in the peritumoral tissue

smooth muscle can be accurately diagnosed as MVI; however, micro- veins have only a thin layer of the outer membrane that contains longitudinally arranged collagen fibers and elastic fibers; thus, staining methods for elastic fibers can be applied for identification, including Victoria blue, orcein, and Elastica van Gieson staining (EVG).

3. Satellite nodules: Satellite nodules usually refers to small tumor foci located in the paracancerous tissue within a distance of ≤2 cm from the primary tumor, and there is no continuity between them (Fig. 7.82). Those lesions adjacent to the main tumor or the capsule of the tumor are often sub-tumor foci. Lesions located in the paracancerous tissue at a distance >2 cm from the primary tumor (Fig. 7.83), particularly cancer nodules with a diameter >2 cm, can be either intrahepatic metastasis of the primary tumor or new tumor foci, which are usually indistinguishable morphologically, and molecular clone detection should be considered to determine the clonal origin and the nature of these lesions.

4. Early hepatocarcinogenesis: Early hepatocarcinogenesis in the precancerous liver tissues are often well-differentiated foci based on the background of cirrhosis and high-grade dysplastic nodules, exhibiting natural transition between carcinoma trabecules and hepatic plates (Fig. 7.83), and they are the pathological basis of multicentric origin for HCC development.
5. Transition: No significant border can be found between the carcinoma cells and normal liver cells in the pericarcinoma tissues due to the transition or replacement growth without fibrous capsule. The only slight difference between them is the cytoplasmic staining and trabecular

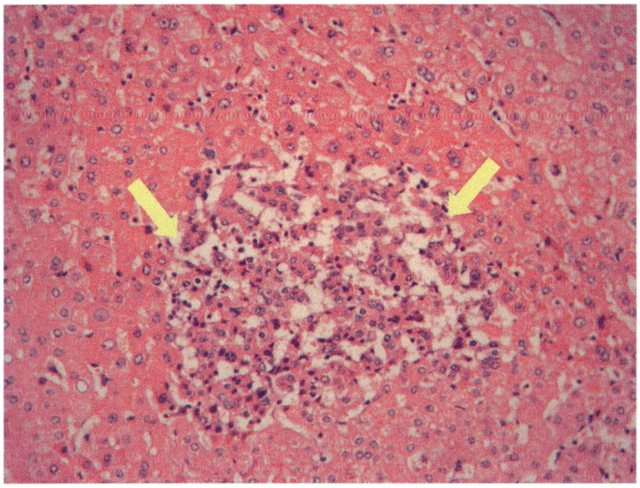

Fig. 7.83 HCC, showing early carcinoma foci inthe peritumoral tissue

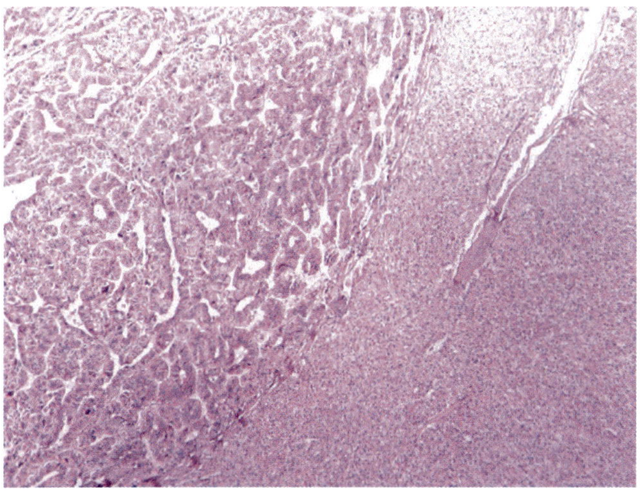

Fig. 7.84 HCC, pseudoglandular pattern with pseudoglandular pattern

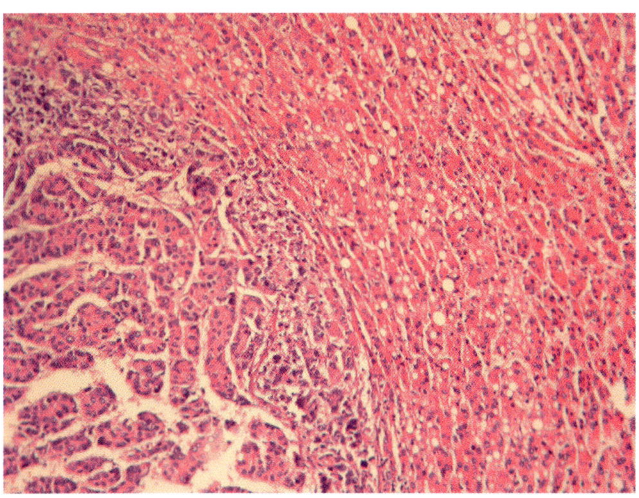

Fig. 7.85 HCC, thin trabecular pattern with thick trabecular pattern

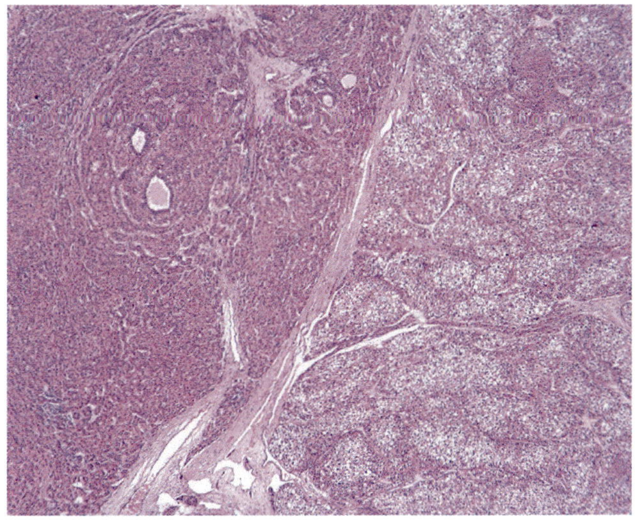

Fig. 7.86 HCC, thick trabecular pattern with thin trabecular pattern

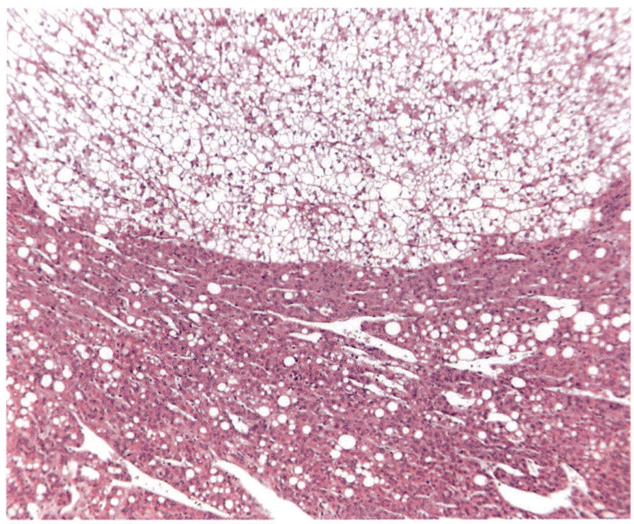

Fig. 7.87 HCC, clear cell type with thin trabecular pattern

width which can be used carefully for identification (Fig. 7.84).

6. Multiple histological structures: We observed that about 30% of HCC contain two or more different histological and cytological types, named as HCC with multiple histological structures (MS-HCC) (Figs. 7.85, 7.86, 7.87, 7.88, and 7.89). This phenotype represents one of the HCC heterogeneous features, and it also suggests polyclonal origins of the tumor cells in HCC. We conducted genomic microsatellite variation pattern analysis on the clonal association in MS-HCC tissues and found at least a part of MS-HCC cases have multicentric origins. Theoretically, this multi-phenomenon of MS-HCC may suggest the formation of multiple subclones due to the

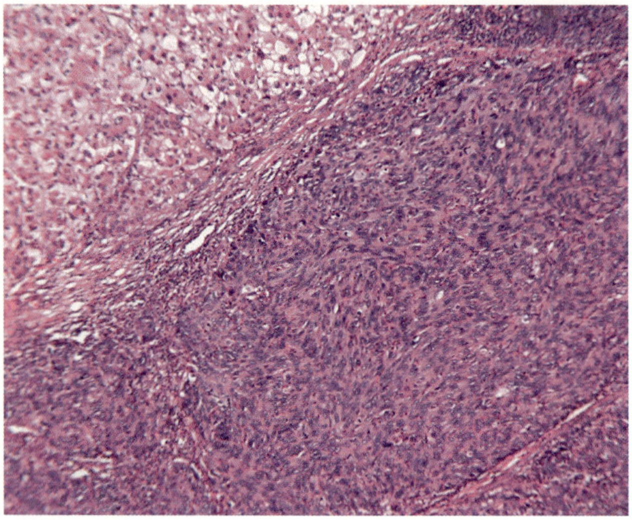

Fig. 7.88 HCC, clear cell type with spindle cell type

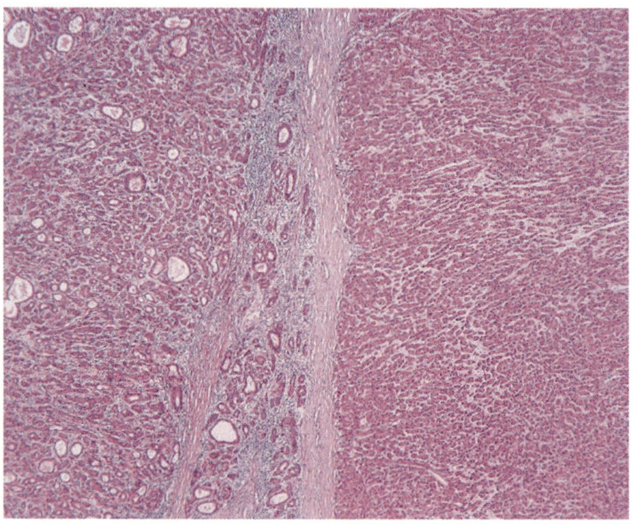

Fig. 7.89 HCC, pseudoglandular pattern with thin trabecular pattern

selection pressure and mutation variations among the carcinoma cells, which may improve the complexity and diversity of biological behaviors as well as the clinical response to the treatment of HCC, and this is worthy of further classification studies [20].

7. Neural invasion: Invasion of neural tissues by HCC can be found occasionally in a few cases (Fig. 7.90a, b), suggesting that HCC may also be disseminated along the nerve sheath.

8. Invasion of hepatic sinusoids: It is caused by the direct invasion of the carcinoma cells into the adjacent hepatic sinusoids to form map-like irregular boundaries due to the absence of capsule around the tumor (Fig. 7.91).

(5) Inclusion body

HCC cells may contain a variety of types of inclusion bodies, which facilitate the diagnosis, and the common types of inclusion bodies mainly have the following two types.

1. Pale bodies: They are oval, pale-stained, eosinophilic bodies in the cytoplasm, and the nuclei were frequently displaced to the periphery by the inclusions (Figs. 7.92 and 7.93) and negative for periodic acid-Schiff (PAS) staining and Masson's trichrome staining. Immunohistochemistry shows they are positive for fibrinogen and electron microscope demonstrated pale bodies containing electron density particles wrapped by a membrane closely related to the dilated rough endoplasmic reticulum, suggesting that pale bodies may be caused by deficient transportation of fibrinogen resulting in its accumulation in cystic endoplasmic reticulum. The occurrence of pale bodies in the HCC cells is of diagnostic significance to some extent.

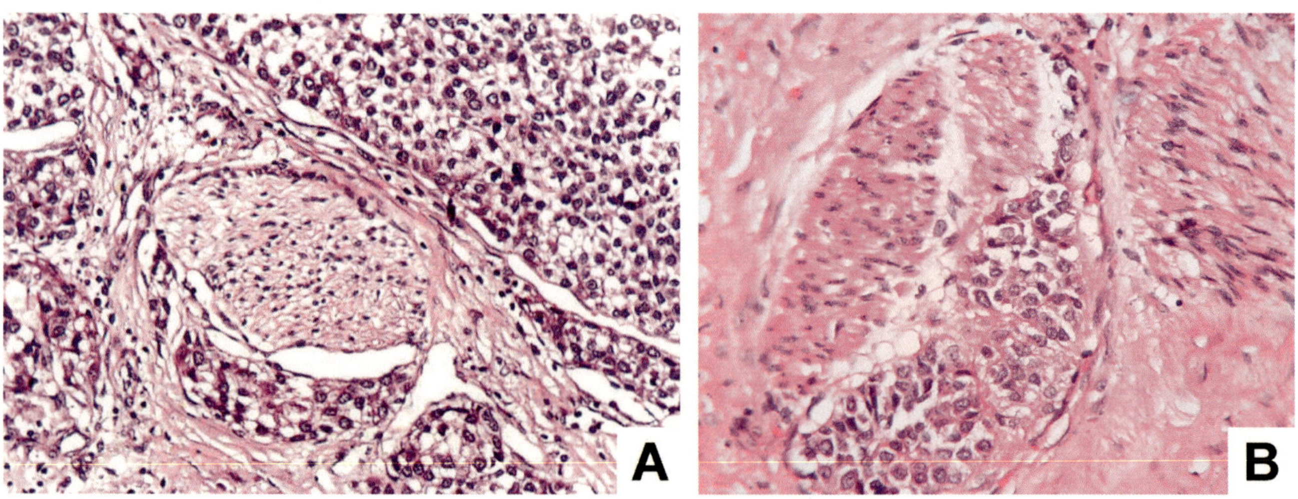

Fig. 7.90 HCC, perineural invasion of HCC cells

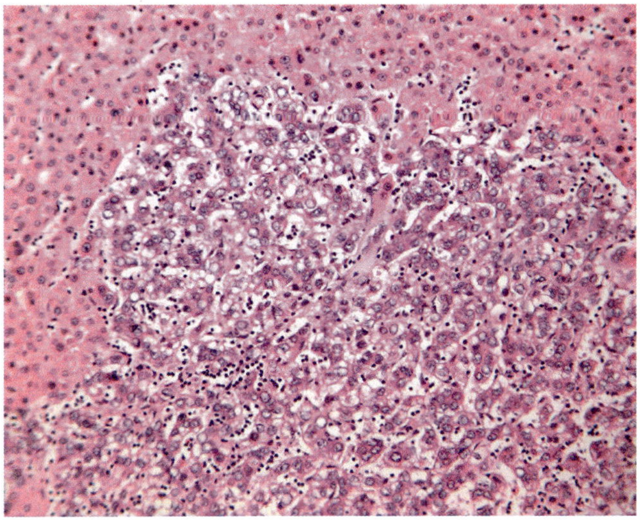

Fig. 7.91 HCC, infiltration of carcinoma cells into the hepatic sinusoids

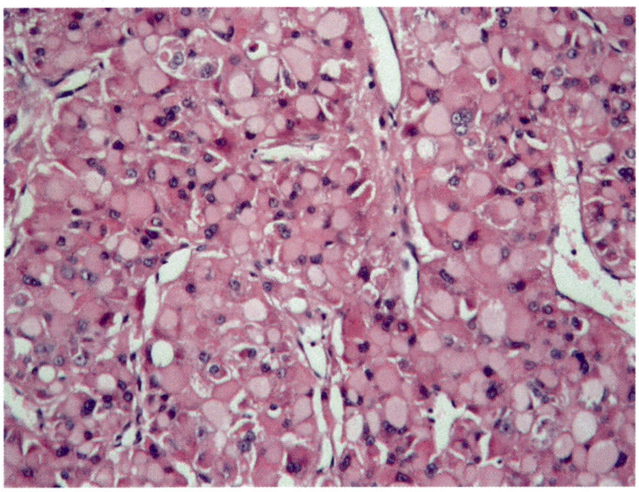

Fig. 7.92 HCC, pale bodies, tumor cells contained intracytoplasmic ground-glass-like pale bodies

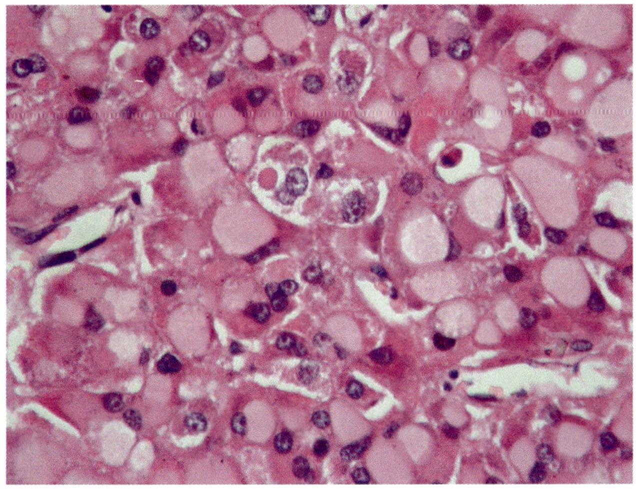

Fig. 7.93 HCC, pale bodies, hepatocytes displayed pale or eosinophilic staining of the cytoplasm with nuclei displacement to the periphery

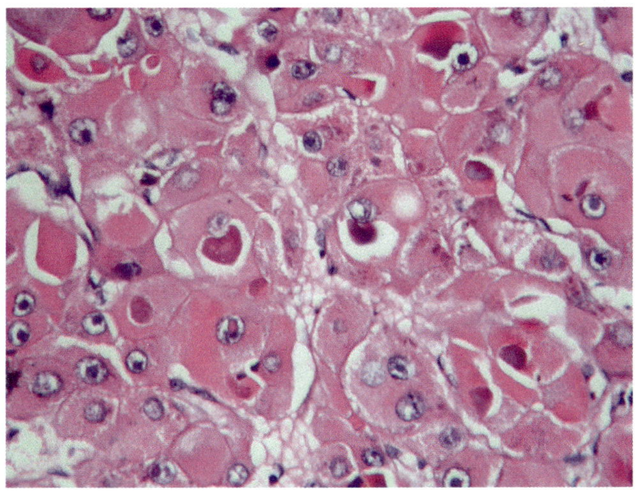

Fig. 7.94 HCC, eosinophilic bodies, intracellular hyaline bodies with surrounding halo

2. Eosinophilic bodies: They are spherical or rod-shaped, homogeneous red-dyed hyaline bodies in the cytoplasm, 2–20 μm in diameter. Small ones are only half the volume of a nucleus, while large ones are 2–3 times larger than a nucleus. The cytoplasm is filled with eosinophilic bodies which are surrounded by halos (Figs. 7.94 and 7.95). They are negative for α1-antitrypsin, CK, and PAS staining, containing components of p62 protein which can enhance the transcriptional activity of liver cells. The major difference between them and Mallory bodies is that the former almost does not contain ubiquitin [21].

We observed that eosinophilic bodies reacted on HBsAg staining (Figs. 7.96 and 7.97), indicating the existence of associated protein components. Under electron microscope, eosinophilic bodies consist of homogeneous granules or reticular electronic density matrix, wrapped in the dilated rough endoplasmic reticulum or the remnants of the endoplasmic reticulum. It has been speculated that eosinophilic bodies are formed by intracellular accumulation of proteins due to abnormal protein secretion or transportation, which is indicative of injured tumor cells [22].

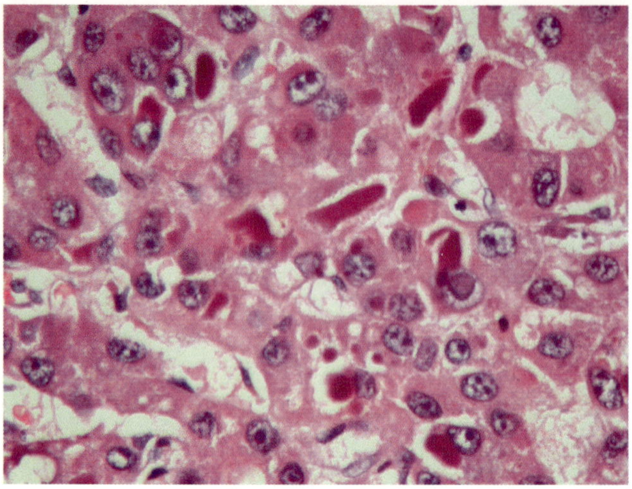

Fig. 7.95 HCC, eosinophilic bodies, intracytoplasmic oval homogeneous eosinophilic hyaline bodies

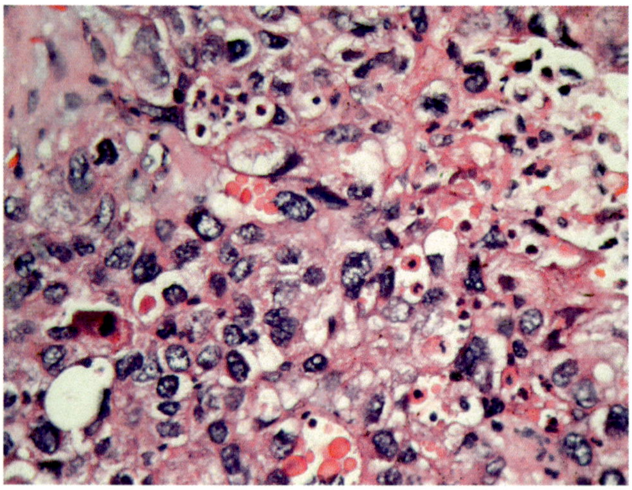

Fig. 7.96 HCC, eosinophilic bodies, intracytoplasmic small round eosinophilic hyaline bodies

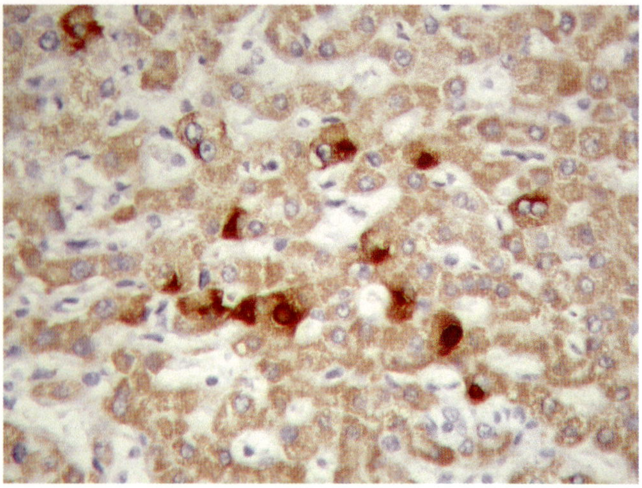

Fig. 7.97 HCC, eosinophilic bodies are positive for HBsAg immunohistochemical staining

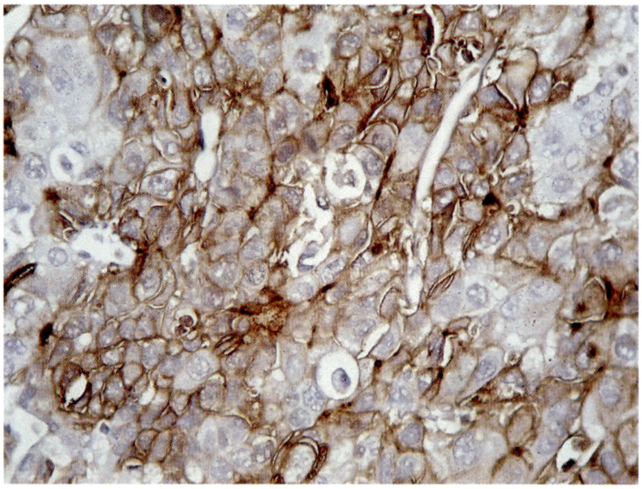

Fig. 7.98 HCC, immunohistochemical staining, a bile canalicular pattern of staining with pCEA

7.1.1.7 Immunohistochemistry

Commonly used markers for liver cells are Hep Par-1, CD10 (Fig. 7.98), pCEA (Fig. 7.99), GPC-3, CD34 (Figs. 7.21 and 7.24), AFP, etc. The former three markers cannot be used to distinguish the nature of liver cells, while the latter three markers are characteristically expressed in HCC tissues. And in differentiation from non-hepatocellular tumors, a combination of liver cell markers is very effective, and positive HBsAg staining is of certain reference value in the diagnosis of HCC (Fig. 7.100). The American Association for the Study of Liver Diseases (AASLD), the European Association of Liver Diseases, and the Panel of International Consensus Group all make the recommendation of diagnostic marker combination for HCC, "GPC-3+HSP70+GS," which has a sensitivity and a specificity of 72% and 100%, respectively [23]. In addition, Yong et al. (2013) recently found high expression of the carcinoembryonic gene SALL4 in 55.6% of HCC tissues, but no expression was detected in pericarcinoma liver tissues and was associated with a poor prognosis. It can be used as a potential diagnostic marker in immunohistochemistry for HCC [24], and the evaluation of the background (inflammation, fibrosis) in the pericarcinoma liver tissue can rely on Masson staining.

7.1.1.8 Differential Diagnosis

The acinar (pseudoglandular)-type HCC should be differentiated from intrahepatic cholangiocarcinoma (ICC) and hepatic metastatic adenocarcinoma (HMA), and the main differential points of the three are shown in Table 7.1. The immunohistochemical features of HCC are shown in Chap. 6 Immunohistochemistry and Special Staining for Liver Tissue.

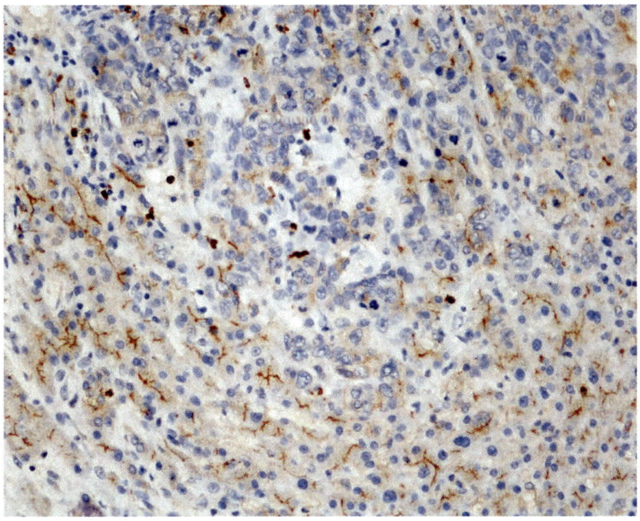

Fig. 7.99 HCC, immunohistochemical staining, a bile canalicular pattern of staining with CD10

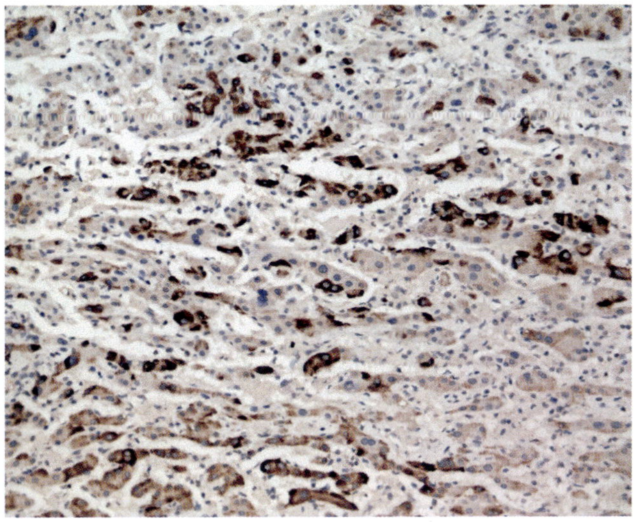

Fig. 7.100 HCC, immunohistochemical staining, showing adjacent non-tumor HBsAg-positive tissue

Table 7.1 Differential diagnosisof acinar HCC, ICC, and HMA

Features	Acinar HCC	ICC	HMA
Clinic			
Elevated serum AFP	Most cases	Some cases	Normal
Elevated serum CA19-9	Normal	Most cases	Normal
Hepatitis history	Most cases	A few cases	Rare
Histology			
Fibrous stroma	No/rare	Rich	Little
Adenoid structure	Cuboidal cells	Cuboidal cells	Cuboidal/columnar cells
Bile secretion	Yes	None	None
Mucus secretion	None	Yes	Yes
Immunohistochemistry			
Hep Par-1 positive	83–93%	Occasionally	Occasionally
GPC-3 positive	50–90%	0	0
CK19 positive	10–20%	85–95%	0–40%
MUC-1 positive	0	65.8–73.8%	50–80%
pCEA staining	Canalicular pattern	Cytoplasmic pattern	Cytoplasmic pattern
CD34 staining	Rich microvessels	Sparse microvessels	Sparse microvessels

7.1.1.9 Assessment of Prognosis and Staging

Many factors have an impact on the prognosis of HCC. And to accurately evaluate the risk of postsurgical recurrence, survival, and prognosis in HCC patients, approximately 20 clinical pathological staging schemes for HCC have been proposed in the current literature, including the following HCC staging systems with great influence, such as the seventh edition of the American Joint Committee on Cancer (AJCC)/The Union for International Cancer Control (UICC) tumor-node-metastasis (TNM) staging system (Table 7.2), Okuda staging, the Cancer of the Liver Italian Program (CLIP) index, the Barcelona Clinic Liver Cancer (BCLC) score, the French staging, the Chinese University Prognostic Index (CUPI), Japan Integrated Staging (JIS), the Tokyo score, etc. The index system is usually composed of serological indexes and pathological parameters (such as tumor size, tumor number, MVI, satellite nodules, differentiation, grading, etc.), while the currently available staging systems in the literature have not received unanimous verdict in the assessment of HCC biological characteristics and prognosis of patients with HCC, each of which has advantages and disadvantages. Kee et al. (2013) identified that the seventh edition of the TNM staging was of better predictive value for the prognosis of HCC than its sixth edition [25]. In view of the high heterogeneity and malignancy of HCC, it is not sufficient to predict its complex biological behaviors based on the limited clinical and pathological indexes. Therefore, several indexes have been included into the staging of HCC, such as serum albumin, bilirubin, vascular endothelial growth (VEGF), and insulin-like growth factor-1 (IGF-1) [26]. It can

Table 7.2 TNM staging of HCC by AJCC (seventh edition)

TNM staging	Features		
T_1	Solitary tumor without vascular invasion		
T_2	Single tumor with vascular invasion or multiple tumors, none more than 5 cm		
T_{3a}	Multiple tumors, more than 5 cm		
T_{3b}	Single tumor or multiple tumors of any size involving a major branch of the portal vein of hepatic vein		
T_4	Tumor with direct invasion of adjacent organs other than the gallbladder or with perforation of the visceral peritoneum		
N_0	No regional lymph node metastasis		
N_1	Regional lymph node metastasis		
M_0	No distant metastasis		
M_1	Distant metastasis		
Staging			
Stage I	T_1	N_0	M_0
Stage II	T_2	N_0	M_0
Stage IIIA	T_{3a}	N_0	M_0
Stage IIIB	T_{3b}	N_0	M_0
Stage IIIC	T_4	N_0	M_0
Stage IVA	Any T	N_1	M_0
Stage IVB	Any T	Any N	M_1

be expected that, with the development of understanding on the biological characteristics of HCC, there will be consistent improvement and perfection in the prognostic evaluation system of HCC, including the international TNM staging.

In addition, Shirabe et al. (2014) proposed that in cases of HCC with the tumor diameter of 3.6 cm, the maximum standard uptake value (SUVmax) of 18F- fluorodeoxyglucose (FDG) in positron emission tomography (PET) was 4.2, and the abnormal prothrombin in serum reached 10 mAU/ml, both of which have the highest sensitivity and specificity in prediction of MVI [27]. Tsujita et al. (2012) proposed the indexes affecting the prognosis of patients with recurrent HCC: ①indocyanine green retention rate at 15 minutes, ②the disease-free interval, ③tumor size, ④portal vein invasion at resection of the primary HCC, ⑤ gender, and ⑥blood loss [28]. Kadalayil et al. (2013) proposed the prognosis indexes for TACE in HCC, including albumin <36 g/dl, bilirubin >17 μmol/L, and AFP >400 ng/ml or the diameter of the primary tumor >7 cm, each of which was recorded as 1 point. The median survival time for patients scoring 0, 1, 2, and >2 points was 27.6 months, 18.5 months, 9 months, and 3.6 months [29], respectively. Furthermore, the molecular typing of HCC will be an important trend for HCC research in the future.

7.1.1.10 Pathological Diagnosis Report

As stated, factors related to the therapeutic effect and survival of patients with HCC include growth pattern, proliferation activity, invasion and metastasis potential, postoperative recurrence risk, and variation of genes and proteins associated with biological characteristics, the main carrier for the above important information is the tumor tissue specimens. Obviously, the traditional pathology focuses on the diagnosis model mainly based on the morphological features of HCC tissues and cells; however, it does not fit the concern about the pathobiological features of HCC in modern hepatic surgery, and new adjustments and supplements in the diagnostic concept, modes, and contents should be made to establish a comprehensive mode of pathological diagnosis based on both pathology and biology, further providing practical pathological information for the improvement of clinical curative effects. This is an important trend for future pathology of hepatic tumors.

Therefore, pathological diagnosis report for HCC should meet the clinical demands and concerns for the assessment of tumor growth pattern, prediction of metastasis and recurrence risk, formulation of individualized treatment strategy and evaluation of prognosis. No uniform standards on the content or format of the pathological diagnosis report for HCC have been determined, and it mainly includes the following aspects depending on the specific circumstances:

① Morphological features related to prognosis, including macroscopic (tumor number, tumor size, gross type, etc.) and microscopic features (histological types, differentiation degree, MVI, satellite nodules, growth pattern, etc.) with attached typical photographs.

② Auxiliary diagnostic criteria, e.g., diagnostic and differential diagnostic evidences based on immunohistochemistry, including dual-phenotype HCC (DPHCC).

③ Characteristics of biological behaviors, e.g., detection results of molecular markers associated with the risk of invasion, recurrence, and prognosis of HCC.

④ Diagnosis of specific lesions, e.g., analysis of the clonal origin of recurrent and multinodular HCC and analysis of genomic instability in precancerous lesions, including high-grade dysplastic nodules, hepatocellular adenoma, etc.

⑤ Analysis on therapeutic sensitivity: Despite several molecular target drugs for HCC at present, screening of sensitive populations and specific molecular targets need further explorations. Furthermore, patients with low expression of miR-26a in HCC tissues treated by interferon were found to have an improved 5-year survival rate from 30 to 65% in the study by the Liver Cancer Institute of Fudan University, suggesting it was a potential pathological marker for evaluating interferon therapy in the future, and more attention should be paid to their further results from multicenter validation study.

⑥ Remarks: Specifications on important morphological and biological indicators, such as tumor invasion, metastasis and prognosis, and differential diagnosis, should be illustrated or supplemented in the remarks to facilitate clinicians' concern and understanding.

7.1.2 Small Hepatocellular Carcinoma

(1) Basic concept of small hepatocellular carcinoma (SHCC)

Early discovery, early treatment, and early cure and the smaller the tumor, the better the therapeutic efficacy have always been the basic principles and the ideal goals of modern surgical oncology. Many studies have suggested that the size of solid tumors can be used as an important reference index to assess the clinical prognosis of the patients. Despite many clinical and pathological factors that affect the malignancy and prognosis of the tumor, tumor size remains the most intuitive and simple index for presurgical assessment on tumorous progression stages. A typical example is the concepts of early gastric carcinoma, small gastric carcinoma, and micro-gastric carcinoma which were proposed 30 years ago and has greatly improved the level of clinical diagnosis and treatment of gastric cancer. In the late 1970s, Chinese scholars represented by academician Prof. Zhao-You Tang and Prof. Meng-Chao Wu first put forward the important concept of SHCC, being the milestone in development of clinical research of HCC into a new era of SHCC. In those days, the understanding of SHCC features in the field of hepatic surgery mainly include the following: 70% of the HCC patients with no obvious clinical symptoms had tumors ≤5 cm in diameter, and more than 70% of the HCC patients with obvious clinical symptoms had tumors >5 cm in diameter. Therefore, the tumor volume of ≤5 cm in diameter is widely accepted as the diagnostic standard for SHCC both at home and abroad. Under the condition of limited diagnostic and treatment techniques of HCC in that time, low rates of diagnosis and surgical resection of SHCC ≤5 cm were observed, and there were even reports in which surgically excised HCC <4.5 cm was called microcarcinoma [30]. And a diameter of 5 cm was still adopted as the pathological staging criteria in the seventh edition of TNM staging of HCC issued by AJCC and UICC in 2009.

On the basis of the study of 500 autopsy cases of HCC pathological specimens, the pathological classification of the "Five Major Types and Six Sub-Types" of HCC was put forward by the Chinese Cooperative Pathology Group of Liver Cancer in 1982, and three nodules ≤3 cm in diameter were called SHCC, which was especially proposed for the first time and was one of the most prominent contributions in the field of pathology of HCC in China. Since then, we have conducted systematic studies on the relationship between HCC size and its pathological biological behaviors based on the rat carcinogenesis model and surgically excised human HCC of different tumor sizes, demonstrating that SHCC ≤3 cm is often DNA diploid dominant, with relatively benign biological behaviors of HCC in the early stage, good prognosis, and low recurrence rate, while LHCC >3 cm is often DNA ploidy dominant, with obvious malignant biological behaviors, high postoperative recurrence rate, and low long-term survival rate. Thus, it has been proposed that HCC which is approximate 3 cm in diameter is in a key period in which its biological characteristics transform from relatively benign nature to marked malignancy, and the early diagnosis and treatment of SHCC can lead to relatively good therapeutic effects based on its pathobiological feature of radical resectability. Right now, BCLC staging system-defined HCC in the early stage may include patients with single or up to three tumor nodules, each ≤3 cm. However, based on the clonal origin theory of multinodular HCC, we think there is a great possibility of intrahepatic metastasis for three tumor nodules ≤3 cm. Therefore, in the *Practice guidelines for the pathological diagnosis of primary liver cancer: 2015 update* issued by the Chinese Pathological Group of Hepatobiliary Tumor and Liver Transplantation, a single tumor with a diameter from >1 cm to ≤3 cm is defined as SHCC.

Based on the statistics of data from the Department of Pathology in our hospital, the proportion of SHCC ≤3 cm treated by surgical resection has continuously increased (Fig. 7.101), and the postoperative survival rate at 5 years was 67.8%. Interestingly, Moribe et al. (2009) detected the methylation of 12 genes in 25 cases of HCC using quantitative methylation-specific PCR (MSP), and the results showed that all the SHCC ≤3 cm contained three gene methylation of RASSF1A, SPINT2, and CCND2, and its specificity, sensitivity, and accuracy were 100%, ≥75%, and 95%, respectively [31]. Llovet et al. (2006) found a successively increasing expression of three-gene spectrum consisting of GPC-3, survivin, and LYVE1 spectrum in dysplastic nodules, SHCC (diameter (2 ± 0.6) cm, ranged 0.9–3 cm) and LHCC, and the diagnostic accuracy of the gene spectrum in the three kinds of lesions reached 94% [32]. These two studies further suggest that there are corresponding molecular variations in the transformation from SHCC (≤3 cm) to LHCC (>3 cm) which is worth further study.

However, no uniform criterion for the tumor volume of SHCC has been accepted at home and abroad, and 5 cm of SHCC in diameter is still in use by many scholars, which is not correspondent to the biological characteristics of early HCC or current clinical techniques in early detection and early diagnosis of HCC. The present international staging systems, such as BCLC and AASLD, defined the early HCC as tumors ≤3 cm and very early HCC as tumors ≤2 cm. Nevertheless, up to now, most studies on SHCC ≤2 cm are based on multicenter joint studies with long-term data collection, and among the cases of surgically resected HCC in centers for hepatic diseases all around the world, reports of SHCC ≤2 cm are still very rare with only a few studies on their biological characteristics (Table 7.3). For instance, Minagawa et al. (2007) collected 2767 cases of ≤2 cm SHCC from 829 units in Japan during a 30-year period. This is a summary of a huge sample, but the actual number of cases in

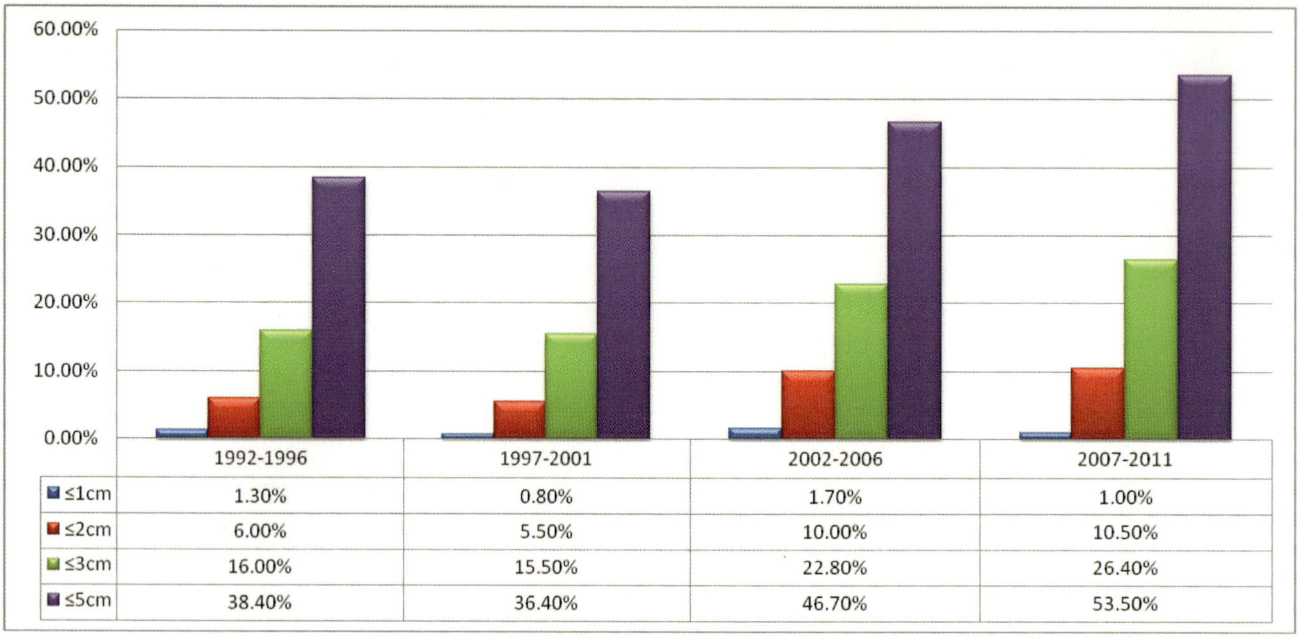

Fig. 7.101 The proportion of SHCC resection in EHBH during the period of 20 years

Table 7.3 Researches on SHCC ≤2 cm in the literature

Authors	Year	Number of cases	Collection period	Number of hospitals
Kondo F et al.	1987	15	10 years	2
Nagao T et al.	1992	23	9 years	1
Nakashima O et al.	1995	27	8 years	1
Takayama T et al.	1998	80	9 years	2
Arii S et al.	2000	1318[a]	8 years	≈800(LCSGJ)
Vauthey JN et al.	2002	57	18 years	4个
Inoue K et al.	2004	70	9 years	2
Ikai I et al.	2004	2320	10 years	≈800(LCSGJ)
Wu FS et al.	2005	45	17 years	1
Ando et al.	2006	91[a]	6 years	1
Minagawa M et al.	2007	2767	6 years	829(LCSGJ)
Forner A et al.	2008	60[a]	>3 years	4
Livraghi T et al.	2008	218 (RFA)	≈11 years	5
Farinati F et al.	2009	65[a]	18 years	10(ITA.LI.CA)
ICGHN	2009	23 (2002)[b]	?	3
		22 (2004)[b]	?	?
Takayama T et al.	2010	1235	3 years	≈800(LCSGJ)
Di Tommaso L et al.	2011	47(liver biopsy)	4 years	2
Yamashita Y et al.	2012	149	16 years	2

LCSGJ Liver Cancer Study Group of Japan, *ICGHN* International Consensus Group on Hepatocellular Neoplasms, *RFA* radiofrequency ablation, *ITA.LI.CA* Liver Cancer Research Group of Italy
[a]Part of the cases have been confirmed by pathological examination
[b]Including hepatic dysplastic nodules

each year for each unit is minimal. Farinati et al. (2009) analyzed the data of 1834 HCC cases (partly confirmed by pathology) during 10 years accumulated by the Cancer of the Liver Italian Program (ITA.LI.CA) and found that cases of ≤2 cm SHCC accounted for only 3%, which could not be analyzed for internal validation due to the insufficient number of cases. Thus, the authors suggested that the tumor volume of ≤2 cm as a criterion for the diagnosis of SHCC is of less staging significance in clinical practice because these cases are few in number.

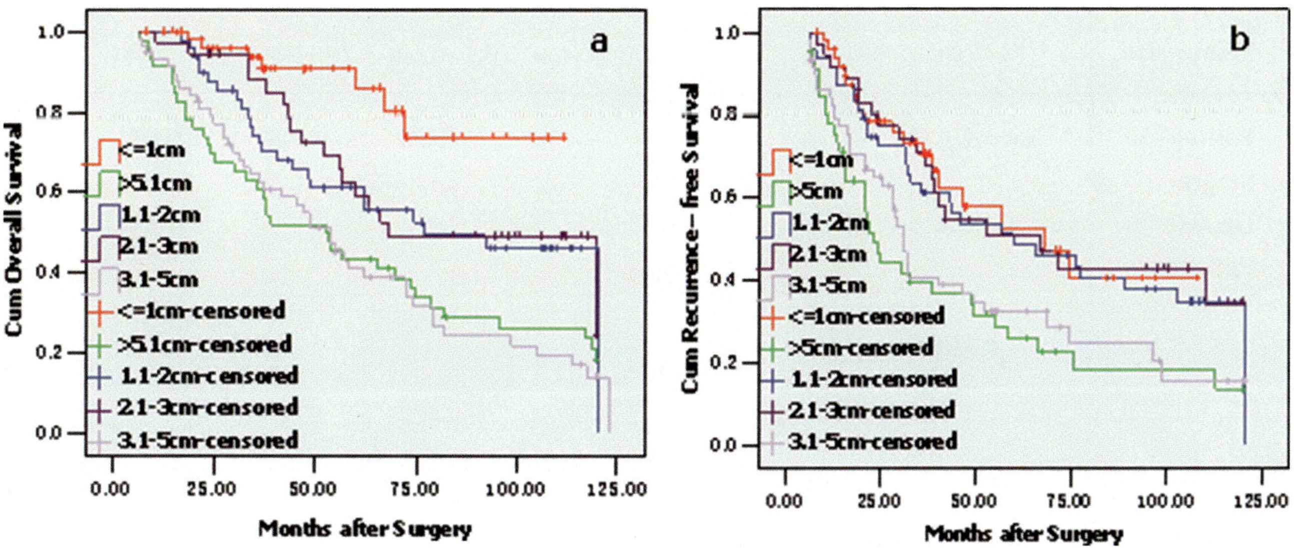

Fig. 7.102 Comparison of the postoperative prognoses among five groups of patients with HCC. (**a**). Overall survival; (**b**). Recurrence-free survival

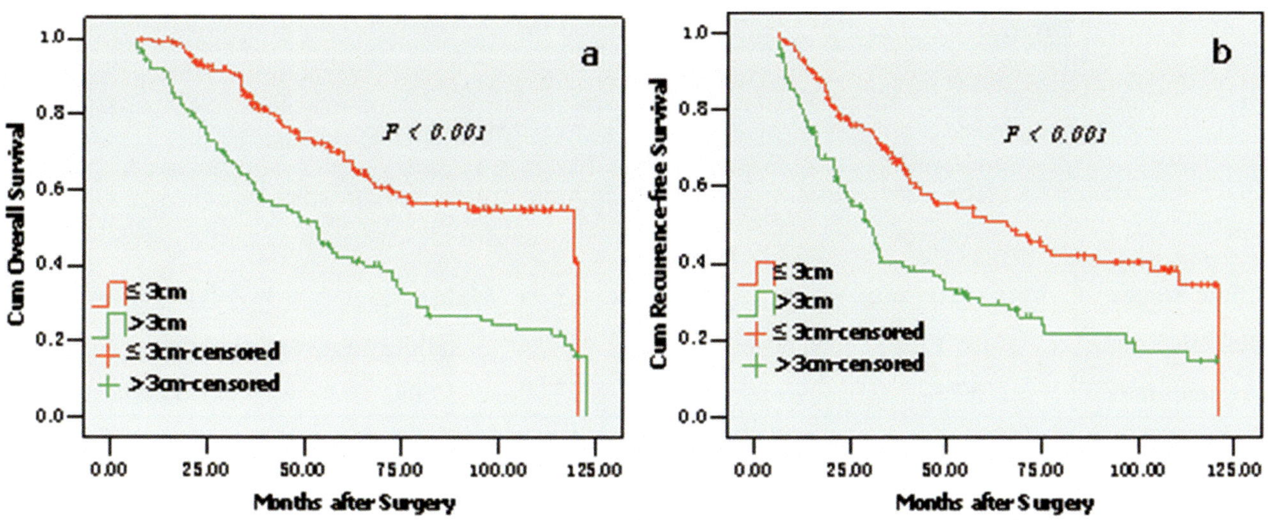

OS	1-yr	3-yr	5-yr	10-yr
SHCC	99.3±0.7%	85.0±3.2%	67.8±4.5%	41.1±12.5%
LHCC	92.3±2.6%	62.9±4.8%	42.3±5.0%	16.2±4.1%

RFS	1-yr	3-yr	5-yr	10-yr
SHCC	93.2±2.2%	67.2±4.2%	52.0±4.9%	34.4±6.0%
LHCC	80.5±3.0%	40.5±5.1%	29.3±4.9%	14.6±4.7%

Fig. 7.103 Comparison of the postoperative prognoses between SHCC group and LHCC group. (**a**). Overall survival; (**b**). Recurrence-free survival

(2) Biological characteristics of SHCC

Many studies have been reported at home and abroad; the long-term survival rate of patients with SHCC is significantly higher than that of LHCC patients, and postoperative recurrence rate was significantly lower than that of LHCC patients. We (2011) conducted a control study of 618 cases of HCC patients, who were divided into five groups according to the diameter of the tumors, ≤1 cm, 1.1–2 cm, 2.1–3 cm, 3.1–5 cm, and >5 cm, and the results showed that no significant difference in pathologic parameters and operative prognosis is found between 1–3 cm and >5 cm groups except the group of patients with tumors ≤1 cm in diameter (Fig. 7.102). However, if the patients were divided into two groups with the tumor diameter of 3 cm as a threshold, there were significant difference in pathologic parameters and operative prognosis between the two groups (Fig. 7.103) [33].

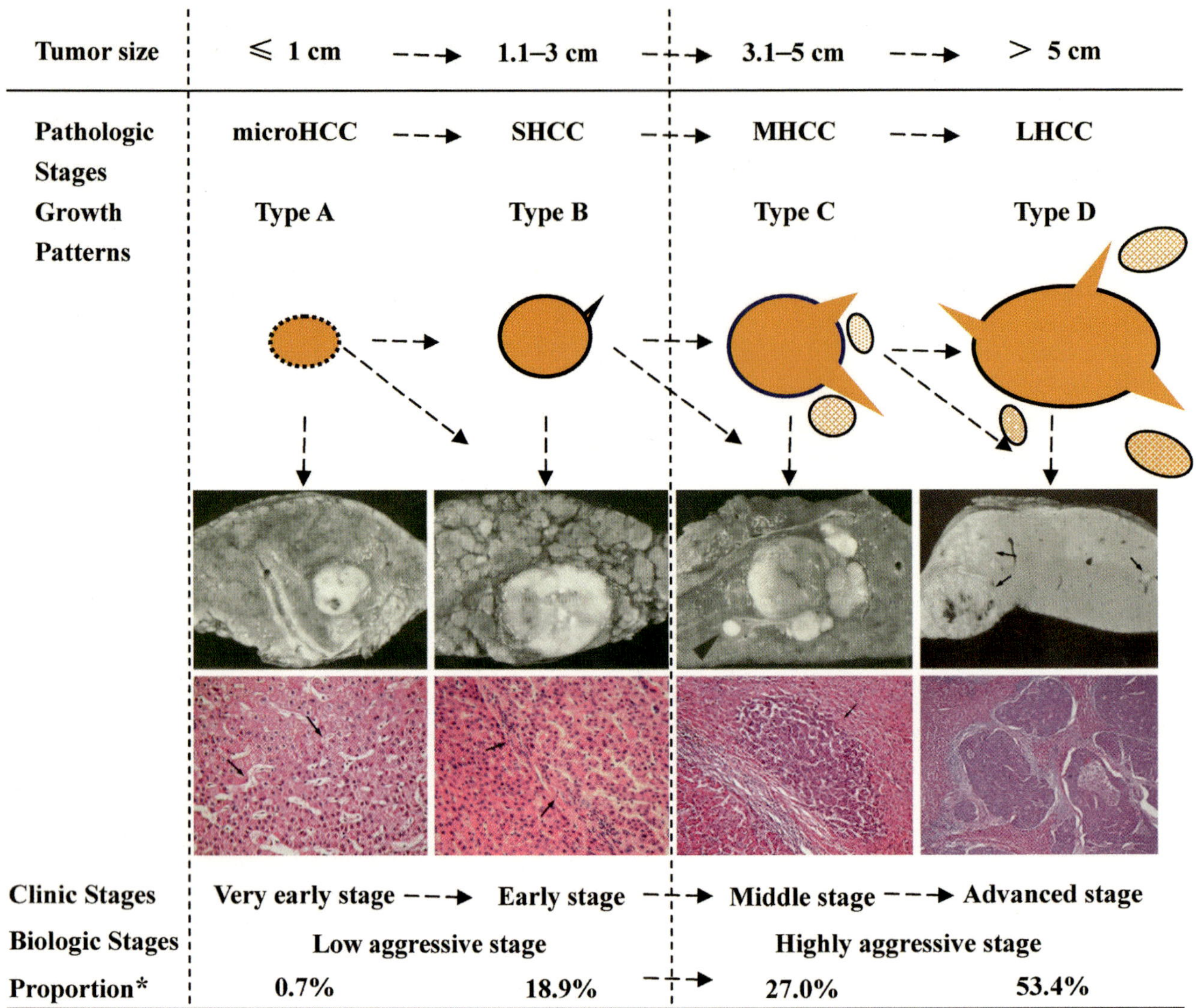

*According to 2 417 surgical resected HCCs from Eastern Hepatobiliary Surgery Hospital in 2007.

Fig. 7.104 EHBH pathological staging of HCC

Based on our observations, the main biological characteristics of SHCC include DNA diploid dominant, relatively slow growth with single and localized nodule, high degrees of differentiation, thin-trabecular type in histology, with or without a fibrous capsule, clear boundaries, rare MVI or satellite focus which are usually found in liver tissues 0.5–1 cm from the surgical margin, high postsurgical survival rate, and low recurrence rate. Tumors larger than 3 cm in diameter have pathobiological indexes which indicate transformation into malignant LHCC in progression, such as significantly increased rates of capsular and microvascular invasion, occurrence of satellite focus, and postsurgical recurrence. Combining our researching results and understanding, the growth and progression of HCC can be generally divided into four stages correspondent to four patterns of tumor growth, including microcarcinoma (≤1 cm, non-capsule stage) with transition between the tumor margin and pericarcinoma liver tissues → SHCC (1–3 cm, capsule formation stage) with dominantly solitary nodular growth, a clear border and an intact capsule in most of the cases, or with capsular invasion in a few cases → medium-sized HCC (3–5 cm, accelerated growth stage) with more extracapsular subcarcinoma foci and increased microvascular invasion → large HCC (>5 cm, malignant advanced stage) with multifocal infiltration in most cases, capsular invasion, MVI, and commonly seen satellite nodules (Fig. 7.104) [33, 34].

(3) Concepts of SHCC and early HCC

Early HCC (EHCC) should be referred to a small and well-differentiated HCC in the early stage of development, with relatively benign biological behaviors, no vascular invasion, and intrahepatic metastasis. However, the current conception and criterion of EHCC and SHCC is not consistent in the world. In BCLC staging classification, three nodules ≤3 cm in diameter were included in the early stage (stage A). However, from the point of view of pathology, three HCC nodules have a great possibility of intrahepatic metastasis, suggesting not in early stage in a biological sense. Nathan et al. (2013) defined EHCC as HCC ≤5 cm in diameter, without metastatic foci, lymph node metastasis, extrahepatic expansion, or invasion of major blood vessels. Sakamoto et al. (1998) defined EHCC as well-differentiated (Edmondson pathological grade I or grade I with grade II in a few region) HCC with negative tumor staining in angiography regardless of the size of the tumor. EHCC was also adopted in the WHO's Pathological Classification of Hepatobiliary Tumors (2010), which was defined as well-differentiated SHCC with a diameter of <2 cm. In general, SHCC refers to a HCC in small size, which is a morphological concept, while EHCC refers to HCC in early stages of tumorigenesis and progression with relatively benign biological behaviors, which is a biological concept. Therefore, it is inappropriate to simply equate SHCC and EHCC, since a few cases of SHCC have malignant biological behaviors including DNA ploidy, capsular invasion, and MVI formation in earlier stages. Table 7.4 shows the differences in criteria of staging systems on SHCC and EHCC in the literature, each of which has a certain influence.

Table 7.4 Criteria on SHCC and EHCC in the literature

Staging system by	Year	Staging	Tumor diameter
CSLC	2001	Ia	≤3 cm
		Ib	≤5 cm
		IIa	≤10 cm
		IIb	>10 cm
BCLC	2003	Very early HCC	<2 cm
		Early HCC	1or 3 nodules, ≤3 cm
IHPBA	2003	T_1	≤2 cm
Llovet et al.	2006	Very early HCC	≤2 cm, MVI(−)
		Early HCC	≤2 cm, MVI(+),or
			2–5 cm, or
			2–3nodules, ≤ 3 cm
LCSGJ	2007	T_1	≤2 cm, MVI(−)
AJCCTNM staging (seventh edition)	2009	T_1	Any size, MVI(−)
		T_2	Any size, MVI(+)
ITA.LI.CA	2009	Early HCC	<5 cm
JSH	2010	Early HCC (SHCC)	≤3 cm, well-differentiated

CSLC Chinese Society of Liver Cancer, *BCLC* Barcelona Clinic Liver Cancer, *IHPBA* International Hepato-Pancreato-Biliary Association, *LCSGJ* Liver Cancer Study Group of Japan, *AJCC* American Joint Committee on Cancer, *AASLD* American Association for the Study of Liver Diseases, *ICGHN* International Consensus Group on Hepatocellular Neoplasms, *ITA.LI.CA* Liver Cancer Research Group of Italy, *JSH* Japan Society of Hepatology

(4) Clinicopathological significance of SHCC

When evaluating the biological characteristics according to the tumor size of HCC, most SHCC ≤3 cm presents relatively benign performances of EHCC in early stage of tumorigenesis and development, with long-term survival rate and low recurrence rate after radical resection, indicating SHCC ≤3 cm has the pathological basis of radical resectability. However, we have found that about 26% of the SHCC contain DNA ploidy, presenting significantly malignant biological behaviors, such as poor differentiation, capsular invasion, and formation of microvascular thrombus, with postsurgical early recurrence; even a microcarcinoma of 0.6 cm in diameter may contain MVI, suggesting that these SHCC have an increased growth activity, and has an accelerated progress of malignancy, which does not belong to the biological category of EHCC. It is certain that part of the LHCC may have the morphological representation of SHCC and the biological characteristics of EHCC, with long-term survival rate and low recurrence rate after radical resection. Thus, SHCC is not completely equal to EHCC in the strict sense. In clinical surgery, the individualized therapeutic strategy for SHCC should be formulated according to the pathological type and growth pattern with a certain extent of surgical resection. Generally, for SHCC ≤1–3 cm in diameter, a retaining resection extension of 0.5–1 cm should be considered, and for HCC larger than 3 cm, it should be >1–2 cm to completely remove possible residual satellite foci or MVI, which also fits in radiofrequency ablation in order to improve the long-term treatment efficacy.

(5) Pathological characteristics of SHCC

7.1.2.1 Gross Features

SHCC is often a solitary nodule in expansive growth. The section of SHCC shows homogeneous and dense tissue, with visible slender radial fibers, similar to the hepatocellular tumor-like nodules, and a clear boundary separating it from the surrounding liver tissue (Fig. 7.105). It can also be in multinodular fusion growth (Fig. 7.106), and approximately 67% of SHCC cases have a complete fibrous capsule. Some SHCC or microcarcinomas have no obvious capsule or continuous capsule, with expansive extrusion boundary, suggesting the capsule is a local defensive reaction during the growth and expansion of the tumor. However,

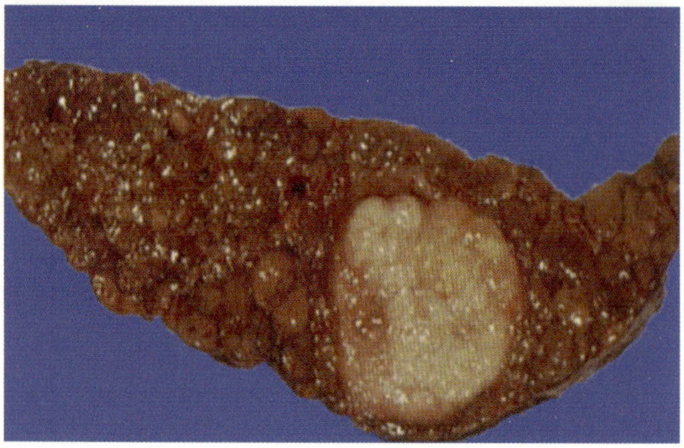

Fig. 7.105 SHCC, a round tumor nodule with clear boundary

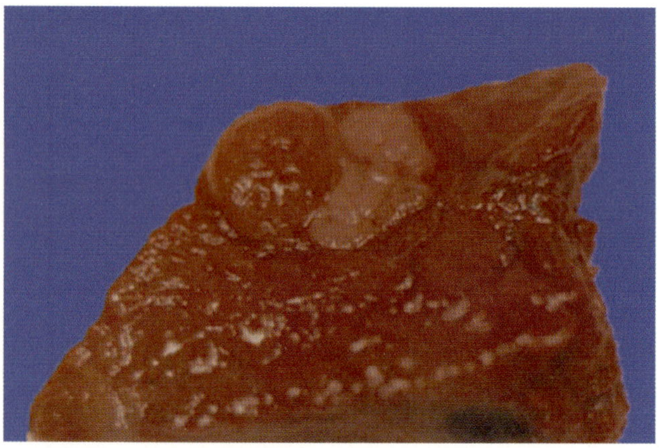

Fig. 7.106 SHCC, two nodules become confluent with clear boundary

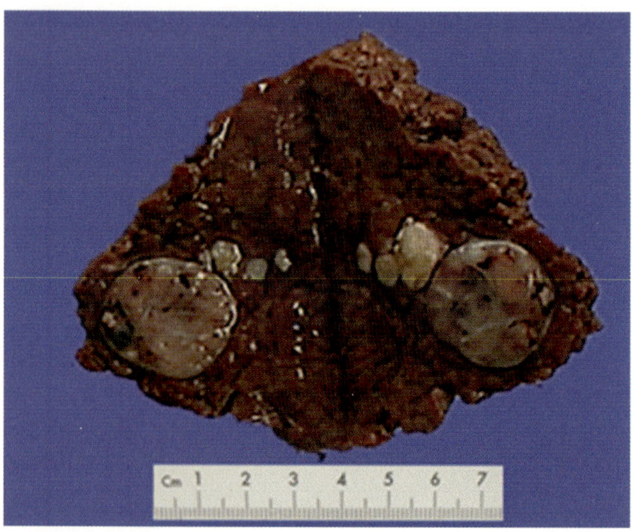

Fig. 7.107 SHCC, several satellite foci in the surrounding cancer tissue

satellite foci and tumor thrombus can be found on the cutting margin of the tumor (Figs. 7.107 and 7.108), and these

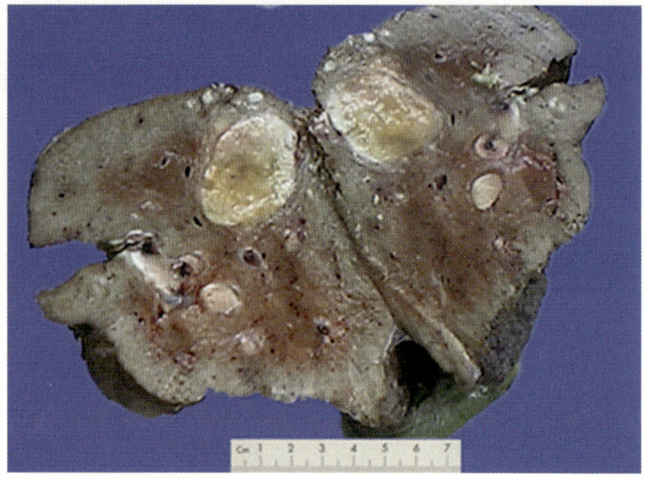

Fig. 7.108 SHCC, multiple satellite foci in the surrounding cancer tissue

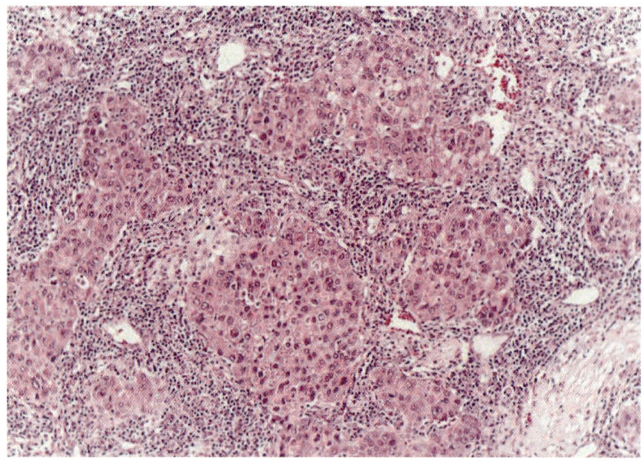

Fig. 7.109 SHCC, large amounts of lymphocytes infiltrated in the tumorous stroma

invasive behaviors become more significant as the tumor increases in size in most cases, especially in LHCC with a diameter>3 cm, in which the occurrence rate of invasion is higher.

7.1.2.2 Microscopic Features

Approximately 60% of SHCC are well differentiated in grade I to grade II (Figs. 7.1, 7.2, 7.3, 7.4, 7.5, 7.6, 7.7, 7.8, 7.9, 7.10, 7.11, 7.12, 7.13, 7.14, 7.15, 7.16, 7.17, 7.18, 7.19, and 7.20), and the cancer cells are consistent in size, with slight nuclear atypia, increased cell density, eosinophilic or basophilic cytoplasm, darker-stained nucleus, slightly increased nuclear to cytoplasmic ratio, and mitotic figures in a few cases. The tumor cells are often arranged in thin trabecules, and the hepatic sinusoid gap increases, with or without pseudoglandular structures. Infiltration of a large number of lymphocytes in the tumor boundary or tumorous stroma (Figs. 7.109 and 7.110) suggests a strong focal immune

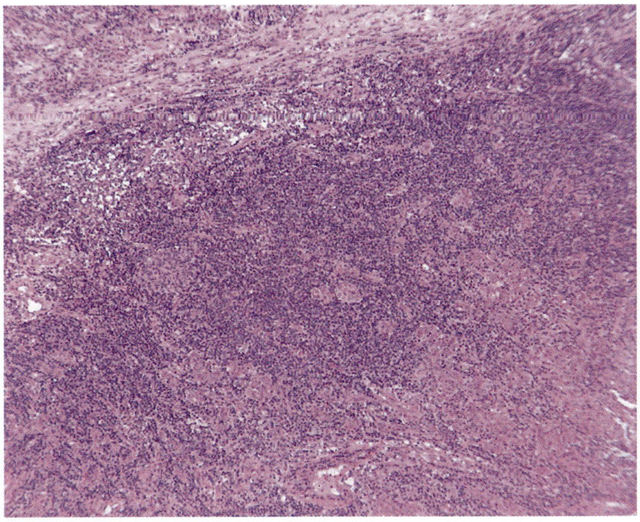

Fig. 7.110 SHCC, a large number of lymphocytes infiltrated at the peripheral region

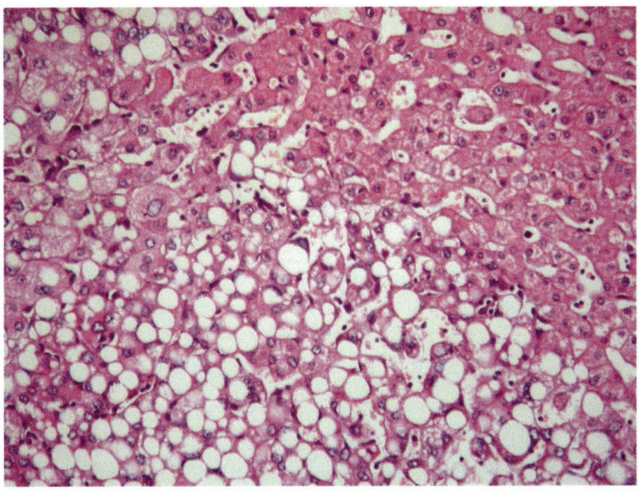

Fig. 7.111 SHCC, steatosis of liver tumor cells

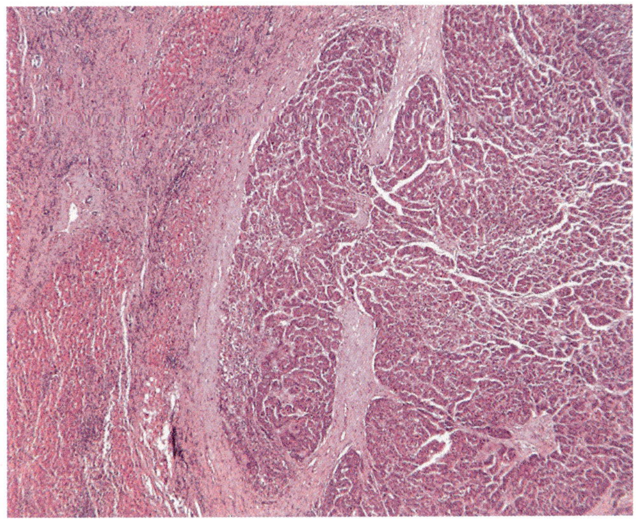

Fig. 7.112 SHCC, capsular invasion and surrounded by fibrous membrane

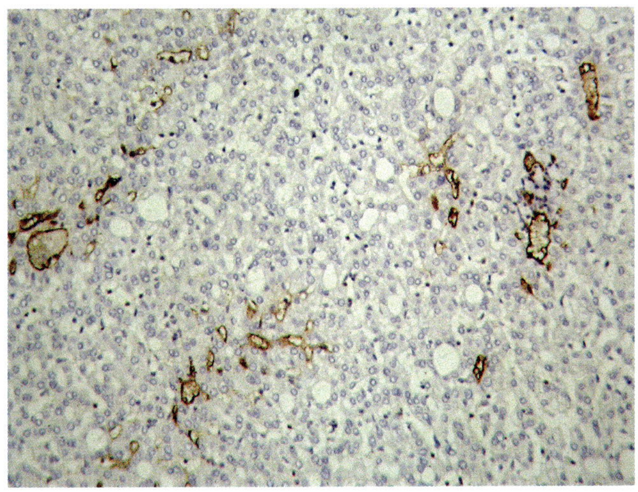

Fig. 7.113 SHCC, immunohistochemical staining of CD34 showing microvascular rarefaction

response in the patient. Portal tracts can also be found in some microcarcinoma, the number of which decreases with the increase of HCC volume, while the number of arterioles increases with the increase of volume of HCC, reflecting the dynamic changes of blood supply pattern during the growth of HCC, and abnormal blood supply in this process may be an important factor leading to high differentiated SHCC, especially microcarcinoma with frequent fatty changes (Fig. 7.111). It should be noted that SHCC with capsular invasion or even invasion into the surrounding liver tissue is not a rare phenomenon (Fig. 7.112) and should be paid careful attention in observation.

7.1.2.3 Differential Diagnosis

Due to the complete envelope in most cases of well-differentiated SHCC or transition between the tumor and the liver tissue without obvious invasion of adjacent liver tissue, it should be well differentiated from hepatocellular nodular lesions, such as hepatocellular adenoma (HCA), high-grade dysplastic nodule (HGDN), hepatic focal nodular hyperplasia (FNH), etc. Cases with obvious fatty degeneration should also be distinguished from hepatic epithelioid angiomyolipoma. Much difficulty exists in the differential diagnosis of small liver biopsy tissues, and examinations such as immunohistochemistry or gene marker detection are beneficial. It is worth noting that well-differentiated SHCC can exhibit untypical "HCC-like microvascular density" in CD34 staining (Fig. 7.113) which may interfere the judgment, and reticular fiber staining is helpful to distinguish normal liver cells and tumor cell nests interspersed in the interstitial fibrous trabecules. The absence of local bile duct reaction in CK7

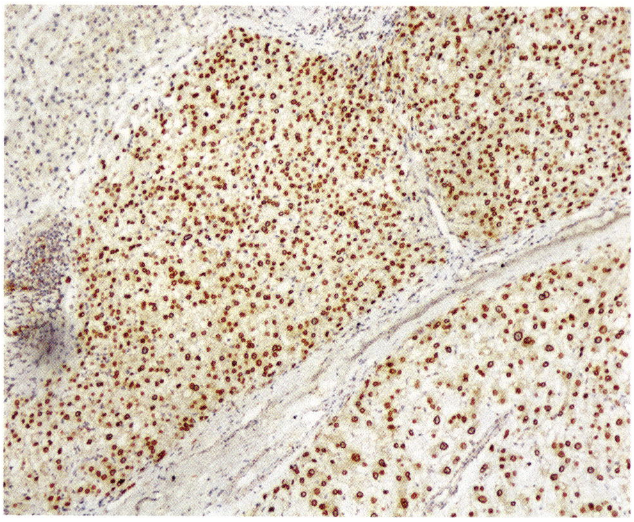

Fig. 7.114 SHCC, immunohistochemical staining of PCNA showing strong positive staining of the nuclei

staining in the surrounding fibrous tissue around the liver cell mass may suggest the stromal invasion of a true tumor. The expression intensity in Ki-67 or PCNA staining (Fig. 7.114) contributes to the assessment of the nature of the tumor. Tremosini et al. (2012) conducted an ultrasound-guided fine needle aspiration biopsy in 60 cases of hepatic nodular lesions with diameter of 5–20 mm, and the tissues are examined using a combined immunohistochemical staining panel of "GPC-3+HSP70+GS"; the result of which with positive staining of two markers facilitates the diagnosis of HCC with sensitivity and specificity of 62% and 100% [35], respectively. However, according to our experience, similar to reports of some other scholars, the sensitivity of GPC-3 for HCC is relatively low (<50%), especially in cases with negative GPC-3 staining, and should be carefully diagnosed. In 2009, 34 famous pathologists from 13 countries and 2 clinicians formed the International Consensus Group for Hepatocellular Neoplasia (ICGHN), and they put forward the consensus of pathodiagnosis of early HCC after 7 years' work, and interstitial infiltration was included as a major criterion for the diagnosis of EHCC or differential diagnosis from high-grade dysplastic nodules [23].

7.1.3 Fibrolamellar Hepatocellular Carcinoma

7.1.3.1 Pathogenesis and Mechanism

Fibrolamellar hepatocellular carcinoma (FL-HCC) was first reported by Edmondson in 1956. Regional differences have been found in the occurrence rates of FL-HCC. It accounts for 1–5% of HCC and is rare in endemic areas of HCC with extremely rare cases found in China. The incidence rate of FL-HCC in the United States is 0.02/100,000 [36]. The expression of TGF-β in FL-HCC cells reaches as high as 82%, which is probably associated with characteristic lamellar fibers, and FL-HCC cells also express cholangiocyte markers such as EMA and CK7, as well as the stem cell markers EpCAM and CK19, suggesting that FL-HCC may derive from hepatic progenitor cell with ductular differentiation potentials. FL-HCC does not contain mutation of CTNNβ or p53 gene, and high expression of Y654-catenin is a suggestion of upregulation of the receptor tyrosine kinase, while some people consider FL-HCC as an independent disease. FL-HCC has not been found to be caused by certain factors or combined with other diseases, and little association was found between it with common factors related to HCC, such as HBV/HCV hepatitis, cirrhosis of the liver, alcohol, or metabolic diseases. Honeyman et al. (2014) conducted whole transcriptome and genome sequencing in FL-HCC and found that in all 15 cases of FL-HCC tissue detected DNAJB1-PRKACA chimeric transcripts, which may be associated with the pathogenesis of FL-HCC but not in conventional HCC and could also be a potential-specific molecular marker in support of the diagnosis of FL-HCC [37].

7.1.3.2 Clinical Features

Typical cases of FL-HCC are often found in adolescents and young adults, aged 5–35 years old (85% at age 35 years or younger) with slightly more women. The clinical symptoms are similar to those of common HCC but often with normal liver function, no history of HBV/HCV infection, and no background of liver diseases such as hepatitis and cirrhosis. The serum AFP is negative in 85–90% of the patients, but serum CEA can be increased. Elevation of serum vitamin B_{12} and capacity of unsaturated B12 binding, transcobalamin, and neurotensin can be discovered in most FL-HCC cases with a relative specificity. Dynamic CT scanning shows lobulated masses with heterogeneity and central scars in the normal livers, and MRI T_2-weighted images show low density with calcification in most cases. In fact, FL-HCC is extremely rare in China or even in Asia. In the study of Malouf et al. (2014), the statistics of 90 cases of FL-HCC in the United States showed that Asians accounted for only 4.4% of the patients [38].

So far, only five cases of typical FL-HCC both clinically and pathologically have been diagnosed in the Department of Pathology of EHBH, Second Military Medical University, and the patients were ages 21.2 years old on average with a male to female ratio of 0.66. The patients had no history of hepatitis, and negative or weakly positive serum AFP was found in 80% of the patients with the mean tumor diameter reaching 13.2 cm (Table 7.5). And the four consultation cases of FL-HCC diagnosed in our hospital concerned patients with a male to female ratio of 1:1 and the average age of 26.8 years old.

Table 7.5 Clinical and pathological characteristics of five cases of FL-HCC

Case	Gender	Age (years)	Reasons for admission	HBV/HCV infection	Serum AFP(μg/ml)	Location	Size (cm)
1.	Female	14	Abdominal pain	Negative	>1000	Left lobe	19 × 16
2.	Female	26	Health check	Negative	4.2	Right lobe	7 × 5.6
3.	Female	32	Abdominal pain	Negative	8.6	Right lobe	15 × 13
4.	Male	20	Health check	Negative	1.2	Right lobe	11.7 × 9.3
5.	Male	14	Abdominal mass	Negative	33.4	Right lobe	13.1 × 12

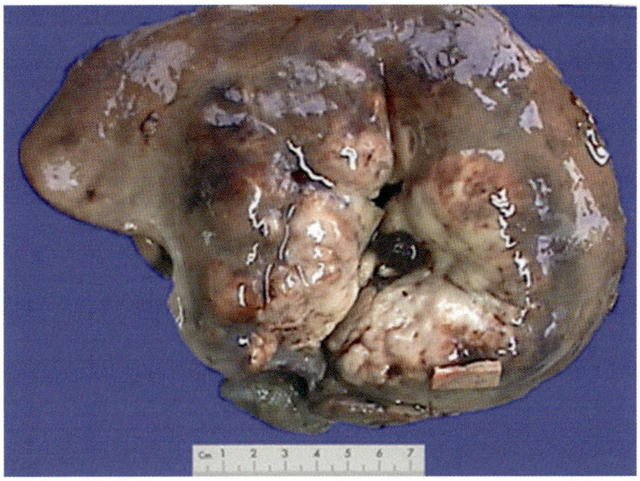

Fig. 7.115 FL-HCC, showing central scar and central depression

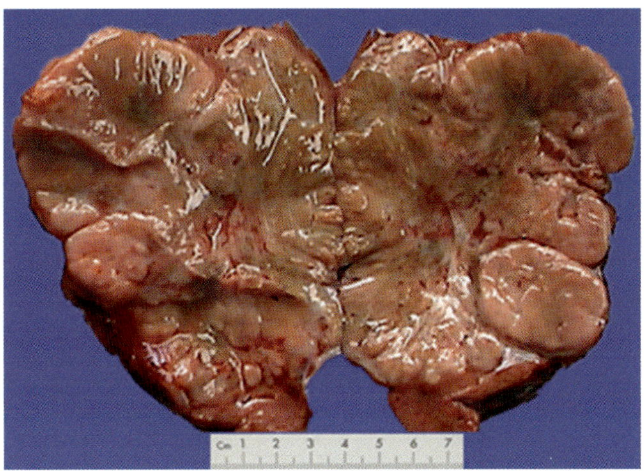

Fig. 7.116 FL-HCC, showing central stellate scar on the cut surface

7.1.3.3 Gross Features

The lesions are located in the left hepatic lobe in more than 50% of the FL-HCC cases, which are often huge in volume with an average diameter of 13 cm ranged 3–25 cm, and great depression can be found in the center due to contraction of the fibrous scar (Case 1, Fig. 7.115). It has been reported resected FL-HCC of 40 cm in diameter and 6000 g in weight, and the patient remains survived 14 years after the surgery. The section of the tumor contained a central or eccentric radial fibrous scar, separating the FL-HCC tissue into multinodular lobulated structure (Case 3) (Case 5, Fig. 7.116), often with an intact capsule and are green in color because of the bile content. Cystic degeneration can be found in huge lesions, and the surrounding liver tissue is often without chronic hepatitis or cirrhosis.

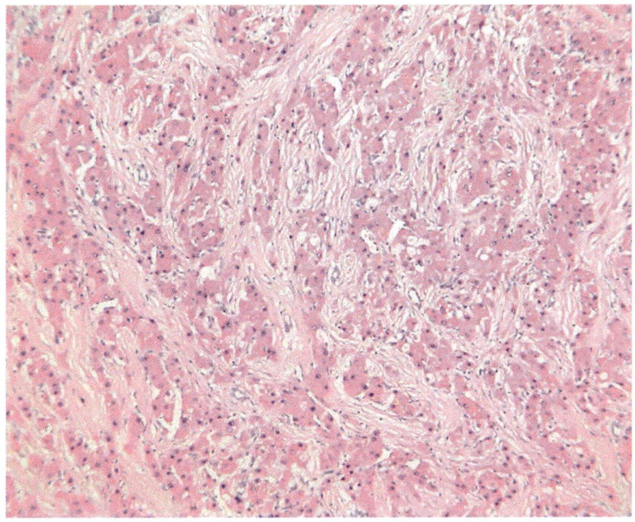

Fig. 7.117 FL-HCC, polygonal cells with granular eosinophilic cytoplasm surrounded by lamellar fibrous bands

7.1.3.4 Microscopic Features

FL-HCC is morphologically characterized by laminated fibrous layers interspersed between the oncocytic polygonal cells. The cancer tissue was arranged in nests or trabecules and surrounded by abundant and dense lamellar fibrous tissue in an orderly form containing collagen of type I, type III, and type V. The cancer cells are often polygonal, large in volume, with obvious and hawkeye-shaped nucleolus, few mitotic figures, strongly eosinophilic granular cytoplasm, and a large number of swelling mitochondria; thus, it is also called eosinophilic HCC with lamellar fibrosis (Figs. 7.117, 7.118, 7.119, and 7.120). The cytoplasm often contains anti-amylase digestion and positive PAS-stained eosinophilic bodies (Fig. 7.121), and about 50% of the cases contain pale bodies (Fig. 7.122) which composed by α1-AT and fibrinogen and are negative for PAS staining and positive for ubiquitin antibody staining. Mucus staining shows the mucus produced by FL-HCC in some cases, which is significantly different from conventional HCC. Rhodanine staining shows

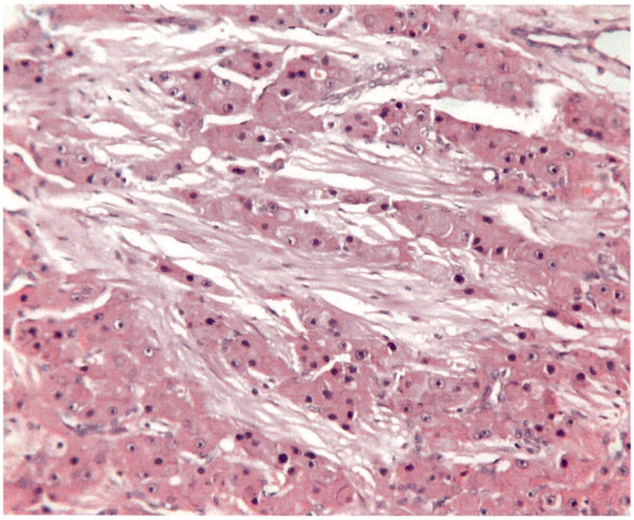

Fig. 7.118 FL-HCC, showing thick fibrous collagen bands in a unique "lamellar" pattern

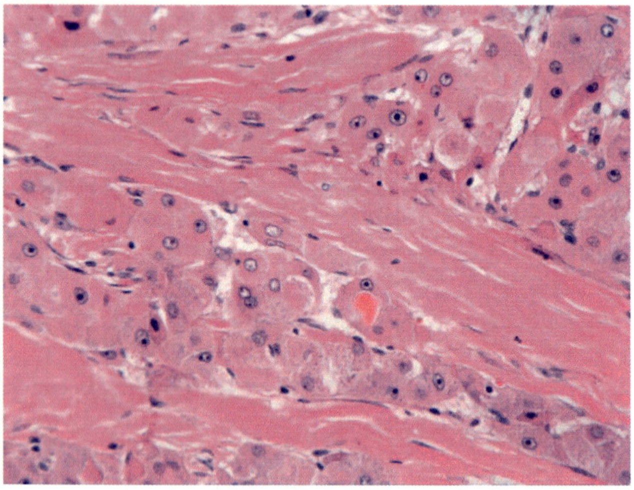

Fig. 7.119 FL-HCC, fibrous collagen bands encircling or surrounding the neoplastic hepatocytes

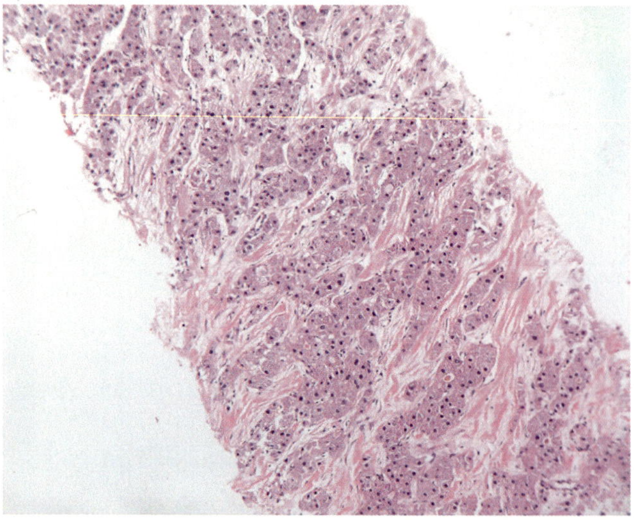

Fig. 7.120 FL-HCC, liver biopsy, showing abundant fibrous collagen bands

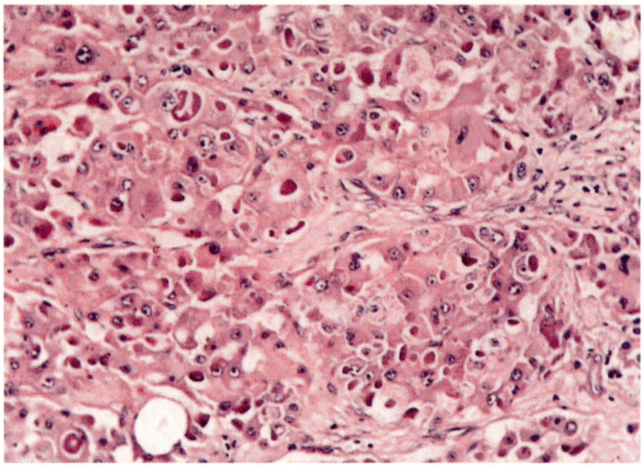

Fig. 7.121 FL-HCC, showing cytoplasmic eosinophilic bodies

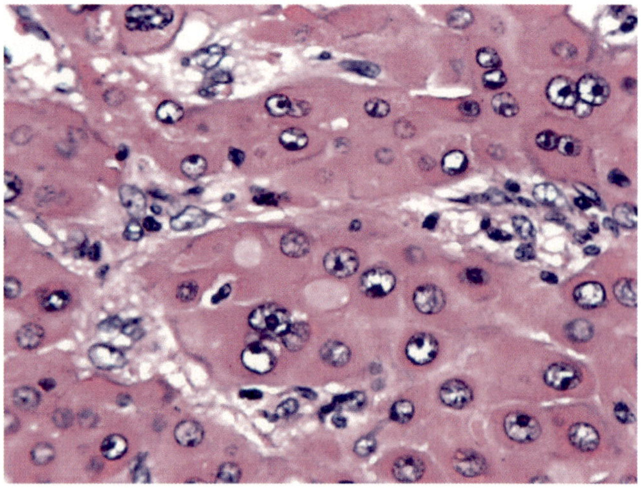

Fig. 7.122 FL-HCC, showing cytoplasmic pale bodies

that most FL-HCC has accumulation of copper-binding proteins. The tumors usually have a complete fibrous capsule on the margin of them.

7.1.3.5 Immunohistochemistry

FL-HCC expresses hepatocellular markers, such as Hep Par-1, pCEA, GPC-3 (Fig. 7.123), CK8 and CK18, as well as bile duct markers CK7 and CK19 (Fig. 7.124). In addition, they are often positive for α1-AT, fibrinogen, C-reactive protein and ferritin staining, and negative for HBsAg staining. CD34 staining displays dense micro-blood vessels. Also, the FL-HCC tissues are found to express neuroendocrine markers, such as Syn, CgA, and NSE. And Malouf et al. (2014) recently found that FL-HCC specifically expressed neuroendocrine protein PCSK1 which was diffusely distributed in the cytoplasm and helpful in diagnosis.

7.1.3.6 Electron Microscopic Observation

It is characterized by the emergence of a large number of back-to-back mitochondria, as well as intracytoplasmic

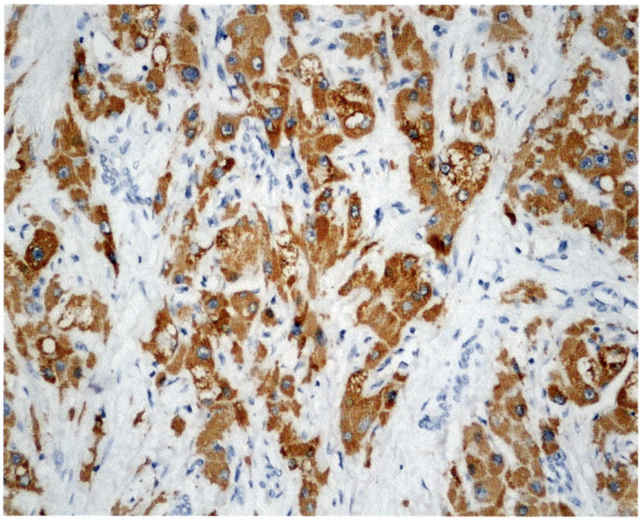

Fig. 7.123 FL-HCC, showing positive immunohistochemical staining of Hep Par-1

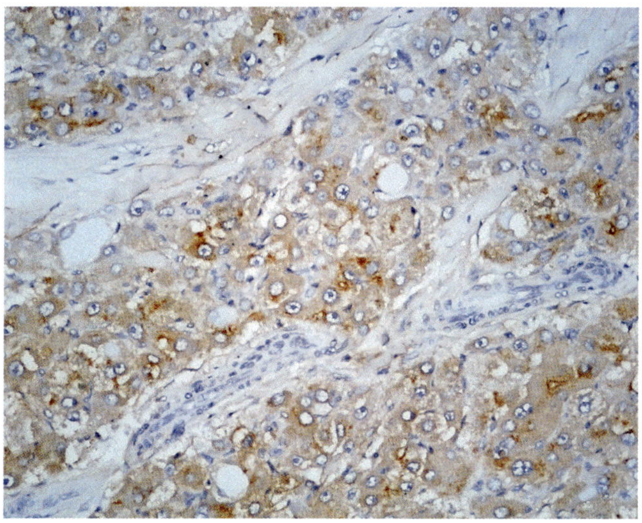

Fig. 7.124 FL-HCC, showing positive immunohistochemical staining of GPC-3

globular hyaline bodies, Mallory bodies, and occasional neurosecretory granules.

7.1.3.7 Differential Diagnosis

FL-HCC should be carefully distinguished from sclerosing or scirrhous HCC. The main differential points between them have been summarized in Table 7.6. Cheuk et al. (2001) reported one case of clear cell-type FL-HCC, but it was negative for both PAS staining and post-diastase digestion PAS staining, suggesting it did not contain glycogen to exclude the diagnosis of clear cell-type HCC.

7.1.3.8 Treatment and Prognosis

Most of the researchers found that the FL-HCC has a high rate of surgical resection and a better prognosis than that of conventional-type HCC, with a 5-year survival rate reaching 30–76%. Younger age, no history of liver diseases, and early stage of tumor may be the important factors for a better prognosis. Kaseb et al. (2013) proposed combined therapy of fluorouracil and interferon was an effective treatment for FL-HCC, which could prolong the survival period of the patients [39]. However, the rate of local lymphatic metastasis in FL-HCC is as high as 40%, and these patients have a poorer prognosis. A study of European Childhood Liver Tumors Strategy Group (SIOPEL) suggested that there was no significant difference of 3-year overall survival rate between FL-HCC and conventional-type HCC (42%:33%) [40].

Table 7.6 Clinicopathological characteristics of FL-HCC and conventional HCC

Features	FL-HCC	HCC
Average age (years)	20–25	55–60
Male to female ratio	1:1	(4–8):1
Liver cirrhosis	None	Common
Serum HBsAg	None	Common
Serum AFP	Negative (most cases)	Positive (30–85%)
Serum vitaminB_{12}	Elevated	Normal
Serum neurotensin	Elevated	Normal
Radial fibrous scar	Common	None
Capsular invasion	Rare	Common
Cholestasis	Common	Yes
Fibrolamellar structure	Yes	None
Eosinophilic cytoplasm	Yes	None
Pale bodies	Common (50%)	Few (<10%)
Tissue calcifications	Common	Few
CK19 positive	23%	5–10%
Surgical resection rate	48–75%	10–20%
Five-year survival after surgery	~75%	~30%

7.1.4 Combined Hepatocellular-Cholangiocarcinoma

7.1.4.1 Pathogenesis and Mechanism

Combined hepatocellular-cholangiocarcinoma (cHCC-CC) is defined as a single tumor composed of both unequivocally HCC and intrahepatic cholangiocarcinoma (ICC) components, also known as hepatocholangiocarcinoma. It has been reported that regional difference exists in the incidence of cHCC-CC in the literature, which ranges from 1.4 to 6.5% accounting for 0.4–14.2% of hepatic tumors. Of all the malignant hepatobiliary tumors diagnosed in our department during the 30 years, cHCC-CC accounted for about 1.67%. Garancini et al. (2014) reported a group of American data and displayed that cHCC-CC accounted for 0.77% of HCC [41].

The histogenesis of cHCC-CC is still not very clear with current hypotheses including the following:

1. Collision tumor: Two independently developed HCC and ICC nodule gradually move closer and eventually merge into one tumor in their growth process. The incidence of liver collision tumor is 0.1–1%. And it is characterized by binocular fusion tumor in morphology with a fibrous capsule separating the two kinds of tumor components, without confusion or transition. And the two components belong to two independent cell clones of different genetic phenotype. However, the so-called collision tumor of the liver is not included in the definition of cHCC-CC proposed by WHO classification.
2. It is generated by differentiation of HCC or CC to another component, due to the finding of intermediate transitional zone between HCC and CC components [42]. But even the degrees of differentiation of cancer cells in the intermediate transitional zone have no significant difference from the surrounding HCC and ICC tissues. In addition, as a mature component of HCC and ICC, the actual incidence rate of cHCC-CC will be a little higher if there is a path for the tumor to transform into another type of tumor via dedifferentiation or transdifferentiation.
3. Bidirectional differentiation of hepatic progenitor cells. Coulouarn et al. (2012) found that two main signaling pathways are activated in cHCC-CC tissues, namely, transforming growth factor-β (TGF-β) and Wnt/β-catenin pathway, and the genetic spectrum variation characteristics are similar to those features of HCC with characteristics of stem cells, including low differentiation degree and poor prognosis, suggesting there is a continuous development among ICC, cHCC-CC, and poorly differentiated HCC [43]. Cai et al. (2012) suggested that HBV infection-induced chronic liver inflammation could activate hepatic progenitor cells, the activity of which was related to the invasion of cHCC-CC and the proliferation of pericarcinoma small bile ducts, and the latter is a useful marker for predicting the risk of recurrence [44]. We had studied both components of the tumor in 16 cases of cHCC-CC via comparison analysis of microsatellite loss of heterozygosity (LOH) frequency in order to investigate the clonal relationship between them. The results showed that the difference rate of LOH model in all the cases of cHCC-CC was less than 30%, indicating that they were both derived from the same clone.

7.1.4.2 Clinical Features

The clinical manifestations, imaging features, and biological characteristics are between those of cHCC-CC and HCC, which are further associated with the proportion of HCC and ICC in the tumor tissues. If the proportion of HCC is larger, the patients will manifest more characteristics of HCC and vice versa. During the 30 years, 563 cases of cHCC-CC have been diagnosed in the Department of Pathology of EHBH with a male to female ratio of 4.86:1 and a median age of 50 years old, and the infection rate of HBV was 76.7%. The typical CT images of cHCC-CC show early enhancement in the peripheral region around the tumor and delayed enhancement of the central region with slight enhancement in peripheral areas. Generally speaking, cases with characteristic images of HCC with elevated serum CA19-9 and cases with characteristic images of ICC with elevated serum AFP, or with both elevation of serum AFP and CA19-9, are possibly cHCC-CC, but pathological examination is necessary to confirm the diagnosis.

7.1.4.3 Gross Features

cHCC-CC is similar to the characteristics of conventional HCC; however, tissue in different texture and color can sometimes be observed, and localized sampling can show different parts characterized by the features of HCC and ICC (Figs. 7.125 and 7.126).

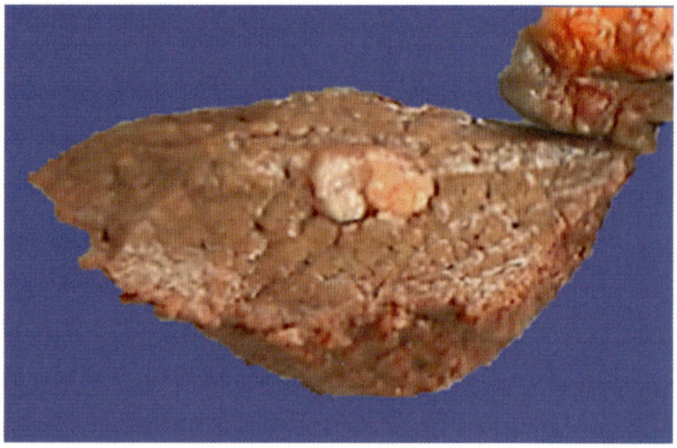

Fig. 7.125 cHCC-CC, no fibrous separation between ICC (nodule with *gray-white color, left*) and HCC (*pale-yellow area, right*)

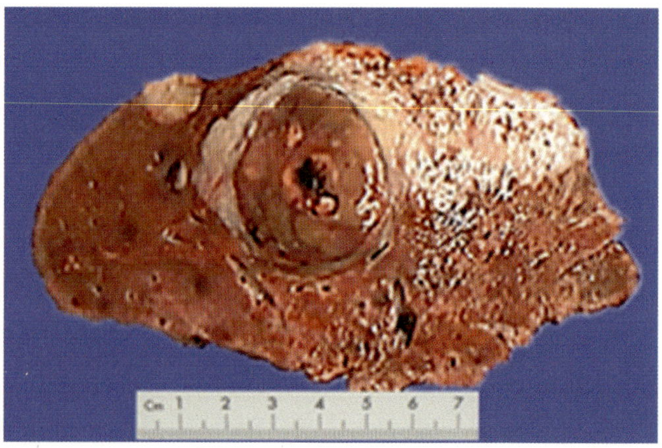

Fig. 7.126 cHCC-CC, no fibrous separation between HCC (*central brown area*) and ICC (*gray-white area* around the tumor periphery)

7.1.4.4 Microscopic Features

(1) Histological classification

1. Allen-Lisa (1949) classification: Type A, characterized by synchronous, separate, and autonomous epicenters of HCC and CC in one liver; type B, comprised of closely admixing distinguished foci of HCC and CC; and type C, consisting of truly combined HCC and CC components originating from the same tumor.
2. Goodman (1985) classification: Type 1 (collision tumor), synchronous or metachronous occurrence of distinct epicenters of HCC and CC in the same liver, which collide each other; type II (transitional tumor), intimate intermingling of two components with actual transition of HCC elements to CC elements in the same tumor; and type III (fibrolamellar tumor), similar to a fibrolamellar HCC but with mucin-producing pseudoglands.
3. WHO (2010) classification: A tumor contains two unequivocal, intimately mixed components of both HCC and CC which only consist of type C in Allen-Lisa classification and type 2 in Goodman classification. It can be divided into two types: ① classical type consists of HCC and ICC, as well as the transition zone between them, and cancer cells in the transition zone have intermediate morphology of liver cells and bile duct cells, similar to stem cells or progenitor cells and ② tumors with the characteristics of stem cells. From the perspective of the WHO criteria as well as the reports in the literature, the stem cell components in the cHCC-CC are mostly distributed in local or marginal parts of the tumors. Furthermore, the HCC and CC themselves have the ability to differentiate into neuroendocrine tissues, and there are reports of collision tumor composed by HCC and neuroendocrine tumors [45, 46]. So, the classification of cHCC-CC with stem cell features should also be consistent with the definition of cHCC-CC by WHO, and further studies are needed to clarify the classification significance of cHCC-CC with stem cell features.

It is worth noting that cholangiocellular carcinoma was once considered as a subtype of ICC; however, WHO described and discussed it as a stem cell subtype of cHCC-CC which can often been discovered in the peripheral regions of the tumor [4]. Based on our own experience, carcinoma of small bile ducts mainly contains tumorous small bile ducts with or without few small HCC nest; thus, actually it does not meet the morphological diagnostic criteria of cHCC-CC by WHO. To understand more on the above condition, more pathological data and in-depth study on the carcinoma of small bile ducts are further needed. And carcinomas of small bile ducts are discussed specifically in the chapter of ICC in this book [47–50].

(2) Histological morphology

The basic feature of cHCC-CC is the defined coexistence of two tumor components of HCC and CC in a liver nodule, each of which expresses its own immunohistochemical phenotype, and both tumorous components can be separated in different regions (Figs. 7.127 and 7.128) or mingled (Figs. 7.129 and 7.130), with no real fibrous capsule to separate them. HCC components are trabecular, pseudoglandular, or dense in structure, with polygonal cancer cells, less interstitial tissue, and lining of sinusoid blood spaces between trabecules, while CC components are associated with gland-like structures, secretion of mucus, lining of cuboidal cancer cells, abundant interstitial fibrous tissue, and transition

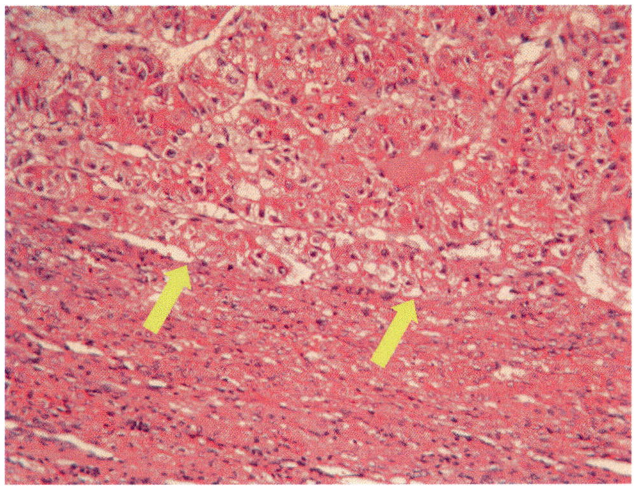

Fig. 7.127 cHCC-CC, ICC (*upper*) and HCC (*below*) closely adjacent

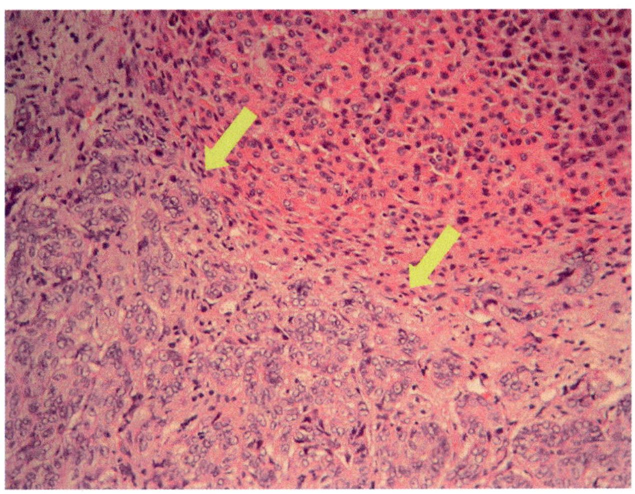

Fig. 7.128 cHCC-CC, HCC (*upper*) and ICC (*below*) closely adjacent

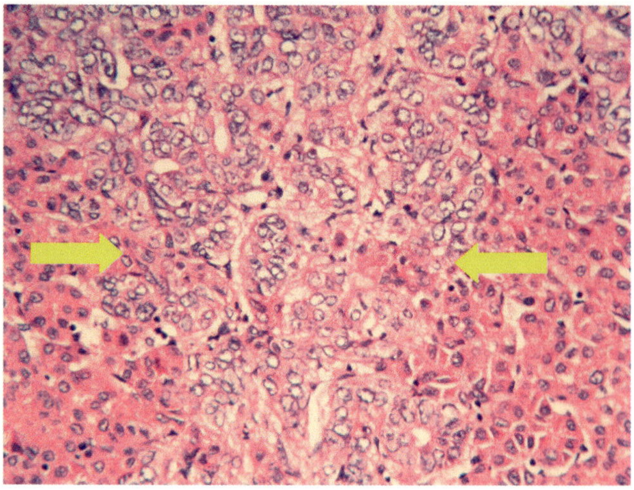

Fig. 7.129 cHCC-CC, ICC (*central area*) and HCC (*peripheral area*) closely adjacent

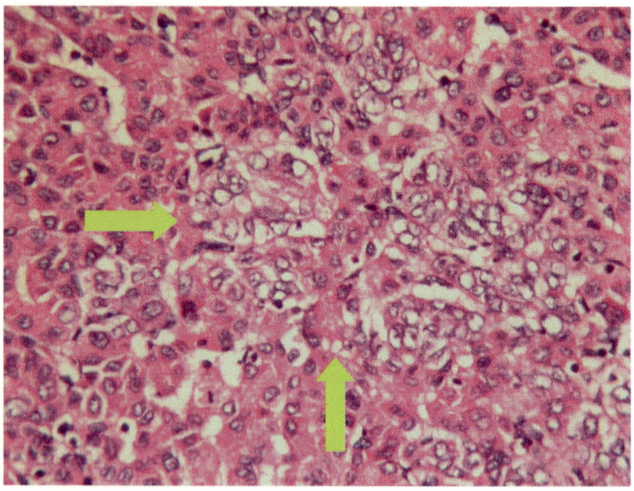

Fig. 7.130 cHCC-CC, ICC (*arrow*) intertwined with HCC components

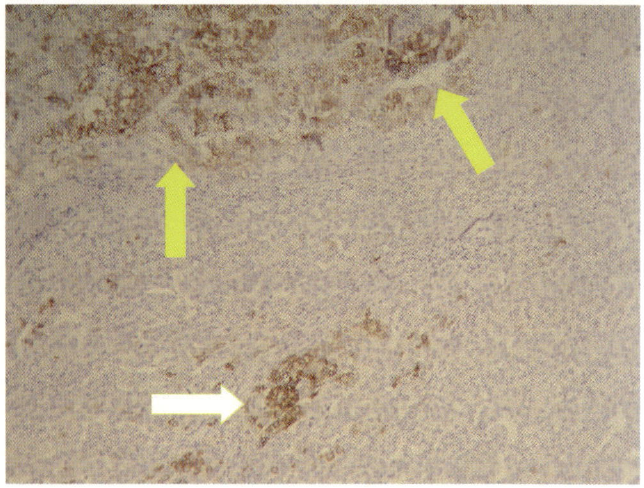

Fig. 7.131 cHCC-CC, showing positive immunohistochemical staining of Hep Par-1 in HCC area (*upper yellow arrow*) and ICC area (*white arrow*)

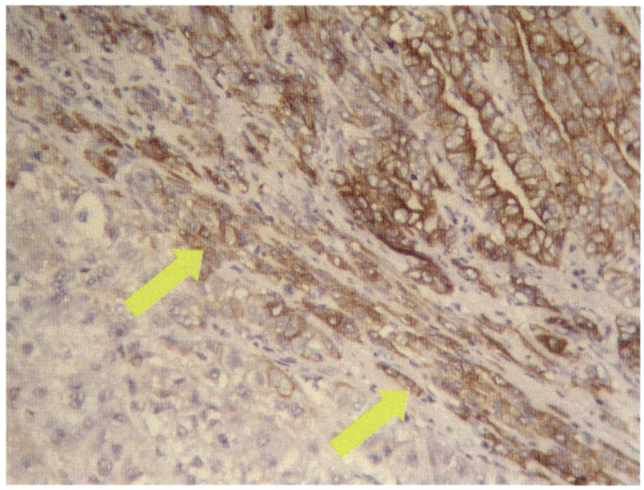

Fig. 7.132 cHCC-CC, showing positive immunohistochemical staining of CK19 in ICC area (*upper right*) and intermediate cells (*arrow*)

between cHCC-CC components can often be observed, though the cancer cells in the transition (intermediate type) may not have the typical morphological and histological features of HCC or CC cells.

There is no definite proportion of the two components in cHCC-CC currently. And to standardize the diagnostic criteria, according to our experience, it should be taken into account that sampling bias and lesion distribution with heterogeneity cannot be totally avoided; the proportion of one of the two tumorous components in cHCC-CC should reach 30–50% or above. For cases with a tumor component accounting for 15–30%, it is determined that this component is the dominant one in cHCC-CC tissues in pathological diagnosis, and if a tumor component is less than 15%, it should be considered to increase the sampling sites and quantity to determine whether it is a true cHCC-CC, or the dominant component should be considered as an independent lesion, and the proportions of the rest should be recorded and illustrated, because these lesions often cannot reflect the unique biological characteristics of cHCC-CC as an independent disease.

7.1.4.5 Immunohistochemistry

cHCC-CC is often characterized by biphasic phenotype, namely, regions of HCC are positive for Hep Par-1 (Fig. 7.131) and GPC-3, with or without staining of CK19 (Fig. 7.132) and CK7 (Fig. 7.133), while CC parts are positive for CK19 (Fig. 7.132), CK7 (Fig. 7.133), and MUC-1, with or without Hep Par-1 staining (Fig. 7.131). The cancer cells in the transition zone can also be examined by CD10 and polyclonal CEA staining, to determine the existence of hepatocellular or cholangiocellular differentiation in these cancer

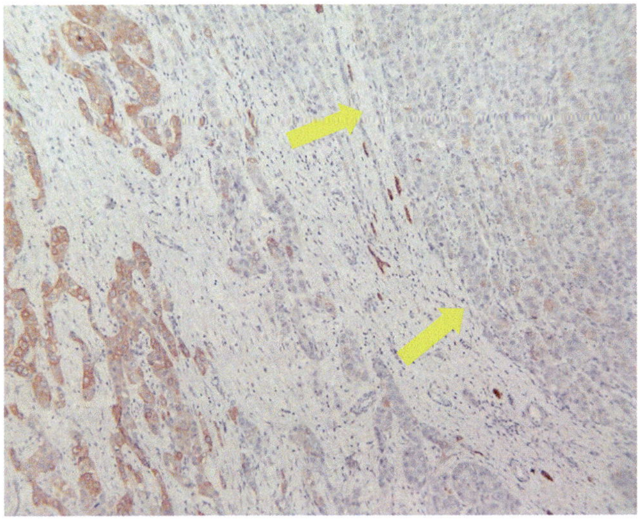

Fig. 7.133 cHCC-CC, showing positive immunohistochemical staining of CK7 in ICC (*below left*) and weak staining of CK7 in HCC cells (*upper right*)

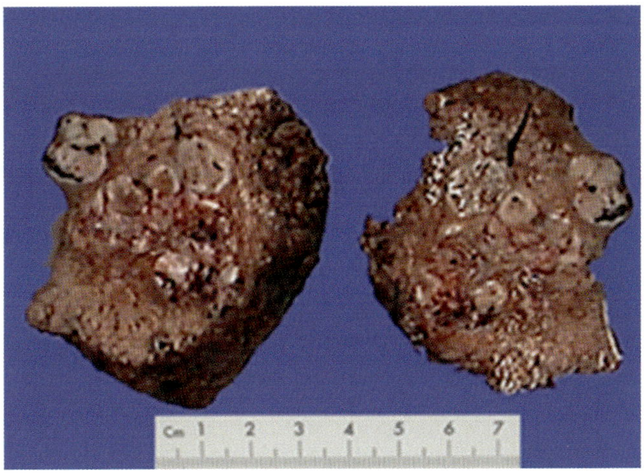

Fig. 7.134 Liver cancer, showing multiple-nodule type, showing multiple ICC and HCC nodules

cells. From the perspective of immunopathological typing, staining of stem cell markers can also be an option, such as CD56, c-kit, CD133, or EpCAM.

7.1.4.6 Differential Diagnosis

The diagnosis of cHCC-CC should the based on the combination of histological and immunohistochemical features of the tumor tissues, and we should pay attention to identification of pseudoglandular tube structures in the HCC tissues from true glandular tubes of CC, as well as collision tumor produced by fusion growth of HCC and CC (Figs. 7.134 and 7.135).

7.1.4.7 Treatment and Prognosis

Overall, cHCC-CC is a type of highly invasive tumors, and its long-term prognosis is poor; thus, surgical resection should be the first therapeutic option which is the principle of the treatment. The data provided by Shanghai Zhongshan Hospital (2012) showed that of the 103 cases of surgical resection cHCC-CC, the cumulative recurrence rates after 1 year, 3 years, and 5 years were 59.3, 85.1, and 98.2%, respectively, and overall survival rates after 1 year, 3 years, and 5 years were 73.9, 41.4, and 36.4%, respectively, suggesting the intermediate biological characteristics and surgical prognosis of cHCC-CC were between those of HCC and ICC [51]. The low long-term survival rate was related to the high recurrence rate (> 50%) after liver transplantation. Park et al. (2013) reported that cases of cHCC-CC had a high recurrence rate 1 year after liver transplantation [52]. Groeschl et al. (2013) provided the statistics of data from the database of "Surveillance, Epidemiology and End Results (SEER)" in the United States, showing that the survival rates 3 years after surgical resection of HCC and cHCC-CC were similar (55%:46%, $P = 0.4$), but the survival rate 3 years after liver transplantation in HCC patients was significantly higher than that in cHCC-CC patients (78%:48%, $P = 0.01$) [53]. Statistics on the data from SEER database was demonstrated by Garancini et al. (2014) showing that the overall survival rate 5 years after surgical resection and the disease-free survival rate reached 41.1 and 52.8%, respectively, suggesting that SEER stage and tumor size of 5–10 cm were independent prognostic factors which had an effect on the 5-year survival rate in these patients [41].

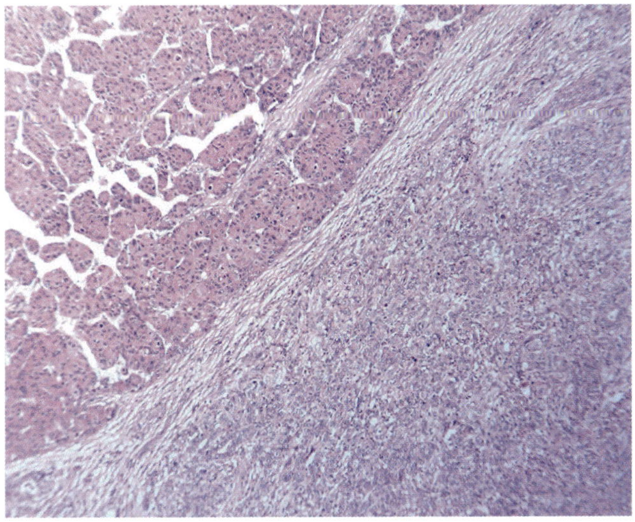

Fig. 7.135 Liver cancer, collision type, showing completed fibrous capsule between HCC area (*upper*) and ICC area (*below*)

7.1.5 Dual-Phenotype HCC

We have noticed in pathological practice that a typical HCC in morphology can express markers of both the liver cell line (e.g., Hep Par-1, CK18, pCEA, etc.) and bile duct cell line (e.g., CK7, CK19, MUC-1, etc.), different from the cHCC-

CC containing both HCC and CC components, and we named it as dual-phenotype HCC (DPHCC) [54]. Clearly, morphopathologically, DPHCC is not completely the same as cHCC-CC.

Based on the analysis on the characteristics of immunohistochemical phenotype, DPHCC accounts for about 5% of HCC. In clinical practice, DPHCC's performance is similar to that of HCC, including a history of HBV or HCV infection, as well as chronic hepatitis and cirrhosis background, and elevation of both serum AFP and CA19-9 can be found in some cases. Histologically, DPHCC represents typical HCC features, such as polygon-shaped cancer cells, trabecular arrangement, sinuses, and pseudoglandular structure. In immunohistochemistry, the carcinoma cells, which express markers of liver cells with canalicular staining pattern for CD10 and pCEA, show the phenotypic characteristics of immunohistochemical proteins in CC (Fig. 7.136). Interestingly, the MVI found in DPHCC tissue maintained the dual phenotype, suggesting it is composed by cell populations with high proliferation and invasion activities (Fig. 7.137). According to our diagnostic criteria, the number of dual-phenotype positive cancer cells should be more than 15%, and they often show high expression of stem cell markers, such as EpCAM. DPHCC showed stronger invasiveness in biological behavior, and the incidence of satellite nodules and MVI is higher than that of common HCC. In the aspect of prognosis, the total survival rate and recurrence rate in patients with DPHCC are significantly poorer than those of the common HCC [54]. And our experimental studies showed that inhibition or upregulation of the expression of CK19 mRNA in HCC cells can markedly affect the proliferation and invasion of cancer cells. We hypothesized that DPHCC is a unique molecular subtype of HCC, originating from hepatic progenitor cells in the liver and maintaining a bidirectional differentiation potential, and it has a higher malignancy due to its dual biological behavior of HCC and ICC (Fig. 7.138). Govaere et al. (2013) also reported a lower invasive activity in the CK19 knockout HCC cell strain, as well as decreased drug resistance to 5-FU and sorafenib, suggesting the multiple drug resistance of DPHCC in clinical treatment [55]. Therefore, the routine pathological diagnosis should contain careful classification of special subtypes of HCC including DPHCC, to provide elaborate pathological information for clinical development of individualized diagnosis and treatment strategies.

7.2 Malignant Bile Duct Tumors

Wen-Ming Cong
Department of Pathology, Eastern Hepatobiliary Surgery Hospital, Second Military Medical University, Shanghai, China

7.2.1 Intrahepatic Cholangiocarcinoma

7.2.1.1 Incidence

According to its anatomical origin, cholangiocarcinoma (CCA) can be divided into intrahepatic type (ICC), perihilar type (pCCA), and distal type (dCCA), accounting for 5–10%, 60–70%, and 20–30%, respectively. These three types of cholangiocarcinomas are all independent lesions and are different from each other in epidemiology, pathological biology, clinical features, therapeutic strategies, and prognosis. The International Liver Cancer Association (ILCA) suggested that the names of Klatskin tumor and extrahepatic cholangiocarcinoma should be deprecated [56]. The term of cholangiocarcinoma usually refers to the malignant tumors of extrahepatic bile ducts, including two major types, namely, hilar cholangiocarcinoma and distal cholangiocarcinoma, while ICC refers to malignant tumors derived from intrahepatic biliary tree cells at all levels, including second-degree bile ducts in the liver adjacent to the hepatic portal, segmental bile ducts, and peripheral glands of the ducts (perihilar ICC), or malignant tumors in the perihepatic regions derived from the epithelium of the subsegmental bile canaliculus (septal bile duct, interlobular biliary canals, and cholangiole) (peripheral ICC) [57].

According to statistics, ICC accounted for 13% of all the tumor-related deaths of 7,600,000 per year in the world. The incidence rates of ICC in different countries vary greatly, and the annual incidence rate is in 113/100,000 in Thailand; 8.75/100,000 in Gwangju, South Korea; 7.55/100,000 in Shanghai, China; 3.4/100,000 in Osaka, Japan; 1.45/100,000 in Singapore; and 2.1/100,000 on average in Western countries including 1.67/100,000 in the United States [56]. Among 40,656 cases of hepatobiliary tumors diagnosed in the Department of Pathology of EHBH, Second Military Medical University during the 30-year period, malignant hepatic tumors accounted for 80%, and the top two tumors are HCC (86%) and ICC (8%), respectively.

7.2.1.2 Etiology and Pathogenesis

There are many known pathogenic factors closely related to the genesis of ICC, many of which are similar to those of HCC, including intrahepatic bile duct stones, chronic cholangitis, HBV/HCV infection, primary sclerosing cholangitis, chronic ulcerative colitis, parasite infection, bile duct malformation (common bile duct cyst and Caroli disease), cirrhosis, congenital hepatic fibrosis, fatty liver, diabetes, obesity, smoking, alcohol abuse, and environmental factors. The total lifetime prevalence rate of choledochal cyst is 5–30%, and the International Agency for Research on Cancer (IARC) listed *Clonorchis sinensis* as a class 1 carcinogen in 2009.

In recent years, the relationship between HBV/HCV infection and ICC has attracted increasing attention. The rate

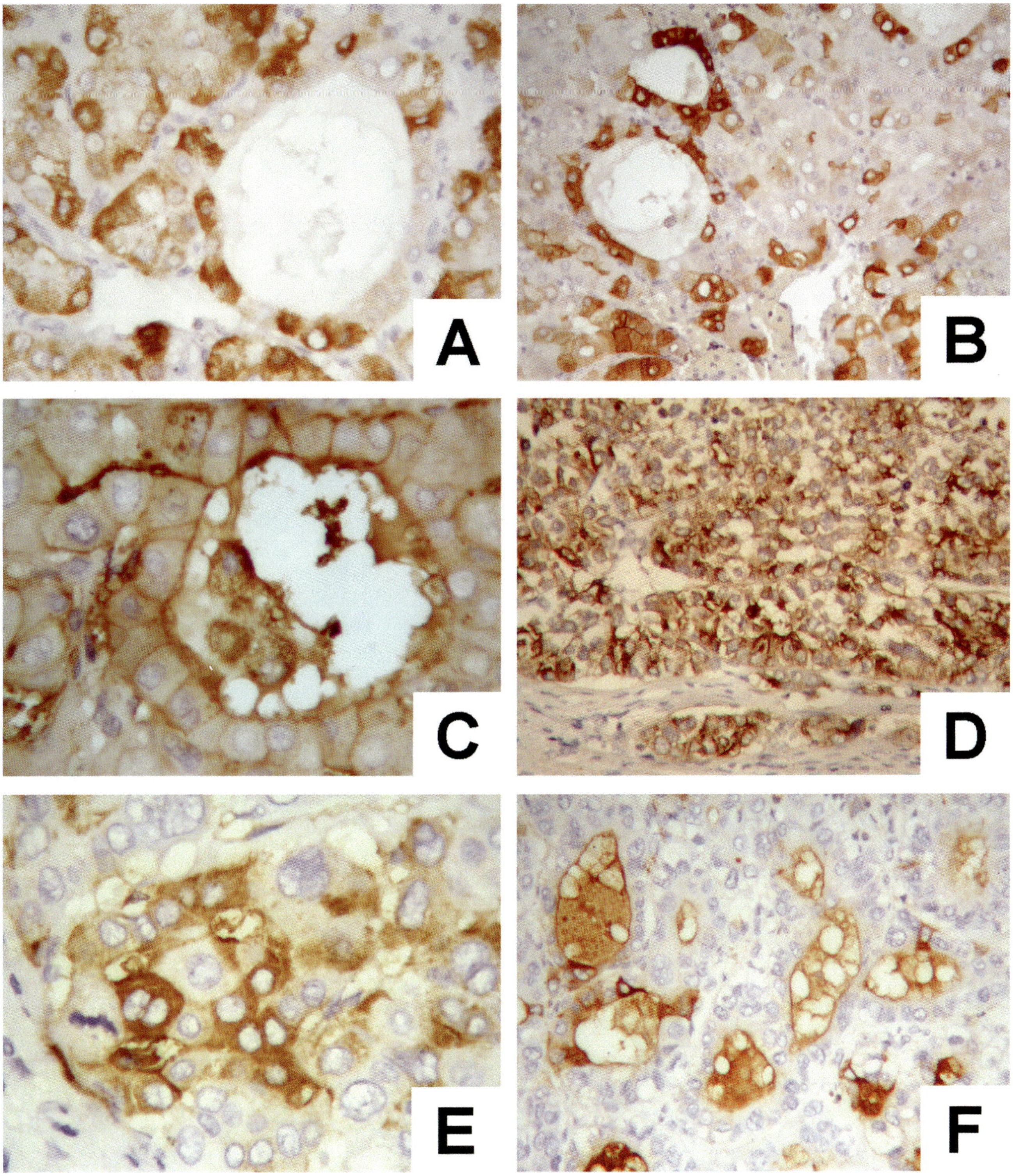

Fig. 7.136 Immunohistochemical staining of sequential series of tissue sections for DPHCC, (**a**) cytoplasmic stained for Hep Par-1; (**b**) cytoplasmic stained for CK19; (**c**) a bile canalicular stained for pCEA; (**d**) cytoplasmic stained for MUC-1; (**e**) cytoplasmic stained for CA19-9; (**f**) cytoplasmic stained for CA19-9

of positive serum HCV in ICC patients in Japan reached 36%, and the risk of developing ICC in patients with HCV-induced hepatic cirrhosis is 1000 times greater than in the general population [58]. Our recent statistics of the ICC cases with surgical resection in the EHBH during a period of nearly 30 years showed that the rates of HBV and HCV

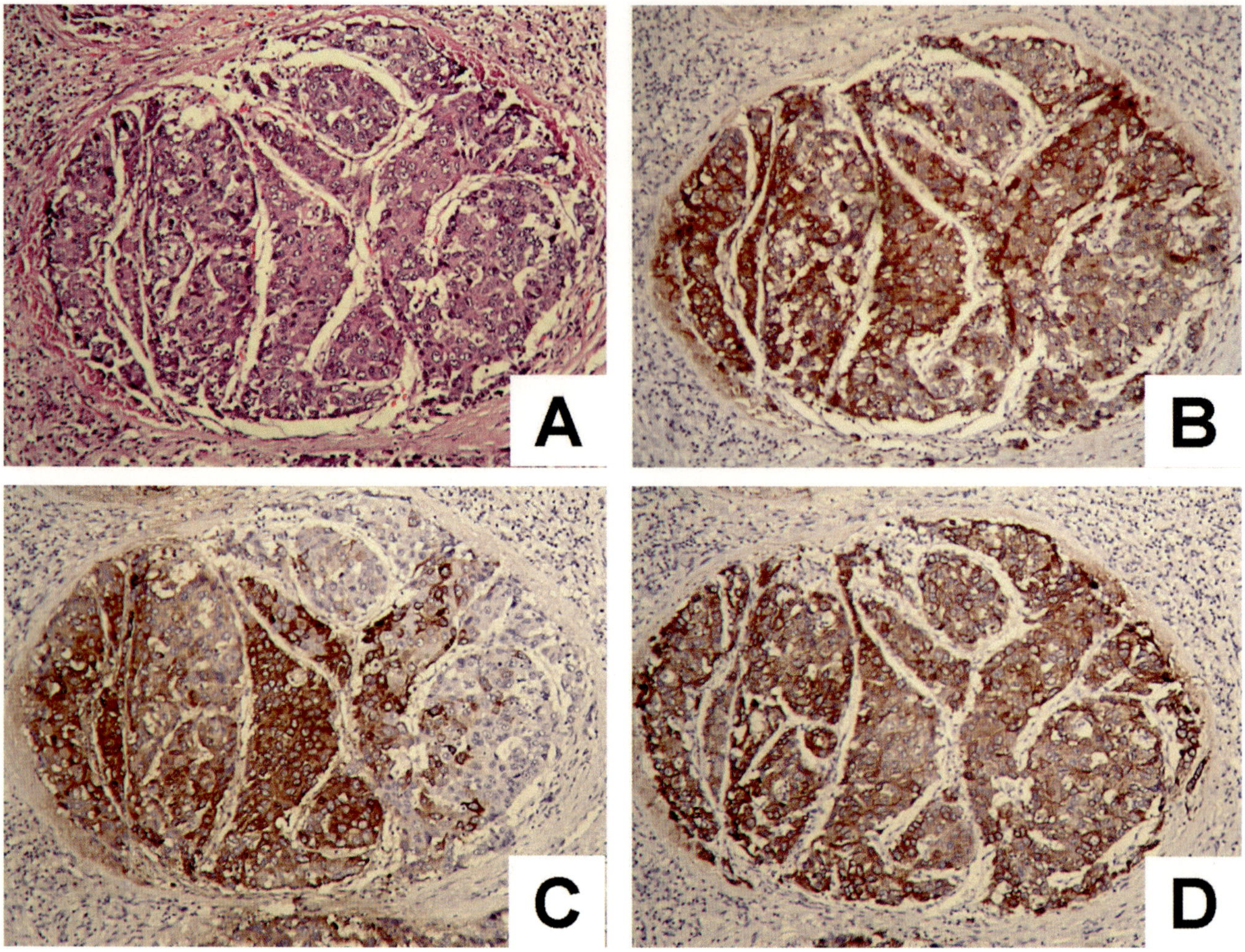

Fig. 7.137 Immunohistochemical staining of sequential series of tissue sections for DPHCC, (**a**) HE-stained section of MVI; (**b**) pCEA-positive immunostaining of the same specimen as A; (**c**) Hep Par-1-positive immunostaining of the same specimen as A; (**d**) CK19-positive immunostaining of the same specimen as A

infection (confirmed via serum and/or immunohistochemical examination) were 47.44% and 9.64%, respectively. Litianyu et al. (2008) found HCV core gene-coding protein (HCVc) can induce transition of the cholangiocarcinoma cells from epithelial to mesenchymal phenotype and significantly promote their motility, invasion, and metastasis. Palmer et al. (2012) conducted a meta-analysis aiming at Western countries showed that the odds ratio (OR, 95% CI ICC) defined risk factors for ICC include liver cirrhosis (22.92, 18.24–28.7), hepatitis type B (5.10, 2.91–8.95), hepatitis type C (4.84, 2.41–9.71), alcohol abuse (2.81,1.52–5.21), type 2 diabetes mellitus (1.89, 1.74–2.07), obesity (1.56,1.26–1.94), and smoking (1.31,0.95– 1.82) [59]. Chinese scholars (2012) reported that the ratio risk (RR, 95% confidence interval) of ICC in hepatitis type B patients was 3.42 (2.46:43.74) [60]. Razumilava et al. (2013) reported that the annual risk of developing cholangiocarcinoma for patients with primary sclerosing cholangitis in Western countries was 0.5–1.5%, and its lifetime incidence rate was 5–10% [61].

From the perspective of development in the study of molecular mechanisms of ICC, technological strategy in many studies on HCC can be applied to the research on ICC, and molecular variation of ICC and HCC is similar, such as the same genomic features and markers in ICC and HCC with poor prognosis, but they also have their own unique characteristics. The author (2001) studied 22 cases of ICC and found the rates of loss of heterozygosity/mutation in four kinds of tumor suppressor genes in ICC tissues were APC (68.8%), DCC (46.2%), OGG1 (41.7%), and p53 (37.5%), respectively, compared with those in HCC: p53 (87.5%), APC (58.8%), OGG1 (50%), and DCC (25%), showing the difference in the type and frequency of genetic mutations, suggesting the synergy of multigenetic mutations played an important role in the multistage development of ICC, and different molecular mechanisms and carcinogenesis pathways may be involved in the genesis of ICC and HCC, respectively [62].

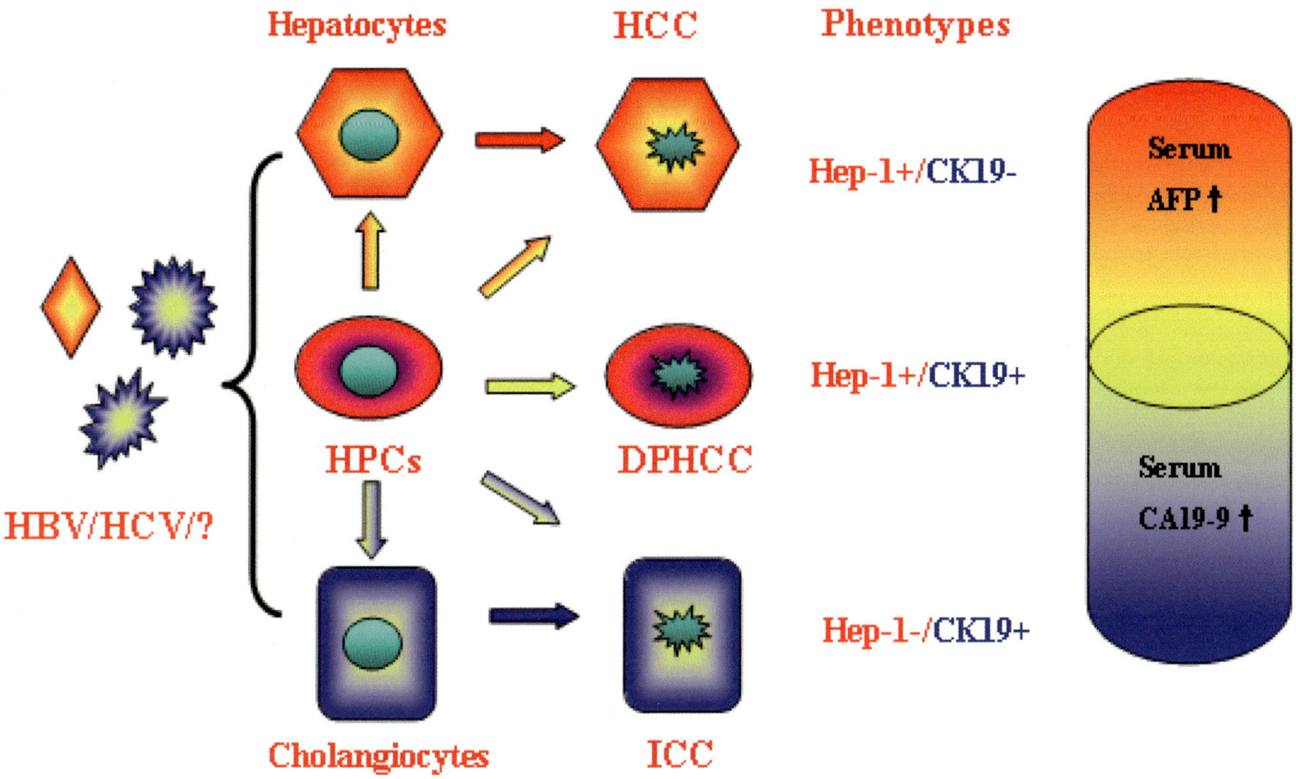

Fig. 7.138 Schematic diagram of the mechanism of DPHCC. HBV/HCV or other pathogenic factors may lead to the malignant transformation of hepatocytes, hepatic progenitor cells (HPCs), and cholangiocytes into HCC, DPHCC, and ICC, respectively. One hallmark of DPHCC cells is a bidirectional differentiation and can open both liver cell genes (e.g., Hep Par-1) and bile duct cell genes (e.g., CK19), and both serum AFP and CA19-9 contents may simultaneously increase (Reprint with permission from Cancer letter, 2015, Vol 368 (1), 14–19)

According to the current understanding, common mutations in cholangiocarcinomas include KRAS (5–54%), TP53 (44%), SMAD4 (17%), and isocitrate dehydrogenases 1 and 2 (IDH1/2, 10–23%), as well as BRAF, NRAS, PI3K, EGFR, MET, PIK3CA (<5%), etc. And common methylated genes include p16^{INK4A} (18–83%), suppressor of cytokine signaling-3 (SOCS-3.88%), RAS-associated domain family 1A gene (RASSF1A, 49%), and p14ARF (25%). Cell membrane receptors of therapeutic significance in molecular target therapies include ERBB2, EGFR, VEGFR, gp130/IL6-R, etc., and downstream signal transduction pathways of therapeutic significance in molecular target therapies include KRAS/MAPK, PI3K-AKT-mTOR, IL-6/STAT, COX-2/PGE2, etc., among which RAS-RAF-MEK-ERK signaling axis stimulates cell proliferation, and PI3K-AKT-mTOR signaling axis promotes cell survival [56, 63, 64].

Researchers have shown that interleukin-6 (IL-6) is one of the key cytokines involved in the carcinogenesis of bile duct epithelial cells and its main functions are as follows:

① It can stimulate the bile duct epithelium and cancer cells to release IL-6 by autocrine or paracrine secretion in situations such as chronic inflammation, cholestasis, and tumor microenvironments, inducing high expressions of inducible nitric oxide synthase (iNOS), leading to high expression of reactive nitric oxide (RNOS), resulting in gene mutation and DNA strand breaks in cells.
② Methylation silencing of SOCS-3 gene can be detected in both cholangiocarcinoma tissues and cells, which can lead to the absence of negative feedback regulation for IL-6 signal transduction pathways, resulting in increased expression of inflammatory molecules and upregulation of Mcl-1 gene which encodes the protein of antiapoptotic Bcl-2, and this can cause resistance to cytotoxic therapies in cholangiocarcinoma.
③ By enhancing the activity of telomerase, inhibiting the shortening of telomere, the cholangiocarcinoma cells can escape senescence.
④ IL-6 can affect the methylation of the promoter regions by regulating the activity of DNA methyltransferase, and overexpression of IL-6 can lead to the methylation of the promoters of a set of genes, such as the methylation of epidermal growth factor receptor (EGFR).
⑤ IL-6 receptor subunits, gp130 and gp130, can be highly expressed by the cholangiocarcinoma cells, which can be combined with IL-6 activating the downstream signal transduction pathways, such as JAK/STAT, PI3K/Akt and MAPK, resulting in the ability of long-term survival and

continuous proliferation in cholangiocarcinoma cells through a series of cascase involving key molecular targets [56, 65, 66].

From the perspective of histogenesis, it was once believed that the ICC could be originated in the bile duct epithelial cells, periductal glandular epithelial cells, and hepatic progenitor cells. But with the application of advanced molecular biological methods, including the recent cell fate tracking technology, new discoveries will change the traditional understanding and theories. Fan et al. (2012) found that under the combined effects of Notch and AKT signal transduction pathways, the well-differentiated mature mouse hepatocytes can also develop ICC via transdifferentiation into bile duct epithelium [67], which helps understand the pathogenesis of ICC in patients with HBV/HCV hepatitis. Notch signaling pathway plays a key role in the development regulation of intrahepatic bile ducts and is closely related to activation of hepatic progenitor cells. Recent studies have shown that mice with expression of Notch-1 can develop ICC [68]. Andersen et al. (2012) found that cholangiocarcinoma with KRAS mutation has drug resistance to tyrosine kinase inhibitor therapy [69]. Oishi et al. (2012) suggested that miR-200 participated in the epithelial-mesenchymal transition (EMT) of ICC, directly targeting neural cell adhesion molecule 1 (NCAM1), and the expression of both molecules is associated with the prognosis, which may be the molecular markers of stem cell-like ICC with high invasion and the potential therapeutic targets [70]. Karakatsanis et al. (2013) found that miR-21 and miR-221 in HCC tissues were significantly upregulated and were related to tumor staging and the prognosis [71]. In addition, the relationship between ICC and gene polymorphism of enzyme systems, which are related to DNA methylation, DNA damage/repair and biliary toxins clearance, has also been highly valued [71]. In a word, although the pathogenesis of ICC is not entirely clear, several important progresses have been made. And a summary of the main knowledge in the pathogenesis of ICC was made in Fig. 7.139, which is also the basis and focus of further study on molecular mechanism of ICC.

7.2.1.3 Pathological Staging of ICC

Currently, it has been recognized that ICC and HCC are different in many aspects, including pathogenic mechanism, histogenesis, biological characteristics, molecular targets, and prognostic risk factors. Therefore, it is necessary to study the clinical pathologic staging system with the characteristics of ICC. The following five staging systems for ICC thoroughly reflect the current understanding of clinical pathological parameters which affects the prognosis of ICC. In the future, it should be considered to add in the indexes which can reflect the mole biological characteristics of HCC.

1. AJCC/UICCTNM-ICC (seventh edition) (2009). According to the number of tumors, invasion of the adjacent tissues, vascular invasion, lymphatic metastasis, and

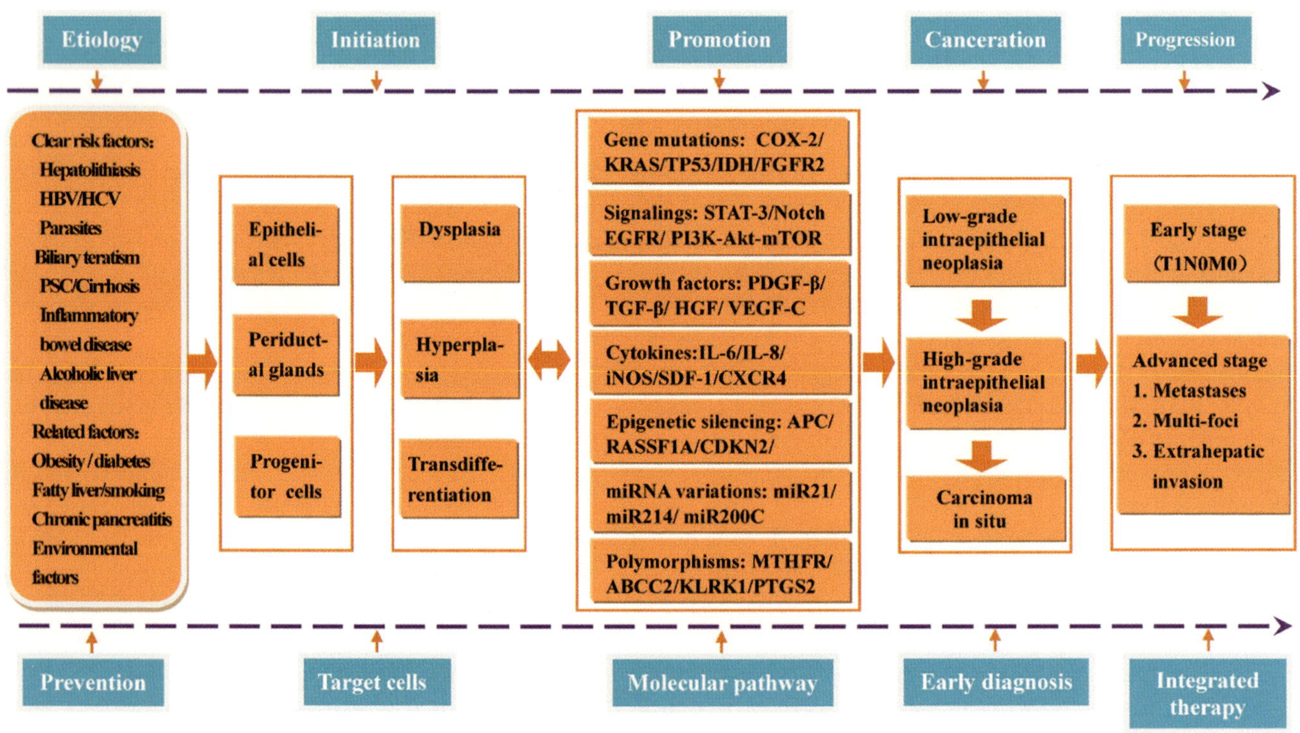

Fig. 7.139 Possible pathogenesis of multiple stages of ICC development

Table 7.7 The seventh AJCC staging system for ICC

TNM staging	Characteristics
T_1	Single tumor without vascular invasion[a]
T_{2a}	Single tumor with vascular invasion[a]
T_{2b}	Multiple tumors, with or without vascular invasion[a]
T_3	Tumor(s) perforating the visceral peritoneum or involving the local extrahepatic structures by direct invasion
T_4	Tumor with periductal invasion[b]
N_0	No regional lymph node metastases
N_1	Regional lymph node metastases[c]
M_0	No distant metastases
M_1	Distant metastases
Staging	
Stage I	$T_1 N_0 M_0$
Stage II	$T_2 N_0 M_0$
Stage III	$T_3 N_0 M_0$
Stage IVA	$T_4 N_0 M_0$, Any T, $N_1 M_0$
Stage IVB	Any T, Any N, M_1

Reprint with permission from Compton, Intrahepatic Bile Ducts, Springer, 2012

[a]Including vascular (portal vein or hepatic vein) and microvascular invasion

[b]Including periductal infiltration and mixed mass periductal invasion type

[c]Distal metastasis (M1) refers to involvement of the abdominal cavity, abdominal aorta, and inferior vena cava

Table 7.8 Nathan's pathological staging for ICC

Staging	Index		
	Microvascular invasion	Multiple tumors	Diameter of the tumors
sT_1	Without	Without	All
sT_2	With	Without	All
	Without	With	All
	With	With	All
sT_3	Invasion of extrahepatic tissues[a]		
Staging			
Stage I	sT_1, N_0, M_0		
Stage II	sT_2, N_0, M_0		
Stage III	sT_3, N_0, M_0, or N_1 M_0 (any sT)		
Stage IV	M_1 (any sT, any N)		

Reprint with permission from Compton, Intrahepatic Bile Ducts, Springer, 2012

[a]Invasion of the gallbladder excluded, invasion of the hepatic artery or vena cava included

distant metastasis, as well as other parameters of ICC, the TNM staging of ICC (including cHCC-CC) (Table 7.7) was proposed. The specifications of several terms are shown as follows: multinodular tumors including multiple primary tumors and satellite nodules, vascular invasion including gross appearance of invasion of portal vein, venous thrombosis and MVI, regional lymphatic metastasis including hepatic hilar lymph nodes with

Table 7.9 TNM staging for ICC by Liver Cancer Study Group of Japan

Staging	T	N	M
Stage I	T_1	N_0	M_0
Stage II	T_2	N_0	M_0
Stage III	T_3	N_0	M_0
Stage IVA	T_4	N_0	M_0
	Or all T	N_1	M_0
Stage IVB	Any T	Any N	M_1

T_1, solitary tumor nodule, diameter ≤2 cm, no serosa invasion of the portal vein, hepatic vein, or bile ducts; T_2, with 2 of the indexes; T_3, with one of the indexes; N_0, no lymphatic metastasis; N_1, any lymphatic metastasis; M_0, no distal metastasis; M_1, distal metastasis

drainage through the right lobe of the liver and hepatic portal areas, peri-duodenal lymph nodes and peri-pancreatic lymph nodes, as well as the lymph nodes of ligamentum hepatogastricum, and distal lymphatic metastasis referring to the involvement of lymph nodes in the abdominal cavity, around the abdominal aorta and inferior vena cava without any definition of the number of lymph nodes, T4 classification simply based on the gross type of ICC. However, whether the periductal infiltrating type is suitable for use as an independent grading index of advanced ICC, and poor prognosis needs to be confirmed by more evidence-based information [72]. The 5-year survival rate of ICC in TNM I stage with R0 resection can reach 40%.

2. Nathan's pathological staging for ICC (2009): Aiming at the problem of insufficient stratification of T stages in TNM staging system, a simplified T staging including core indexes was proposed, including vascular invasion, number of the tumors, and extrahepatic metastasis. Although the rate of lymphatic metastasis in ICC cases reached 32% which was an independent predictor for poor prognosis in ICC, it is not included in this index system, since lymph node dissection has not yet been included into routine operation of ICC (Table 7.8) [73].

3. Liver Cancer Study Group of Japan (LCSGJ) (2003) staging for ICC LCSGJ divided ICC into three gross types, including mass-forming (MF), periductal-infiltrating (PI), and intraductal-growing (ID) types, and in view of rare cases of the latter two types of ICC, the TNM staging proposed by LCSGJ is only for mass-forming-type ICC (Table 7.9) [74].

4. Fudan's prognostic scores for ICC (2013): A 5-score staging system consisting of five parameters with five points for each of them, including serum alkaline phosphatase (ALP), CA19-9, number of tumors, maximum diameter of the tumors, and tumor types, screened from 244 patients.

Table 7.10 Fudan's prognostic scores for ICC

Factors	Score		
Serum ALP (U/l)			
≤147.0	0		
>147.0	1		
Serum CA19-9 (μg/l)			
≤37.0	0		
>37.0	1		
Tumor number			
Single	0		
Multiple (≥2个)	1		
Maximum tumor diameter (cm)			
<10	0		
≥10	1		
Tumor boundary			
Clear	0		
Unclear	1		
Risk grouping	End index	Risk ratio (95% confidence interval)	*P*
Low risk	0	1	0.01
Moderate risk	1	2.001 (1.180–3.394)	<0.001
High risk	2	3.719 (2.179–6.347)	<0.001
	3	5.456 (3.162–9.413)	<0.001
Very high risk	4	12.255 (6.344–3.556)	<0.001
	5	27.519 (9.944–79.152)	<0.001

The score of 0, 1, 2–3, and 4–5 indicates low, moderate, high, and very high risk, respectively (Table 7.10), and the 5-year survival rates of patients with the above corresponding scores are 48.6%, 25.6%, 10.3%, and 0, respectively [75].

5. EHBH's prognosis assessment for ICC (2013): In EHBH, based on the pathological analysis of 367 cases of surgically resected ICC, a nomograph was proposed consisting seven parameters, including serum CEA, CA19-9, vascular invasion, lymphatic metastasis, direct invasion and local metastasis, number of tumorous nodules, and diameter of the tumors. The value of each parameter can be calculated through their conversion into counts listed on the first line, and the added numerical value of a patient should be marked on the chart of total index value. And it can be used to evaluate the prognosis of a patient conveniently and intuitively by comparison of the added numerical value and the 3-year and 5-year survival rates (Table 7.11) [76].

According to a study on postsurgical information of 67 cases of ICC in EHBH of Second Military Medical University, it was shown that 22 cases (32.8%) had lymphatic metastasis and the metastasis rate of primary tumors in the left lobe of the liver was 47%, which was significantly higher than that of the right lobe of the liver (18.2%). In addi-

Table 7.11 Nomograph of prognosis assessment of ICC in EHBH

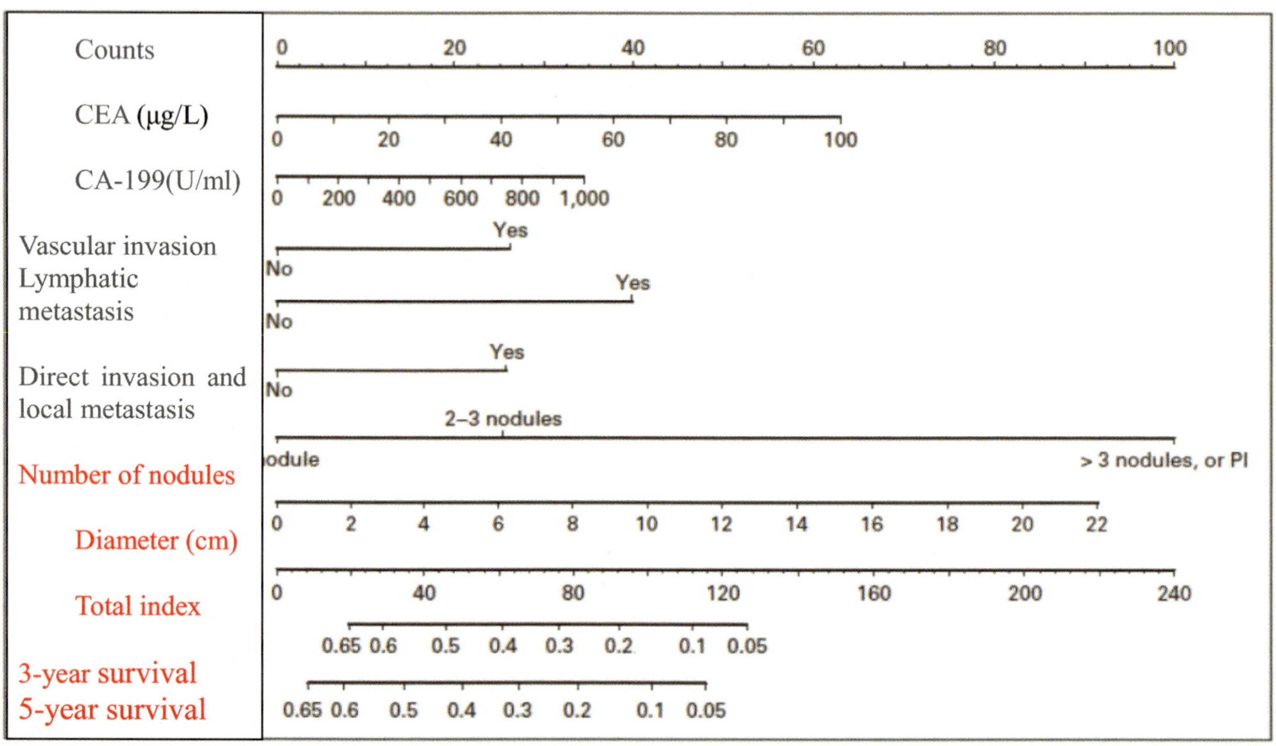

tion, skipping lymphatic metastasis has also been observed in these cases, of which the metastasis rate of lymph nodes on ligamentum hepatoduodenale was the highest, indicating the lymph nodes on ligamentum hepatoduodenale can be regarded as the sentinel lymph nodes in ICC [77].

7.2.1.4 Clinical Features

Of all the 2602 cases of ICC diagnosed in the Department of Pathology of EHBH during the 30 years, the patients were 53.35 years old on average with the male to female ratio of 2.22:1. The clinical features of peripheral ICC are not specific, and obvious symptoms were found in early stage, while patients with progression ICC may exhibit clinical manifestations similar to those of HCC, including hepatomegaly, pain in the hepatic zone, decreased apatite, weight loss, fatigue, abdominal distension, and abdominal mass. Biliary obstructive jaundice was rare. The diagnostic sensitivity and specificity of significantly higher serum CA19-9 levels (>100 U/ml) were 89% and 86%, respectively. The sensitivity of CEA was 30%, and the sensitivity of intraductal ultrasound was 89–95%. About 25% of ICC patients had elevated serum AFP levels to different degrees, especially in patients with chronic viral hepatitis and cirrhosis patients. Ultrasound type B shows ICC as intrahepatic hypoechoic mass with smooth and irregularly thickened margins. Dynamic CT images display gradual enhancement or delayed enhancement of ICC lesions [78, 79].

7.2.1.5 Gross Features

ICC lesions are often found in the left lobe of the liver, with a diameter of 2–15 cm, and the sections are usually gray white, homogeneous, and tender in texture, with less hemorrhage and necrosis. Most cases have no fibrous capsule, showing an invasive border, and the liver tissues often contain cholestasis and little cirrhosis.

The gross morphology of ICC is similar to that of HCC with its own characteristics, which can be roughly divided into the following nine gross types:

1. Mass-forming type: It is the most common type (> 85%), forming masses or nodules in the liver parenchyma, and the tumors are gray white, dense, and tender in texture because of fibroconnective tissues, often with no fibrous capsule (Fig. 7.140), prone to intrahepatic metastasis.
2. Periductal-infiltrating type: The tumors do not form masses but expand to both sides along the wall of bile ducts, resulting in thickened wall of the involved bile ducts, luminal stenosis, and dilatation of peripheral bile ducts (Fig. 7.141), and tumors often invade the liver parenchyma along the portal vein or disseminate along the interlobular biliary canals in the portal area leading to portal lymphatic metastasis in the liver.
3. Intraductal growth type: Polypoid or papillary tumors grow and protrude into the lumen of bile ducts, with or without invasion of the bile duct wall (Fig. 7.142).
4. Superficial spreading type: The cancer cells are arranged in a micropapillary structure, which only invade and grow in the epithelial layer of the bile duct with no invasion of the bile duct wall (Fig. 7.143).
5. Multinodular type: The tumor is composed by a number of tumor nodules which can grow in confluent multinodular pattern (Fig. 7.144). And stones can be found in the bile ducts in cases with secondary carcinoma derived from the bile duct stones (Fig. 7.145).

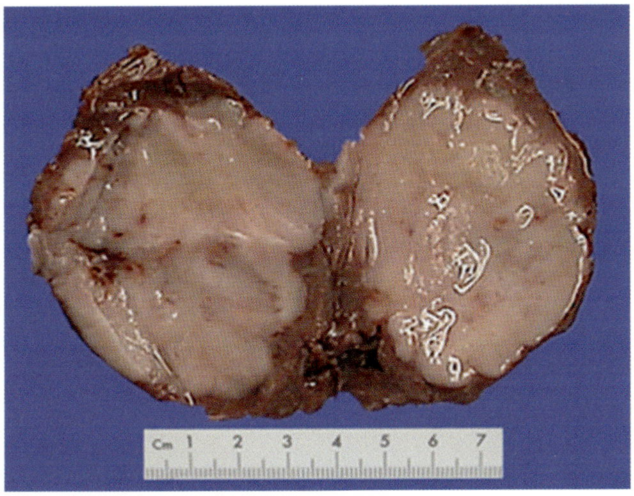

Fig. 7.140 ICC, mass-forming type, *gray-white* tumor with tough and dense connective tissue

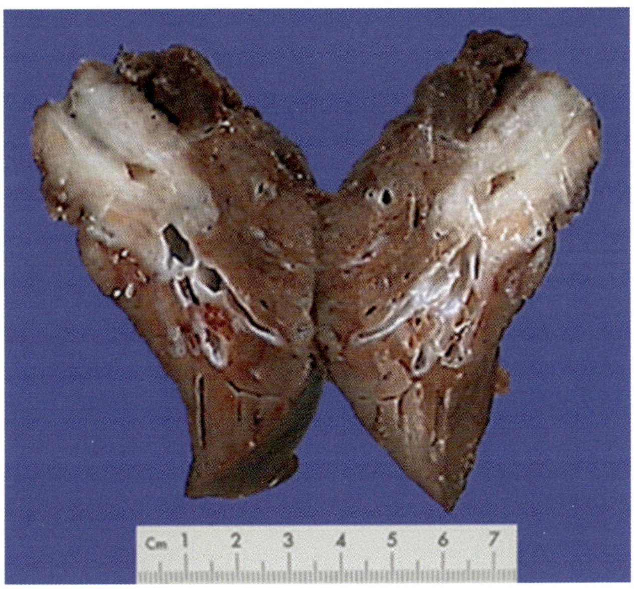

Fig. 7.141 ICC, periductal-infiltrating type, tumor growing along the bile duct

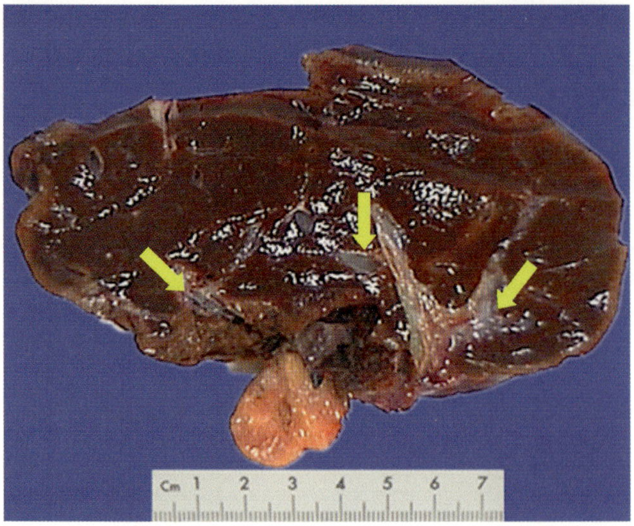

Fig. 7.142 ICC, intraductal growth type, bile duct filled with *gray* and *white* jelly-like tumor tissue

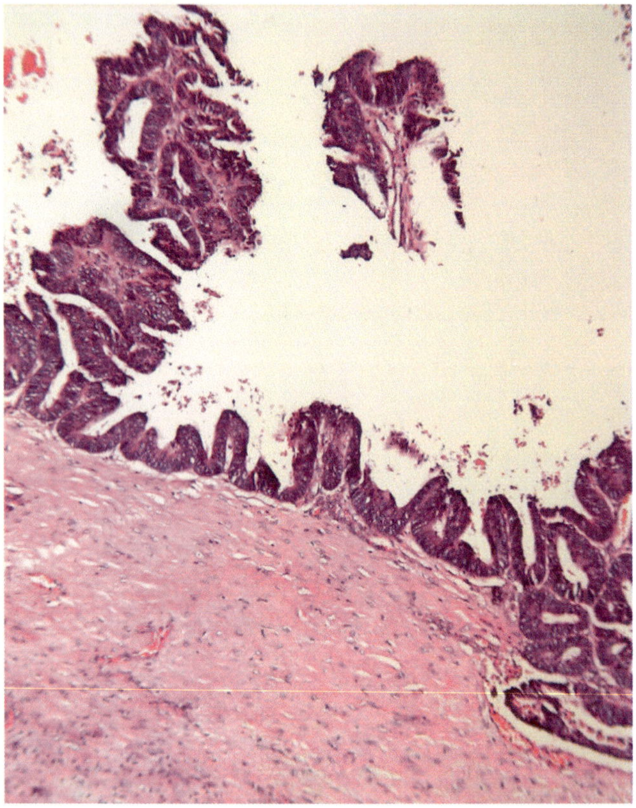

Fig. 7.143 ICC, superficial spreading type, tumor infiltrating through the mucous layer

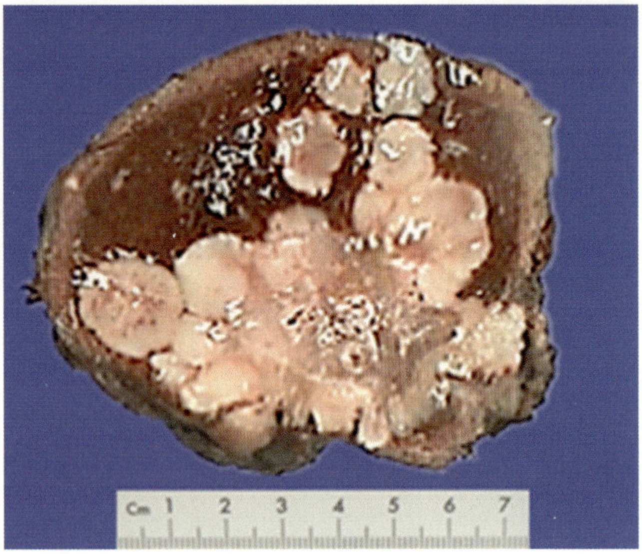

Fig. 7.144 ICC, multinodular type, nodules enlarge and become confluent

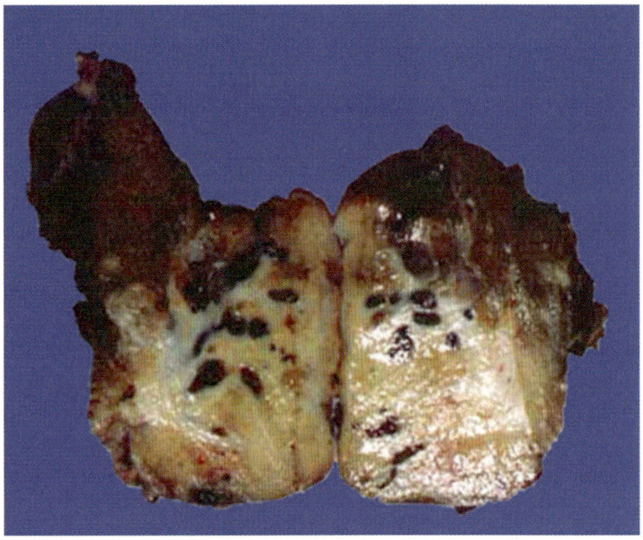

Fig. 7.145 ICC, mass-forming type, showing calculus of the bile duct

6. Diffuse type: The tumor shows multiple nodules in diffuse growth and distribution in the liver (Fig. 7.146).
7. Massive type: The diameter of the tumor reaches >10 cm (Fig. 7.147).
8. Small carcinoma type: The diameter of the tumor is ≤3 cm (Fig. 7.148).
9. Mixed-type combinations of the above types: It has been pointed out that ICC ≥5 cm is an important index to predict MVI and poor differentiation of ICC cells [80].

7.2.1.6 Microscopic Features

ICC lesions are mostly moderately or well-differentiated tubular adenocarcinoma, and the size of tumorous glands is associated with the grade of the branches in the biliary tree. In general, central-type ICC mainly involves grade 1–3

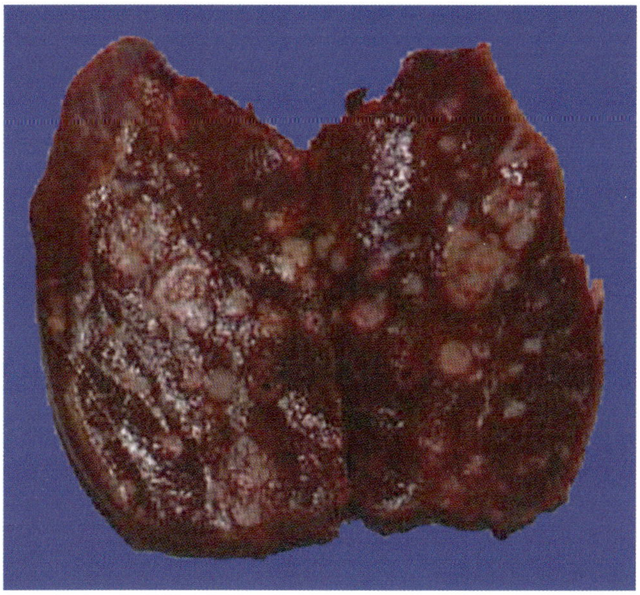

Fig. 7.146 ICC, diffuse type, tumor nodules scattered throughout the liver parenchyma

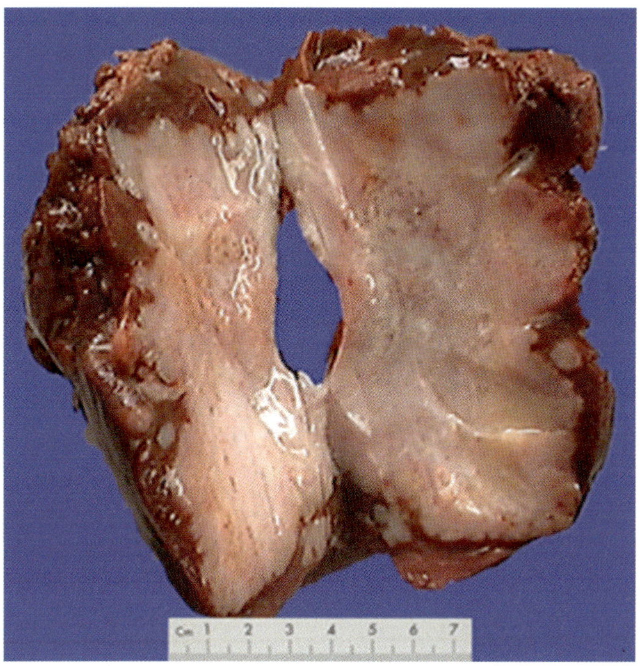

Fig. 7.147 ICC, massive type, a huge mass >10 cm with the boundary not well defined

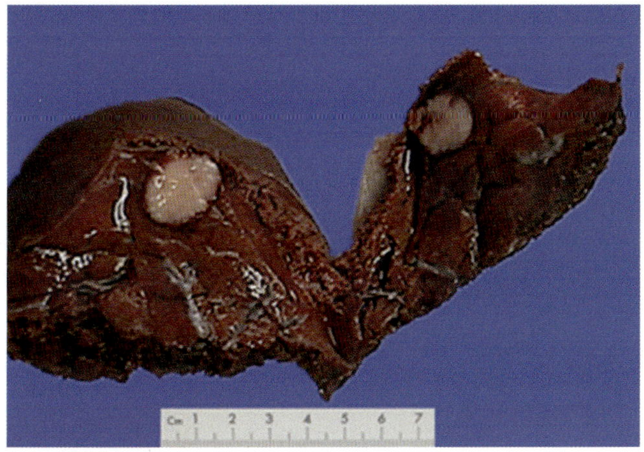

Fig. 7.148 ICC, small ICC, a small nodule <3 cm with a clear boundary

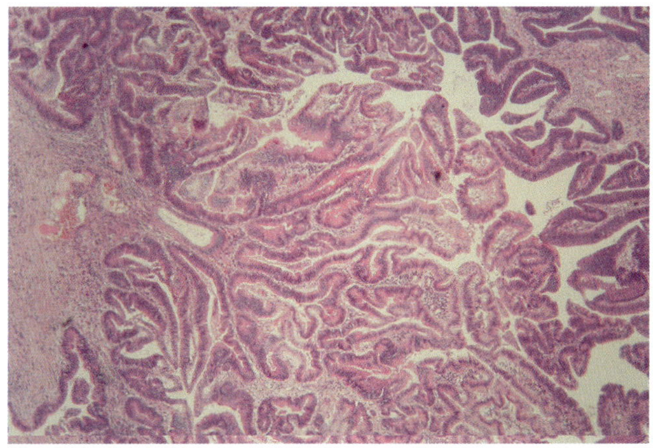

Fig. 7.149 ICC, papillary adenocarcinoma in the bile duct with the bile duct wall infiltration

major branches of the bile ducts, and the large glands in the tumor consisting of tall columnar cells are multicapillary and grow invasively along the bile duct wall (Fig. 7.149). Gradual transition between the cancer tissue and intraepithelial neoplasia of epithelium of the bile ducts in different degrees can be found in some cases (Fig. 7.150). Intraductal-type ICC is characterized by inward growth of the tumor in the bile ducts, with tumorous glands filling the lumen, but no obvious invasion of bile duct wall is observed (Fig. 7.151). Peripheral-type ICC mainly involves the septal bile duct and interlobular bile ducts, and the cancer cells are cuboidal, with tumorous glands sized between the major bile ducts and bile canaliculi, while different diameters of the bile ducts can be found on the same slice (Fig. 7.152). The fibrous interstitial tissue varies according to different density of the glands (Fig. 7.153). Cholangiocarcinoma of bile canaliculi (cholangiocellular carcinoma) originating in the canals of Hering is a special subtype of ICC, with tumorous glands composed of small cuboidal cells and small and regular lumens, which may be similar to the proliferated small bile ducts, and it is rich in fibrous stroma (Fig. 7.154). It is specifically discussed in Part 4 of this section.

It is worth noting that highly cystic dilatation of the glands in ICC cases is sometimes observed in our experience, which connects to each other to form patch-like structure. The cancer cells are small and cuboid in a monolayer arrangement along the luminal surface, like expansive microvascular net-

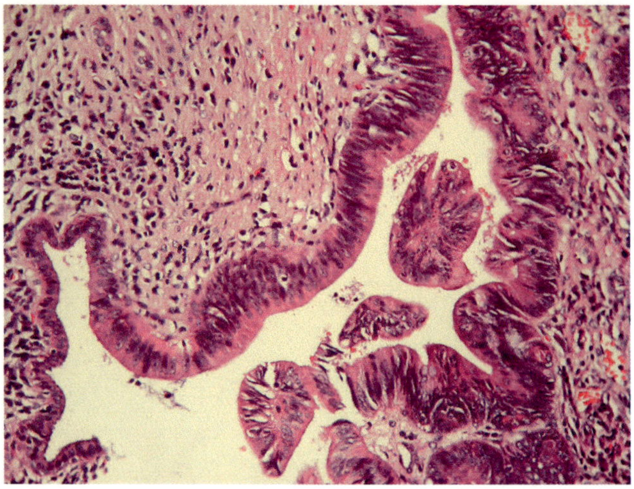

Fig. 7.150 ICC, showing the transition from low-grade to high-grade intraepithelial neoplasia to microinvasion

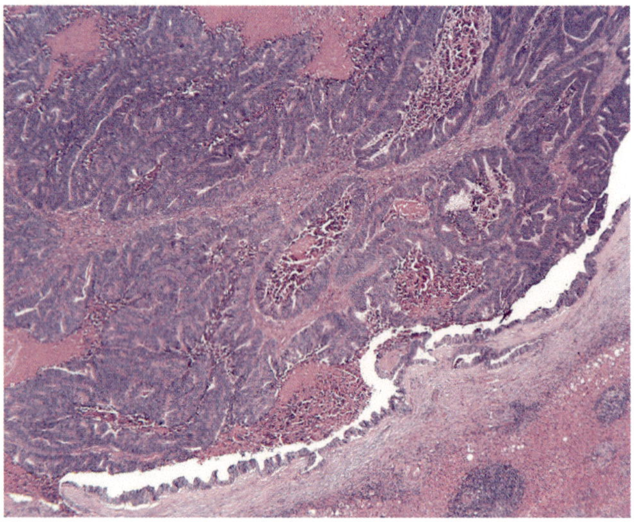

Fig. 7.151 HCC, intraductal growth type, adenocarcinoma spreads intraluminally within the dilated bile ducts

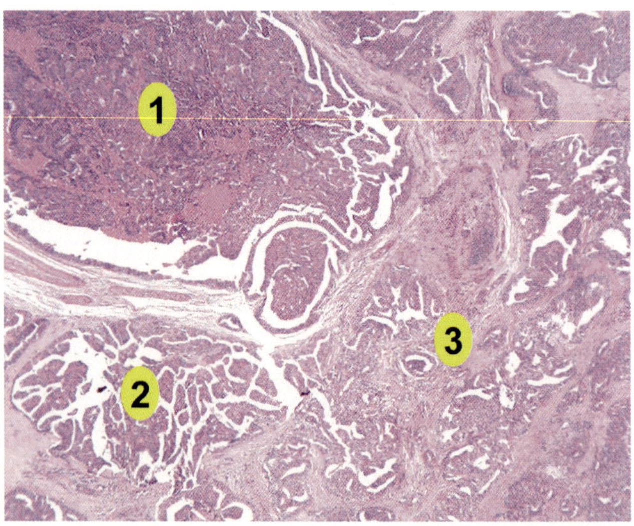

Fig. 7.152 ICC, showing large-sized (*1*), medium-sized (*2*), and small- sized (*3*) bile duct carcinoma

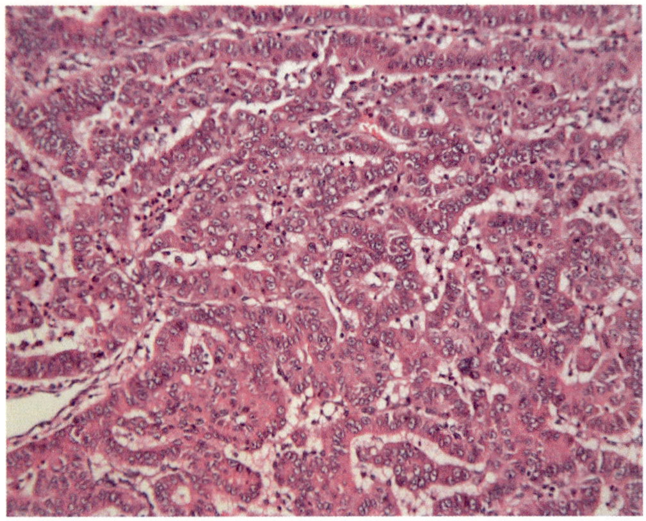

Fig. 7.153 ICC, papillotubular adenocarcinoma without fibrous stroma

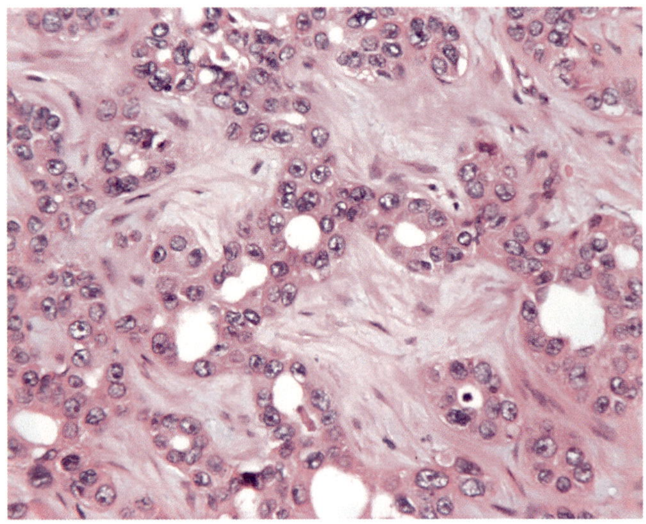

Fig. 7.154 ICC, well-differentiated adenocarcinoma with abundant fibrous stroma

work (Figs. 7.155, 7.156, 7.157, 7.158, 7.159, and 7.160). These cases need special and careful differentiation from hemangioma, hemangioendothelioma or angiosarcoma, etc.

Recently, Liau et al. (2014) divided ICC into two types according to the relationship between immunohistochemical features and location of the ICC lesions:

① Bile duct type is characterized by the tall columnar tumor cells arranged in a large glandular pattern, with high expression of S100P, TFF1, and AGR2, and 23% of the cases contain KRAS gene mutation.
② Cholangiolar type is characterized by the cuboidal to low columnar tumor cells that contain scanty cytoplasm with high expression of N-cadherin, and only 1% of the cases contain KRAS gene mutation, and IDH1/2 gene mutation

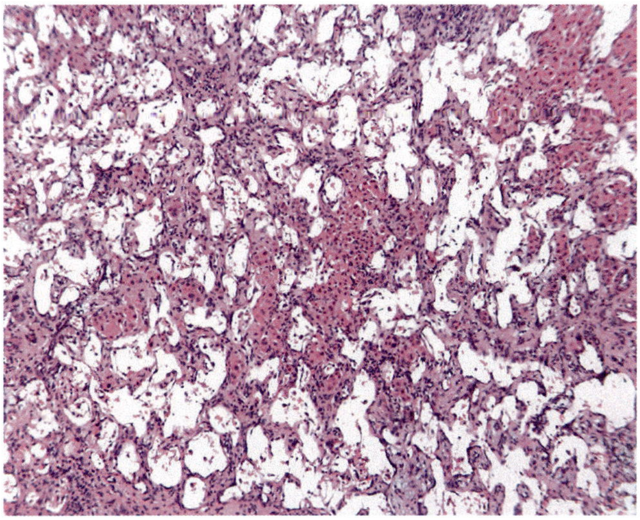

Fig. 7.155 ICC, cystically dilated adenocarcinoma mingled with residual liver tissue

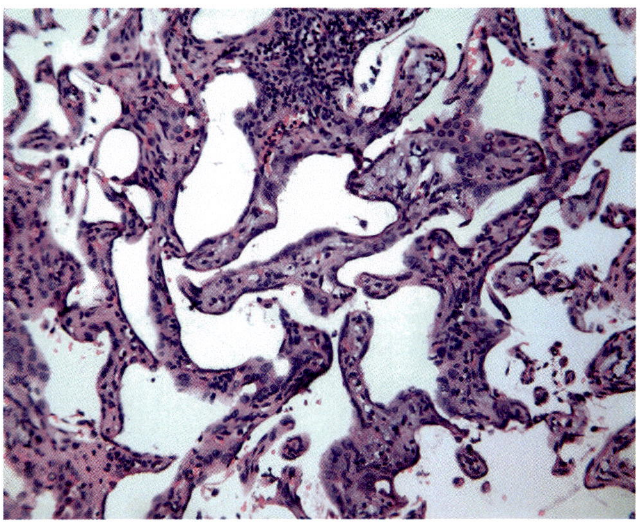

Fig. 7.156 ICC, cystically dilated glands lined with cuboidal tumor cells

rate and postoperative 5-year survival rate were both significantly higher than those in bile duct-type ICC [81].

Poorly differentiated cholangiocarcinoma cells are fusiform or round, with poor adhesion, loosely arranged in patches similar to spindle cell sarcoma (sarcomatous carcinoma), a few visible distorted glands with small lumen, insignificant glandular structure, and mitotic figures (Fig. 7.161). Mucous lakes can be found within the glandular lumen due to large amounts of mucus, and AB or PAS staining is of diagnostic significance which can display the neutral or acidic mucus in the cytoplasm, while the cancer cells do not secrete bile (Fig. 7.162). Streak or trabecular structure

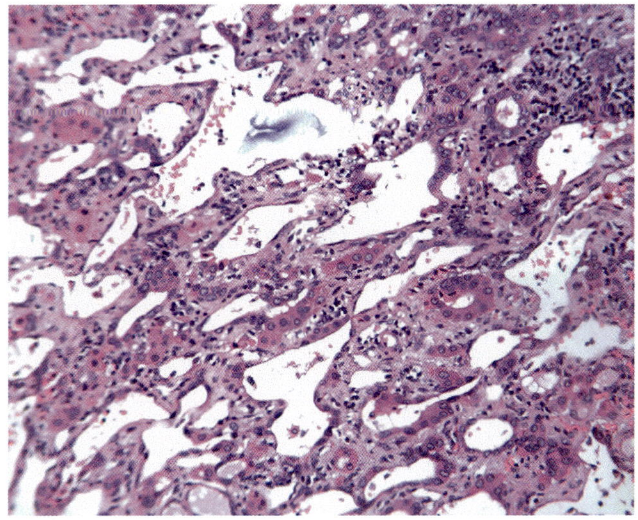

Fig. 7.157 ICC, cystically dilated adenocarcinoma mingled with tubular adenocarcinoma

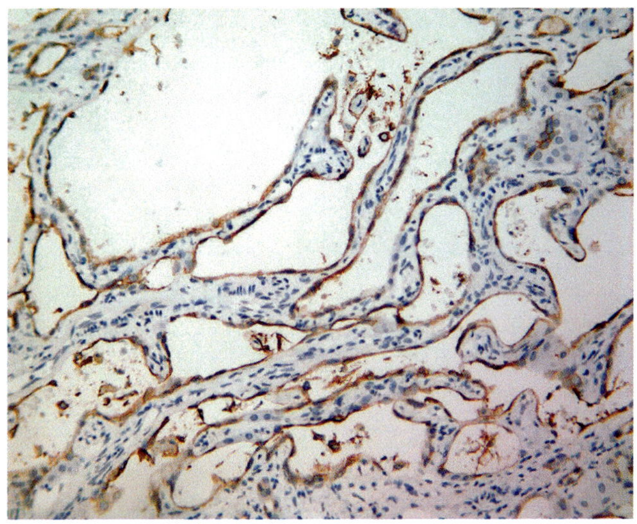

Fig. 7.158 ICC, showing positive immunohistochemical staining of CK7 in cystically dilated adenocarcinoma cells

can also been seen in the tumor (Fig. 7.163), as well as schistosome eggs (Fig. 7.164). The central region of ICC tissues often contains abundant fibrous stroma with a small amount of lymphocytes, and cancer cells in the peripheral zone grow aggressively. Cases with little fibrous stroma and solid trabecular or nest arrangement should often be differentiated from trabecular HCC, and cases with invasion of the periductal glands and their lumens should be differentiated from reactive hyperplasia of the periductal glands.

7.2.1.7 Biological Characteristics

ICC tissues often do not have a fibrous capsular and show a map-like boundary with an irregular shape. Patterns of infil-

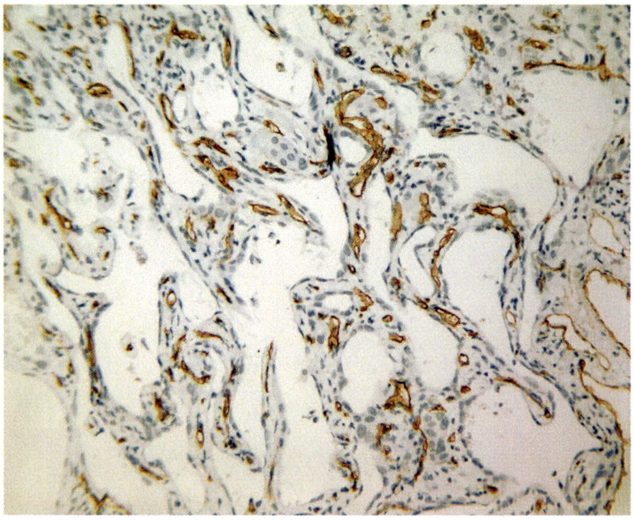

Fig. 7.159 ICC, showing negative immunohistochemical staining of CD34 in cystically dilated adenocarcinoma cells

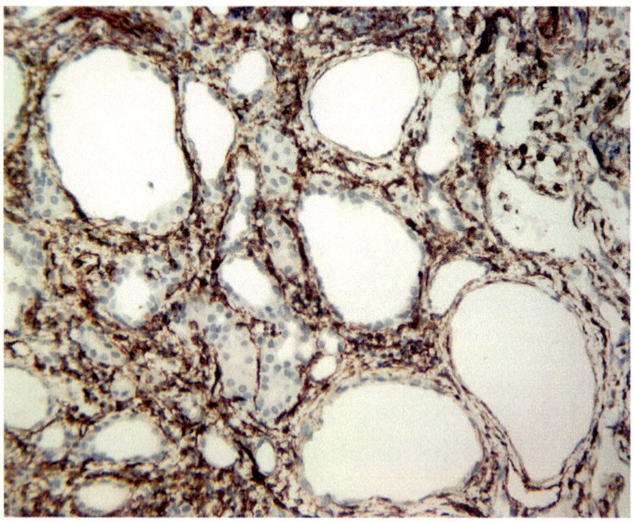

Fig. 7.160 ICC, showing negative immunohistochemical staining of vimentin in cystically dilated adenocarcinoma cells

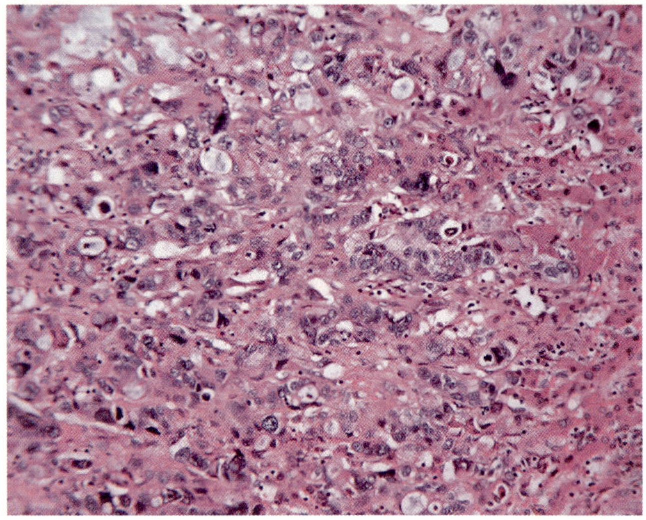

Fig. 7.161 ICC, poorly differentiated adenocarcinoma with obscure glandular structures

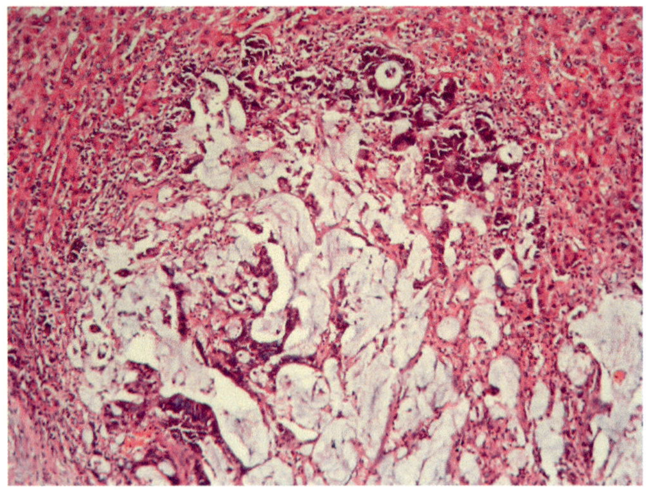

Fig. 7.162 ICC, poorly differentiated adenocarcinoma with mucous lake formation

tration and metastasis of ICC cells include direct invasion of the adjacent liver sinusoids (Fig. 7.165), formation of subfoci or satellite nodules (Fig. 7.166), invasive growth into the liver tissue (Fig. 7.167 and 7.168), skipping metastasis along the portal tracts (Fig. 7.169), invasion of the portal vein branches (Fig. 7.170), formation of cholangiocarcinoma thrombi in lymphatic vessels (Figs. 7.171 and 7.172), nerve tissues (Fig. 7.173), and adjacent pericancerous liver tissues (Fig. 7.174). Different pathological types of ICC present different invasion patterns, leading to different clinical outcomes. For example, the best prognosis is found in cases with intraductal growth-type and superficial spreading ICC, and mass-forming ICC has a better prognosis compared to periductal infiltrating-type ICC. Invasion of the portal vein and lymphatic invasion are often found in adenocarcinoma, while adenosquamous carcinoma, squamous carcinoma, and mucoepidermoid carcinoma usually metastasize into the lung and other organs. Undifferentiated carcinoma tends to metastasize in the liver. Ji et al. (2012) reported that the clinical prognosis of ICC is related to the gross type and stage of ICC, of which intraductal growth type > mass-forming type and periductal-infiltrating type > mixed type; however, histological type has nothing to do with the prognosis [82]. Aishima et al. (2007) found that the prognosis of hepatic perihilar ICC was significantly poorer than that of peripheral ICC, and intrahepatic metastasis is an independent prognostic factor of perihilar-type ICC, while lymphatic metastasis is an independent prognostic factor of peripheral ICC [57].

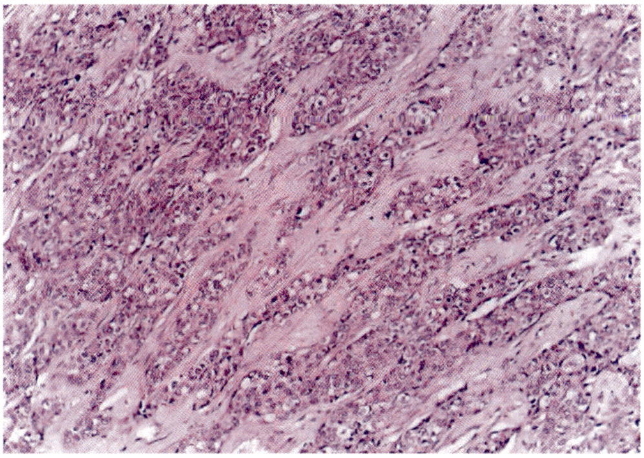

Fig. 7.163 ICC, poorly differentiated adenocarcinoma arranged in cords with abundant fibrous stroma

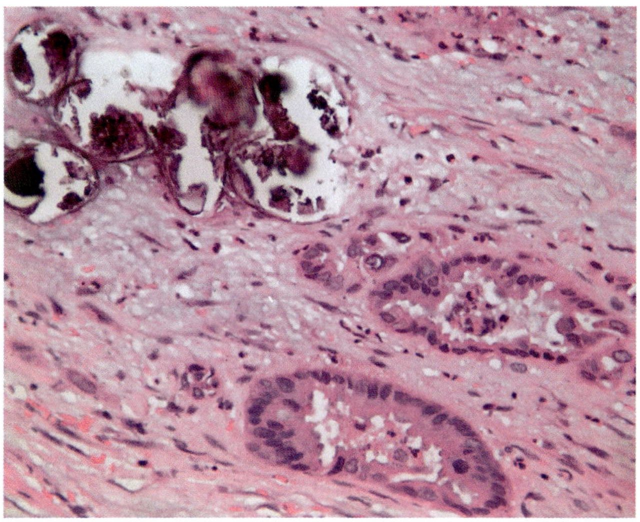

Fig. 7.164 ICC, showing calcified schistosomal egg in ICC tissue

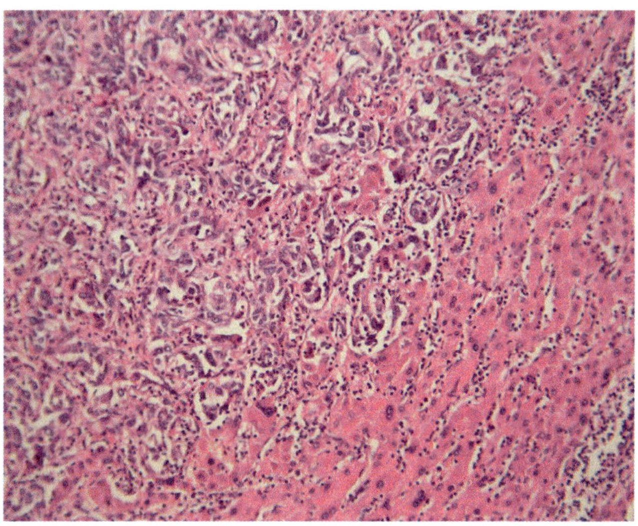

Fig. 7.165 ICC, invasive growth of cancer cells along liver sinus

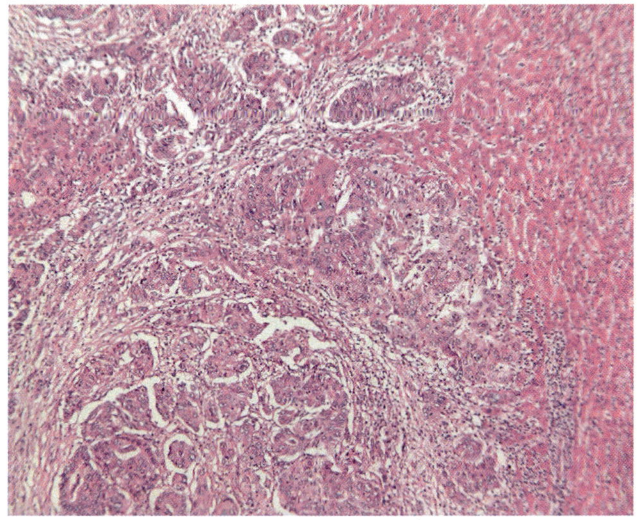

Fig. 7.166 ICC, cancer foci in adjacent liver tissue

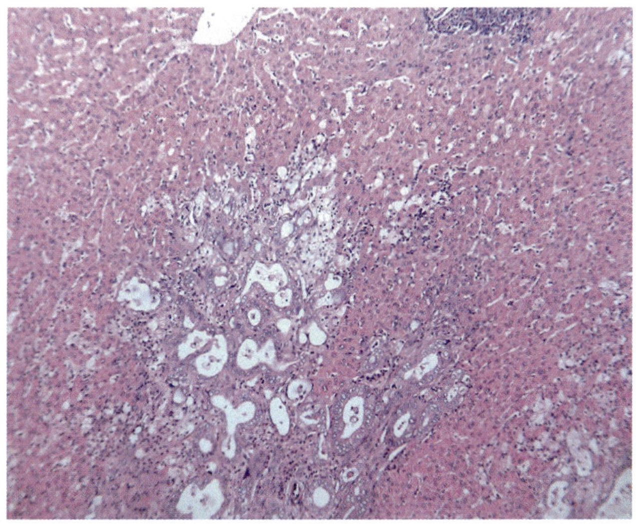

Fig. 7.167 ICC, multiple foci of malignant growth

ICC has abundant fibrous stroma containing complex components, such as blood vessels, lymphatic vessels, various mesenchymal cells, and inflammatory cells, and lymphatic invasion is an important biological characteristic of ICC. Aishima et al. (2008) studied immunohistochemical staining for lymphatic specific marker, D2–40, in 88 cases of ICC tissues, and the results showed that 38 cases (43%) had lymphatic invasion, of which invasion of pericancerous tissues, marginal, and central regions of the tumor accounts for 63%, 79%, and 24%, respectively. In undifferentiated ICC, the lymphangiogenesis is more active in the pericancerous and the marginal regions of the tumor compared to that in the central regions. And lymphatic collapse is often observed in the central regions due to the rapid growth of the tumor, while the peripheral lymphatic lumen is often in the open state which is a high-risk area of lymphatic invasion. The

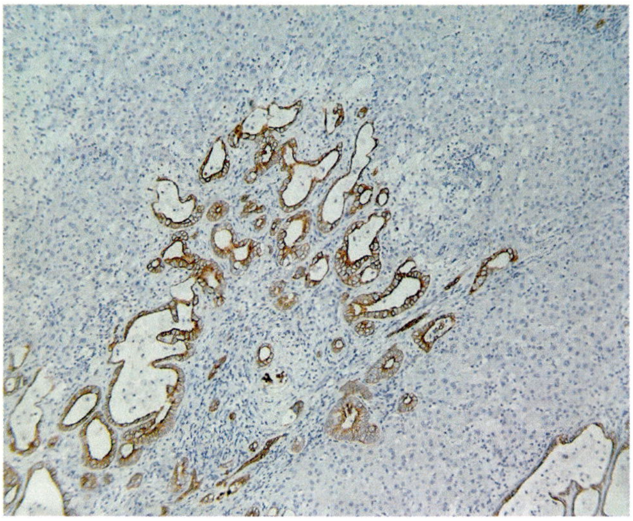

Fig. 7.168 ICC, CK7 immunohistochemical staining of the same specimen as Fig. 7.167

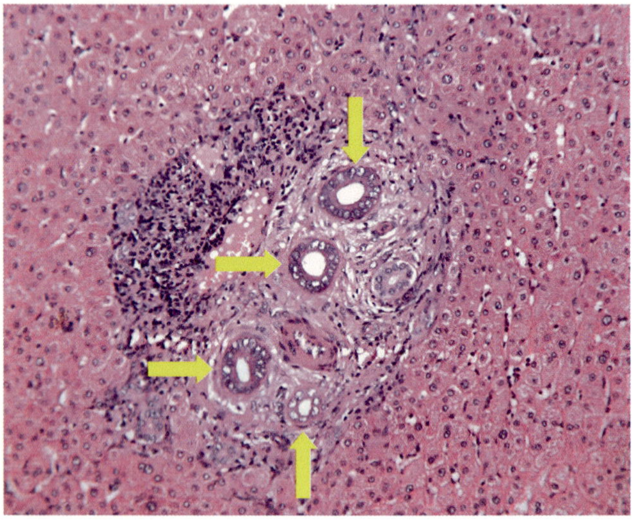

Fig. 7.169 ICC, showing skip metastases through liver portal tracts

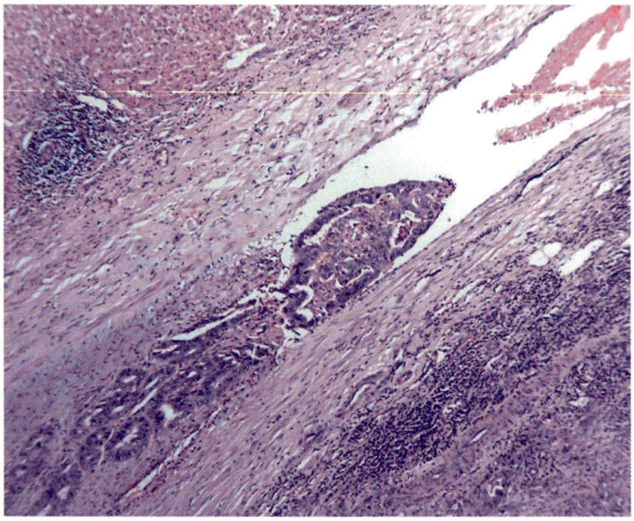

Fig. 7.170 ICC, tumor invasion of the branches of the portal vein

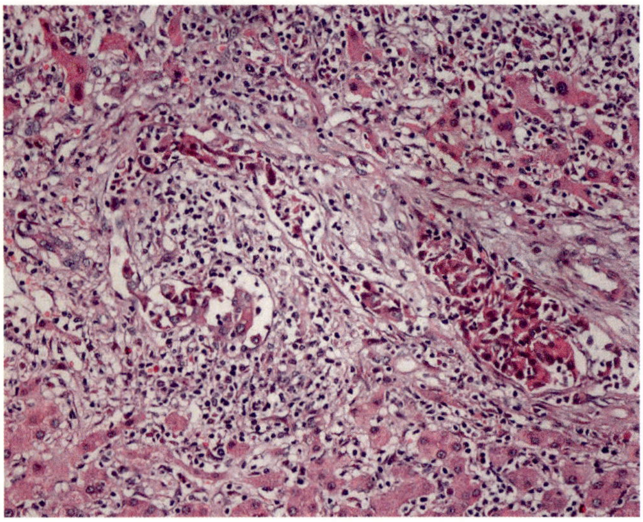

Fig. 7.171 ICC, invasion of tumor cells into lymphatic vessels

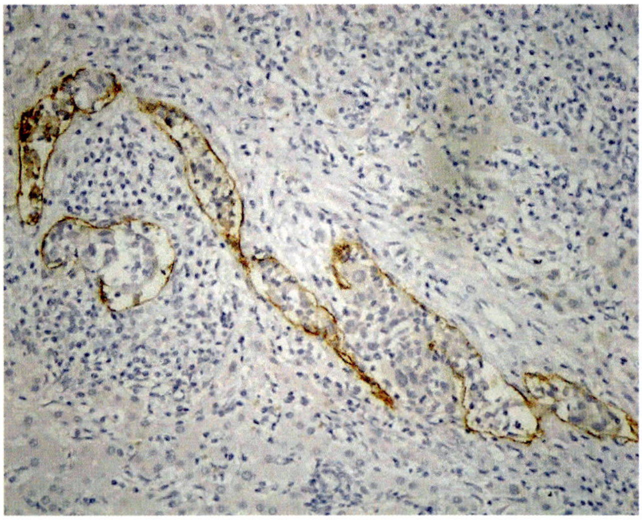

Fig. 7.172 ICC, immunohistochemical staining of D2–40 showing lymphatic invasion

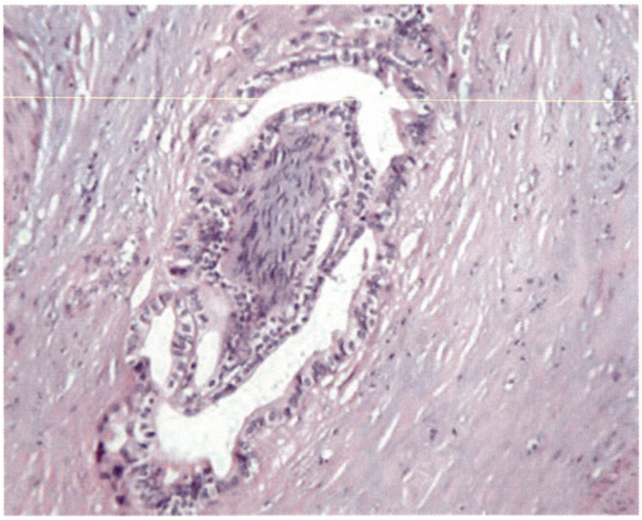

Fig. 7.173 ICC, perineuronal invasion

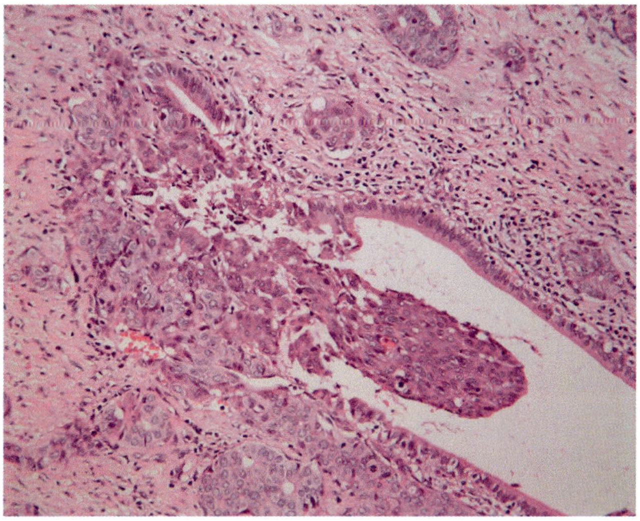

Fig. 7.174 ICC, invasion of tumor cells into the bile ducts

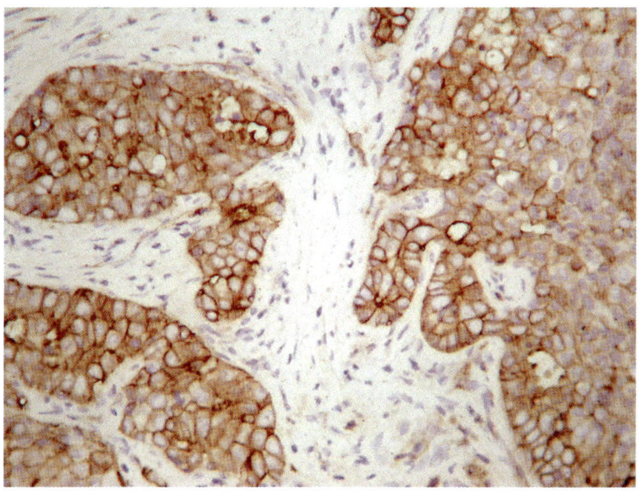

Fig. 7.175 ICC, showing positive immunohistochemical staining ofAQP-1

low density in the center of the tumor was significantly related to the marked lymphatic invasion rate. It has been shown in multivariate analysis that the expression of vascular endothelial growth factor-C (VEGF-C), histological differentiation, and lymphatic metastasis are independent prognostic factors [83], and microscopic observation showing negative tumor cells on the resection margin is also an important indicator of good prognosis.

7.2.1.8 Immunohistochemistry

ICC tissues are positive for bile duct epithelial markers, such as CK7, CK19, AQP-1 (Fig. 7.175), and MUC-1, and bile duct epithelial staining is helpful to find the microglandular infiltration which cannot easily be observed on common HE sections under the light microscope (Fig. 7.176). Our previous studies showed that ICC was positive for CK19 in 92.5% cases and MUC-1 in 73.8% cases [84]. Positive and focal expression of CK20 can be found in ICC, but its diffuse expression is more often in gastrointestinal metastatic adenocarcinoma in the liver. And combination of CK20 with CK7/CK19 markers contributes to the differential diagnosis of these two tumors. Positive expressions of epithelial cell adhesion molecule (EpCAM) and neural cell adhesion molecule (NCAM) suggest the tumor may originate from liver progenitor cells. Aishima et al. (2011) proposed that the expressions of S100P and ezrin protein increase successively in low-grade intraepithelial neoplasia and high-grade intraepithelial neoplasia, and the nuclear expression of S100P in peripheral-type ICC was associated with vascular and lymphatic invasion, indicating a poor prognosis [85]. Trabecular ICC should be differentiated from HCC, and liver cell marker staining may be helpful in the differential diagnosis, such as CD10 (Fig. 7.177) and Hep Par-1. CD34 staining can show the loose and disorder arrangement of micro-blood vessels (Fig. 7.178). Podoplanin, which is expressed in lymphatic endothelial cells, can be specifically recognized by D2–40 monoclonal antibody, and therefore it is useful in the observation of lymphatic invasion in the tumor. Ruys et al. (2014) demonstrated a meta-analysis and suggested that EGFR, MUC1, MUC4, and p27 proteins are useful markers for prognosis evaluation of ICC [86].

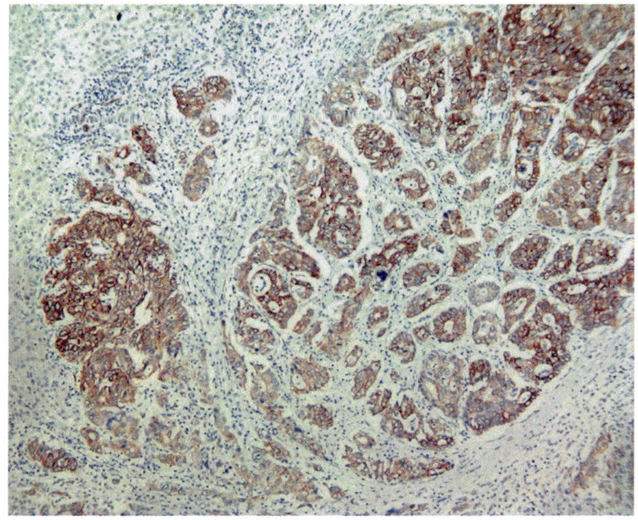

Fig. 7.176 ICC, showing positive immunohistochemical staining of CK19

7.2.1.9 Precancerous Lesions

From the histopathological perspective, the major precancerous lesions associated with the occurrence of ICC include the following three types:

1. Biliary intraepithelial neoplasia (BilIN): This is often flat lesions derived from the bile duct epithelium without

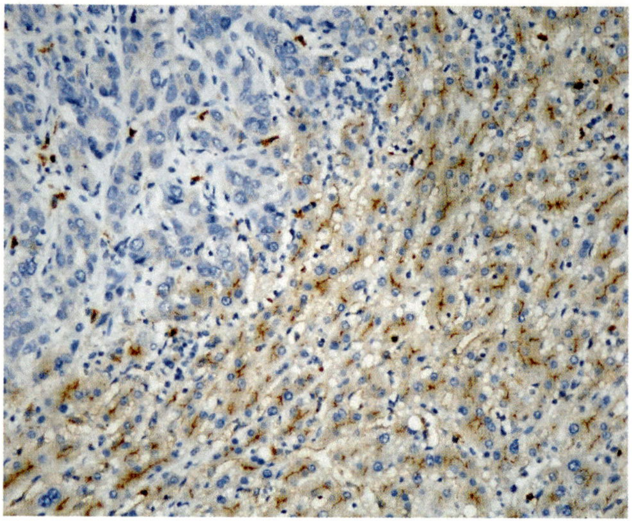

Fig. 7.177 ICC, showing negative immunohistochemical staining of CD10 (*upper left*)

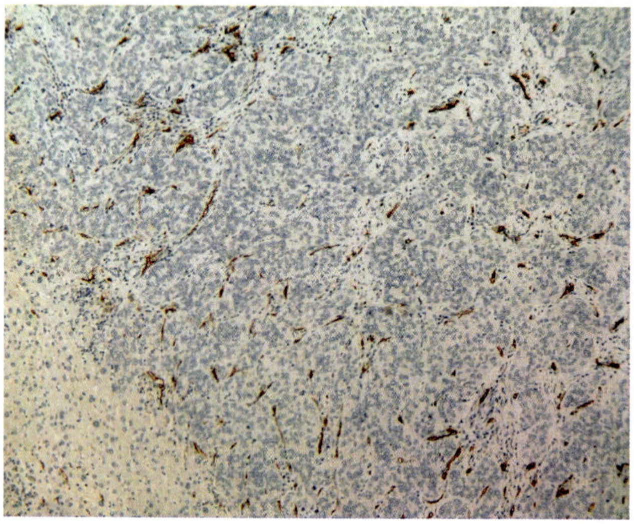

Fig. 7.178 ICC, CD34 staining showing sparse and disordered blood microvessels

mass formation, and BilIN-1, BilIN-2, and BilIN-3 are equivalent to low, moderate, and high-grade atypical hyperplasia, while BilIN-3 is equivalent to carcinoma in situ [4, 87].

2. Intraductal papillary neoplasms of the bile ducts (IPNB): IPNB may arise from the biliary epithelium in the extra- or intrahepatic large bile duct or peribiliary glands. They are intraductal tubular and papillary tumors, divided into four histological subtypes including pancreatobiliary type, intestinal type, gastric type, and oncocytic type. IPNB can evolve into papillary carcinoma (invasive), infiltrating ductal adenocarcinoma, and mucinous (colloid) adenocarcinoma [87]. In the WHO classification, IPNB is classified into low-grade IPNB (with low- or intermediate-grade intraepithelial neoplasia or borderline lesions), high-grade IPNB (with high-grade intraepithelial neoplasia, noninvasion or in situ papillary adenocarcinoma), and invasive IPNB with invasion of the bile duct wall and the surrounding liver tissue [88].
3. Biliary mucinous cystic neoplasms (MCNB): They can progress into invasive ductal adenocarcinoma and mucinous carcinoma (colloid carcinoma) [4, 87]. See the specific contents in the related chapters of this book.

7.2.1.10 Differential Diagnosis

Pseudoglandular HCC is similar to ICC, thick trabecular HCC, and trabecular ICC with little fibrous stroma in histological and cellular morphology; thus, it is difficult to identify these lesions, and the differential diagnosis should be relied on immunohistochemistry. Generally, HCC cells are positive for Hep Par-1, arginase-1, and GPC-3, and specifically showing a typical capillarization by CD34 staining, while they are negative for CK19/CK7/MUC-1. However, ICC cells are positive for CK19 and negative for Hep Par-1 and GPC-3. Besides, specialized canalicular staining pattern, probably due to cross-reactivity to biliary glycoprotein 1 present in bile canaliculi, can be marked on the membrane of the liver cells (such as CD10 and pCEA), which is beneficial in the identification. Nishino et al. (2008) screened three genes with specifically high expression in ICC tissues: insulin-like growth factor binding protein 5 gene (IGFBP5), biglycan, and claudin-4, by series analysis of gene expression (SAGE) and DNA chip analysis, and immunohistochemistry showed that claudin-4 was highly expressed in ICC tissues, while it was negative in HCC tissues, which was helpful in differential diagnosis. In addition, it was also noted that the ICC should be differentiated from extrahepatic metastatic adenocarcinomas [89].

7.2.1.11 Treatment and Prognosis

Surgical excision should be the first choice when designing the treatment strategy for ICC, which can improve the average survival period to 2 years. The mean survival time was only 9 months in nonsurgical cases; however, the long-term prognosis is not satisfactory due to the high malignancy and frequent recurrence of ICC. A large number of researches reported that the 5-year survival rate after ICC resection was 25–40%. Becker et al. (2008) demonstrated a retrospective analysis on the data from United Network for Organ Sharing (UNOS) database and showed that the 1-year and 5-year survival rates after liver transplantation were 74% and 30% [90], respectively, based on the 280 cases of ICC cases from 1987 to 2005. Ji et al. (2012) reported that the median survival time of ICC patients with radical resection (30 cases) and liver transplantation (10 cases) were 13 months and 3 months [82], respectively. ICC recurrences are mainly found in the liver, and extrahepatic recurrence is found in only 20–30% of the recurrent cases. Radiofrequency ablation (RFA) has an effectiveness of 90–100% for small tumors (< 3 cm), with the median overall survival time of 33–38.5 months, 1-year survival rate of 84.6 100%, and 3-year survival rate of 43.3–83.3%. And in accordance with the recommendations of the ILCA guidelines, all patients with radiotherapy and chemotherapy of ICC should be diagnosed based on the definite pathological evidence before these treatments [56].

To date, clinical targeted drug trials involving molecular targets, including VEGFR, EGFR, PDGFR, mTOR, and BRAF, can potentially provide valuable molecular targeting therapies for ICC in the future. Andersen et al. (2012) found that lapatinib could inhibit the expression of EGFR and HER2 in cholangiocarcinoma cells and the growth of these cancer cells, so the patients may benefit from the treatment of dual-targeting tyrosine kinase inhibitor (TKI); however, ICC cases with KRAS mutations are resistant to TKI treatment [69]. Once the therapeutic molecular targets for ICC are identified, molecular pathology will become the mainstay of molecular targeting therapy.

7.2.2 Bile Duct Cystadenocarcinoma

7.2.2.1 Pathogenesis and Mechanism

Bile duct cystadenocarcinoma is often derived from the malignant transformation of ovarian stroma in biliary cystadenoma, choledochal cyst, or biliary cystadenoma, while hepatic cirrhosis, chronic cholangitis, HBV infection, and intrahepatic bile duct stones can cause chronic inflammation of peribiliary glands, and the malignant transformation of which may result in bile duct cystadenocarcinoma and is the risk factor [91].

The 2010 version of WHO histological classification adopted the term of mucinous cystic neoplasm synonyms (MCN), among which noninvasive MCN and bile duct cystadenoma refer to the same tumor. According to the degree of dysplasia of MCN cells, MCN can be divided into noninvasive MCN with low-grade, intermediate-grade, and high-grade dysplasia. If there is a component of invasive carcinoma in MCN, the diagnosis should be MCN-associated invasive carcinoma, with tubular and papillary adenocarcinoma as the most common type, which can be classified into the category of intraductal papillary neoplasms of the bile ducts (IPNB) [88].

7.2.2.2 Clinical Features

A total of 56 cases with biliary cystadenocarcinoma have been diagnosed in the Department of Pathology of EHBH, Second Military Medical University, and women accounted for 96.4%, while men accounted for only 3.6%. The patients were 53.4 years old on average, who manifested right upper abdominal discomfort, abdominal pain, or abdominal mass in most cases, and elevated serum levels of CEA and CA19-9 were found in the majority of these patients, while their serum AFP were negative.

7.2.2.3 Gross Features

The tumors were spherical, often larger than 10 cm with an average diameter of 7.3 cm, with a smooth surface, a fibrous pseudocapsule, and the section showed cystic and solid or multilocular cystic mass with a smooth inner wall, or a granular or papillary ridges, containing mucoid or even jelly material, or thin yellow-brown protein solution in the cavities (Figs. 7.179 and 7.180).

7.2.2.4 Microscopic Features

The cystic walls were lined with epithelial cells which were cuboidal or columnar, with eosinophilic cytoplasm, a nucleus located in the basal part of the cell. The mucinous epithelium usually supported by an ovarian stroma. High-grade cystadenocarcinoma cells lost the cellular polarity with significantly nuclear atypia, arranged in multilayers, and active pathological karyokinesis. These tumor cells can be arranged in papillary structures to form cystic papillary adenocarcinoma (Fig. 7.181). The basement membrane of the cyst wall can be lined with mucus-secreting cells with expanded glandular cavities containing mucus and necrosis, which is the feature of cystic mucinous adenocarcinoma (Fig. 7.182). In some part of the tumor, various differentiations could be discovered, such as squamous cell carcinoma, adenosquamous carcinoma, and spindle cells (sarcomatoid) differentiation, and the tumor tissue could invade the ovarian stroma, the latter of which can also develop malignancy.

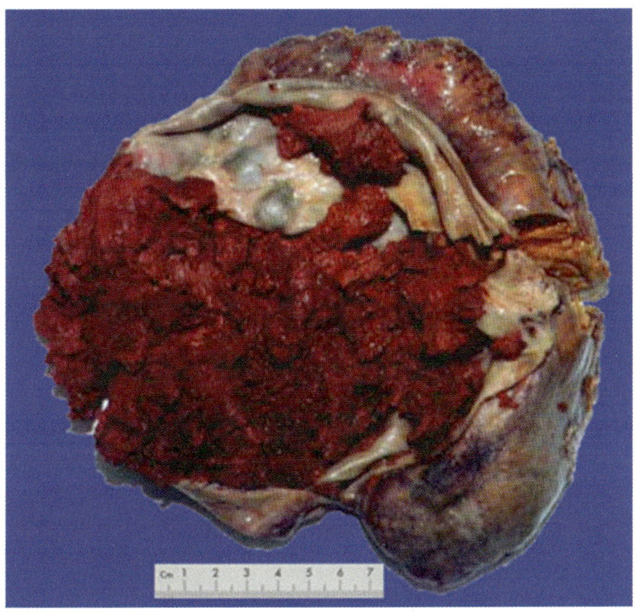

Fig. 7.179 Bile duct cystadenocarcinoma, severe and extensive necrosis

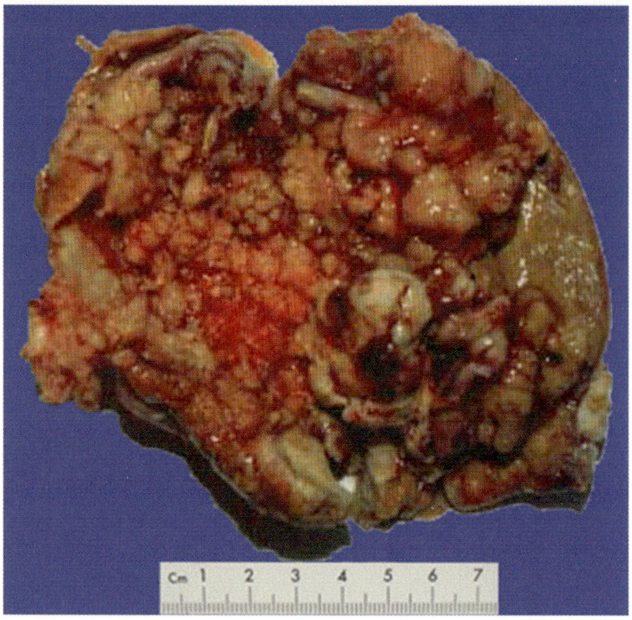

Fig. 7.180 Bile duct cystadenocarcinoma, papillary nodules of varying sizes persisting throughout the surface of the cyst wall

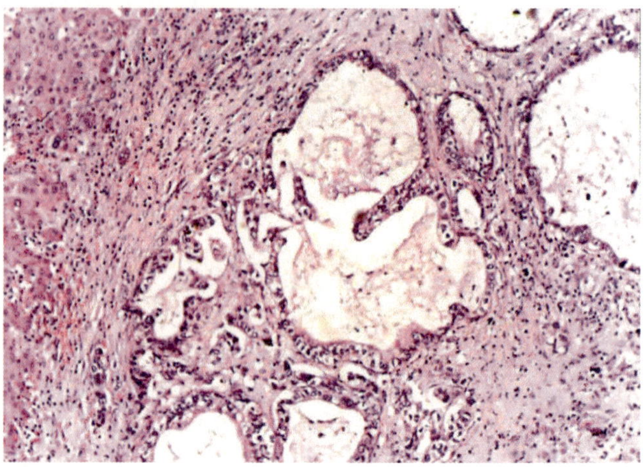

Fig. 7.181 Bile duct cystadenocarcinoma, cancer cells arranged in papillary structures

7.2.2.5 Immunohistochemistry

The cancer cells were positive for CK19, CK7, EMA, and CEA, and the spindle ovarian stroma was positive for vimentin, SMA, desmin, estrogen, and progesterone receptors.

7.2.2.6 Differential Diagnosis

The difference between biliary cystadenocarcinoma and cystadenoma lies in the invasive features of the former, including obvious atypia or pleomorphism, invasion of the cystic wall, or the surrounding liver tissues, and biliary cystadenocarcinoma can grow aggressively along the sinusoids of the liver, bile ducts, and nerve tissues. For patients with a history of biliary cystadenoma or biliary cystadenoma with-

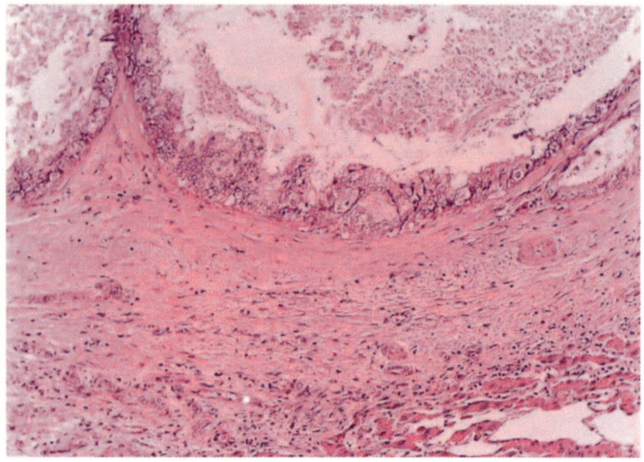

Fig. 7.182 Bile duct cystadenocarcinoma, cancer cells were cubic or columnar without ovarian-like stroma

out complete surgical resection, it should be noted that the biliary cystadenoma can develop malignancy.

7.2.2.7 Treatment and Prognosis

Surgery resection of bile duct cystadenocarcinoma receives a better therapeutic effect than that of intrahepatic cholangiocarcinoma, and its 5-year disease-free survival rate is 25–100% [92]. The female patients with ovarian-like stroma have a more benign clinical course, and surgical resection is followed by good outcome. However, the male patients without ovarian-like stroma have a faster progression of bile duct cystadenocarcinoma, which is prone to develop intrahepatic metastasis, and the prognosis is poor [93]. To prevent the occurrence of bile duct cystadenocarcinoma, laparoscopic resection of cystic tumors in the liver can be operated under the guidance of liver biopsy when necessary, and if the biopsy tissue is diagnosed as simple benign hepatic cyst, the tumor can be partly removed, while cases diagnosed as cystadenoma should receive complete resection.

7.2.3 Mucin-Producing Intrahepatic Cholangiocarcinoma

Most of intrahepatic or extrahepatic bile duct tumors produce mucus in the tumor cells or tumor tissues; however, large amounts of jelly myxoid fluid can obstruct the bile ducts in some cases, leading to obstructive jaundice, cholangitis, or biliary obstructive dilation, clinically known as mucus biliary syndrome, and this kind of bile duct tumors is collectively referred to as mucin-producing ICC or mucin-producing bile duct tumors (MPBTs).

Shibahara et al. (2004) divided MPBTs into two histological subtypes, which have overlap between them.

1. Columnar type: The tumor is similar to microvillous adenoma of small intestine or low papillary structure containing one to a few layers of columnar cells. The epithelium of the tumor consists of pseudostratified columnar cells, with basophilic cytoplasm, column-shaped nuclei, and small nucleoli. The columnar-type adenocarcinoma is positive for MUC-2 and has a high positive expression of Ki-67 as shown in immunohistochemistry. It can metastasize directly along the mucosa and lymph nodes with a poor prognosis in the patients.
2. Cuboidal type: It is a tumor with pancreatic ducts and/or eosinophil cells, based on which it can also be divided into pancreatic duct type and eosinophilic cell type. The former is rich in micropapillary with complex dendritic branches, while the latter contains cuboidal cells with eosinophilic and granular cytoplasm forming intraepithelial compartments and grows in cribriform architecture. The cubic adenocarcinoma is positive for MUC-6 and MUC-4 in immunohistochemistry [94].

Nine cases of surgically excised MPBTs were reported in 2014, with six female and three male patients who were 57.9 years old as the median age. Among which, five cases were intrahepatic bile duct MPBTs, including three cases of serous cystadenoma, two cases of mucinous cystadenoma, and the other four cases were extrahepatic bile duct MPBTs including one case of papillary adenocarcinoma, one case of papillary adenoma with canceration, one case of mucinous cystadenocarcinoma, and one case of tubular adenoma. All these patients survived to date [95].

7.2.4 Special Types of Intrahepatic Cholangiocarcinoma

(1) Cholangiocellular carcinoma (CLC)

CLC, also known as small bile duct carcinoma, was first reported by Steiner and Higginson in 1959, specifically refers to adenoma derived from small bile ducts or the canals of Hering, characterized by well-differentiated tubular adenocarcinoma, and is sometimes similar to hyperplasia of the small bile ducts or reactive hyperplasia of small bile duct histologically, which belongs to the special types of ICC. To distinguish it from conventional ICC, CLC was once used in the pathological diagnosis. In the 2010 edition of the WHO *Histological Classification of the Liver and Intrahepatic Bile Duct Tumors*, it was suggested that the CLC tissues containing residual liver cell masses can be defined as a special subtype of cHCC-CC. As HCC component or hepatocellular differentiation in CLC tissues can be seldomly observed, it should be carefully not to confuse them.

CLC lesions are often located in the peripheral regions of the hepatic lobes, and their gross appearances are similar to that of common types of ICC. The cross sections are grayish white in color, lobulated in shape, and often without hemorrhage or necrosis, and the tumors usually have a capsule with an unclear boundary. Under the microscope, the CLC cells are small and cuboidal, similar to the epithelial cells of small bile ducts, consistent in size, with a little cytoplasm, increased karyoplasmic ratios, and ovoid nuclei and rare mitotic figures. These cancer cells are arranged in small tubular, solid cords or branched structures, with abundant fibrous stroma of hyaline degeneration or collagen degeneration (Figs. 7.183 and 7.184), which is similar to reactive hyperplastic small bile ducts at low magnification (Fig. 7.185) and should carefully distinguished. The author has also found CLC derived from

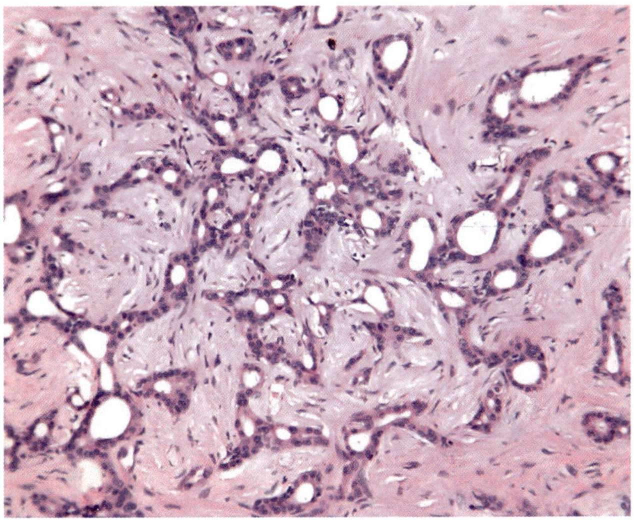

Fig. 7.183 CLC, cancer cells arranged in small glandular tubes or anastomosing pattern

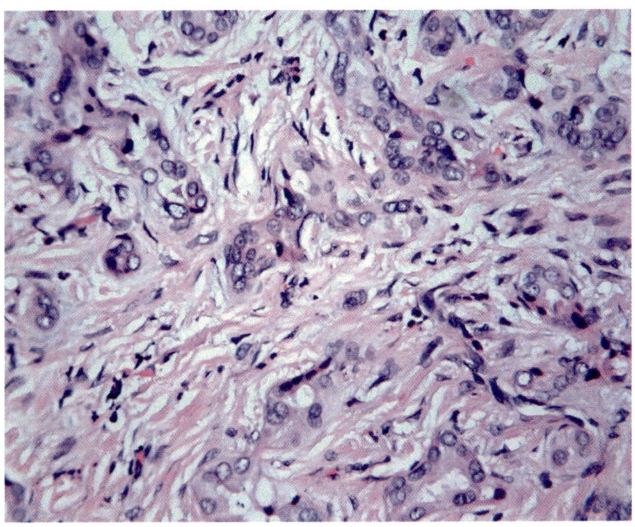

Fig. 7.184 CLC, small cancer glands resembling cholangioles

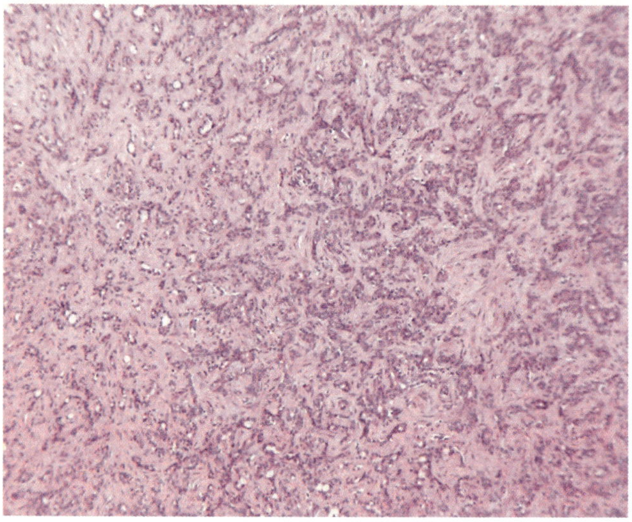

Fig. 7.185 CLC, showing a tubular, cord-like, anastomosing pattern resembling proliferative small bile ducts

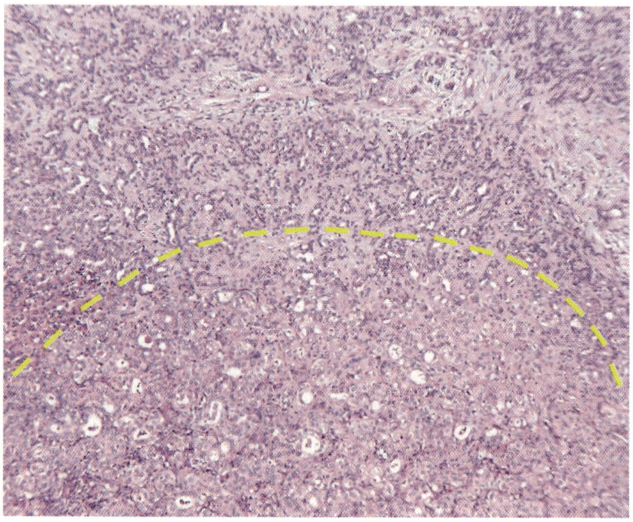

Fig. 7.186 CLC, CLC (*upper*) accompanied with bile duct adenoma (*below*)

canceration of cholangioadenoma, with both components connected closely with a transition zone (Fig. 7.186).

Sasaki et al. (2014) found high expression of EZH2 in all CLC cases and no expression of EZH2 in cholangioadenoma and reactive hyperplasia of small bile ducts, while high expression of p16^{INK4a} was found in all the cases of reactive hyperplasia of small bile ducts and 81% of the cholangioadenoma cases, which was expressed only in 12% of the CLC lesions, and it can be used in the differential diagnosis in immunohistochemistry [96]. The immunohistochemical features of CLC are similar to those of ICC, and positive staining of stem cell markers and neural cell adhesion molecule (NCAM) suggest it originates from the hepatic progenitor cells. CLC is considered to be derived from progenitor cells with ductular differentiation in the liver, so it has strong invasiveness and recurrence rate. Kannmoto et al. (2008) reported nine cases of CLC patients with five cases (56%) of HCV infection, one case (11%) of HBV infection, and the postoperative survival time was 1–72 months [97].

(2) Lymphoepithelioma-like carcinoma (LELC)

LELC is characterized by undifferentiated carcinoma complicated by large amounts of dense lymphoplasmacytic stroma. Hepatic LELC is extremely rare, with 16 cases of lymphoepithelioma-like intrahepatic cholangiocarcinoma (LEL-ICC) and 10 cases of lymphoepithelioma-like hepatocellular carcinoma (LEL-HCC) reported in the English literature till now [98, 99]. A total of 11 cases of hepatic LELC have been diagnosed in the Department of Pathology of EHBH, Second Military Medical University, since 2007, including nine cases located in the right lobe and two cases in the left lobe of the liver, with a male to female ratio of 8:3, an average age of 51.7 years (35–62), and the tumor sizes ranged 1.7 cm × 1.9 cm–10.2 cm × 6.3 cm. The vast majority of these cases were bile duct type, of which only one case was HCC with a small amount of areas of lymphoepithelioma-like carcinoma. Either LEL-ICC or LEL-HCC, most of these cases were complicated by EBV infection or positive EBER in situ hybridization, but in EBV-negative hepatic LELC, HBV- or HCV-related cirrhosis can be found in the surrounding liver tissues in most cases, suggesting that HBV or HCV infection may also be related to the occurrence of hepatic LELC.

The tumors are often found in the elderly with slightly more female patients, solitary, with clear boundaries and complete fibrous capsules, and hepatic cirrhosis can be found in the patients with chronic HBV/HCV infection. According to the microscopic features, LELC can be divided into two basic types:

1. LEL-ICC: It is composed by poorly differentiated adenocarcinoma with dense stroma containing mature lymphocytes and plasma cells, with visible lymphoid follicles (Fig. 7.187). The proportion of adenocarcinoma varies a lot (Figs. 7.188 and 7.189), but the density of lymphoplasmacytes is significantly larger than that of adenocarcinoma components. Immunohistochemistry shows that adenocarcinoma is positive for P53, CK7, CK19, and EMA, while undifferentiated carcinoma is focally positive for CK7 and CK19, both components of adenocarcinoma and undifferentiated carcinoma are negative for Hep Par-1, CK20, vimentin, and AFP, and the interstitial lymphoplasmacytes are mixed polyclonal cell populations, including CD8-positive T cell as the dominant cell type [98].

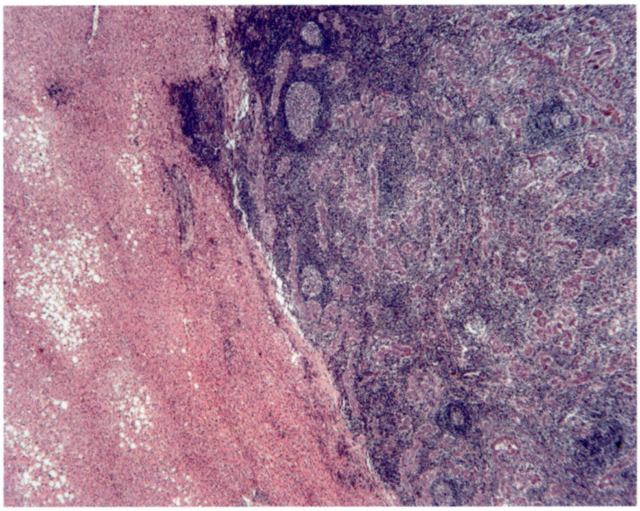

Fig. 7.187 LEL-ICC, abundant lymphoid infiltrate inside adenocarcinoma tissue with lymphoid follicular formation

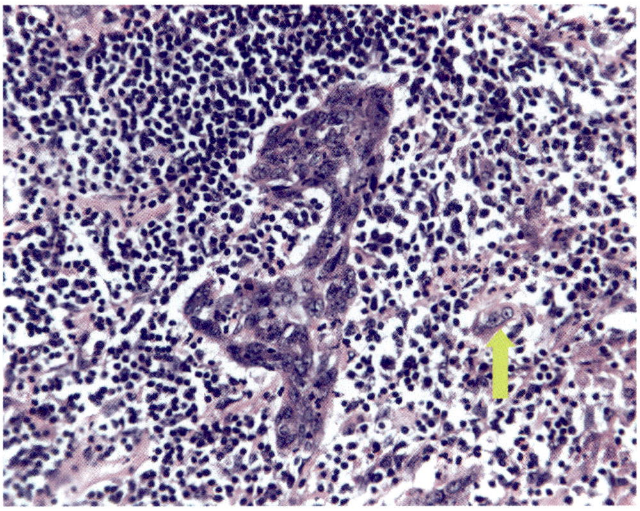

Fig. 7.188 LEL-ICC, poorly or undifferentiated adenocarcinoma cells (*arrows*) with conspicuous lymphoid stroma

2. LEL-HCC: Undifferentiated carcinoma components are arranged in focal or trabecular structures, with eosinophilic cytoplasm, large nuclei, and prominent nucleoli, which are similar to undifferentiated HCC, and the interstitial infiltration of a large number of lymphocytes and plasmacytes can be observed. Immunohistochemistry shows that the cancer cells are positive for Hep Par-1 and GPC-3 positive, and CD34 staining displays that the capillary tumor tissue may not be typical. Due to the immune barrier and inhibition on the growth and invasion of the tumor cells by CD8-positive T cell-mediated cytotoxicity, rare microvascular invasion can be found in LEL-HCC. Its overall postoperative survival time is longer than that in conventional HCC [99, 100].

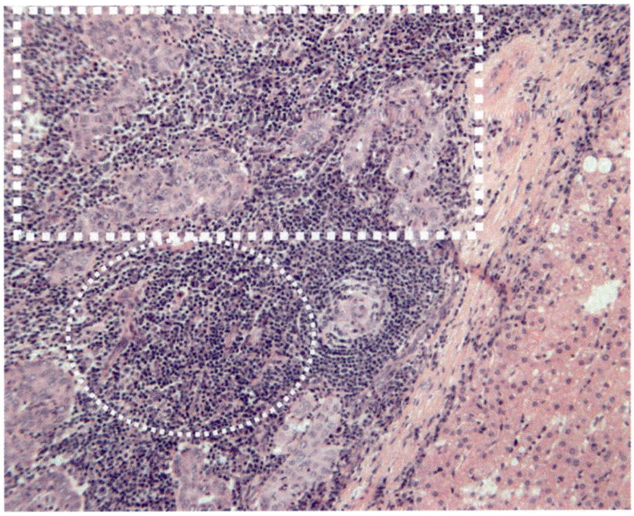

Fig. 7.189 LEL-ICC, tubular adenocarcinoma (*box*) accompanied with undifferentiated adenocarcinoma (*circle*)

(3) Mucoepidermoid carcinoma

7.2.4.1 Pathogenesis and Mechanism

The disease is often found in the salivary glands, and other possible locations include the thyroid, esophagus, respiratory tract, breast, and pancreas, with hepatic mucoepidermoid carcinoma as a very rare type, which is usually believed to originate from the end branches of intrahepatic bile ducts or canceration of cholangiocytes, and it is a special type of ICC [4]. The pathogenesis of hepatic mucoepidermoid carcinoma is unknown. It is generally believed that it may be related to secondary canceration of biliary epithelial squamous metaplasia derived from congenital choledochal cyst, *Clonorchis sinensis* infection, and intrahepatic bile duct stones and sclerotic cholangitis may induce squamous metaplasia and lead to adenocarcinoma.

7.2.4.2 Clinical Features

Arakaw et al. (2008) collected the data of 17 cases of hepatic mucoepidermoid carcinoma, with ten male and seven female cases, with an average age of 60 (35–81) years old. And common clinical manifestation includes abdominal pain, weight loss, upper abdominal discomfort, abnormal liver function, obstructive jaundice, etc. The serum CEA, CA19-9, and alkaline phosphatase are elevated, while serum AFP is negative [101].

7.2.4.3 Gross Features

The tumor is a solitary mass, round or oval, and large in volume with a diameter of 1.5–18 cm and 8.4 cm on average. The section is grayish white, showing cystic cavities of varying sizes which contain milky white translucent mucus, and satellite lesions can be found in the surrounding liver tissues of cases with intrahepatic metastasis.

7.2.4.4 Microscopic Features

The tumor was composed by mucus-secreting cells, squamous cells, epidermoid cells, and polygonal intermediate cells (basaloid cells) arranged in interlacing pattern to form nest structures according to the different proportions. The mucus-secreting cells in the solid nests can form cystic structures lined by cuboidal epithelium or columnar mucous secretory epithelium, and the cavities contain mucus. The squamous cells can have intercellular bridges with keratinization. According to the proportion of intracystic components in the tumor tissue, nerve invasion, tumor necrosis, nuclear mitotic figures, and differentiation degree, the mucoepidermoid carcinoma can be divided into high and low differentiated types. In general, high-grade differentiation mucoepidermoid carcinoma grows slowly, with infrequent metastasis, and is mainly composed of mucous cells which form adenoid structures. The tumor contains well-differentiated squamous cells and fewer intermediate cells, with a high rate of postoperative survival. However poorly differentiated mucoepidermoid carcinoma grows rapidly, with a high extrahepatic metastasis rate, and is mainly composed by solid nests of squamous cell and intermediate cells. These tumors have few mucous-like cells and cystic cavities, with poorly differentiated squamous cell, higher degree of malignancy, and neural invasion.

7.2.4.5 Immunohistochemistry

Epidermoid cells are positive for P63, CK5, CK6, and CK7 staining, and mucous cells are positive for periodic acid-Schiff (PAS) reaction and PAS staining. Positive Her-2/neu suggests higher degree of malignancy and a poor prognosis.

7.2.4.6 Differential Diagnosis

We must first rule out extrahepatic metastasis of mucoepidermoid carcinoma, and simple squamous cell carcinoma, mucus secretion cells, or cystic cavity structures can be found via expanded sampling, the latter of which is positive for Alcian blue and PAS staining [102].

7.2.4.7 Treatment and Prognosis

The biological behaviors of hepatic mucoepidermoid carcinoma are complicated with high malignancy. Widely extrahepatic metastasis is often found in the patients with this tumor, which has a recurrence trend and leads to poor outcomes; thus, multidisciplinary therapies should be attached much attention.

(4) Squamous cell carcinoma

The tumors originate from intrahepatic bile duct epithelium, which develops epithelial squamous metaplasia, due to stimulation of chronic inflammation caused by intrahepatic bile duct stones and nonparasitic cysts, further leading to canceration. So far, the domestic and foreign literature reported about 50 cases of this tumor, and the majority of the patients are the elderly, with a history of intrahepatic bile duct stones or hepatic cyst [103, 104]. The tumors are grayish white and solid masses with a diameter of 1–14 cm and often an incomplete cystic wall, invading the surrounding liver tissue. The cystic cavities contain brown liquid. Histologically, the carcinoma tissues present nest structures, and the cancer cells are distributed in a mosaic arrangement, with visible keratin cells and intercellular bridges (Figs. 7.190, 7.191, 7.192, and 7.193), and squamous epithelial metaplasia of the involved bile ducts or cysts can also be observed.

Prior to the diagnosis of this disease, it is the first step to exclude hepatic metastasis of squamous carcinoma. And if the hepatic squamous carcinoma invades the surrounding liver tissues, it is prone to metastasis and postoperative recurrence with a poor prognosis. Liver transplantation has been

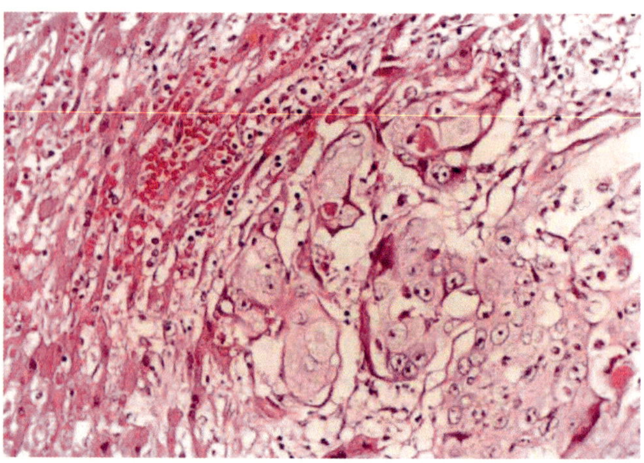

Fig. 7.190 Hepatic squamous cell carcinoma, polygonal tumor cells with keratinization and intercellular bridges

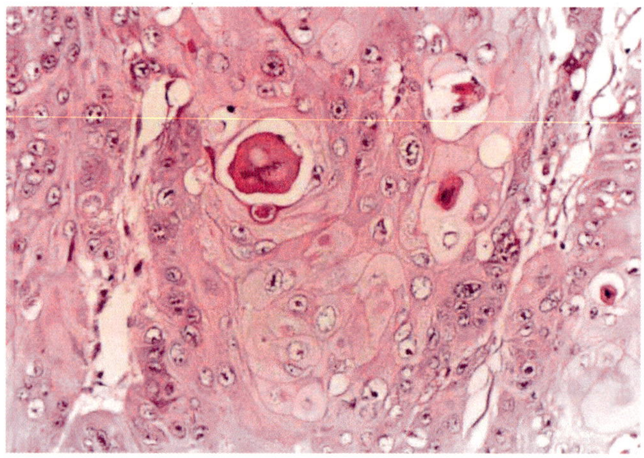

Fig. 7.191 Hepatic squamous cell carcinoma, malignant squamous cells with keratinization and intercellular bridges

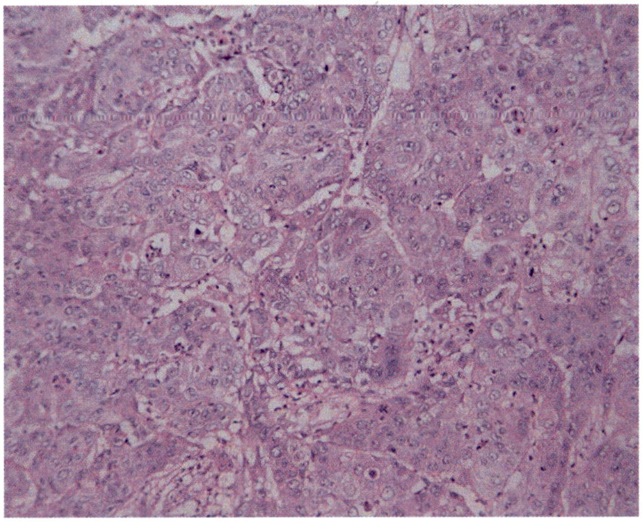

Fig. 7.192 Hepatic squamous cell carcinoma, squamous cell carcinoma composed of irregular nests or cords of polygonal cells

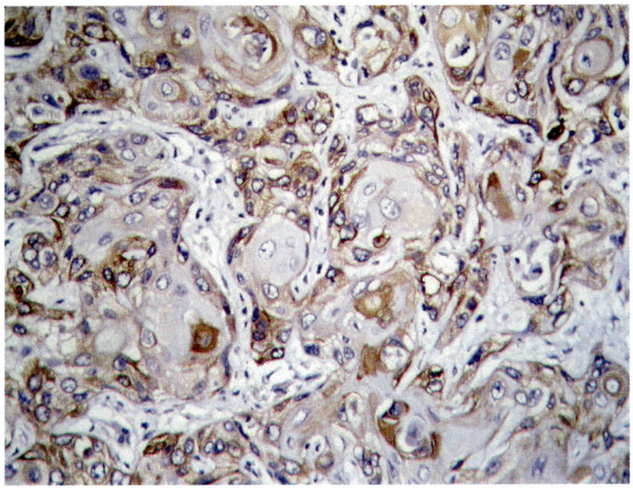

Fig. 7.193 Hepatic squamous cell carcinoma, showing positive immunohistochemical staining of CK19

reported in the treatment of this disease with relatively good effects [105].

(5) Adenosquamous carcinoma

Hepatic adenosquamous carcinoma accounts for 2–3% of ICC cases, and about 60 cases have been reported in the literature [106, 107]. The tumor is composed of adenocarcinoma and squamous carcinoma with a transitional zone between the two components, each of which accounts for more than 30%. Although hepatic mucoepidermoid carcinoma is suggested to be a synonym for hepatic adenosquamous carcinoma, the latter of which is essentially a kind of mixed tumor, lacking in the nest structures mixed up by mucinous, intermediate cells, and squamous cells, which are found in the mucoepidermoid carcinoma. And it was pointed out in the 2010 version of WHO Histological Classification of Hepatic and Intrahepatic Bile Duct tumors that differential diagnosis should be made between adenosquamous carcinoma and mucoepidermoid carcinoma. Hepatic adenosquamous carcinoma is prone to vascular, cholangical, and lymphatic invasion and is suggested to have a significantly higher malignant potential compared to adenocarcinoma. On the whole, patients with hepatic adenosquamous carcinoma have a poor prognosis [106].

(6) Epithelial-myoepithelial carcinoma

Donalh et al. first made the description of epithelial-myoepithelial carcinoma in 1972, and this is a variant of clear cell carcinoma of parotid gland. Tsuneyma et al. (1999) reported a case of hepatic epithelial-myoepithelial carcinoma in a 67-year-old male patient, who received a surgical resection of a subcapsular tumor, which was 3 cm in diameter in the right lobe of the liver. Liu Yong et al. (2006) reported a case of a 37-year-old woman who received a surgical resection for a 10 cm epithelial- myoepithelial carcinoma in the right hepatic lobe. Under the microscope, it presented the basic characteristics of epithelial-myoepithelial carcinoma: the tumor was composed by the inner layer of ductular epithelial cells and the outer layer of myoepithelial cells, forming a typical dual-tubular structure [108, 109]. The immunohistochemistry staining shows that the epithelial cells are positive for CK and EMA, and myoepithelial cells are positive for SMA, S-100, P63, and GFAP.

(7) Clear cell carcinoma

It is a rare histological variant of ICC, and more than ten cases have been reported to date. In histology, it is a tubular or papillary adenocarcinoma composed of clear cells, with abundant fibrous stroma, and the cancer cells express bile duct epithelial markers, such as CK7 and CK19, and may contain glycogen in the cytoplasm, which is positive for PAS staining. CD56 is often expressed in reactive hyperplasia of bile duct and cholangioadenoma tissues. However, Haas et al. (2007) found that CD56 was also expressed in three cases of clear cell ICC, suggesting that clear cell carcinoma of the bile duct may derive from the reactive hyperplasia of bile duct or biliary hamartoma-like lesions [110]. Its postoperative prognosis is relatively good [111].

(8) Papillary cystic tumor

Also known as solid-pseudopapillary tumor, solid and papillary epithelial neoplasm, or solid cystic tumor, papillary cystic tumor is a borderline tumor originating in the pancreas, and there are few primary hepatic papillary cystic tumors, with only two cases reported [112, 113]. Hepatic solid-pseudopapillary tumor is similar to its counterpart in the pancreas with the same name in clinical features, tumor number, characteristics under the microscope, ultrastructure, and histogenesis, suggesting that this tumor may originate from pluripotent stem cells, which differentiated into pancreatic acinar cells and ductular cells [112].

Pancreatic solid-pseudopapillary tumor is often found in young or middle-aged women, and the two reported cases of hepatic solid-pseudopapillary tumor concerned female patients as well who were aged 41 and 56 years old, respectively. One patient presented with abdominal pain and abdominal distension, while the other patient had no specific clinical symptoms and was only discovered in physical examination. The former patient had two lesions located separately in the right and left lobe of the liver, the sizes of which were 30 cm × 27 cm × 7.5 cm and 5.5 cm × 4.0 cm × 2.5 cm, respectively. And the cross sections of the tumors showed multicystic structures with hemorrhage and necrosis. The tumor tissues were found to be arranged in two forms under the microscope. In the first form, the cancer cells were high cuboidal with homogeneous cytoplasm and lobulated nuclei or nuclei with nuclear grooves, arranged in 2–3 layers surrounding the slender fibrovascular axis, forming papillary structures. In the other form, the tumor cells are polygonal in solid growth pattern, with consistent size, microcystic degeneration, and no pancreatic invasion. The pancreatic solid-pseudopapillary tumor is positively stained in immunohistochemistry investigations of α1-AT, AACT, NSE, and vimentin.

This tumor belongs to the category of borderline lesions, and the patients received surgical resection with no information of long-term follow-up. However, the patients with pancreatic solid-pseudopapillary tumors were treated with satisfactory outcomes after complete surgical resection [113].

7.3 Vascular and Lymphatic Tumors

Hui Dong
Department of Pathology, Eastern Hepatobiliary Surgery Hospital, Second Military Medical University, Shanghai, China

7.3.1 Angiosarcoma

7.3.1.1 Pathogenesis and Mechanism

Angiosarcoma was previously known as "Kupffer cell sarcoma," and it is clear that the tumor is derived from endothelial cells of blood sinuses, also known as hemangioendothelial sarcoma. It has been estimated that about 200 cases of angiosarcoma of the liver are newly diagnosed around the world each year, and 10–20 new cases are diagnosed in the United States each year, with the incidence rate of (0.14–0.25)/1000000. From January 1982 to June 2014, a total of 18 cases of hepatic angiosarcoma resected have been diagnosed in the Department of Pathology, Eastern Hepatobiliary Surgery Hospital, Second Military Medical University. And among the more than 30 thousand cases of primary hepatic malignant tumors treated with resection during the same period, hepatic angiosarcoma accounted for 0.06% [5], ranking fifth among all the malignant mesenchymal tumors in the liver. And under the following circumstances, the risk of developing hepatic angiosarcoma in adults increases: ① liver cirrhosis, found in about one-third of adult patients, including liver cirrhosis induced by hemoglobin pigmentation; ② exposure to vinyl chloride; ③ exposure to thoria, when the angiosarcoma can be mixed with HCC and/or cholangiocarcinoma; and ④ exposure to arsenic agents. There are 58–75% of the cases belonging to idiopathic ones, the etiology of which is still unclear.

7.3.1.2 Clinical Features

Among the 18 cases of hepatic angiosarcoma in Department of Pathology, Eastern Hepatobiliary Surgery Hospital, Second Military Medical University, the male to female ratio was 1:0.8, and the average age was 54.6 (28–78) years old. Most patients had early manifestations, such as abdominal pain, nausea, loss of appetite, fatigue, weight loss, anemia, fever, hepatomegaly, and late symptoms and signs, such as jaundice, ascites, and splenomegaly. A few cases had the initiative symptom of rupture and hemorrhage of the tumor, as well as severe hypoglycemia. Besides, most patients had abnormal serum bromsulphalein (BSP) retention, elevated alkaline phosphatase, and prolonged prothrombin time. There may be some symptoms and signs which are related to the mechanism, such as vinyl chloride-related splenomegaly and hypersplenism and thorium-related atrophy of spleen. According to the literature, 65% of the angiosarcoma patients have significant clinical symptoms, such as abdominal pain, hepatomegaly, or abdominal effusion, and others are abdominal hemorrhage (15%), splenomegaly (15%), and distant metastasis (9%) [114, 115]. Hepatic artery angiography is of important significance in the diagnosis of hepatic angiosarcoma, demonstrating flow from the center to small blood vessels lake, with contrast of the central few-blood-vessel region in the background of the peripheral vascular staining, and the involved hepatic arteries are often compressed by the tumor.

7.3.1.3 Gross Features

The tumors are usually multiple nodules in varying sizes, often 4–20 cm in diameter, while the diameter of a single tumor reach larger than 10 cm. The tumors are poorly cir-

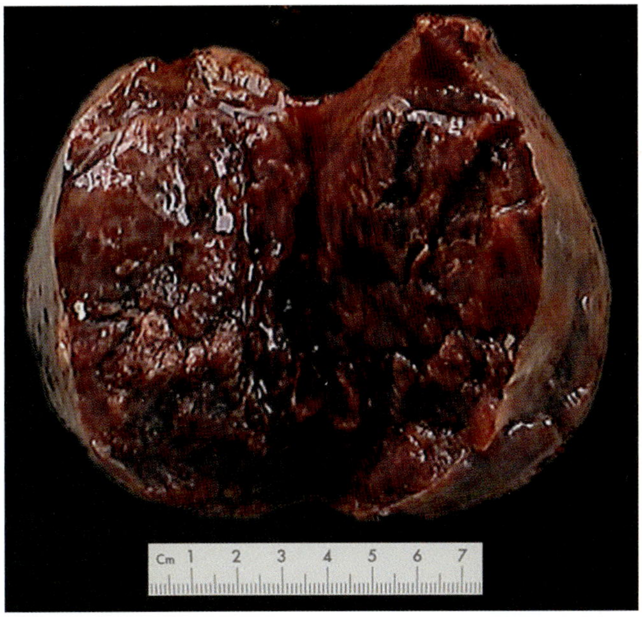

Fig. 7.194 Hepatic angiosarcoma. The cross sections of the tumors are often *dark red* and honeycomb-like cavities containing blood, with obvious hemorrhage and necrosis

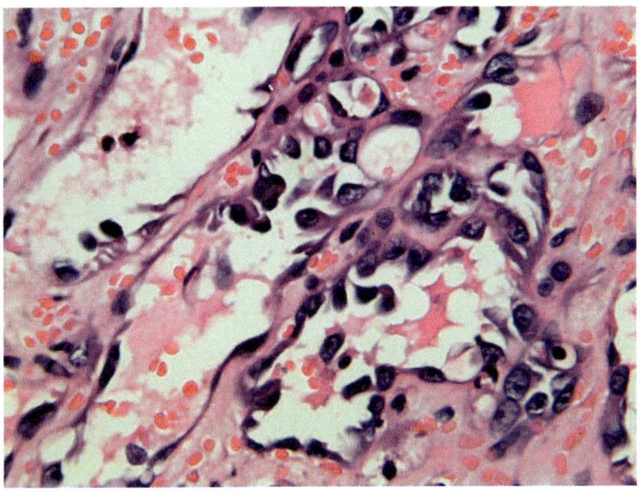

Fig. 7.195 Hepatic angiosarcoma. The tumor tissues have an flake architecture or sinusoid cavities varying in size, lined with single or multiple layers of irregular tumor cells, which are arranged as hobnail-like pattern, with large hyperchromasia nuclear

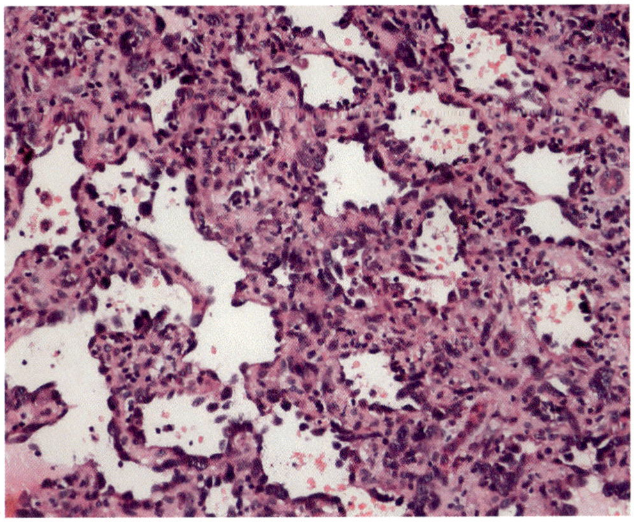

Fig. 7.196 Hepatic angiosarcoma. The tumor cell is irregular, lining in the inner surface of the cavities, which are arranged as hobnail-like pattern, with large hyperchromasia nuclear

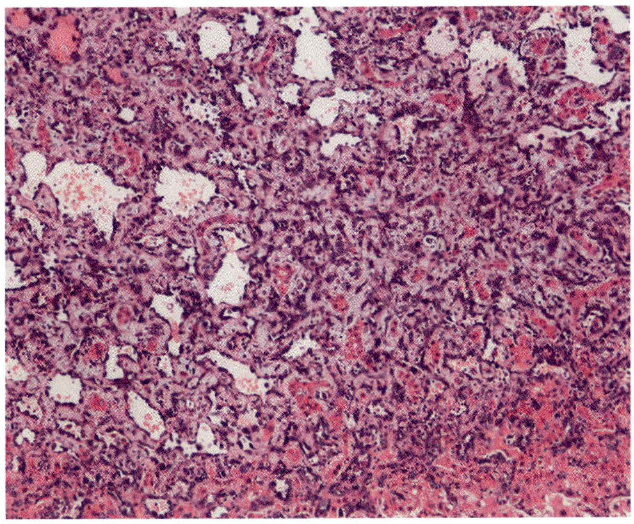

Fig. 7.197 Hepatic Angiosarcoma. Residue hepatic islets are visible in the rapidly growing tumor tissues

cumscribed with tumor cells involving the whole liver. The cross sections of the tumors are often dark red and honeycomb like, with obvious hemorrhage, necrosis, calcification, and cystic degeneration (Fig. 7.194). Cases of hepatic angiosarcoma associated with thorium dioxide poisoning often contain hepatic fibrosis.

7.3.1.4 Microscopic Features

Have an architectural pattern that varies from sponge like to solid or pseudopapillary, lined with single or multiple layers of tumor cells, which are spindle or pleomorphic, with slightly eosinophilic cytoplasm, spindle, polygonal, or multiple nucleoli with hyperchromasia, mitotic activity, and nuclear irregularity/pleomorphism. The hobnail-like tumor cells can be hung on the walls of blood vessels (Figs. 7.195 and 7.196). Meganucleus and phagocytosis can be observed in a few tumor cells. The tumors have no complete capsule and spread along the epithelium of the sinusoids and terminal branches of the hepatic veins and portal veins. They can grow on the hepatic plates in a frame or sheet-like pattern, inducing the dissociation of the hepatic plates, atrophy, or disappearance of the liver cells. Furthermore, visible residual liver cell cords can be found in the rapid growing tumor tissues (Fig. 7.197). The tumor cells proliferate to form intralu-

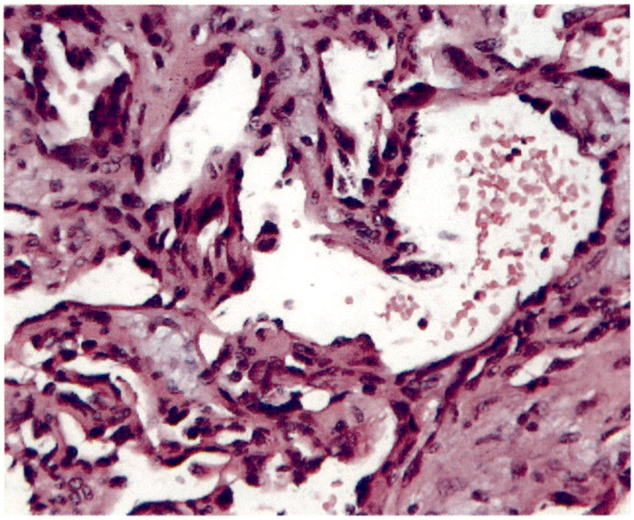

Fig. 7.198 Hepatic angiosarcoma. The tumor cells proliferate to form intraluminal papillae, the vascular cavity was lined with pleomorphic neoplastic cells

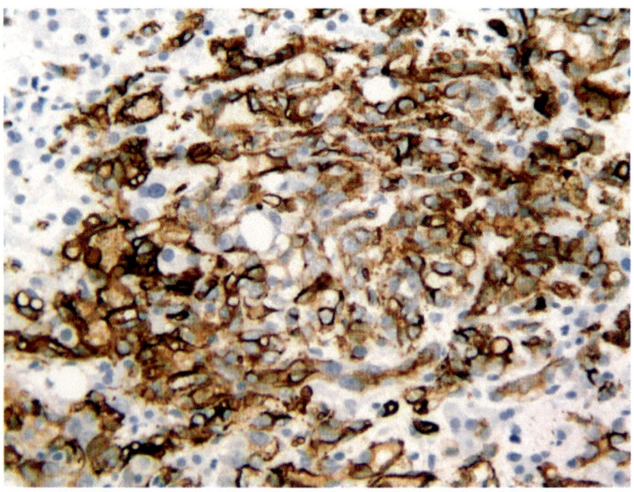

Fig. 7.199 Hepatic angiosarcoma. CD34 is positive in tumor cells

minal papillae (Fig. 7.198), containing blood clots and cellular debris within the vascular channels. Visible extramedullary hematopoiesis and infarction can also be found in the tumor, and nodular masses can be formed when a large number of tumor cells proliferate, resembling fibrosarcoma. Reticular fiber staining shows that the tumor cells are located in the inner side of the reticular fiber ring without reticular fibers between the tumor cells.

Dimashkieh et al. [116] reported a pediatric case of hepatic-rich cell sarcoma with a vortex pattern of arrangement, and the tumor cells were Kaposi-like spindle cells, suggesting that the histological morphology of hepatic angiosarcoma in children is different from that in the adults.

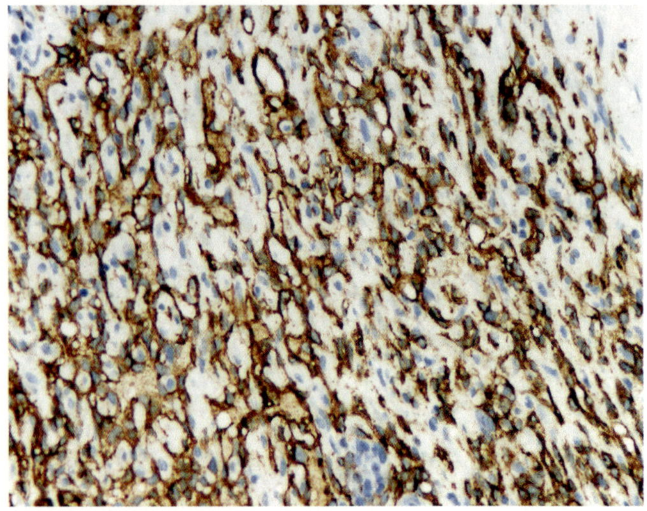

Fig. 7.200 Hepatic angiosarcoma. CD34 is positive in tumor cells

7.3.1.5 Immunohistochemistry

The tumor cells are positive for vimentin, F-VIII, and CD34 (Figs. 7.199 and 7.200) and negative for desmin, AFP, CK, and CEA.

7.3.1.6 Differential Diagnosis

It has been reported that only about 50% of angiosarcoma cases were correctly diagnosed. Angiosarcomas are extremely variable in differentiation, ranging from well-differentiated lesions that may be difficult to distinguish from hemangiomas or hepatic peliosis, to exclusively spindled lesions resembling sarcoma, hepatic yolk sac tumor or purely epithelioid lesions easily mistaken for primary or metastatic carcinoma. Epithelioid angiosarcomas are composed of sheets of epithelioid endothelial cells with abundant eosinophilic cytoplasm. Such lesions should be distinguished from epithelioid hemangioendothelioma (EHE); the former has more nuclear atypia, mitotic activity, necrosis, and hemorrhage.

7.3.1.7 Treatment and Prognosis

The angiosarcomas are highly aggressive and rapidly progressive, with fewer opportunities for resection, and the overall prognosis is poor. It is reported in the literature [117] that the treatment effects for hepatic angiosarcoma is unsatisfactory, with the majority of patients died of liver failure, abdominal bleeding, or disseminated intravascular coagulation (DIC) 6 months after their diagnosis of angiosarcoma. Only 3% of these patients had a survival period of more than 24 months. Of the 18 cases of hepatic angiosarcoma diagnosed in the Department of Pathology, Eastern Hepatobiliary Surgery Hospital, Second Military Medical University, the median survival time of the patients was 12 months, including one patient treated with both surgical resection and postoperative chemotherapy, who is still alive with survival time

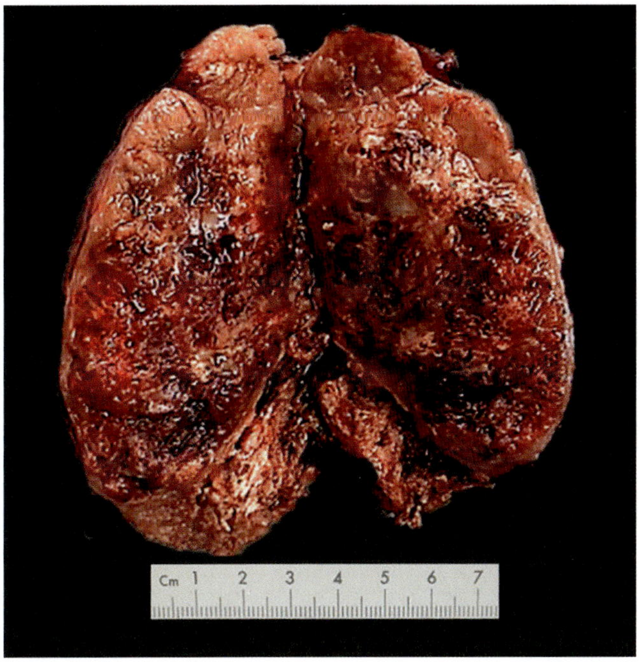

Fig. 7.201 Hepatic malignant hemangiopericytoma. The appearance of necrosis and hemorrhage in the tumor

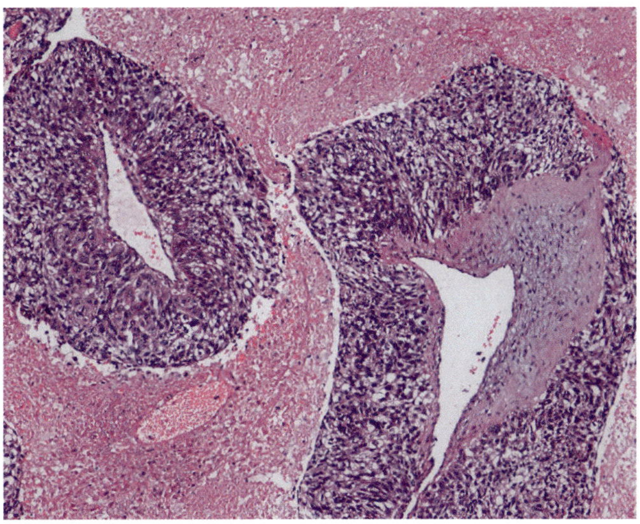

Fig. 7.202 Hepatic malignant hemangiopericytoma. Shows a staghorn or slit like vasculature with perivascular hyalinization, around which are arrayed spindled cells

longer than 10 years. Due to its relative resistance to radiation, surgical resection with chemotherapy is helpful to prolong the survival period for patients with angiosarcoma.

7.3.2 Malignant Hemangiopericytoma

7.3.2.1 Pathogenesis and Mechanism

Malignant hemangiopericytoma is very rare and often found in the lower limbs, pelvic cavity, retroperitoneal region, neck, etc., and there have been around 12 cases with hepatic involvement reported in the literature. It is generally considered to originate from pluripotent mesenchymal stem cells in the peripheral vascular areas, and their pathogenesis is partly associated with the exposure to high concentration of vinyl chloride in the working environment.

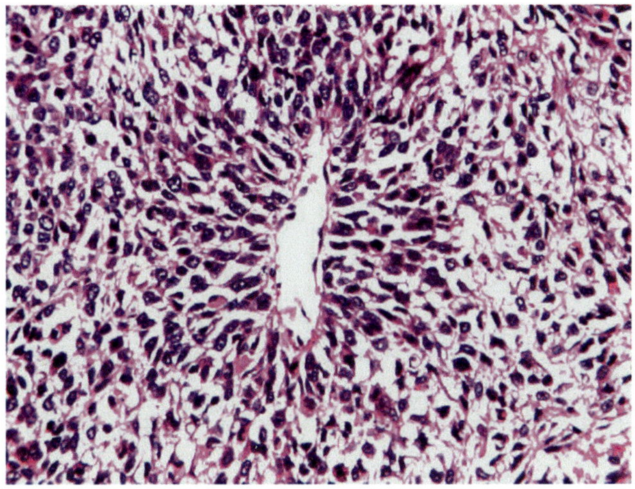

Fig. 7.203 Hepatic malignant hemangiopericytoma. The tumor cells arranged as radiation surrounding slit like vasculature

7.3.2.2 Clinical Features

Three cases of hepatic malignant hemangiopericytoma have been diagnosed in the Department of Pathology, Eastern Hepatobiliary Surgery Hospital, Second Military Medical University, and the patients were all male, and their average age was 52 years old. The liver was occupied by the mass, causing local discomfort and hepatic vein compression syndrome, and some patients manifested Budd-Chiari syndrome. A small number of patients had hypoglycemia which returned to normal after the resection of the tumor. Imaging showed that the tumors were rich in blood vessels, accompanied by central necrosis and clear boundaries.

7.3.2.3 Gross Features

The tumors are often large in volume, with a diameter of up to 20 cm and well delineated. The cut surface is fleshy, light brown, and cystic which is similar to cystadenocarcinoma, and the appearance of necrosis and hemorrhage in the tumor is often suggestive of malignancy (Fig. 7.201).

7.3.2.4 Microscopic Features

Hemangiopericytoma shows a staghorn or slit-like vasculature with perivascular hyalinization, around which is arrayed spindled to ovoid cells (Figs. 7.202 and 7.203). These vascular walls have an intact basement membrane, lined by a single layer of endothelial cells. The tumor cells were spindled or short fusiform with unclear boundaries, round

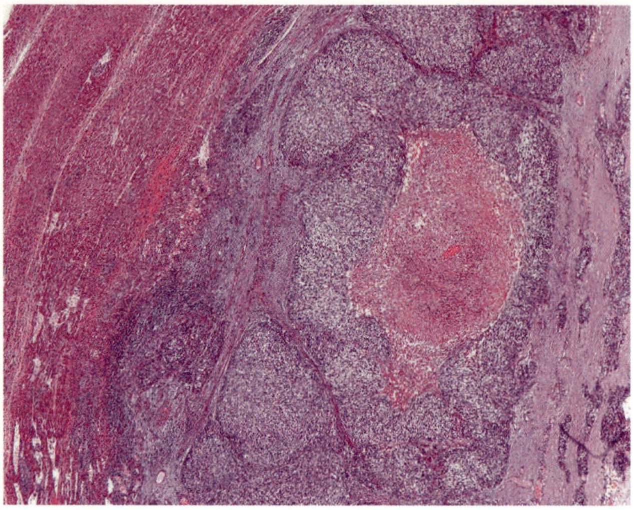

Fig. 7.204 Hepatic malignant hemangiopericytoma. Tumor cells infiltrate into the adjacent hepatic tissue

nuclei, smooth chromatin, and different degrees of nuclear atypia. Reticular fiber staining shows reticular fibers parallel with the arrangement of tumor cells, and the tumor cells produce abundant reticular fibers to form a grid. Biological behaviors of hepatic hemangiopericytoma can be divided into malignant, benign, or intermediate type, with slow growth in most cases. Malignant hemangiopericytoma are hypercellular lesions that usually display nuclear pleomorphism, hyperchromasia, areas of tumor necrosis, and/or increased mitotic activity (≥4 mitoses/10 HPF), including atypical mitoses and infiltrative growing into the surrounding liver tissue (Fig. 7.204).

7.3.2.5 Immunohistochemistry

No special markers are found, and the tumor cells are positive for vimentin and negative for F-VIII and desmin.

7.3.2.6 Differential Diagnosis

It should be noted that the hepatic malignant hemangiopericytoma should be differentiated from hepatocellular carcinoma, angiosarcoma, hepatoblastoma, and intrahepatic cholangiocarcinoma.

7.3.2.7 Treatment and Prognosis

Malignant hemangiopericytoma is 12%. Lymphatic metastasis is the main spread path. Once diagnosed, the tumor should be treated with wide surgical excision, combined with chemotherapy and radiotherapy. According to our experience, the patients of the two cases with hepatic malignant hemangiopericytoma had recurrent tumors 43 months and 84 months after postsurgery protocol chemotherapy, respectively, suggesting that it is highly aggressive and is not sensitive to chemotherapy.

7.3.3 Epithelioid Hemangioendothelioma

7.3.3.1 Pathogenesis and Mechanism

Epithelioid hemangioendothelioma (EHE) is a low-grade vascular tumor and was once named as histiocytoid hemangioendothelioma, sclerosing endothelioid angiosarcoma, sclerosing interstitial vascular sarcoma, or pseudocartilagenous sarcoma. Weiss and Enzinger (1982) first reported EHE of soft tissue and pointed out that it was an intermediate tumor between benign hemangioma and angiosarcoma. Ishak et al. (1985) first reported hepatic EHE. From January 1982 to June 2014, a total of 20 cases of hepatic EHE with surgical resection in the Department of Pathology, Eastern Hepatobiliary Surgery Hospital, Second Military Medical University, accounted for 0.07% of more than 30 thousand cases of primary malignant hepatic tumors surgically excised during the same period. Of all these 20 cases, three cases (15%) were HBsAg positive (Table 7.14), revealing the potential relationship between HBV infection and EHE which needs further studies. Some cases may be associated with the history of oral contraceptives, and individual cases of EHE have also been discovered after the exposure to vinyl chloride. Mendlick et al. (2001) found nonrandom translocation of chromosome in EHE, namely, t(1; 3)(p36.3;q25).

7.3.3.2 Clinical Features

Mehrabi et al. [118] reviewed the 402 cases of hepatic EHE and found the male to female ratio was 1:1.5, with an average age of 41.7 years (3–86). And of the 20 cases of hepatic EHE diagnosed in the Department of Pathology, Eastern Hepatobiliary Surgery Hospital, Second Military Medical University, the male to female ratio was 1:1.5, and the average age was 47.5 (20–71) years. Most of these patients had no specific clinical symptoms, and about 40% of them were discovered by accident. The common clinical manifestations include right upper abdominal pain and discomfort, weight loss, and hepatosplenomegaly, and a small number of cases had jaundice or occasional hemoperitoneum caused by tumor rupture. Some patients may present with liver failure or the Budd-Chiari syndrome. Two-thirds of the patients had elevated serum alkaline phosphatase levels, and some patients had elevated serum CEA, while only a small number of patients presented increased peripheral white blood cell count. Serum AFP was negative in most of the patients. In an imaging study, MRI is superior to CT, with some relatively specific performances, such as single or multiple nodules with tumor fusion, or location of hepatic surface underneath the hepatic capsule. Characteristic images of EHE on MRI are lesions with low signals on T1-weighted sequences, heterogenous high signals on T2-weighted sequences. Halo signals with low signals around the lesions can be seen, and enhanced MRI shows high-intensity signals at the periphery of the lesions with a hypodense center

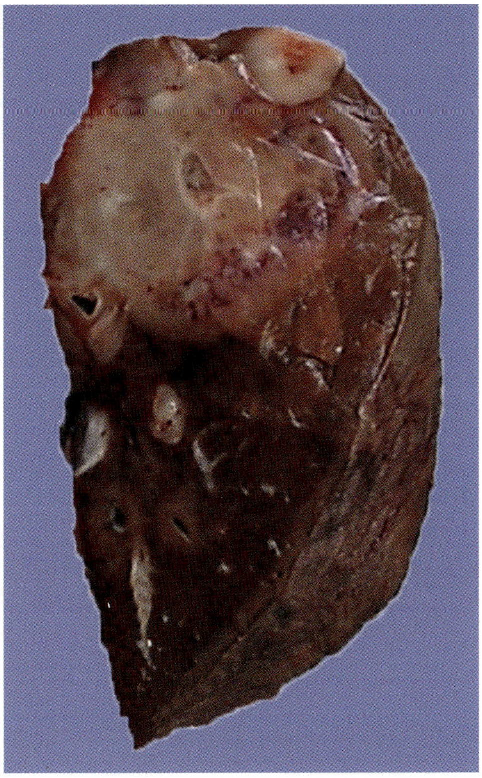

Fig. 7.205 Hepatic epithelioid hemangioendothelioma. The tumor is a *pale white*, dense and hard rubber-like nodule

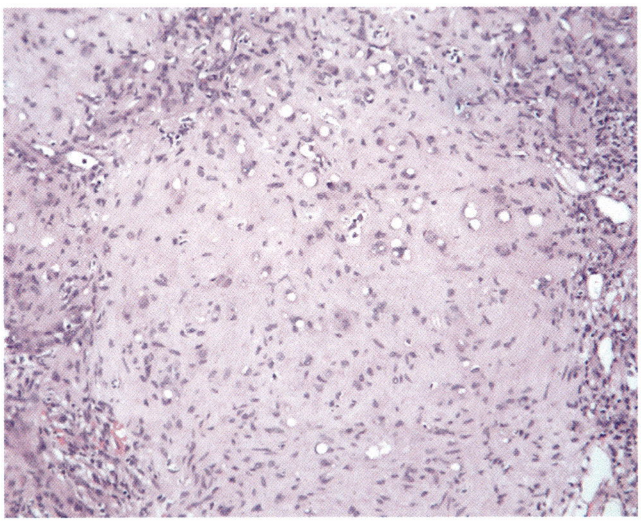

Fig. 7.206 Hepatic epithelioid hemangioendothelioma. Fibrous stroma is abundant in hypocellular area, epithelioid neoplastic cells are distributed sparsely

in portal venous phase. Signs such as capsular retraction can be observed in cases with lesions adjacent to the capsule. But these images are similar to those of metastatic tumors in the liver, and it is difficult to make the differential diagnosis;

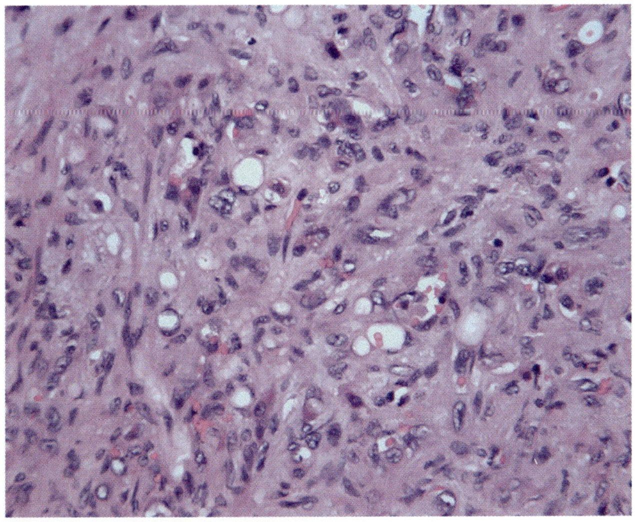

Fig. 7.207 Hepatic epithelioid hemangioendothelioma. Signet ring cell-like structures representing tumor cells with intracytoplasmic lumina, unsymmetric nuclei, occasionally containing solitary red blood cell

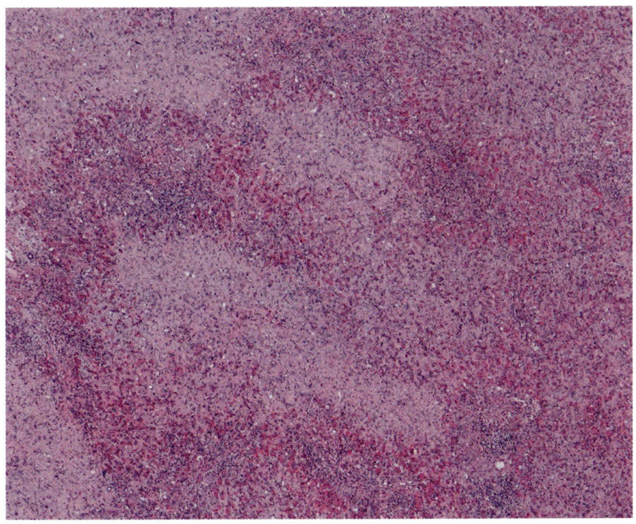

Fig. 7.208 Hepatic epithelioid hemangioendothelioma. The epithelioid cells infiltrated preexisting sinusoids with a patchy pattern

thus, definite diagnosis of EHE depends on pathological examination.

7.3.3.3 Gross Features

Among the 20 cases of EHE diagnosed in the Department of Pathology, Eastern Hepatobiliary Surgery Hospital, Second Military Medical University, 16 cases (76.1%) were multiple lesions (2–5) with diameters ranging from 0.2 to 14 cm and distributed in the whole liver. The cut sections were grayish white or brownish yellow. The tumors were dense and hard with focal calcific and gritty areas (Fig. 7.205). HCC was

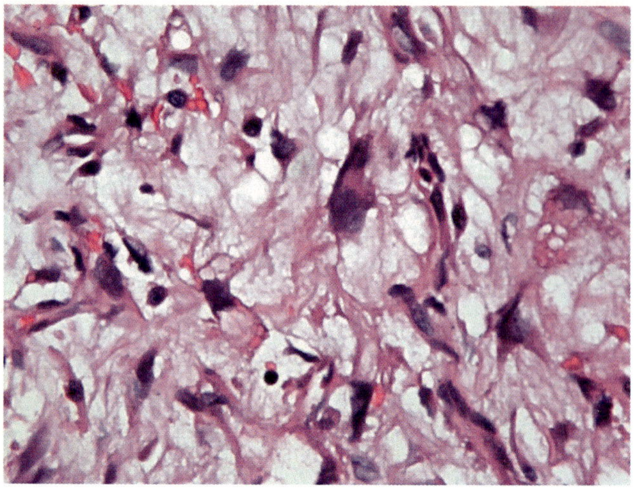

Fig. 7.209 Hepatic epithelioid hemangioendothelioma. Showing stellate or spindle dentritic cells with finger-like protrusions of cytoplasm

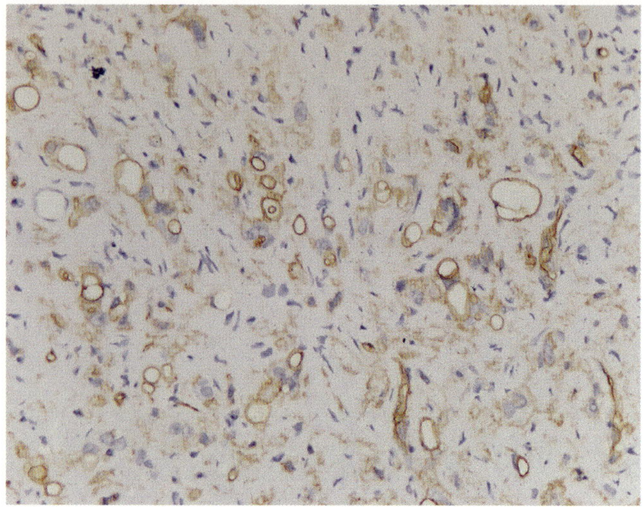

Fig. 7.211 Hepatic epithelioid hemangioendothelioma. CD34 is positive

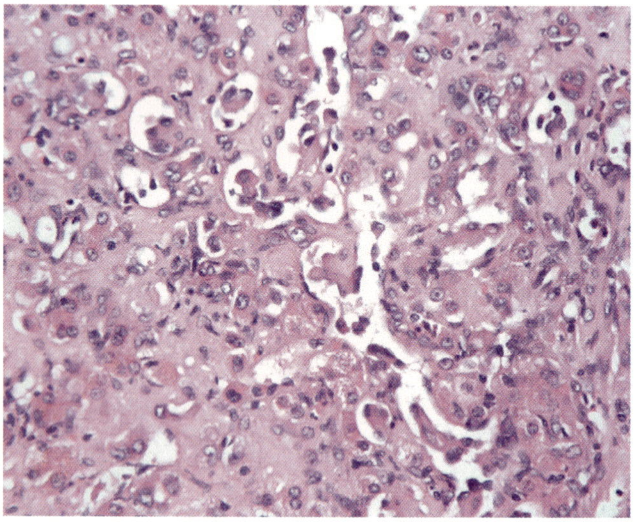

Fig. 7.210 Hepatic epithelioid hemangioendothelioma. Papillary pattern of neoplastic cells in the hepatic sinusoid

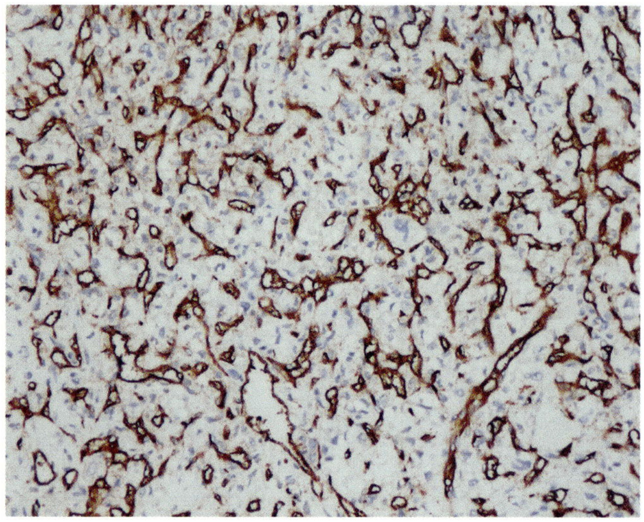

Fig. 7.212 Hepatic epithelioid hemangioendothelioma. Intensive CD34 positive neoplastic vasculature in adjacent liver tissue

found in three cases of EHE, and the HCC nodules were all larger in diameter and complicated with cirrhosis.

7.3.3.4 Microscopic Features

"Ribbon" structure: The tumor nodules with the central fibrosis and sclerosis are hypocellular at the center (Fig. 7.206) and cellular at the periphery. The tumor cells are mainly epithelioid, found in all EHE tissues. Epithelioid cells were medium to large, rounded or variable in shape, and had an eosinophilic cytoplasm and vesicular nuclei with small, inconspicuous nucleoli. Signet ring cell-like structures represent tumor cells with intracytoplasmic lumina, unsymmetric nuclei, occasionally containing solitary red blood cell (Fig. 7.207) negative for mucicarmine, showing that they are intracellular vascular cavities. The epithelioid cells infiltrated preexisting sinusoids (Fig. 7.208), terminal hepatic venules, and portal vein branches, and they can form tumor thrombi in the terminal hepatic veins and portal vein branches, causing completely organized occlusion of theses vascular cavities.

In addition, about 16% of the EHE was comprised predominantly of "dendritic" cells with spindle or stellate shapes, multiple interdigitating processes, and a pale eosinophilic cytoplasm, abundant collagen matrix with myxoid degeneration. In cases in which the dendritic cells predominated, cells with intracytoplasmic vacuoles were less frequent (Fig. 7.209). Overall, 58% of hepatic EHE cases show no mitoses, and 29% of hepatic EHE have <2 mitoses/10

HPF, while only 13% cases of hepatic EHE >2 mitoses/10 HPF. It is worth noting that tumor cells sometimes infiltrate hepatic sinusoids, leading to dilated hepatic sinusoids, and they further form papillary pattern in the hepatic sinusoid, which are similar to adenoid architectures (Fig. 7.210).

7.3.3.5 Immunohistochemistry

The tumor cells are positive for endothelial cell markers with a high positive rate, such as F-VIII, CD34 (Figs. 7.211 and 7.212), CD31, and vimentin, while SMA is only positive in a few cases.

7.3.3.6 Electron Microscopic Observation

The tumor cells have characteristics of endothelial cells, such as basement membrane, pinosome, cytoplasmic Weibel-Palade bodies and a large number of intermediate filaments.

7.3.3.7 Differential Diagnosis

For EHE with plenty of stromal fibrosis, much attention should be paid to its differentiation from fibrosarcoma. And for cases with papillary invasion of hepatic sinusoids, EHE should be distinguished from metastatic adenocarcinoma. EHE with signet ring-like epithelioid cells must be differentiated from metastatic signet ring cell carcinoma, while the latter is negative for CD34, CD31, and F-VIII staining, and mucus staining shows cytoplasmic mucus rather than a true vascular cavity. And angiosarcoma has no intracellular vacuole or dense stromal fibrosis or sclerotic area.

7.3.3.8 Cytogenetic Characteristics

EHE can contain amplification of t(1;3)(p36.3;q25) and t(10;14)(p13;q42), as well as 11 (q13–13q14) and 12 (Q11 to q21), or loss of 11 (q21 to qter) [119]. Cao Yan et al. reported that the genetic changes of pulmonary EHE mainly involve multiple chromosome small fragments (<10 MB), and the changes include more amplification of chromosomal fragments and less loss of these fragments [120].

7.3.3.9 Treatment and Prognosis

EHE grow slowly, with less aggresive in biological behavior, less vascular invasion, low extrahepatic metastasis rate (about 27%), and a better prognosis than that of hepatic angiosarcoma. EHEs have a certain resistance to radiotherapy and chemotherapy; thus, surgical resection should be the first choice in the treatment with the postoperation survival time reaching 5–28 years. Liver transplantation is beneficial in cases involved. In rare cases, recurrent tumors can be discovered in the allograft. Nuclear mitotic figures, nuclear atypia, and density of tumor cells are related to the prognosis to a certain degree, while patients with mitotic figures >2/10 HPF have a poor prognosis. Follow-up of a group of 137 patients showed that 43% of these patients had 5-year survival period, and over 20-year survival was found in seven cases. Of the 20 cases of EHE diagnosed in our hospital, the median postoperative survival time was 87 months, with the longest survival period of more than 2 years. And the five deaths included three cases complicated by hepatocellular carcinoma, cholangiocarcinoma, and nail thyroid carcinoma, respectively, suggesting that EHE patients with malignant tumors have a poor prognosis.

7.3.4 Kaposi Sarcoma

7.3.4.1 Pathogenesis and Mechanism

Kaposi sarcoma (KS) was first reported by Moritz Kaposi in 1872, and it is a malignant tumor composed of spindle cells and slit-like vascular channels. In recent years, it has been found that the tumor expresses VEGFR, confirming its origin of lymphatic or vascular endothelial cells, and it is a multicenter hemangioendotheliosarcoma. According to different causes, KS can be divided into four subtypes: classic type or Mediterranean KS, African or endemic KS, iatrogenic or transplant-related KS, and epidemic or AIDS-related KS. And the histopathological features of all these four types of KS are always the same regardless of clinical scenario. AIDS-related KS is induced by infection of human immunodeficiency virus (HIV) and human herpesvirus type 8 (HHV-8) or Kaposi sarcoma-associated herpesvirus [121, 122]. In patients with Kaposi sarcoma, the positive rate of HHV-8 DNA was 80–100% in the tumor tissues. And it has been reported that the incidence of hepatic KS was 0.12–2.16% after organ transplantation.

7.3.4.2 Clinical Features

The disease is more common in patients with acquired immune deficiency syndrome (AIDS) (> 90%) and organ transplantation, so the patients often manifest symptoms associated with T cell immunodeficiency in severe AIDS, such as fever, weight loss, systemic lymphadenectasis, and combining with other infections of protozoan, fungal, and viral, causing abdominal pain, hepatomegaly, etc.

7.3.4.3 Gross Features

Hepatic KS lesions have a characteristic distribution, most of which are multiple, scattered, different in size, tan and brown cavernous lesions, with the portal area as the center and unclear boundaries, and often 1–2 cm in diameter, which are similar to the morphology of hematoma or hemangioma.

7.3.4.4 Microscopic Features

Kaposi sarcoma is characterized by proliferation of spindled tumor cells, irregular slit-like vascular channels, extravasated red blood cells, and hemosiderosis. Chronic inflammation is common and a helpful diagnostic clue. The lesions mainly involve the portal and periportal areas, showing spin-

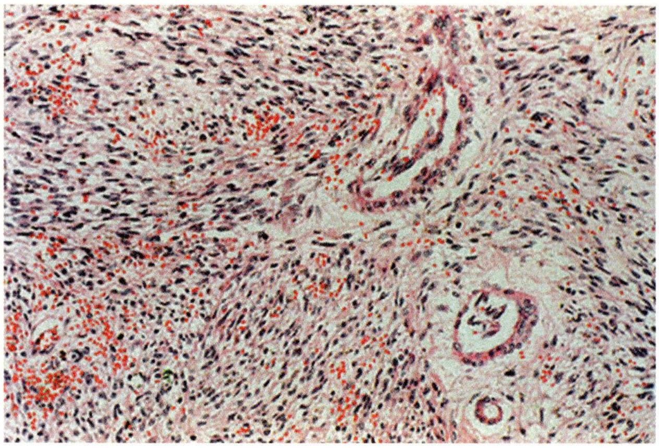

Fig. 7.213 Hepatic Kaposi sarcoma. Showing spindled tumor cells, slit capillary cavities and red blood cell spillover outside the cavities

dle cellular nodules, and abundant slit capillary cavities interlacing in the nodules (Fig. 7.213). Most cases contain eosinophilic bodies which are positive for PAS staining, and the tumor cells often invade the muscular layer of the portal vein wall, the surrounding liver sinusoids, and hepatic plates.

7.3.4.5 Immunohistochemistry

The spindle cells are positive for CD31, CD34, and F-VIII staining, and AIDS-related KS is positive for anti-KSHV nuclear antigen.

7.3.4.6 Electron Microscopic Observation

Visible cytoplasmic Weibel-Palade bodies

7.3.4.7 Differential Diagnosis

Current reports in domestic literature concerned classic KS in the skin, posttransplantation KS, and AIDS-related KS, and the differential diagnosis of all the four subtypes of KS should be based on the combination of clinical history and serum HIV detection. In addition, differentiation from vascular tumors, such as hepatic angiosarcoma and infant hemangioendothelioma, should be carried out by integrated investigation of the history, serum HIV testing, gross, and microscopic characteristics.

7.3.4.8 Treatment and Prognosis

Hepatic KS can metastasize via hematogenous and lymphatic systems with a poor prognosis. In cases with liver transplantation-related KS, it is reported that early diagnosis and timely reduction of immunosuppression have significant therapeutic effects.

7.3.5 Lymphoma

7.3.5.1 Pathogenesis and Mechanism

Since Ata and Kamal reported the first case of primary hepatic lymphoma (PHL) in 1965, about 100 cases have been reported in the literature, accounting for 0.4% of all the cases of extranodal lymphoma. According to the report by Bronowick [123], HCV infection rate was 9–42% in patients with PHL in Western countries, suggesting that HCV infection may be the main cause of PHL. Studies have shown that chronic HCV infection can lead to persistent monoclonal amplification of intrahepatic lymphocytes and inhibition of apoptosis, which proceed to malignant transformation to induce PHL. HCV-induced PHL may be realized by the following indirect ways: ① continuous stimulation of multiclonal proliferation of B lymphocytes, leading to the transformation of monoclonal amplification of B lymphocytes; ② induced translocation of t(8;14), resulting in overexpression of antiapoptosis gene Bcl–2, monoclonal IgH gene rearrangements; and ③ HCV virus core and/or NS5 protein-induced transcriptional regulatory changes of P21, P53, H-ras, etc.

A total of 35 cases of PHL were diagnosed in the Department of Pathology, Eastern Hepatobiliary Surgery Hospital, Second Military Medical University, from January 1982 to June 2014, which ranks second of all malignant hepatic mesenchymal tumors in our hospital, second to undifferentiated embryonal sarcoma, in which 12 cases (34.3%) were HBsAg positive and only 1 case (2.9%) was complicated with HCV infection. HBV and HCV are both considered to belong to the type of lymphotropic virus. Sekiguchi et al. [124] reported a case of a young male patient who developed PHL 7 months after the onset of acute hepatitis B. Therefore, we speculate that HCV has a limited role in the pathogenesis of Chinese PHL, while HBV can be integrated into the genome of intrahepatic lymphocytes, which induces clonal proliferation and mutation of lymphocytes, resulting in PHL. HBV infection plays an important role in the pathogenesis of PHL, especially in Chinese PHL. In addition, patients with long-term use of cyclosporine after liver transplantation, systemic lupus erythematosus, autoimmune liver disease, and exposure to hazardous chemicals can also develop PHL.

7.3.5.2 Clinical Features

Among these 35 cases of PHL diagnosed in the Department of Pathology, Eastern Hepatobiliary Surgery Hospital, Second Military Medical University, the average age of the patients was 52.6 years ranged from 17 to 79 years, with a male to female ratio of 2.5:1. The common clinical symptoms were fever, emaciation, weight loss, and night sweats, all of which are the so-called "type B symptoms" of lymphoma. And 56% of the patients had right upper abdominal pain or discomfort, 82% of patients had hepatosplenomegaly, or liver masses found in physical examination. Most cases had elevated serum lactate dehydrogenase (LDH), which may indicate a poor prognosis, and LDH can be used as a reference marker for the diagnosis and therapeutic assessment. Liver dysfunction to different degrees can also

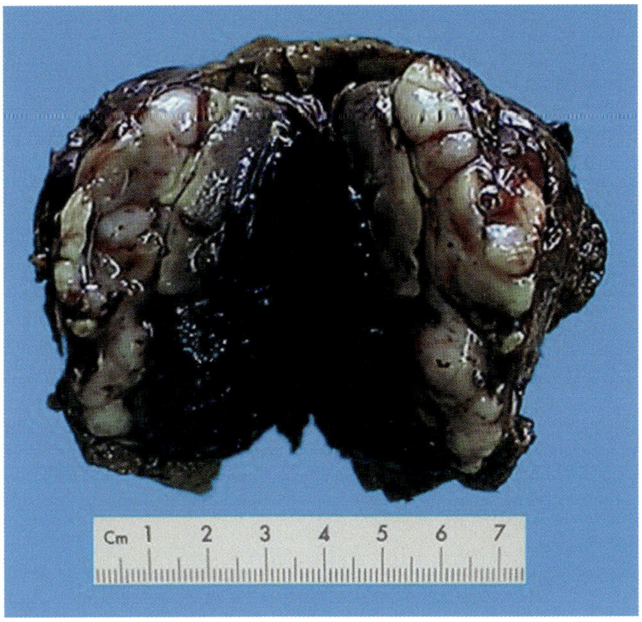

Fig. 7.214 Hepatic primary B-cell lymphoma. The tumor is gray-white, partial hemorrage and necrosis

Table 7.12 Histological classification of hepatic lymphoma

Classification	Number of cases
Diffuse large B cell	41 (46%)
Pleomorphic small cell	5 (6%)
Hepatosplenic T cell lymphoma	4 (5%)
Diffuse histiocytic	4 (5%)
Combined diffuse mixed large and small cell	3 (3%)
Lymphoma of mucosa-associated lymphoid tissue	3 (3%)
Diffuse small non-cleaved	3 (3%)
Lymphoblastic	3 (3%)
T zone	2 (2%)
Diffuse immunoblastic	2 (2%)
Small lymphocytic	2 (2%)
Follicular small cleaved cell	1 (1%)
Diffuse small cleaved cell	1 (1%)
Mantle cell lymphoma	1 (1%)
Anaplastic large cell lymphoma	1 (1%)
T-cell rich B-cell lymphoma	1 (1%)
Lymphoplasmacytoid	1 (1%)
Centrocytic	1 (1%)
Diffuse large non-cleaved cell	1 (1%)
Diffuse undifferentiated	1 (1%)
Diffuse poorly differentiated lymphocytic	1 (1%)
Unclassified	2 (2%)

be discovered. Haide et al. [125] reported that PHL could manifest fulminant liver damage. B-ultrasound study shows hypoechoic or isoechoic mass. Computed tomography images display homogeneous areas with decreased density in the enhanced scanning. Magnetic resonance imaging

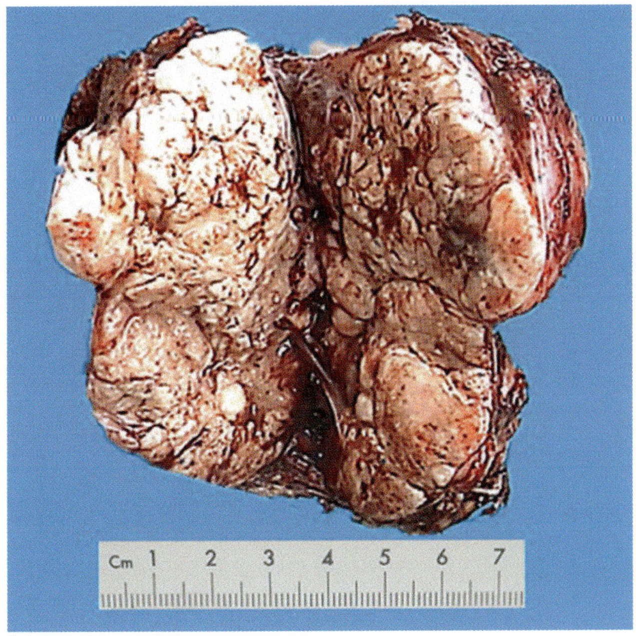

Fig. 7.215 Hepatic primary T-cell lymphoma. Huge, gray-white lobulated nodule

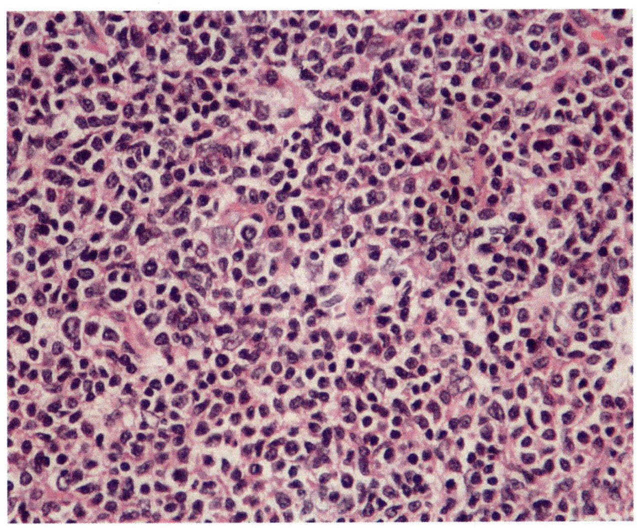

Fig. 7.216 Hepatic primary B-cell lymphoma. Large tumor cells is distributed diffusely

shows abnormal signals, including low-signal areas on T1-weighted imaging with high-signal areas in anaplasia zone of hemorrhage or necrosis, and high signals on T2-weighted imaging. However, the clinical and imaging findings of PHL cannot be used as evidence to differentiate it from other primary or metastatic hepatic tumors.

7.3.5.3 Gross Features

Larger than 5 cm, without encapsulation, but their margins are generally well defined. Typical primary hepatic lym-

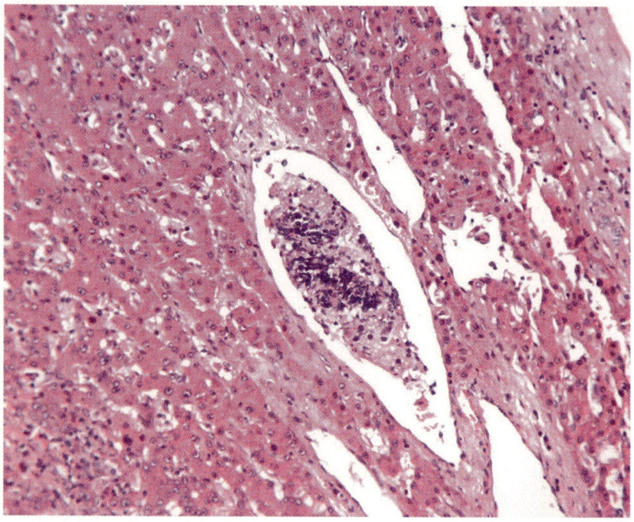

Fig. 7.217 Hepatic primary B-cell lymphoma. Microvascular invasion

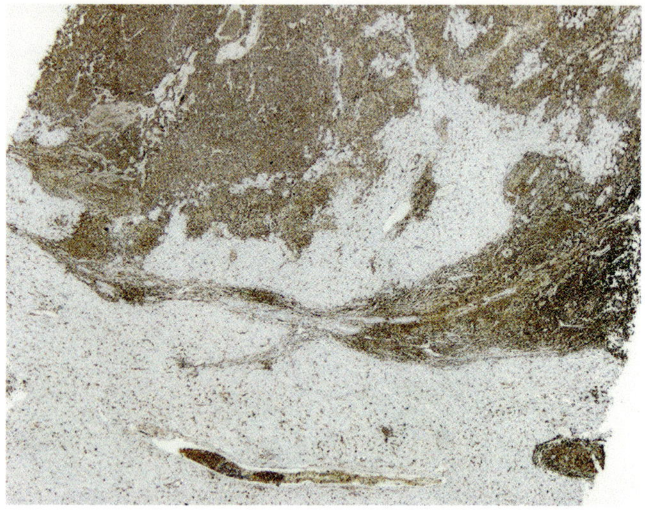

Fig. 7.218 Hepatic primary B-cell lymphoma. CD20 is positive, infiltrating into the adjacent liver tissue

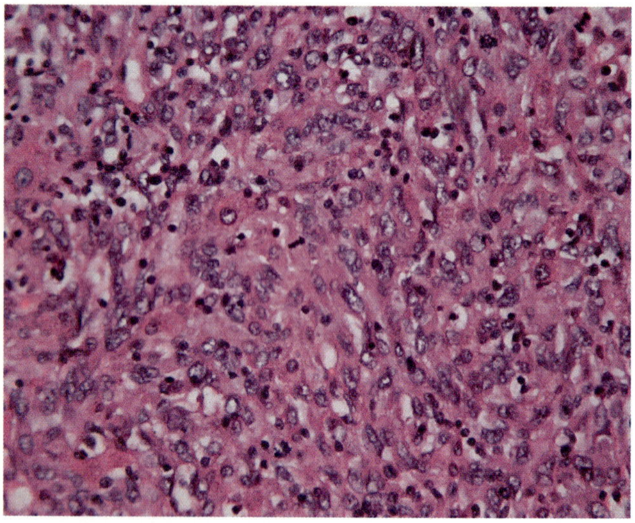

Fig. 7.219 Hepatic primary T-cell lymphoma. Conspicuously atypic neoplastic cells with active mitotic figures

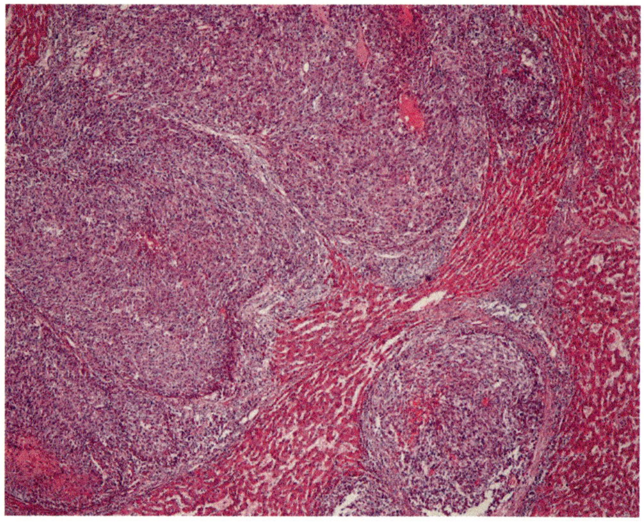

Fig. 7.220 Hepatic primary T-cell lymphoma. Tumor grows in multinodular pattern

phoma may contain red-colored irregular congestive zone around the yellow-white nodules (Figs. 7.214 and 7.215).

7.3.5.4 Microscopic Features

Lei et al. (1998) reviewed the 90 cases of PHL reported in the literature and found more than 20 histological types of PHL, including B cell-type, T cell-type, and non-B- and non-T-type PHL, accounting for 62, 30, and 8% of all the cases, respectively (Table 7.12) [126]. So far among all reports of PHL concerned non-Hodgkin's lymphoma, the most common types of lymphoma are diffuse large B cell lymphoma (DLBCL), T cell lymphoma, and lymphoma of mucosa-associated lymphoid tissue.

1. Diffuse large B cell lymphoma: This type of lymphoma consists of large and round cells arranged diffusely, with abundant cytoplasm, large nuclei, clear nuclear membranes, and prominent and eosinophilic nucleoli, and the mitotic figures can be easily observed (Fig. 7.216). The tumor cells grow diffusely along the hepatic plates or hepatic sinusoid with visible outline of liver lobules in the tumor tissues, with or without invasion of the portal vein (Fig. 7.217). They may also show a solid nodular growth pattern without residual liver tissue or portal areas. The tumor cells are positive for B cell-related antigens in immunohistochemistry, such as CD20 (Fig. 7.218).

2. T cell lymphoma: The tumor cells were relatively monotonous and medium in size with a rim of pale cytoplasm

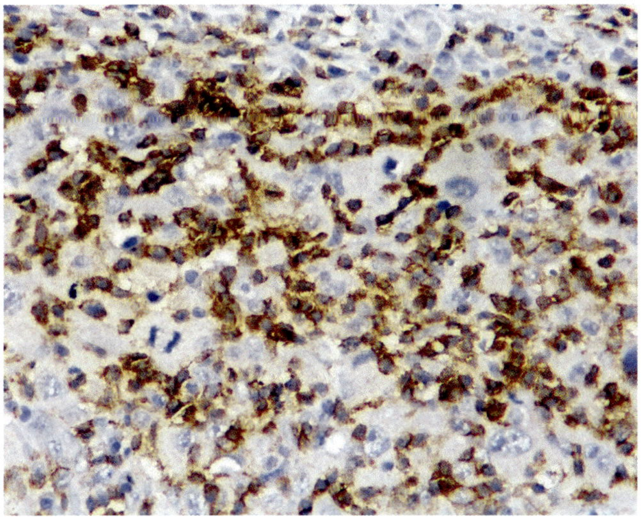

Fig. 7.221 Hepatic primary T-cell lymphoma. CD45RO staining is positive

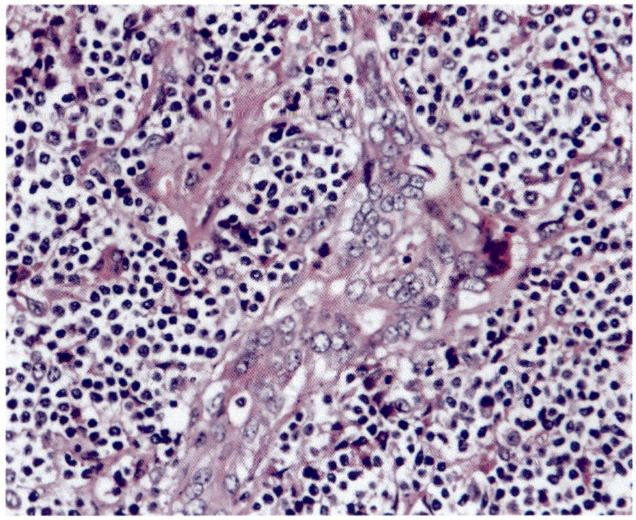

Fig. 7.222 Hepatic mucosa-associated lymphoid tissue lymphoma. Neoplastic cells infiltrated into the epitheliam of the bile duct

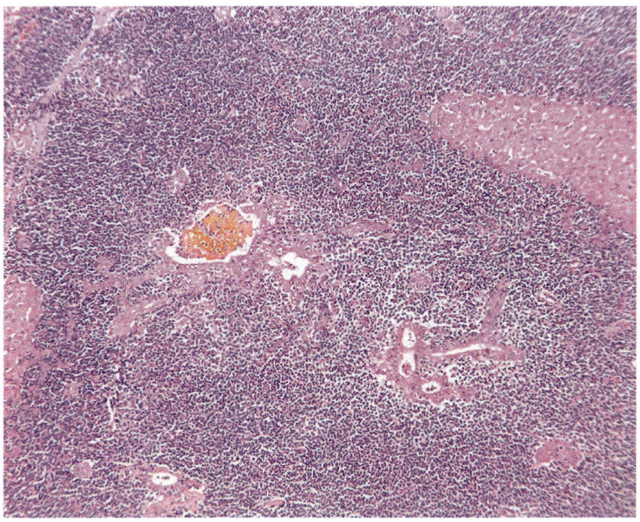

Fig. 7.223 Hepatic mucosa-associated lymphoid tissue lymphoma. Neoplastic cells infiltrated into the gland and the adjacent hepatic tissues

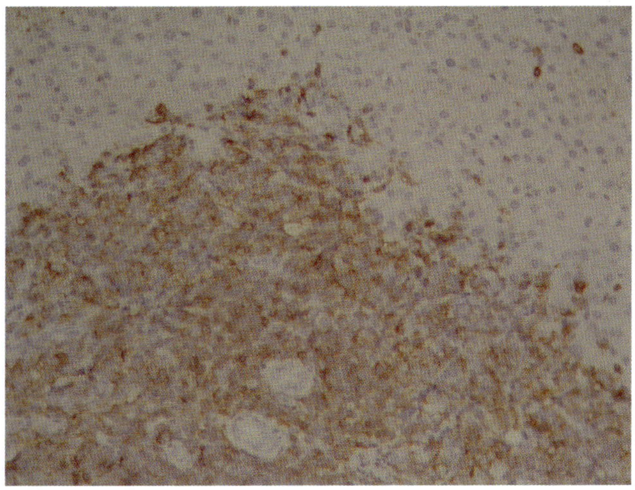

Fig. 7.224 Hepatic mucosa-associated lymphoid tissue lymphoma. CD20 staining is positive

and small basophilic nucleoli (Fig. 7.219), with no capsule, and it tends to infiltrate into portal areas and hepatic sinusoids (Fig. 7.220), showing positive stains for CD45RO (Fig. 7.221).

3. MALT lymphoma: It belongs to extranodal marginal zone B cell lymphoma, first put forward by Isaacson et al. (1983), who first reported hepatic MALT in 1995. More than ten cases of hepatic MALT lymphoma have been reported in the domestic and foreign literature. Some cases are complicated by EBV and HCV infection, as well as cases with primary biliary cirrhosis. And molecular biological studies have found that 60% of the cases have trisomy of chromosome 3 and 25–50% of cases contain chromosome translocation of t(11;18)(q21;q21) and t(3;14)(q27;q32), whereas, there was no t(11;18) chromosomal translocation in the highly aggressive lymphoma. Recent studies have suggested that CD40 signaling and Th2-type T cytokines play an important role in the development of MALT lymphoma.

MALT lymphoma is a low-grade malignant lymphoma, with slow growth and indolent clinical course, and is often

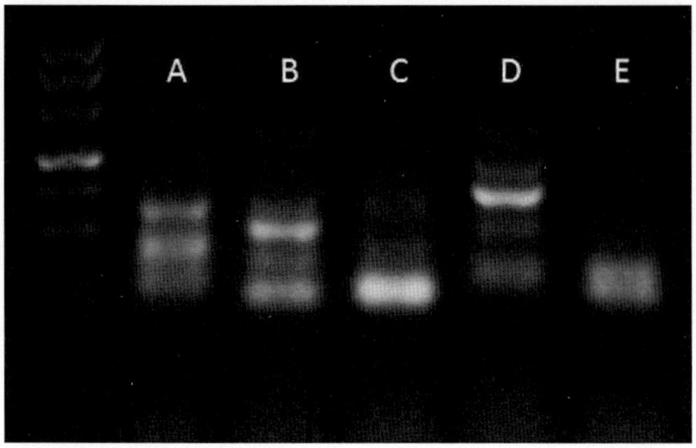

Fig. 7.225 Hepatic mucosa-associated lymphoid tissue lymphoma. IgH gene rearrangement: *A* VH-FR1 –JH(−) IgK gene rearrangement: *D* Vk-Jk(+) *B* VH-FR2 –JH(−) *E* Vk-intron-Kde(−) *C* VH-FR3 –JH(−)

accidentally discovered with no obvious clinical symptoms and normal liver function. Grossly, the tumor is 2–7.5 cm in diameter, pale gray or grayish red in color, and moderately hard in texture. The main points in pathological diagnosis include:

① Lesions with the portal area as the center consist of marginal B cells (i.e., centrocytic cells), monocytic B cells of varying amounts, small lymphocytes, plasma cells, and scattered immunoblastic and centroblastic cells, and some tumor cells can be signet ring like.
② Invasion of centrocytic cells and destruction of the bile duct epithelium form lymphatic epithelial lesions (Figs. 7.222 and 7.223).
③ The immune phenotype was CD20 (Fig. 7.224) positive, CD5, CD10, D1 cyclin, and CD23 negative, and 75% of the cases had IgH gene rearrangement (Fig. 7.225). The prognosis of this type treated with surgery has a good prognosis, and the tumor is sensitive to radiotherapy; however, it has a potential to develop into a highly malignant MALT lymphoma.

7.3.5.5 Differential Diagnosis

According to statistics, more than half of the cases of lymphoma can involve the liver in its late stages; therefore, metastatic hepatic lymphoma should be excluded before PHL was diagnosed. The diagnosis of primary hepatic lymphoma should be based on the following:

① Clinical symptoms were caused by liver disease.
② There was no distant lymphatic disease or lesions of related tissues and organs at confirmed diagnosis.
③ No bone marrow or peripheral blood cells of leukemia, and it is worth noting that there have been cases of leukemia with hepatic infiltration forming occupying lesions in the liver reported in the literature.
④ Extrahepatic metastasis of lymphoma was excluded in all the clinical, laboratory, imaging, pathological, and intraoperative examination.

7.3.5.6 Treatment and Prognosis

It is generally believed that the prognosis of PHL is better than that of HCC. The treatment of PHL is often surgery combined with chemotherapy or radiotherapy, and it needs to be combined with the specific circumstances of the patient to determine the personalized treatment strategy. Of all the 35 cases of PHL diagnosed in the Department of Pathology, Eastern Hepatobiliary Surgery Hospital, Second Military Medical University, the postoperative median survival period of the patients was 26.6 months, with the longest median survival period of 31.7 months found in patients with diffuse large B cell lymphoma. And one patient of PHL with surgical resection and postoperative chemotherapy was found to have a postoperative survival period of over 10 years till now, indicating that surgical resection should be preferred in the treatment of PHL, combining with postsurgical therapies, such as chemotherapy, radiotherapy, Chinese medicine, or immune therapy. And CHOP regimen is the standard chemotherapy for diffuse large B cell lymphoma. It has been found in the literature that patients of PHL treated with simple excision, simple chemotherapy, surgery combined with chemotherapy, and chemotherapy combined with radiotherapy had median survival periods of 22 months, 6 months, 13.6 months, and 27.5 months, respectively; however, the patients treated by palliative therapy had a median survival period of only 0.7 month.

Supplementary: Hepatosplenic T Cell Lymphoma

Hepatosplenic T cell lymphoma (HSTCL) was first described by Farcet et al. in 1990, was classified into special subtypes of peripheral T cell lymphoma by WHO, and is an independent lesion. T cell receptor (TCR) is a heterodimer composed of α and β chains or γ and δ chains. T cells with αβ chains of TCR constitute the majority of mature T cells in the peripheral blood, and they are positive for CD4 or CD8, while the T cells with TCR-γδ chains are negative for both CD4 and CD8, mainly distributed in the red pulp of the spleen, the sinusoids and perisinusoidal space of the liver, bone, and lymph nodes. Thus, HSTCL are mainly γδ type, including rare αβ type.

HSTCL are often found in young men clinically with an average of 35 years; however, cases involved 1–10-year-old children have features of strong invasion, rapid progression, and poor prognosis. The patients primarily manifest the type B symptoms of lymphoma, splenomegaly (100%), hepatomegaly (88%), and selective bone marrow involvement (53–86%). Most of the cases do not have nodular masses, but there are reports of multiple solid lesions with low density in the liver, the basic histological features of which are as follows: infiltration of tumorous T lymphocytes in hepatic sinusoids, red pulp of the spleen, bone marrow sinusoids, and lymph nodes. The tumor cells are often medium and rarely large in size with moderately pale eosinophilic cytoplasm, obscure boundaries, with round or oval nuclei, clear nuclear membrane, slightly dispersed chromatin, and small or inconspicuous nucleoli. Mitotic figures were not easily detected. And immunohistochemistry shows that the neoplastic cells are positive for CD2, CD3, CD43, and TCRγδ and negative for CD4 and CD8. Some neoplastic cells are positive for cytotoxic granule-associated protein TIA-1, while they are negative for perforin and granzyme B, suggesting that these tumor cells derive from immature peripheral γδT cells, but it has also been reported that neoplastic γδT cells can express granzyme B, as well as cytotoxicity. The neoplastic cells are rearranged in TCRγ TCRδ gene rearrangement.

1. Liver: It is characterized by aggregation and infiltration of lymphoid cells into expanded hepatic sinusoids, with varying numbers of lymphoid cells, which can sometimes be mistaken as inflammatory lesions in the liver, so it is also called as sinusoidal T cell lymphoma. It can also form multiple small ocupying lesions in the liver parenchyma, containing residual liver cell islet, and infiltration of neoplastic cells in the portal area to different degrees.
2. Spleen: The lymphoid cells mainly infiltrate into the cord and sinuses of the red pulp of the spleen, with expanded red pulp zone, dilated medullary sinuses, damage, atrophy, or disappearance of the white pulp, with or without extramedullary hematopoiesis.
3. Bone marrow: More than half of the patients had bone marrow involvement, which manifested that neoplastic cells infiltrated into bone marrow stroma and sinuses.
4. The counts of whole peripheral blood cells decrease. Neoplastic cells of medium or large in size can be observed, with moderate to rich granular basophilic cytoplasm and irregular nuclei.
5. Lymph nodes: The submandibular lymph nodes, mesenteric lymph nodes, and supraclavicular lymph nodes can be involved, which show dilation of the subcapsular lymph sinuses, containing infiltration of medium-sized lymphoid cells, and the structure of the lymph nodes can be completely destroyed.

7.3.6 Follicular Dendritic Cell Tumor

7.3.6.1 Pathogenesis and Mechanism

Follicular dendritic cell tumor (FDCT) was reported for the first time by Monde et al. in 1986, also known as follicular dendritic cell sarcoma. Dendritic cells are normal cellular components in follicular germinal centers, so two-thirds of the cases are found in lymph nodes; FDCT is occasionally found in extranodal sites, such as the ampulla, pancreas, spleen, and liver. Due to its postsurgical recurrence, this disease is considered to be a tumor of low-grade malignant potential or low-grade malignancy, rather than inflammatory lesions. A total of six cases of primary hepatic FDCT have been reported in the literature (Table 7.13). The majority of hepatic FDCT cases are positive for EBV-encoding RNA (EBER) in situ hybridization analysis, suggesting that the occurrence of the disease is closely related to EBV infection.

7.3.6.2 Clinical Features

Patients with hepatic FDCT are all females, with a mean age of 51 (35– 68) years. Clinical manifestations include upper abdominal distention, mild fever, weight loss, mild anemia, and polyclonal hypergammaglobulinemia. Individual patients have increased peripheral eosinophilia, which turns to normal after tumor resection. Ultrasonography and CT studies show low-density masses in the liver.

7.3.6.3 Gross Features

Hepatic FDCT lesions are large, with an average diameter of 13.1 (20–9.5) cm, grayish white, soft, with hemorrhage and necrosis, clear boundaries, with or without pseudocapsule.

7.3.6.4 Microscopic Features

The tumor cells are ovoid or plump spindled shape, with eosinophilic cytoplasm, obscure boundaries, and large and conspicuous nuclei which are ovoid or spindled, sparse chromatin, and fine and clear nuclear membrane, with central nucleoli. And multinucleated, bizarre nucleus or Reed-Sternberg-like cells can be found in the tumor tissue, without obvious atypia or mitotic figures. The tumor cells are arranged in sheets, short fascicles, storiform, or radiation structures. Sparse nonneoplastic inflammatory cells could

Table 7.13 Clinicopathological features of six cases of primary hepatic FDCT

Case	Age	Gender	Location	Diameter (cm)	EBV	Prognosis
1	35	Female	Right	20	Positive	Recurrence after 30 months
2	68	Female	Left	11	Positive	Has survived for 2.5 years
3	37	Female	Right	14.5	Positive	Already survived for 2 years
4	57	Female	Left	9.5	Positive	Already survived for 3 years
5	51	Female	Left	12	Positive	Already survived for 1 year
6	58	Female	Right	11.5	Positive	Already survived for 1 year

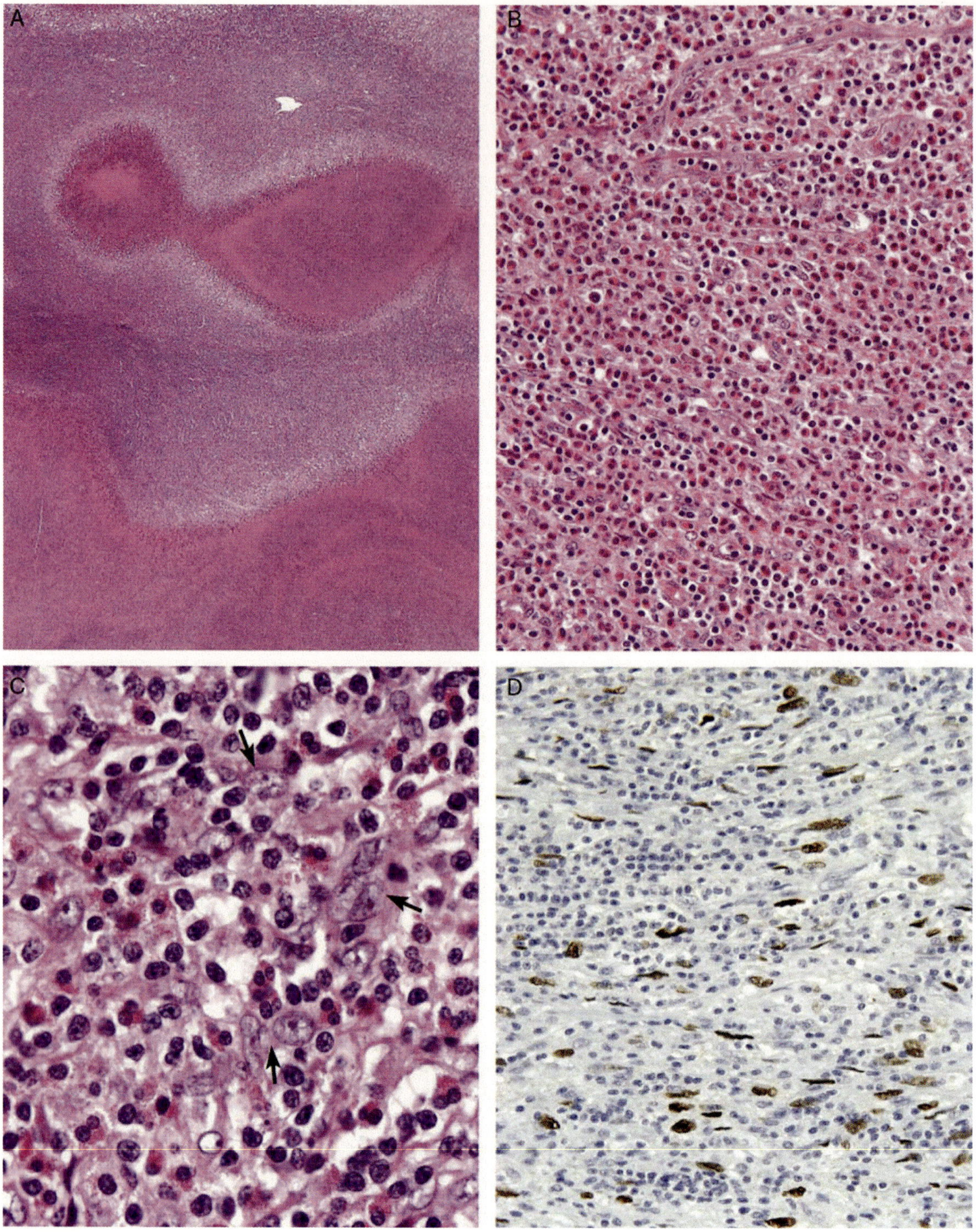

Fig. 7.226 Hepatic inflammatory pseudotumor-like follicular dendritic cell tumor. (**a**) Large necrotic eosinophilic abscesses are seen. (**b**) A heavy infiltration of eosinophils is evident. (**c**) Scattered tumor cells, including multinucleated ones (*arrows*), are interspersed within the inflammatory infiltrate. (**d**) The tumor cells are remarkably highlighted by in situ hybridization for EBV-encoded RNAs. They exhibit a range of nuclear atypia

also be found in the tumor. And the higher the grade of atypia of the neoplastic cells, the higher the grade of malignancy of the tumor.

Inflammatory pseudotumor-like FDCT (IPT like FDCT) is more often seen in the liver and spleen and is considered to be a special type of FDCT [127]. IPT-FDCT is more common in women, often associated with EBV infection, and clinical symptoms are commonly observed. Diffusely distributed tumor cells and a large number of mature plasma cells are mixed together in the tumor (Fig. 7.226), sometimes with infiltration of plenty of eosinophils, non-caseating epithelial granuloma like-cells, and Langhans giant cells. Furthermore, homogeneous coagulative necrosis, interstitial collagen fibrous tissue, or hyaline degeneration can also been discovered, with thickened vascular wall which is deposited by eosinophilic fibrinogen, similar to the histological performance of inflammatory pseudotumor.

7.3.6.5 Immunohistochemistry

The tumor cells are positive for follicular dendritic cell markers, such as CD21 and CD35, which are most commonly used in practice, CD23 with relatively low positive rate, CNA.42 with high sensitivity but low specificity, and other FDC antigens including clusterin, KiM4p, and KiFDRC1p can be expressed, while IPT-FDCT is sometimes positive for SMA, HHF-35, S100, CD68, as well as immunohistochemistry test for EBV-LMP1 or in situ hybridization of EBV-encoding RNA (EBER).

7.3.6.6 Differential Diagnosis

IPT-FDCT should be differentiated histologically from inflammatory pseudotumors, epithelial granulomatous lesions, and solitary necrotic nodules, and the findings of spindle cells, expression of FDC antigens, and EBV help to confirm the diagnosis. In addition, Hodgkin's lymphoma and malignant fibrous histiocytoma also need to be differentiated from FDCT.

7.3.6.7 Treatment and Prognosis

On the whole, the local recurrence rate of FDCT is 36%, and the metastasis rate is 28%. FDCT has lower grade of malignancy than lymphoma, which is similar to low-grade malignant tumors of the soft tissue. Moreover, the malignancy of the hepatic FDCT seems to be lower than that of FDCT in other sites, with a relatively slow clinical process. Ge et al. (2014) reviewed the cases of hepatic IPT-like FDCT reported in the literature, in which metastasis and recurrence occurred in four cases after the initial treatment and peritoneal recurrence occurred 8 and 108 months after the treatment, respectively, in two cases. The total recurrence rate is 11.8%, and the mortality rate is 2.9% [128].

7.3.7 Extramedullary Plasmacytoma

Wen-Ming Cong and Qian Zhao
Department of Pathology, Eastern Hepatobiliary Surgery Hospital, Second Military Medical University, Shanghai, China

7.3.7.1 Pathogenesis and Mechanism

Plasmacytoma or myeloma is divided into intramedullary and extramedullary categories. Schriddel et al. (1905) first described extramedullary plasmacytoma (EMP). Cases of solitary EMP in locations other than hematopoietic tissues in the bone marrow account for 3%, 90% of which occur in abundant lymphoid tissues, such as the head and neck, upper respiratory tract, and oral cavity, while only about 10% of the cases are found in the digestive tract, and the brain and thyroid are less involved. Weichhold et al. (1995) reported the first hepatic EMP, and there are six cases of hepatic EMP reported in the literature till now. Currently, the biological characteristics of primary hepatic EMP are poorly understood.

According to the reports in the literature [129–131], the diagnosis criteria of primary EMP should include the following: ① the lesions are monoclonal proliferation of plasma cells confirmed by histopathology, immunopathology, and molecular pathology; ② patients have no systemic diseases (hypercalcemia, renal failure, anemia, or bone lesions), with normal bone marrow and no evidence of multiple myeloma; and ③ monoclonal immunoglobulin levels in serum and urine are normal.

7.3.7.2 Clinical Features

Lee et al. (2007) reported one case of hepatic solitary EMP, concerning a 60-year-old male patient with a 2 cm × 2 cm mass in segment VI of the liver found in imaging. MRI showed a low-signal lesion on T1-weighted imaging and a high-signal lesion on T2-weighted imaging. CT showed a hypervascular tumor, with low density in portal venous phase. Other examinations demonstrated normal results, such as hepatic and renal function, bone marrow, serum calcium, β-2 microglobulin, immunoelectrophoresis of serum, and urine proteins [132].

7.3.7.3 Gross Features

Cut section is grayish yellow or grayish red. And hemorrhage and necrosis are common. The tumors have obscure boundaries from the surrounding tissues, often without encapsulation, or with a pseudocapsule, and they infiltrated into the surrounding liver tissue.

7.3.7.4 Microscopic Features

The tumor is a solitary lesion consisting of tumor cells with characteristics of plasma cells. The cells are often mature plasma cells and proplasmacytes (immature plasma cells) arranged in clusters or strip structures. The tumor cells similar to mature plasma cells are well differentiated, while those similar to plasmablasts of different degrees are poorly differentiated, containing tumor giant cells or immunoblasts with dual, multiple, or multilobular nuclei, atypia, no radiation arranged chromatin, thickened nuclear membrane, prominent nucleoli, and conspicuous nuclear mitotic figures. PAS staining shows the Russell bodies in the cytoplasm, and Congo red staining shows amyloid substances in the stroma tissues. The tumor has no capsule and can infiltrate into the portal tract and the adjacent liver tissue.

7.3.7.5 Immunohistochemistry

Monoclonal nature of the plasma cells can be further confirmed by PCR gene rearrangement or in situ hybridization analysis, and VS38 monoclonal antibody expression can be a confirmation of the plasmacytic differentiation.

7.3.7.6 Differential Diagnosis

1. Multiple myeloma with involvement of the liver: The diagnosis of isolated hepatic EMP should be made by bone marrow biopsy, bone X-ray, serum and urine immunoelectrophoresis, etc., to exclude multiple myeloma or other locations of the plasma cell tumor invasion of the liver.
2. Hepatic pseudotumor/reactive plasmocytoma/plasma cell granuloma: These tumors may contain a large amount of plasma cells and should be differentiated. Hepatic pseudotumor is not only complex in the composition of inflammatory cells but also rich in fibrous stroma tissue, as well as multiple thick-walled blood vessels with hyaline degeneration, and its plasmacytic component is multiclone.
3. Diffuse large B cell lymphoma/Burkitt lymphoma: When EMP is poorly differentiated, it should be distinguished from lymphoma. The latter is positive for LCA and CD20 while negative for VS38.
4. Posttransplantation lymphoproliferative disorders (PTLDs): It has been reported that EMP-like PTLDs can occur in the solid organs, such as the liver, even 7 years after the transplantation, with abundant lymphocytic components. Some cases were related to EBV infection, and the reduction of immunosuppressive agents is helpful for the regression of the tumor.

7.3.7.7 Treatment and Prognosis

It is a low-grade malignant tumor and highly sensitive to radiotherapy. Currently reported cases of hepatic EMP were often treated with surgical resection, and for those with positive margin, adjuvant radiotherapy should be considered. And for those with unresectable lesions, chemotherapy and local radiotherapy can achieve better therapeutic effects. The prognosis of the patients is relatively good, with a 10-year survival rate up to 70%, and less than 30% of the cases may progress to a systemic disease [133].

7.3.8 Histiocytic Sarcoma

Histiocytic sarcoma (HS) is a rare malignant proliferative disease of histiocytes, which is characterized by mature histiocytes in both morphology and immunohistochemistry. And the diagnosis of HS mainly depends on the confirmation of differentiation of the histiocytes and exclusion of other poorly differentiated malignant tumors, such as lymphoma, carcinoma, sarcoma, melanoma, etc. About one-third of HS cases are found in the lymph nodes, and about one-third in the skin, and other one-third in extranodal sites (mainly in the gastrointestinal tract), while cases have occasionally been reported in other locations, such as the central nervous system, spleen, bone marrow, nasal cavity, lung, thyroid gland, and bile duct [134]. There were two cases of hepatic HS, one case in Chinese (unpublished) and the other in English [135].The latter concerned a patient with chronic Langhans cell histiocytosis of the skin, Rosai-Dorfman disease, and lymphoma in the splenic marginal zone, followed by sudden occurrence of hepatic HS and subsequent death in a short term.

Microscopically, the tumor had obscure boundary with the surrounding liver tissues, and it grew in an invasive growth pattern. The tumor cells were diffusely distributed with poor adhesive ability in most areas, round or oval in shape and large in volume with abundant eosinophilic cytoplasm. Some of them contain vacuoles or are filled with microvacuoles. The nuclei are large, round or oval, vacuolated, with visible deviated nuclei, visible enlarged nucleoli, and conspicuous mitotic figures. Focal multinucleated giant cell tumor can be observed with visible phagocytosis of red blood cells in the cytoplasm of part of the tumor giant cells (hemophagocytic phenomenon). And a large number of reactive cells are commonly seen in the background, including small lymphocytes, plasma cells, neutrophils, and eosinophils. Obvious hemorrhage can be found in local regions of the tumor, as well as foci of necrosis.

Immunohistochemistry shows that the tumor cells are strong positive for one or more histiocytic markers, including CD68, lysozyme and CD163, and S-100 (scattered positive). While they are negative for Hep Par-1, AFP, broad spectrum of CK, langerin, CD1a, CD30, CD31, CD21, CD23, DOG-1, MPO, CAM 5.2, ALK, HMB45, melan-A, CK5/6, and myoglobin. And the nonneoplastic cells in the background are positive for LCA, CD3, CD20, and MPO, and Ki-67 proliferation index varies greatly in different cases. Interestingly, some HS lesions are found in patients with B cell lymphoma (especially follicular lymphoma) or precursor B cell-type acute lymphoblastic leukemia, and IGH/BCL2 gene fusion [136] and monoclonal rearrangement of IGH and TCRγ [137, 138] can be found in molecular pathological study. HS should be distinguished from follicular dendritic cell sarcoma and dif fuse large B cell lymphoma.

Histiocytosarcoma is generally a highly aggressive tumor, with poor response to treatment. Most patients (70%) are diagnosed at advanced stages, and 60–80% of the patients die of its progression. It seems that several factors play an important role in the prognosis of HS. The most important factor is the site and stage of the disease. For instance, the clinical course of HS in the central nervous system and disseminated disease is most aggressive. The second factor for prognosis is the size of the tumor. The patients with large primary tumors (>3.5 cm) appear to have a poor prognosis and short survival period. In addition, proliferation index of tumor cells has a certain impact on the prognosis of the patients [139]. Currently, no standard therapeutic strategy has been formulated for histiocytosarcoma, and comprehensive treatment based on surgery combined with chemotherapy is helpful. Patients with HS have a poor overall prognosis, and the average survival period was reported to be 4–24 months [138].

7.4 Muscular, Fibrous, and Adipose Tumors

7.4.1 Leiomyosarcoma

7.4.1.1 Pathogenesis and Mechanism

Hepatic sarcoma accounts for 0.5–1% of the hepatic malignant tumors. According to the statistics of data on surgically resected hepatic lesions in Eastern Hepatobiliary Surgery Hospital, Second Military Medical University, from January 1982 to December 2011, a total of 11 cases of primary hepatic leiomyosarcoma (LMS) have been found, accounting for 5.59% of all 185 cases of 12 types of hepatic nonepithelial malignant tumors (Table 7.14). By 1992, there are more than 60 cases of hepatic LMS reported in the English literature, and it is estimated that there are more than 100 cases have been reported, not including more than 50 cases of primary LMS in the hepatic circular ligament and the inferior vena cava, and more than 10 cases have been found in domestic reports. The pathogenesis of hepatic LMS is not clear, and previous reports of "leiomyosarcoma" in the literature concerned children with AIDS and patients treated by immunosuppressive agents, while now it is considered to be a kind of EB virus-associated smooth muscle tumor (EBV-SMT) [140], which actually includes malignant leiomyosarcoma and has become the second most common malignant tumor in AIDS on children or can be found in patients using immunosuppressive agents after transplantation or immunosuppressive diseases such as autoimmune diseases and common immunodeficiency syndrome. The histological origin of hepatic LMS is still unknown, and it presumably originates from smooth muscle in parts of the liver, such as smooth muscle cells of intrahepatic portal vein, bile duct and hepatic ligamentum teres, or myoblasts, intrahepatic pluripotent stem cells which might be the common origin of mesenchymal tumors in the liver.

7.4.1.2 Clinical Features

In the 11 cases of LMS diagnosed in the Department of Pathology, Eastern Hepatobiliary Surgery Hospital, Second Military Medical University, five are males and six are females, with an average age of 50.2 years ranged from 31 to 74 years, with 27.27% of the patients complicated with HBV infection. Three cases were discovered by physical examination. The tumors are usually large when patients come to the clinic, and two-thirds of the patients have pain in the hepatic zone with discomfort, nausea, poor appetite, and weight loss

Table 7.14 Clinical and pathological characteristics of 12 types of malignant mesenchymal tumors in the liver

Pathological type	Number of cases	Male	Female	Proportion	Age (years)	Diameter of the tumor (cm)	HBV infection
Undifferentiated sarcoma	39	30	9	0.21	5–70, 36.0 ± 22.2	4–25, 12.6 ± 4.9	15
Lymphoma	35	25	10	0.19	17–79, 50.9 ± 16.4	1–20, 8.4 ± 5.1	12
Malignant fibrous histiocytoma	29	22	7	0.16	5–71, 47.6 ± 11.8	3–28, 9.9 ± 5.8	14
Epithelioid hemangioendothelioma	20	8	12	0.11	20–80, 50.2 ± 15.4	2–10, 4.8 ± 2.3	3
Hemangioendothelioma angiosarcoma	18	10	8	0.10	4–78, 52.2 ± 17.8	2–14, 8.8 ± 3.5	2
Infantile hemangioendothelioma	12	6	6	0.06	5–61 months (38.8 ± 24.8)	1.4–11.7 (4.7 ± 2.5)	0
Leiomyosarcoma	11	5	6	0.06	31–74, 50.2 ± 13.7	2–23, 10.5 ± 6.4	3
Fibrosarcoma	9	5	4	0.05	34–61, 50.9 ± 10.0	1–14, 9.9 ± 3.8	3
Liposarcoma	3	0	3	0.02	26–43, 34.7 ± 8.5	5–17, 9.7 ± 4.2	0
Malignant hemangiopericytoma	3	1	2	0.02	44–61, 52.7 ± 8.5	7–13, 10.3 ± 3.1	1
Malignant mesothelioma	3	1	2	0.02	41–58, 50.0 ± 8.5	7–22, 12.3 ± 8.4	1
Malignant peripheral nerve sheath tumor	3	1	2	0.02	37–52, 46.7 ± 8.4	4–20, 12.0 ± 8.0	0
Total	185	114	71	1	4–80, 46.2 ± 17.3	1–28, 9.9 ± 5.3	54

in 50% of the patients, with or without abdominal swelling or lump, tenderness, and percussion pain in the hepatic zone, all of which are nonspecific. Some patients have early manifestations of hepatic abscess, such as night sweats, mild fever, fatigue, or emaciation, and ascites, edema of lower extremities, and cachexia are found in advanced hepatic LMS. Skin metastasis of LMS is found in a few cases as the first sign, and Budd-Chiari syndrome is observed in LMS with invasion or origination of the hepatic vein or inferior vena cava.

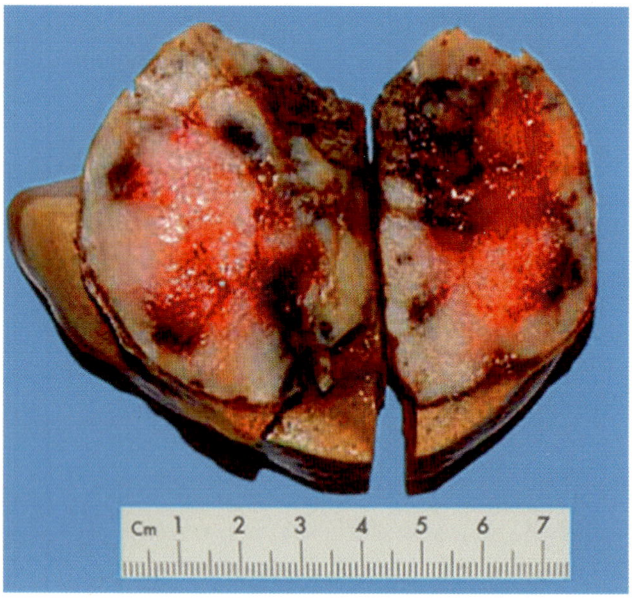

Fig. 7.227 Hepatic leiomyosarcoma. The cross sections of the tumors were multi-colored ranging from *gray* to *grayish brown*, fish-like and soft in texture, with local foci of hemorrhage and necrosis

Laboratory examination shows no specific tumor markers to assist the diagnosis of primary hepatic LMS. More than 50% of the patients present increased lactate dehydrogenase, and a small number of patients have mildly abnormal liver function, while elevated blood bilirubin, prolonged coagulation time are found in advanced cases. Imaging of hepatic LMS on CT and MRI are nonspecific, usually showing rich vascular manifestations. CT images show large heterogeneous hypodensities with clear boundaries with enhancement in the lesions or surround them or cystic masses with enhancement of the thick wall. MRI T1-weighted imaging shows homogeneous or heterogeneous low-density masses, while T2-weighted imaging shows high-density masses, with visible capsules in some cases.

7.4.1.3 Gross Features

Of the 11 cases of LMS diagnosed in the Department of Pathology, Eastern Hepatobiliary Surgery Hospital, Second Military Medical University, 55% (6/11) of the lesions were located in the right lobe of the liver, with a mean diameter of 10.5 + 6.4 (ranged 2–23) cm, and 36.4% of them were multiple nodules. The cross sections of the tumors were multicolored ranging from gray to grayish brown, fish-like and soft in texture, with local foci of hemorrhage and necrosis (Fig. 7.227) or cystic degeneration and no encapsulation, but the boundaries were clear. Some cases contained multinodular lesions, and tumor thrombus can be sometimes found in the portal area and branches of the hepatic portal vein.

7.4.1.4 Microscopic Features

Hepatic LMS and LMS of other deep organs are similar in morphology. Well-differentiated or low-grade LMS mainly consist of spindle cells arranged in intersecting fascicles with

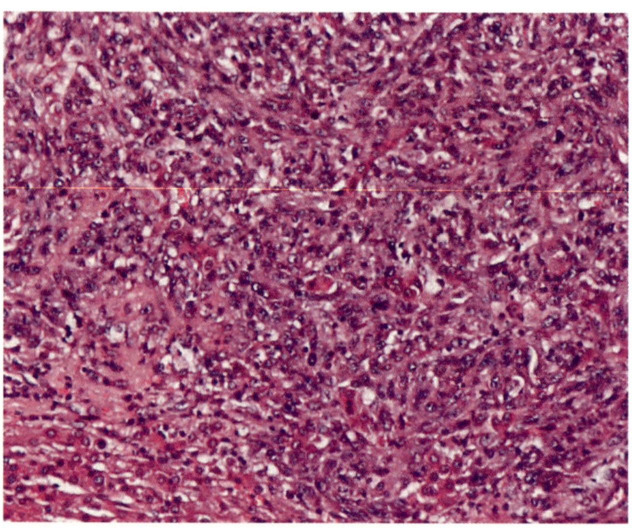

Fig. 7.228 Hepatic leiomyosarcoma. Spindle shaped neoplastic cells arranged in intersecting fasciclesi

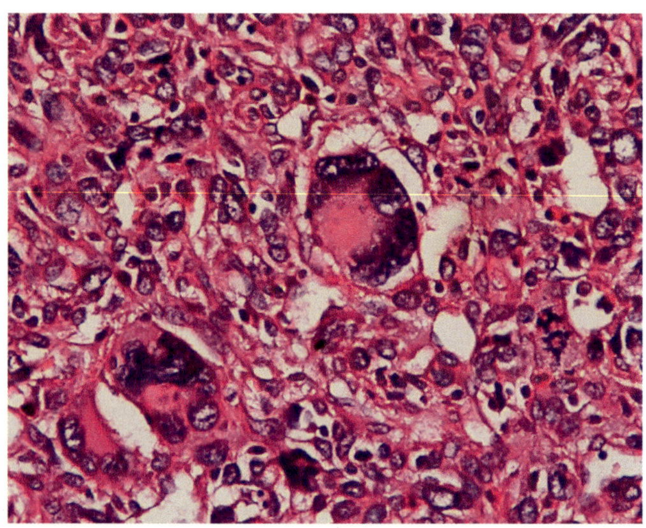

Fig. 7.229 Hepatic pleomorphic leiomyosarcoma. Tumor giant cells with pleomorphic nuclei

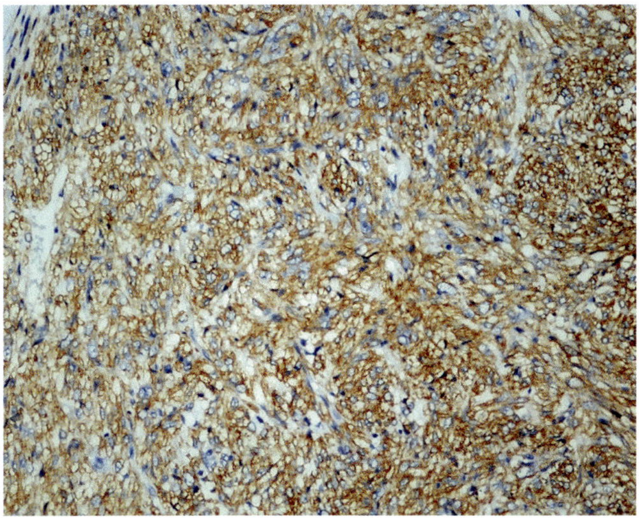

Fig. 7.230 Hepatic pleomorphic leiomyosarcoma. SMA staining is positive

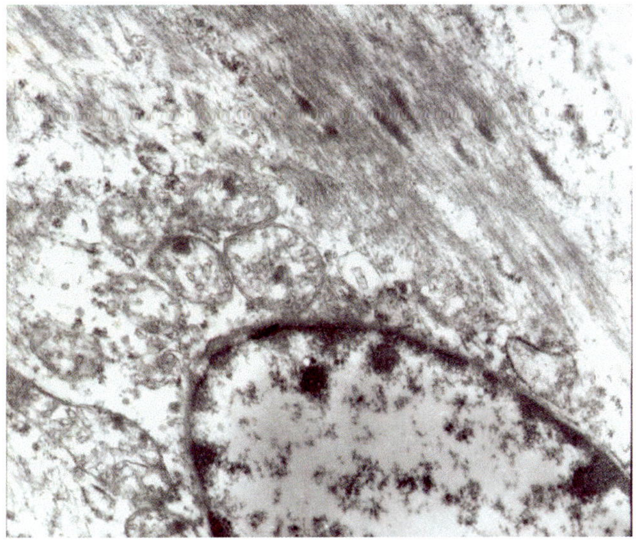

Fig. 7.231 Hepatic leiomyosarcoma. Tumor cells are filled with numerous well-oriented, thin (6–8 nm) myofilaments

clear cell boundaries, pale eosinophilic cytoplasm, numerous well-oriented myofibrils longitudinally placed parallel lines running the length of the nucleus. The cytoplasm of these cells is red in Masson staining, yellow in VG staining, and blue in PTAH staining. The nucleus of the tumor cells in LMS is "cigar shaped" and blunt-ended, hyperchromatic staining, coarse chromatin (Fig. 7.228), and small vacuoles. In some smooth muscle cells, a PAS-positive vacuole is seen at one end of the nucleus, causing a slight indentation which is of diagnostic significance. Mitotic figures more than 5/10 HPF suggest increased malignancy. Poorly differentiated LMS cells are diffuse in arrangement, with nonsignificant fascicle structures, and the cells are pleomorphic (pleomorphic LMS), with or without eosinophilic granular tumor-like cells and tumor giant cells (Fig. 7.229) which are stronger in proliferative activity and invasive biological behaviors. Mucinous LMS presents obvious stroma mucus secretion, while epithelioid LMS cells were obviously epithelioid with tumor cells of round, polygonal, or short spindled, and their cytoplasm is often pale stained or transparent. Silver staining showed the longitudinal distribution of reticular fibers between the fascicles of tumor cells without wrapping around individual cells.

In addition, the recently proposed EB virus-associated smooth muscle tumors (EBV-SMT) is considered to be an independent type, often demonstrating multifocal growth and budding into the vicinity of small blood vessels, and intersecting fascicles of well-differentiated smooth muscle cells can be seen in the lesions.

7.4.1.5 Immunohistochemistry

SMA (Fig. 7.230), muscle-specific actin (HHF35), actin, vimentin, and desmin staining are positive, while CK and EMA can also be positive in epithelioid LMS, which are usually visible in the perinuclear regions possibly due to the presence of keratin 8 and 18. Recently, 1H1 has been reported to be a relatively specific marker for identification of smooth muscle cells. And H-caldesmon can be used to distinguish smooth muscle cells and myofibroblast, while it is positive in 40% of LMS.

7.4.1.6 Electron Microscopic Observation

Differentiated leiomyosarcomas have deeply clefted nuclei and numerous well-oriented myofilaments and dense bodies, dense plague and extracellular basal lamina surrounding the cell membrane (Fig. 7.231). The pinocytotic vesicles and intercellular bridge are conspicuous. On the other hand, poorly differentiated tumors show a loss of myofilaments as rough endoplasmic reticulum, and free ribosomes assume greater prominence.

7.4.1.7 Differential Diagnosis

LMS accounts for 2–9% of all soft tissue sarcomas, and the predilection sites include the uterus, gastrointestinal tract, inferior vena cava, and peritoneal regions; thus, it should be excluded that LMS originates from extrahepatic metastasis in the first place. Well-differentiated LMS should also be distinguished from benign hepatic leiomyoma, and deep LMS often contains more than 5/10 HPF of mitotic figures and/or larger than 5 cm in diameter, apart from atypia and infiltrating growth pattern. Besides, hepatic LMS should also be distinguished from spindled cell tumors, such as hepatic embryonal rhabdomyosarcoma (ERMS), fibrosarcoma (FS), malignant fibrous histiocytoma (MFH), and malignant peripheral nerve sheath tumor (MPNST). Differential diagnosis mainly depends on the morphological features of the

Table 7.15 Clinical and pathological characteristics of five types of malignant mesenchymal tumors in the liver

Key points	LMS	ERMS	FS	MFH	MPNST
Average age (years old)	57	3	55	55	62.5
Male proportion (%)	45	87.5	67	53	100
Cellular morphology	Long spindled	Polymorphism	Spindled	Polymorphism	Long spindled
Nuclear morphology	"cigar shaped" with both blunt ends	Spindled, round	Spindled, both tapering ends	Polymorphism	Round, spindled
Arrangement	Intersecting fascicles	Diffuse	Herring bone	Radiating storiform	Paliform, swirl
Positive immunohistochemical staining	SMA/vimentin / desmin	Myoglobin/ vimentin/desmin	vimentin	vimentin/ACT/CD68	S-100/MBP
Features under electron microscope	Smooth muscle cell	Striated muscle cell	Fibroblast	Multiple cells	Nerve sheath cell
Rate of metastasis (%)	40.9	40	33	34	—
Rate of tumor rupture (%)	0	—	14	0	—
Resection rate (%)	50	—	31	77	—

Table 7.16 Comparison of fusion rate of PAX3-FKHR or PAX7-FKHR between ARMS and ERMS

	ARMS		ERMS	
Literature	PAX3-FKHR	PAX7-FKHR	PAX3-FKHR	PAX7-FKHR
Barr [149]	16/21 (76%)	2/21 (10%)	1/30 (3%)	1/30 (3%)
De Alava [150]	7/13 (54%)	2/13 (15%)	0/9 (0)	0/9 (0)
Downing [151]	20/23 (87%)		2/12 (17%)	
Arden [152]	8/13 (62%)	1/13 (8%)	0/11 (0)	0/11 (0)
Total	51/70 (73%)	5/47 (11%)	3/62 (5%)	1/50 (2%)

cells and combination of immunohistochemical staining, and the key points for differential diagnosis are summarized in Table 7.15.

7.4.1.8 Treatment and Prognosis

All the LMS lesions are similar in biological behavior with highly invasive growth, regardless of their locations. Hepatic LMS can metastasize to the lung, peritoneum, pancreas, and pleura, which is of poor prognosis, and the resection rate is about 50%. Patients without any treatment often died within 1 year after the diagnosis, and their 5-year survival rate was 29%. Tumor size, necrosis, vascular invasion, age of the patient, and nuclear mitotic figures are related to the differentiation and prognosis of the tumor. The combination of surgical treatment and chemotherapy can prolong the average survival period of hepatic LMS patients to 3.3 years, while combination of chemotherapy and radiotherapy could raise the postoperative 5-year survival rate to 53% for patients with LMS originating from the inferior vena cava.

Usually, EBV-SMT is multifocal lesions with better prognosis than traditional LMS, and its histological features are of little significance with the prognosis. In the published literature, only 35% of the EBV-SMV patients died, and most of the deaths were caused by other diseases, such as opportunistic infection, rather than SMT. In the reported 36 cases with treatment data, surgical resection was still the main treatment method, while in two cases with solitary EBV-SMT, radical surgical resection and active antiretroviral therapy led to complete remission of the disease [140]. And for cases diagnosed as EBV-SMT with LMS, the patients should be treated with chemotherapy, radiotherapy, and other adjuvant therapies; however, EBV-SMT shows tolerance to cytotoxic chemotherapy. Furthermore, improving the immune status can improve the prognosis of the patients with EBV-SMT.

7.4.2 Rhabdomyosarcoma

7.4.2.1 Pathogenesis and Mechanism

The liver tissue did not contain striated muscle cells; thus, rhabdomyosarcoma (RMS) in the liver parenchyma may derive from pluripotent stem cells existing in the portal area. The etiology of RMS is unknown. Genetic factors are implicated by the rare occurrence of the disease in siblings [141], at the same time, the occasional presence of the tumor at birth [142], and the association of the disease with other neoplasms in the same patient. It has been reported that RMS is related to a variety of genetic diseases, such as hereditary nephroblastoma, familial polyposis, multiple lentigines syndrome, neurofibromatosis type 1, and a variety of congenital anomalies. The majority of alveolar RMS (ARMS) cases have chromosome translocation of t(2;13)(q35;q14), forming PAX3-FKHR fusion gene on chromosome 13 and FKHR-PAX3 fusion gene on chromosome 2, and the former is more sensitive and specific for RMS detection. Another ARMS sub-type has the chromosomal translocation of t(1;13)(p36;q14), forming PAX7-FKHR, and it is likely that the fusion proteins that result from the translocations involving these genes aberrantly regulate a common set of target genes involved in the pathogenesis of ARMS. Barr et al. [143] conducted a fusion gene detection in RMS tissues using RT-PCR, showing 35 cases (59%) with PAX3-FKHR fusion, 11 cases (19%) with PAX7-FKHR fusion, and 13 cases (22%) without detectable fusion gene. Overall, more than 80% of the histologically diagnosed ARMS cases contained PAX3-FKHR or PAX7-FKHR fusion (Table 7.16) with poor prognosis [144].

Embryonic RMS (ERMS) has different cytogenetic changes compared to ARMS, demonstrating loss of heterozygosity of multiple linkage loci on chromosome 11p15.5 [145], causing secondary inactivation of tumor suppressor genes, including human tyrosine hydroxylase gene [146] or GOK [147] or trisomy chromosome 8 [148]

Primary hepatic RMS is very rare, and 46 cases have been reported in foreign literature. Schoofs et al. [153] reported 1 case and reviewed 12 cases of hepatic primary RMS, finding 5 cases of pleomorphic RMS (PRMS), 2 cases of ERMS, 2 cases of ARMS, and 4 cases of undifferentiated type, as well as PAX3/FOXO1A gene fusion. Fourteen cases have been found in domestic literature since 1982, of which six cases occurred in children.

7.4.2.2 Clinical Features

Primary hepatic RMS occurs mainly in young male children under 3 years of age, with the biliary tree as one of the most common predilection sites in children RMS, accounting for 1% in all children RMS cases. And the tumors are found at birth in about 2% of them. Adult hepatic RMS affected patients 34–76 years of age. PRMS is the common type in adult patients. ERMS (mainly botryoid RMS) is the primary type of RMS involving the bile duct. One case was diagnosed as hepatic ERMS in Eastern Hepatobiliary Surgery Hospital, concerning a female patient 57 years of age. Patients with hepatic RMS often clinically manifest intermittent jaundice, with or without abdominal distention, hepatomegaly, pain in the hepatic zone and discomfort, fever, weight loss, and so on. Budd-Chiari syndrome can occur in cases with invasion of the hepatic vein which have a worse prognosis. Serum AFP was negative, but it has been reported in one case of adult hepatic RMS that serum AFP reached to 167.7 μg/L. CT images showed that RMS has a mass of low density, with no enhancement, clear boundary, central necrosis, and local calcification. MRI T1-weighted images show a hypodense signal, while T2-weighted images show hyperdense signal. Ultrasound type B shows no specific signs.

7.4.2.3 Gross Features

The tumor contains multiple or solitary lesions with varying sizes, and single nodule is 8 (3–14) cm in diameter on average. The cross section of the tumor is often light yellow or grayish white, fish-like with glistening (Fig. 7.232), colliquative necrosis, and cyst formation, or mucus in cases containing much amounts of collagenous or myxoid stroma, without obvious capsule. RMS deriving from bile ducts presents grape-like or polypoid growth of tumor tissue in multiple

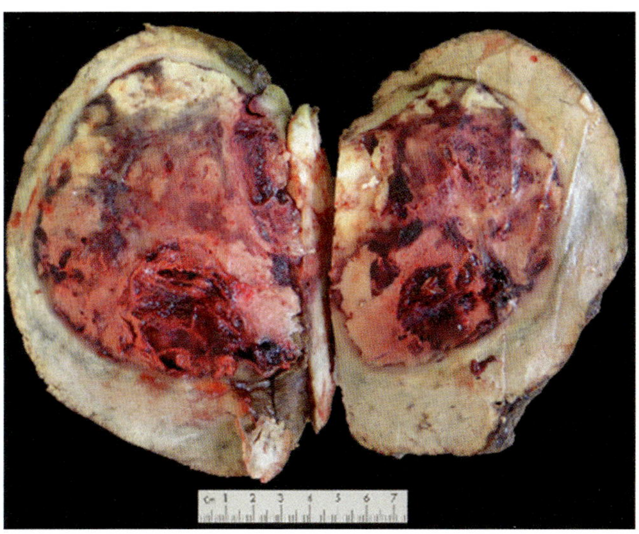

Fig. 7.232 Hepatic rhabdomyosarcoma. The cross section of the tumor is multi-colored, with thin capsule, extensive haemarrhage and necrosis, non-cirrhotic surrounding liver tissues

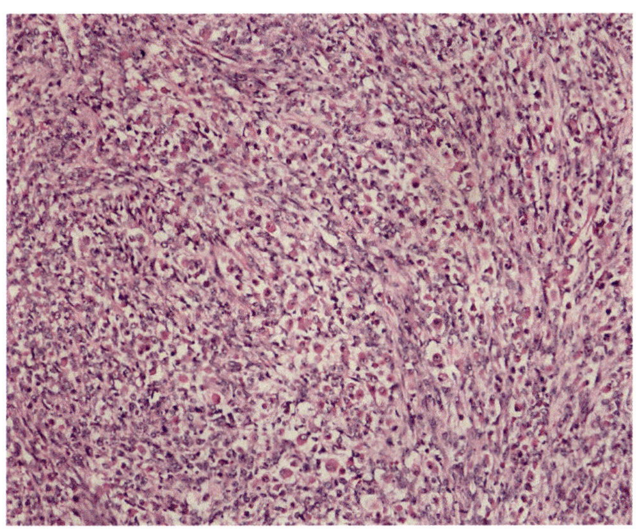

Fig. 7.233 Hepatic rhabdomyosarcoma. The tumor cells can be spindled, small round, oval shaped, arranged as cord or sheet

bile duct branches, with thickened bile duct wall, luminal stenosis, and well circumscribed, which is confined in the lumen.

7.4.2.4 Microscopic Features

1. ERMS is the most common, accounting for approximately 49% of all RMS. Tumor tissue is composed of varying degrees of cellularity with alternating densely packed, hypercellular areas, and loosely textured myxoid areas, with largely varying morphology of tumor cells, which are associated with the number and differentiation of rhabdomyoblasts. The tumor cells can be spindled, small round, oval, strap, racquet shape, tadpoles, or spider-like with abundanteosinophilic cytoplasm (Fig. 7.233), and 50–60% of the cases show cross striations or longitudinal striation in PATH staining; the cytoplasm of these large round or oval rhabdomyoblast-like cells contains granular material or deeply eosinophilic masses of stringy or fibrillary material concentrically arranged near or around the nucleus. Their nuclei are small and deviated, with abundant nuclear chromatin, conspicuous nuclear membrane, and prominent nucleoli. The dedifferentiated rhabdomyoblasts contain dark-red cytoplasm with hyalinization and pyknotic nuclei without cross striations, with small amounts of stromal collagen and varying quantity of mucus-like substance. Biliary RMS grows around the bile ducts with direct connection to dense tumor cells and normal biliary mucosal epithelium, while the deep layer of the tumor cells is separated by the loose myxoid stroma containing rich acidic and sticky polysaccharide, accompanied by infiltration of inflammatory cells, necrosis, and hemorrhage.
2. ARMS is the second common subtype, accounting for approximately 31%, that consists of a large number of poorly differentiated small round or oval tumor cells showing central loss of cellular cohesion and formation of irregular "alveolar" spaces or arranged as papillary, nested, or diffuse pattern, surrounded by a framework of dense and hyalinized fibrous septa. Floating immature rhabdomyoblasts and degenerated tumor cells can be found in irregularly dilated gland cavities. Multinucleated giant cells with pale cytoplasm but without cross striations are a prominent and diagnostically important feature. The giant cells have multiple, peripherally placed nuclei, and pale-staining or weakly eosinophilic cytoplasm, without cross striations. The tumor cells grow surrounding vascular channels, forming radial pseudorosette structure, with rare immature osteoid or chondroid tissues.
3. PRMS is a rare variant of rhabdomyosarcoma that almost always arises in adults older than 45 years of age, mainly containing tumor giant cells with abnormal nucleus and abundant eosinophilic cytoplasm (Fig. 7.234). Rhabdomyoblasts can also be seen, which are racket shaped and tadpole shaped, but they are larger with more irregular outlines compared to ERMS tumor cells. And phagocytosis by tumor cells was seen in a few cases.
4. Sclerosing RMS: Tumor cells are round or oval, with irregular nuclear contours, and a small amount of eosinophilic cytoplasm. The neoplastic cells are divided into lobules, small nests, microalveoli, and even single-file arrays by an abundantly hyalinized, eosinophilic to basophilic matrix which is characteristic, often accounting for more than 50% of the tumor.

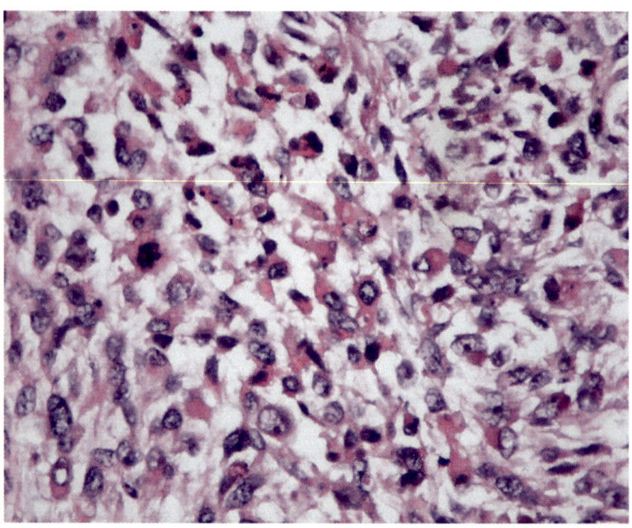

Fig. 7.234 Hepatic rhabdomyosarcoma. The tumor cells contain abundant eosinophilic cytoplasm with visible mitotic figure

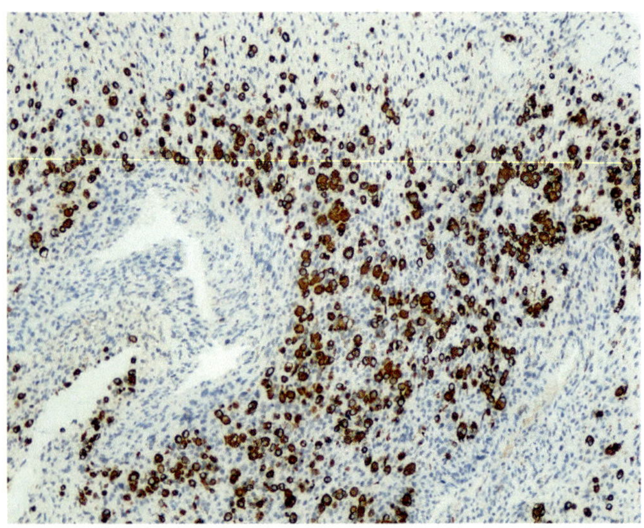

Fig. 7.235 Hepatic rhabdomyosarcoma. Desmin stain is positive

7.4.2.5 Immunohistochemistry

Most of the RMS lesions are positive for myogenic markers, such as desmin (Fig. 7.235), SMA, actin, and myoglobin (Fig. 7.236), while a few ARMS can also be positive for a broad spectrum of CK. There are reports that almost all RMS are positive for MyoD1 (myogenic transcription factor, whose gene is located on chromosome 11p3-5) monoclonal antibody, which is of high diagnostic value, but a few other sarcomas can also be positive, such as LMS. In addition, PRMS shows NSE positive. Recently, Rudzinski et al. [144] selected four antibodies, namely, myogenin, AP2beta, NOS-1, and HMGA2, to determine the presence or absence of ARMS fusion gene using tissue microarray method, and poor prognosis was found in RMS cases without fusion gene. Heerema-McKenney et al. [154] also reported diffusely strong expression of myogenin is an independent prognostic factor for poor prognosis of RMS.

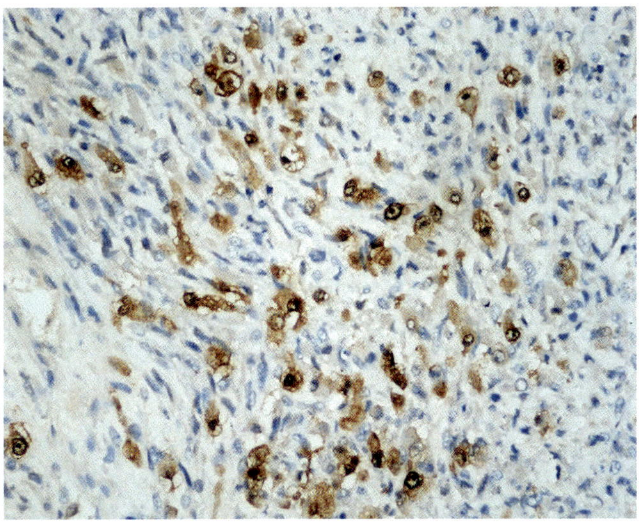

Fig. 7.236 Hepatic rhabdomyosarcoma. Myoglobin stain is positive

7.4.2.6 Electron Microscopic Observation

The tumor cells contain numerous mitochondria and formation of myomere composed of Z-band material and thick or thin filaments.

7.4.2.7 Differential Diagnosis

First of all, metastatic RMS should be excluded, and ARMS should be differentiated from epithelial tumors and a variety of small round tumors, while PRMS need to be distinguished from malignant fibrous histiocytoma. The comprehensive diagnosis is based on the combination of morphological, immunohistochemical, and molecular pathology features.

7.4.2.8 Treatment and Prognosis

Hepatic RMS can be treated by surgical resection combined with chemotherapy, and the postoperative survival is correlated to the TNM staging of the tumor. Neville et al. [155] investigated the presurgical staging of 139 cases of children RMS and their prognosis, showing that postsurgical 3-year survival rate was 55%, and the overall survival rate was 70%. The main factors affecting the prognosis include ① age < 10 years; ② tumor diameter < 5 cm, histological botryoid-type RMS; ③ no local or distant metastasis; and ④ radical resection of the tumor with negative surgical margin. Histologically, the prognosis of botryoid-type RMS and spindle RMS is reported to be the best, after which is that of ERMS, while the prognosis of ARMS and undifferentiated RMS is the worst.

7.4.3 Fibrosarcoma

7.4.3.1 Pathogenesis and Mechanism

So far, more than 40 cases of primary hepatic fibrosarcoma (FS) have been reported in the literature, the pathogenesis of which is unknown. Among the nine cases of primary hepatic FS diagnosed in the Department of Pathology, Eastern

Table 7.17 Clinical features of nine cases of hepatic fibrosarcoma

Case	Gender	Age	Tumor diameter (cm)	Location	HBsAg	Serum AFP (μg/L)	Symptoms and sings
1	Female	53	12	Right	+	1000	Right upper abdominal pain for 1 month
2	Male	45	7.5	Right	–	5.5	Found in physical examination
3	Male	38	14	Right	–	2.7	Chronic diarrhea for 3 months and mild fever for 10 days
4	Male	61	12	Right	–	15.3	Right upper abdominal pain and discomfort, mild fever for more than 1 month
5	Male	57	10	Right	+	20.3	No positive sign
6	Male	50	1.4	Left	+	3.9	None
7	Female	59	11.6	Right	–	3.3	Distension and pain in the hepatic zone
8	Female	34	10	Right	–	4.3	Recurrent reversal right abdominal pain with fever and fatigue
9	Female	61	9.7	Right	–	1.1	Right upper abdominal pain

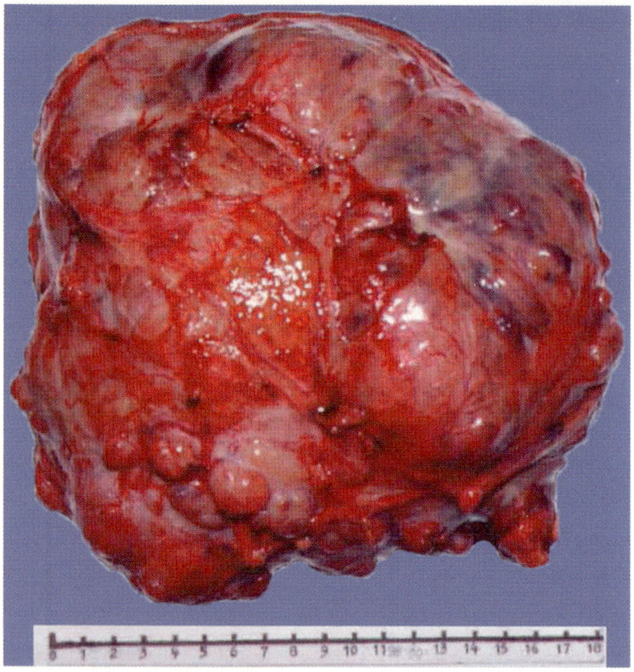

Fig. 7.237 Hepatic fibrosarcoma. The surface of the tumor appears as nodular pattern

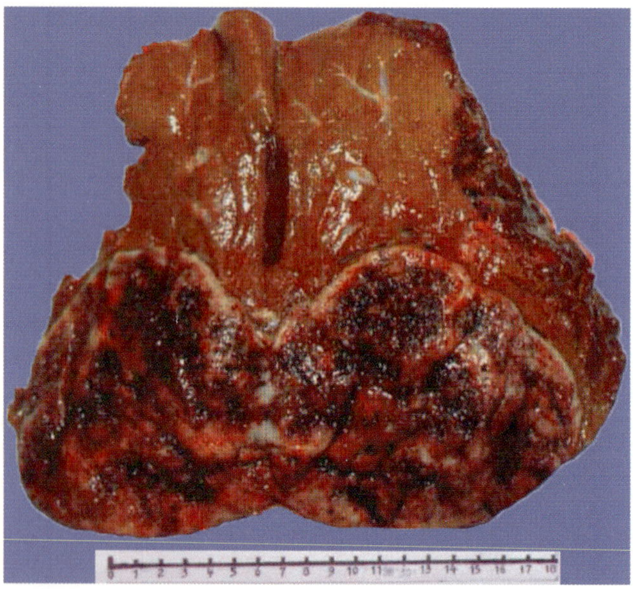

Fig. 7.238 Hepatic fibrosarcoma. The cut section is *gray-red* fleshy with conspicuous hemarrage and necrosis

Hepatobiliary Surgery Hospital, Second Military Medical University, serum HBsAg positive rate was 33.3%, of which two cases were complicated by liver cirrhosis and the etiological relationship between them needs further study. Multiple speculations on the histogenesis of primary hepatic FS have been proposed, such as perivascular and lymphoid connective tissue, cirrhosis connective tissue, vascular smooth muscle cells, or periportal fibrotic tissue, or directly originating from the pluripotent stem cells in the liver.

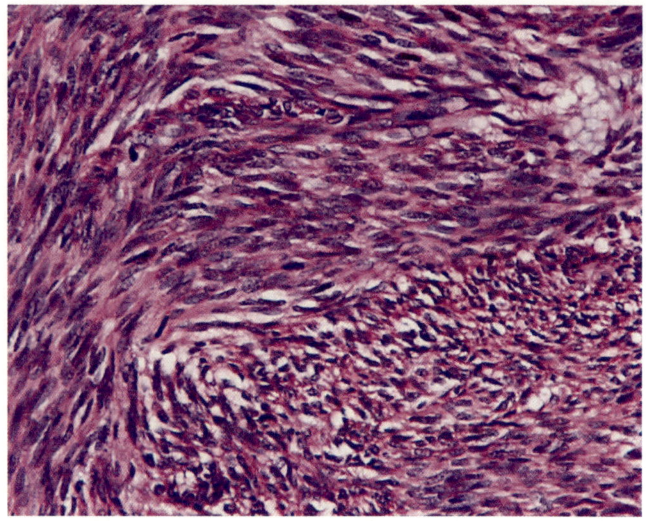

Fig. 7.239 Hepatic fibrosarcoma. Tumor cells are spinded with sharp ends nuclei

Low-grade fibromyxoid sarcoma contains chromosome translocation of t(7;16)(q33;p11) or redundant chromosome loop consisting of chromosomal material on chromosome 7 and 16; chimeric FUS/CREB3L2 fusion transcripts can be detected by RT-PCR or FISH in the tumor. Infantile FS of soft tissue has reverse translocation of t(12;15)(p13;q25), causing gene fusion of NTRK3 and ETV6 or trisomy on chromosome 8, 11, 17, and 20.

7.4.3.2 Clinical Features

According to the data collected in Eastern Hepatobiliary Surgery Hospital, Second Military Medical University (Table 7.17), hepatic FS is commonly found in the elderly with an average age of 51 years (ranging from 34 to 61 years), and male patients are slightly predominated (male to female ratio of 5:4) (information in the literature accounting for 85%). The main clinical manifestations are abdominal pain, distension, weight loss, and right upper abdominal mass, while 22% (2/9) of the cases in the group of patients had liver cirrhosis. Serum CEA, CA19-9, and AFP levels are generally normal; however, among three patients with a history of hepatitis B, two cases had elevated serum AFP and were confirmed to have HCC via postoperative pathological examination. CT showed that hepatic FS are hypodense masses with irregular margin and peripheral nodular enhancement is found in arterial phase. Hepatic artery angiography shows that blood vessels are rich in the tumor.

7.4.3.3 Gross Features

The tumors are often solitary nodules, more often found in the right lobe of the liver (Fig. 7.237), which are larger in

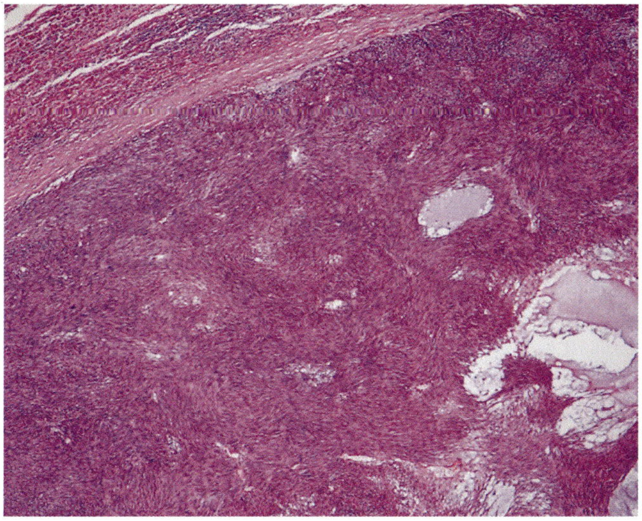

Fig. 7.240 Hepatic fibrosarcoma. The tumor cells are arranged in characteristic herringbone, feathery or fasciculated structures with myxoid stroma and incomplete capsule

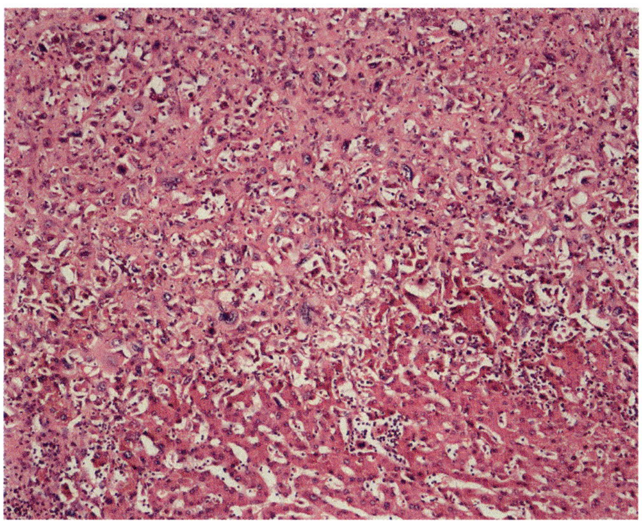

Fig. 7.241 Hepatic fibrosarcoma. Poorly differtiated tumor cells infiltrate into hepatic sinus

volume and the average diameter is 9.9 (1–14) cm with a lobulated surface. The cross sections are gray white or tan yellow and fleshy, soft to firm, and rounded or lobulated, while hemorrhage, necrosis, and cystic degeneration can occur in two-thirds of the tumors (Fig. 7.238). The cut section of myxoid fibrosarcoma is translucent, partly or completely encapsulated. Approximately, a third of all cases contain multiple nodules or satellite lesions, as well as invasion of the portal vein. And three cases contain multiple lesions (2–4 tumors) among the present nine cases of hepatic FS.

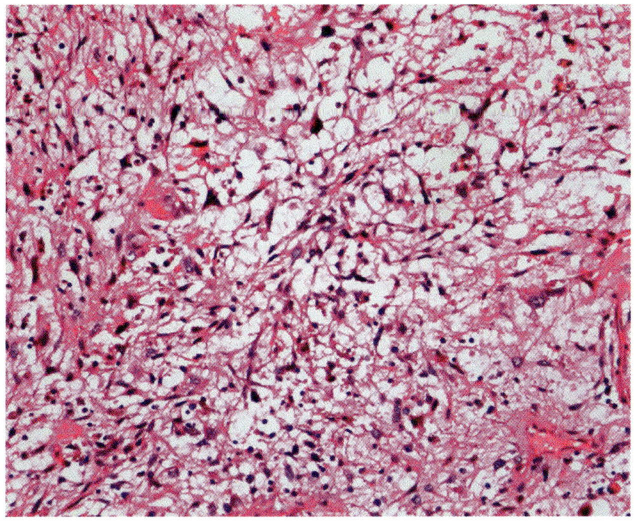

Fig. 7.242 Hepatic myxofibrosarcoma. Stellate tumor cells and curvilinear capillaries are seen in the myxoid stroma

7.4.3.4 Microscopic Features

1. Classic FS: The tumor mainly consists of fibroblast-like spindled cells which vary little in size and shape with scanty cytoplasm (Fig. 7.239) and arranged in characteristic herringbone, feathery, or fasciculated structures (Fig. 7.240), with fusiform nucleus which has both pointed ends and abundant chromatin. Nuclear mitotic figures are easily seen. Local chondrometaplasia or osseous metaplasia can be observed. Poor differentiated tumors are characterized by densely packed pleomorphic tumor cells with thick nuclear chromatin, clear nucleoli and active mitosis, as well as necrosis, less collagen and invasion of the tumor into adjacent hepatic sinus (Fig. 7.241). Silver staining shows that the tumor cells are surrounded by reticular fibers, while Azan-Mallory staining shows a large number of mature collagen in the extracellular spaces of the tumor cells.
2. Myxofibrosarcoma: This kind of tumors consists of different proportions of myxoid components, also known as myxoid malignant fibrous histiocytoma, and at present, there are no uniform diagnostic criteria. Some authors suggested that the diagnosis of myxofibrosarcoma should be made if mucus components accounted for at least more than 50%. It is divided into low, moderate, and high malignant subtypes based on the proportion of mucus composition. Low-grade tumors contain scarce tumor cells, and myxoid component is predominated, characterized by curvilinear capillaries (Fig. 7.242). The tumor cells are arranged around the vessel lumen, and vacuolated cells contain acidic mucus, while rare mitosis can be found. Highly malignant myxofibrosarcoma contains visible focal myxoid stroma and pleomorphic tumor cells

which are similar to malignant fibrous histiocytes, as well as visible multinucleated giant tumor cells and bizarre nucleated giant cells, with visible mitotic figures.

3. Sclerosing epithelioid fibrosarcoma: This type is rarely seen in the liver and only one case has been reported in the literature [156] so far. The tumor was located in the liver with invasion into adjacent soft tissue, including the wall of the inferior vena cava and diaphragm. The tumor was composed of uniform rounded or polygonal epithelioid cells with pale eosinophilic cytoplasm, which are arranged in cords, sheets, or nests, with round nuclei, mild pleomorphism with rare mitosis, and large amounts of hyalinized stroma in the surroundings.

7.4.3.5 Immunohistochemistry

So far, there is no FS specific marker, so the diagnosis is based on exclusion. The tumor cells are only positive for vimentin, while they are negative for epithelium, muscle, reticulum lymphoidal cell, histocyte, and nerve tissue-associated antibodies. Stromal expression of type I and type IV collagen has been observed. Another tumor with low malignancy included in the 2013 WHO classification of soft tissues, known as low-grade fibromyxoid sarcoma, focally expresses SMA and occasionally expresses CD34 or desmin, while both S-100 and EMA staining are negative. Sclerosing epithelioid FS can express Bcl-2 (90% of all the cases), CD99, P53, S-100, EMA (50% of all the cases), and CK (10%), while CD34, CD45, desmin, SMA, and HMB45 staining are all negative. Myxofibrosarcoma occasionally expresses SMA.

7.4.3.6 Differential Diagnosis

First of all, metastatic FS and other spindle cell tumors should be excluded, and classic FS needs to be differentiated from monophasic synovial sarcoma and MPNST, and the differentiation with other hepatic spindle mesenchymal tumors is shown in Table 7.15. Sclerosing epithelioid FS needs to be distinguished from signet ring cell carcinoma, sclerosing lymphoma, epithelioid synovial sarcoma, clear cell sarcoma, MPNST paraganglioma, and extraskeletal osteosarcoma. And comprehensive diagnosis should be made combining clinical history, clinical manifestations, immunohistochemical features, and molecular pathology.

7.4.3.7 Treatment and Prognosis

Hepatic FS tend to metastasize to the lung, adrenal gland, pancreas, bone, lymph nodes, skin, gallbladder, omentum, jejunum, etc., and the patients can survive up to 5 years after surgical resection or radiotherapy. According to the literature [156], peritoneal recurrence occurred 7 months after surgical resection of sclerosing epithelioid FS in the liver, which ceased to grow after systemic chemotherapy of doxorubicin and ifosfamide, and no new metastatic lesions were found, and a second surgical resection of retroperitoneal tumor was conducted, and a 6-month follow-up postoperation confirmed no recurrence.

7.4.4 Liposarcoma

7.4.4.1 Pathogenesis and Mechanism

In adult malignant tumors of soft tissues, liposarcoma is the second common malignant tumor after malignant fibrous histiocytoma, accounting for 16–18% of all soft tissue malignant tumors, and is found mainly in the retroperitoneal space, deep soft tissue of the trunk and adipose tissue of the limbs. Primary hepatic liposarcoma is rare, and 13 cases have been reported up to 2008 in the English literature. The author has found four cases of hepatic liposarcoma in clinical practice, accounting for 8.9% of all malignant mesenchymal tumors (Table 7.14). It is generally believed to be derived from pluripotent mesenchymal cells surrounding blood vessels or cavities; thus, the tumor can be composed by adipocyte cells in different differentiation stages, and hepatic liposarcoma may derive from primitive mesenchymal stem cells.

Table 7.18 Clinical features of four cases of hepatic liposarcoma

Case	Gender	Age (years old)	Location	Diameter (cm)	Ultrasound type B examination
1	Female	43	Left lobe	5	Disorderly low-echo area
2	Female	26	Right lobe	17	Sightly high-echo area
3	Male	46	Left lobe	7	High-echo area
4	Female	35	Right lobe	6.5	Low-echo area

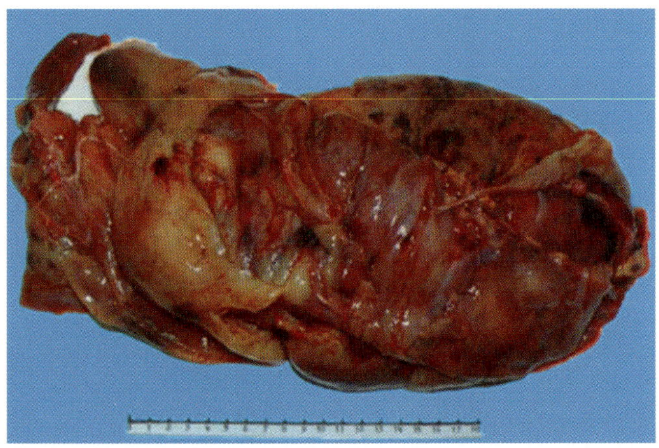

Fig. 7.243 Hepatic liposarcoma. The tumor is *gray-yellow* with expanded lobular surface

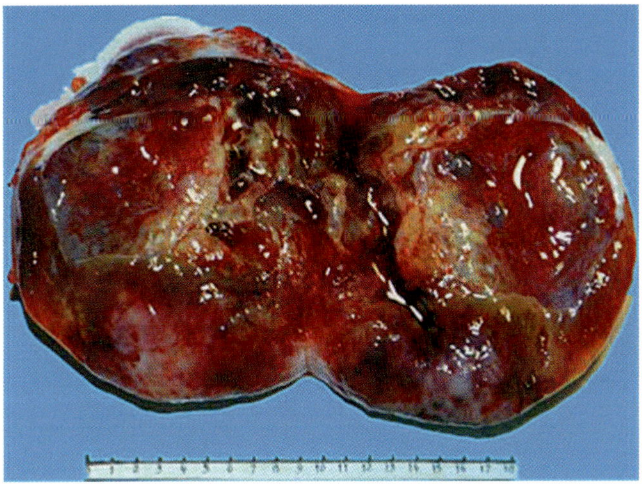

Fig. 7.244 Hepatic liposarcoma. The tumor is *grayish yellow*, translucent, gelatinous, and glossy

7.4.4.2 Clinical Features

Patients of hepatic liposarcoma: It is reported in the literature that the patients of hepatic liposarcoma are approximately 50 years old (ranged from 28 months to 86 years old). Of all the four cases of primary hepatic liposarcoma diagnosed in our department, the male to female ratio was 1:3, and their average age was 37.5 (ranged 26–46 years) years (Table 7.18). Main clinical manifestations include a huge right upper abdominal mass which increases rapidly in size, with pain in the hepatic zone, decreased appetite, and weight loss, while pitting edema of the lower extremity, hydronephrosis complicated by infection due to compression of the kidney and ureter can occur in a few individual patients.

7.4.4.3 Gross Features

The tumor is often large in volume, and the average diameter is 8.9 cm in cases diagnosed in the Department of Pathology, East Hepatobiliary Surgery Hospital, Second Military Medical University. The largest tumor reported in the literature was 27 cm × 15 cm × 15 cm. The tumors are often nodular or lobulated, with necrosis and hemorrhage to different degrees, a slim capsule or pseudocapsule, well-defined margin, visible satellite lesions in some cases, and no cirrhosis in the surrounding liver tissue. The tumor cross section shows largely varying morphology which is associated with different tumor types. For well-differentiated tumors, the cross sections are similar to that of a lipoma (Fig. 7.243). Myxoid liposarcoma is grayish yellow, translucent, gelatinous, and glossy (Fig. 7.244). While pleomorphic liposarcoma is fish-like, complicated by hemorrhage, necrosis, and cystic degeneration, occasionally with visible bone and cartilage.

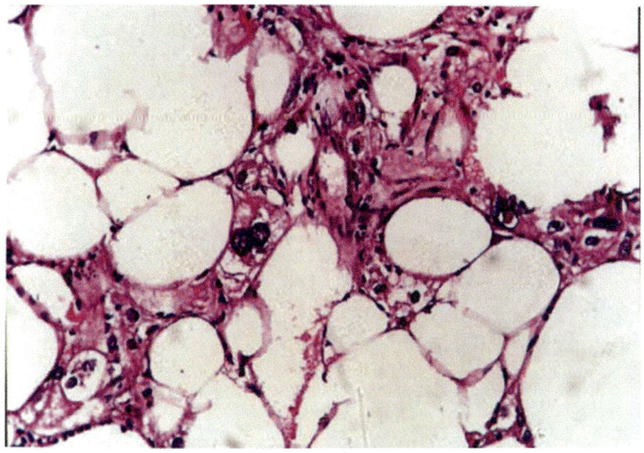

Fig. 7.245 Hepatic liposarcoma. Mature mono-bubble-like fat cells and lipoblasts are seen

7.4.4.4 Microscopic Features

The tissue of liposarcoma is characterized by combination of all cells during the development of adipocytes, including primitive mesenchymal cells, lipoblasts, and well-differentiated fat cells. Thus, the tumor tissue contain adipocytes in various stages of differentiation and varying degree of atypia, such as mononuclear and polynuclear giant lipoblasts, which are large with lobulated nucleus and multinuclei, a hyperchromatic indented or sharply scalloped nucleus, obvious nucleoli, varying sized vacuoles within cytoplasm, sometimes eosinophilic hyaline bodies in the cytoplasm. Mature fat cells are large in size, round in shape, and contain a single large fat vacuole in the cytoplasm, with the nucleus in a crescent shape due to compression. According to the 2013 WHO classification of soft tissues, there are five common histological types of liposarcoma showing as follows:

(1) Well-differentiated liposarcoma/atypical lipomatous tumor

There are three basic types: adipocyte type (lipoma-like type), the inflammatory type, and sclerosing type, the former is more common.

1. Lipoma-like liposarcoma: Most lipoma-like liposarcomas are composed of relatively mature mono-bubble-like fat cells, which is similar to lipoma, while these tumor cells are inconsistent in size and shape compared to normal fat cells, with mild atypia and deep staining of the nuclei, and hyperchromatic stromal cells can be found in fibrous septa, as well as multinucleated stromal cells or lipoblasts (Fig. 7.245) in some cases; however, lipoblasts are not requisite for the diagnosis of liposarcoma.

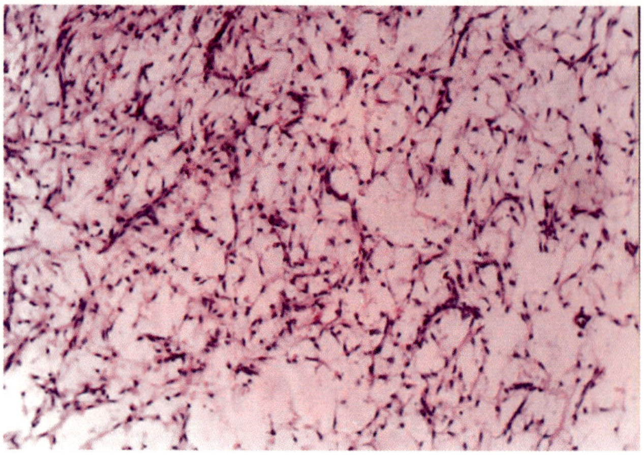

Fig. 7.246 Hepatic myxoid liposarcoma. Stellate or fusiform tumor cells are distributed sparsely in the myxoid stroma

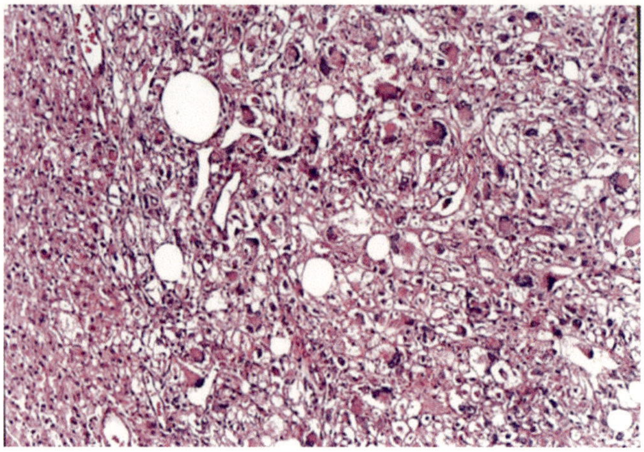

Fig. 7.248 Hepatic pleomorphic liposarcoma. Atypia neoplastic tumor cells are mingled with differentiated lipocyte

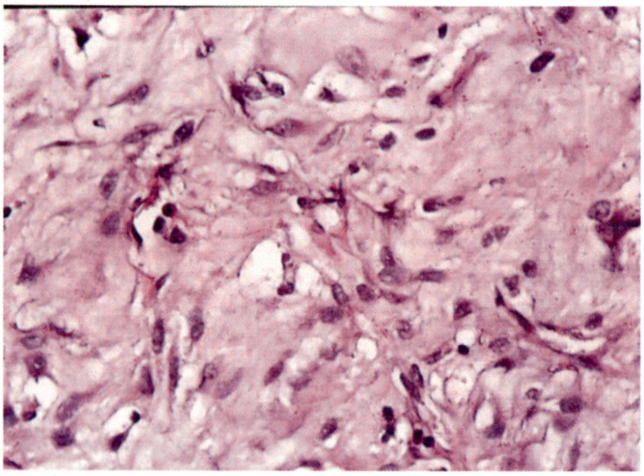

Fig. 7.247 Hepatic myxoid liposarcoma. Immature lipoblast can be found in the myxoid strom

2. Sclerosing liposarcoma: On the basis of lipoma-like liposarcoma, fibrous tissues proliferate obviously in the tumor, which are often slender fibrils and scattered with mature adipocytes and bizarre multinucleated hyperchromatic stromal cells, while lipoblasts are rarely seen outside the region of fat cells. Sometimes the tumor is composed predominantly by fibrotic components, and the fatty components are so rare as to require extensive sampling of the tissue.
3. Inflammatory liposarcoma: Inflammatory liposarcoma is a rare subtype of liposarcoma and commonly found in retroperitoneal region, demonstrating infiltration of a large number of chronic inflammatory cells, of which the fatty ingredients are sometimes very difficult to find and the infiltrated lymphocytes and plasma cells were polyclonal. A few cases are T cell based. For cases with fewer fatty components, deformed and multinucleated stromal cells are helpful in the diagnosis.

(2) Myxoid liposarcoma

Myxoid liposarcoma is the second most common subtype, accounting for 30–35% of all liposarcomas, and is mainly composed of three components: ① mild spindle cells or small round cells, including primitive mesenchymal cells and lipoblasts in various stages of differentiation, the former of which are stellate or fusiform, while the latter are bubble or a signet ring cell (Figs. 7.246 and 7.247); ② a delicate plexiform capillary vascular network; and ③ myxoid matrix, composed of hyaluronic acid, which can form mucus lake, with little atypia and few mitotic figures. It is easy to identify multivacuolar and univacuolar lipoblasts especially prominent at the periphery of the tumor nodules which is of diagnostic value. Myxoid or round cell liposarcoma shares molecular genetic change, suggesting that they are different histological morphology of the same tumor.

Myxoid liposarcoma has two main chromosome translocations: fusion of DDITC gene on t(12;16), 12q13 and FUS gene on 16p11, and t(12;22), which is a fusion of DDIT3 with EWS gene on 22q12. DDIT3 gene promotes the inhibition of growth, and loses its antiproliferative activity when translocated. Tripsy chromosome 8 is the second most common nonrandom chromosomal changes.

(3) Pleomorphic liposarcoma

This is a rare type of liposarcoma, as well as a highly malignant pleomorphic sarcoma with capability of lipid generation, which is characterized by:

① Visible lipoblasts with atypia in various stages of development, such as spindle-shaped, round, and polygonal cells; large in volume, with hyperchromatic and irregularly shaped or fan-shaped nuclei; multivesicular cyto-

Table 7.19 Differential diagnosis of malignant tumors with cytoplasmic vacuoles

Type of tumor	Vacuoles	Pathological characteristics
Liposarcoma	Lipid	Compressed by the lipid to be forked tail, crescent or splayed in shape, and is positive for fat and S-100 staining
Epithelioid hemangioendothelioma	Immature vascular lumen	With obvious vascular differentiation, without nuclear compression by the vacuoles, visible red cells in the lumen, and positive for CD34 and factor VII.
Leiomyosarcoma	Glycogen	With perinuclear vacuoles, and can be positive in PAS and SMA staining.
Rhabdomyosarcoma	Glycogen	Perinuclear vacuoles without nuclear compression, and is positive in PAS staining, while few degenerative fatty vacuoles can also be found, and are positive for desmin and Actin.
Malignant fibrous sarcoma	Glycoprotein	Without nuclear compression by the vacuoles, with diversity in the types of cells, and is negative for S-100 and lipid, while mucus staining shows positive result
Malignant melanoma	Undefined	No nuclear compression and positive for S-100 and HMB-45
Signet ring cell lymphoma	Immunoglobulin or glycoprotein	With translucent or eosinophilic cyplasm and is positive for PAS and LCA

plasm; and nuclei contain pseudo-inclusion bodies or multinucleated tumor giant cells and deformed nucleated tumor cells

② The absence of mucus in the tumor

③ Visible PAS-positive eosinophilic hyaline droplets in the cytoplasm (Fig. 7.248)

About two-thirds of the cases are composed by highly atypical and pleomorphic spindle-shaped cell and scattered or plary lipoblasts, while less than one-third of the cases are composed by highly atypical and pleomorphic cells, epithelioid cells, and scattered lipoblasts, and a small number of cases have a morphological overlap with moderate to high-grade malignant myxoid FS, but the former contain lipoblasts.

(4) Dedifferentiated liposarcoma (DDLPS)

Accounting for 10%, DDLPS is a higher-grade of neoplasm and tends to recur and metastasize. Histologically, dedifferentiated liposarcomas were defined as well-differentiated liposarcomas juxtaposed to areas of high-grade nonlipogenic sarcoma, usually resembling either a fibrosarcoma, malignant fibrous histiocytoma, or rhabdomyosarcoma. Extensive sampling is needed to prevent omission of any tumor components. Coindre et al. (2003) reported 25 cases of retroperitoneal MFH, 17 cases of which were confirmed as DDLPS after comprehensive analysis via immunohistochemistry, molecular pathology, and histological pathology [157]. Thus, for retroperitoneal tumors or hepatic MFH, extensive sampling and careful investigation for well-differentiated liposarcoma are the key points for the diagnosis of DDLPS.

(5) Mixed-type liposarcoma

Mixture of different components of myxoid or round cell liposarcoma, atypical lipomatous tumors (well-differentiated liposarcoma), DDLPS, or pleomorphic liposarcoma has a variety of morphological characteristics of various kinds of liposarcomas.

7.4.4.5 Immunohistochemistry

S-100 staining is positive, and MDM2 and CDK4 are nuclear positive [157], while myogenic and epithelial markers are negative.

7.4.4.6 Differential Diagnosis

About 10% of the metastatic liposarcomas are found in the liver; thus, hepatic metastatic liposarcoma should be excluded in the differential diagnosis. In addition, it should also be distinguished from tumors with cytoplasmic vacuoles (Table 7.19).

7.4.4.7 Treatment and Prognosis

It is 40–90%, while the metastatic and recurrent rate is 20–50%. And the prognosis for well-differentiated and myxoid liposarcomas is better than that of highly malignant round cell myxoid liposarcomas (round cells accounting for more than 25%) or pleomorphic liposarcoma. Thus, comprehensive treatment with adjunctive therapies including chemotherapy and radiotherapy needs to be undertaken for highly malignant liposarcoma or non-radical excised liposarcoma.

7.4.5 Malignant Fibrous Histiocytoma

Hui Dong and Wen-Ming Cong
Department of Pathology, Eastern Hepatobiliary Surgery Hospital, Second Military Medical University, Shanghai, China

7.4.5.1 Pathogenesis and Mechanism

Malignant fibrous histiocytoma (MFH) was first reported by O'Brien and Stout in 1964, and primary hepatic MFH was first reported in 1985. Thirty-six cases were reported in the English literature and 76 cases were reported in the Chinese literature by 2008 [158]. A total of 29 cases of MFH have been diagnosed in the Department of Pathology, Eastern Hepatobiliary Surgery Hospital, Second Military Medical University, accounting for 18.2% of all malignant mesenchymal tumors in the liver diagnosed in our hospital and ranking the third (Table 7.14). In the previous literature, MFH was also known as malignant fibrous xanthoma or fibrous xanthosarcoma. The term of undifferentiated pleomorphic sarcoma was proposed by WHO classification for soft tissues, which equal to pleomorphic MFH, referring to MFH without defined differentiation via comprehensive examinations in histology and immunohistochemistry.

The histogenesis of MFH is still not defined, and the current hypothesized histological derivations include histiocytes, some of which gain the characteristics of fibroblasts, enabling them to be facultative fibroblasts with the features of nerve sheath cells, smooth muscle cells, and other mesenchymal cells; multipotential mesenchymal cell, which has the ability of diverse differentiation, and hepatic MFH may derive from stem cells in the liver parenchyma. So far, the most well-defined etiology is radiation, and some sporadic cases of MFH are associated with exposure to benzoic acid, while in the 29 cases of hepatic MFH diagnosed in the Department of Pathology, Eastern Hepatobiliary Surgery Hospital, Second Military Medical University, 48.3% have a history of HBV infection, the relationship between HBV infection and hepatic MFH needs further investigation.

7.4.5.2 Clinical Features

Among the 29 cases of hepatic MFH diagnosed in the Department of Pathology, Eastern Hepatobiliary Surgery Hospital, Second Military Medical University, elderly, young, and children patients can all be affected with an average age of 47 years and the male to female ratio of 3.14:1. Li et al. [159] reported 7 cases of hepatic MFH diagnosed in his hospital and at the same time reviewed the 27 cases of hepatic MFH in the literature, finding that the average age of the patients was 57.6 years with no obvious gender predominance (18 male cases and 16 female cases). The clinical manifestations include abdominal distension, abdominal discomfort, fatigue, pain in the hepatic zone, fever, weight loss, etc., similar to those of liver abscess or HCC, and a few cases may manifest general malaise, anorexia, and weight loss. Occasionally, peripheral white cell counts (including neutrophils and eosinophilic granulocytes) abnormally elevate in some end-stage patients, but serum AFP and CA19-9 are normal. In terms of imaging features, ultrasound often displays hypoechoic masses or thick-capsuled and anechoic masses in cases with diffuse necrosis. CT shows hypodense lesions with irregular margins, and irregularly enhanced thick capsule of lesions can be observed in a few cystic masses. Arteriography shows the image of the peripheral tumors without central trophic artery. Hepatic MFHs have no specific features in imaging, which can only suggest whether they are malignant or invade into the adjacent organs, as well as whether there is metastasis or recurrence in the follow-up.

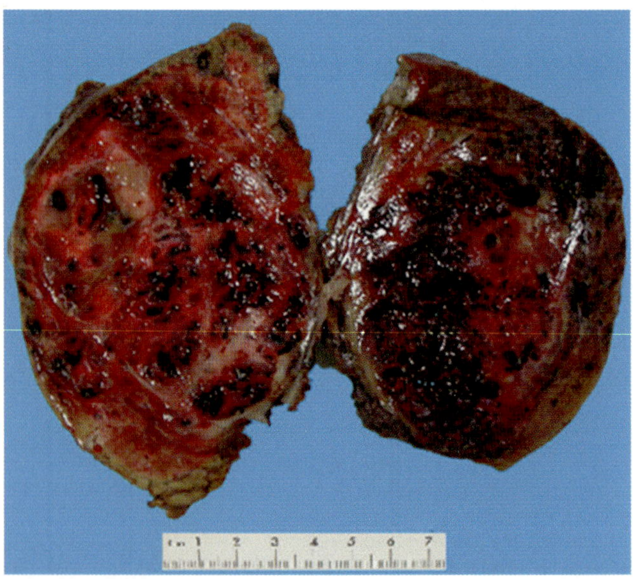

Fig. 7.249 Hepatic malignant fibrous histiocytoma. The tumor cross sections are multi-colored with hemorrhage and necrosis, and infiltration into the border

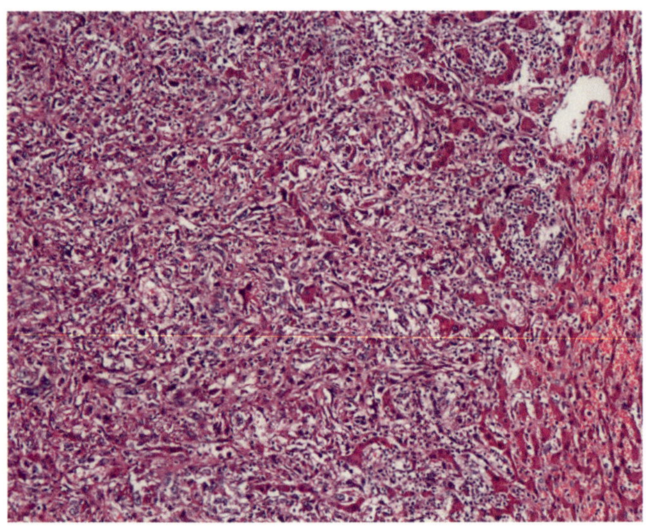

Fig. 7.250 Hepatic malignant fibrous histiocytoma. Storiform arrangement of spindled neoplastic cells infiltrated into the hepatic sinus with the background of inflammation and remaining a few hepatic cells

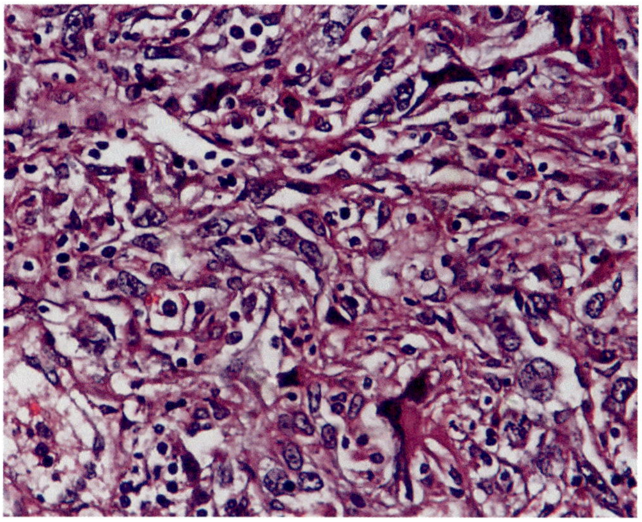

Fig. 7.251 Hepatic malignant fibrous histiocytoma. Showing tumor giant cells with bizzare nuclei and inflammatory cells (high magnification of previous figure)

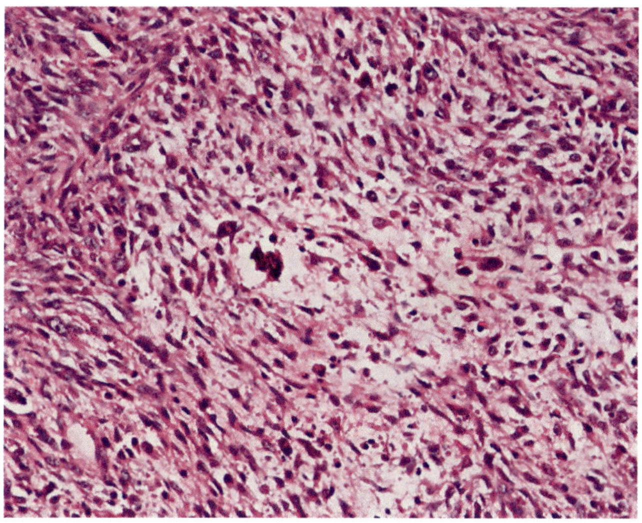

Fig. 7.252 Hepatic malignant fibrous histiocytoma. Tumor cells are spindled with background of myxoid stroma

7.4.5.3 Gross Features

The tumors are round or multinodular. Li et al. reported that 91% of the cases are solitary tumors with an average diameter of 12 cm (ranged 5.5–20 cm) [159]. Of the 29 cases of hepatic MFH diagnosed in Eastern Hepatobiliary Surgery Hospital, Second Military Medical University, 25 cases (86.2%) are solitary lesions, and the average diameter of the tumors is 9.9 cm (ranged 3–28 cm). The tumors are soft and cystic, and the cross sections are fine and smooth, fleshy, gray white, gray yellow, or tan in color, with or without hemorrhage and cystic degeneration and infiltration into the border (Fig. 7.249).

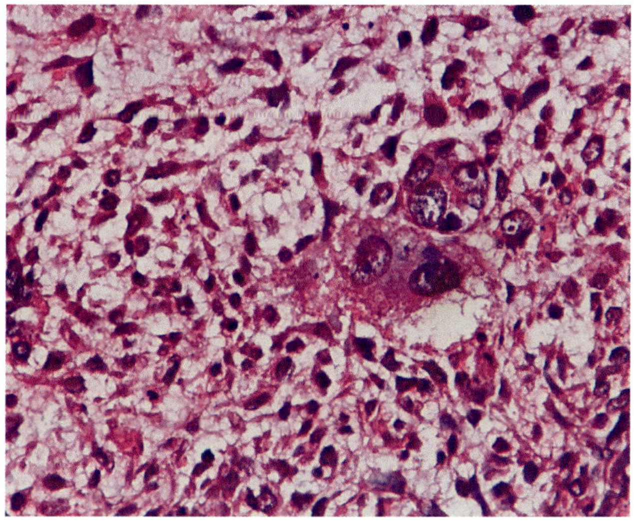

Fig. 7.253 Hepatic malignant fibrous histiocytoma. Spindled tumor cells and tumor giant cells mingled with inflammatory cells

7.4.5.4 Microscopic Features

The histological morphology of hepatic MFH is similar to that of soft tissue MFH; highly pleomorphic tumor cells and their storiform growth pattern are two important microscopic features. MFH contains complex cellular components, pleomorphic tumor cells, and diverse tissue structure, which are the basic characteristics of the tumor. The tumor cells are fusiform, round, oval or bizarre shaped. Only less than 5% of the cells can be suggestive of the histogenesis of the tumor, and various tumoral components can be assembled differently resulting in several subtypes; the histological types of MFH found in soft tissue can also be observed in hepatic MFH.

1. Storiform-pleomorphic type: The most common type, found in 90% of primary hepatic MFH, is arranged in highly pleomorphic shapes with transition between storiform and pleomorphic regions. The tumor cells consist of plump spindle fibroblasts, round or oval histiocytes, giant cells, xanthoma cells, and inflammatory cells. Storiform arrangement of fibroblasts is the main feature (Fig. 7.250).These tumor cells are pleomorphic with obvious atypia and numerous mitotic figures and secondary elements including chronic inflammatory cells, such as lymphocytes, plasma cells, and eosinophilic granulocytes, which are blended with tumor cells (Fig. 7.251).

Li et al. (2008) classified hepatic MFH into three grades of differentiation [159]:

Grade I: fusiform tumor cells contain mild pleomorphic nuclei, which are distributed loosely and sparsely in the myxoid stroma with mucinous degeneration, and mitotic figure is rare (<5/10 HPF), while there is no necrosis.

Grade II: fusiform tumor cells with pleomorphic irregular nuclei, which grow in diffusely storiform pattern with locally visible multinucleated giant cells and mitotic figure of (10–12)/10 HPF, or cells with atypia mitosis, and area of tumoral necrosis is about 20%.

Grade III: the tumor cells are disorderly arranged with pleomorphic multiple hyperchromatic nuclei, mitotic figures of more than 20/10 HPF, commonly visible atypical nuclear mitosis, necrosis of more than 20% of the tumor, and bizarre giant nuclear cells are often found.

2. Myxoid type: About 10% of hepatic MFHs are myxoid type, also known as myxoid FS, which is mildly malignant. The tumor tissue composed of cellular area and myxoid area. The former has the histological structure similar to that of storiform MFH, while the latter contains sparse cells with spindle cells and stellate cells loosely distributed in the myxoid matrix (Figs. 7.252 and 7.253), which is confirmed as acid polysaccharides by histochemical staining. Obvious vascular proliferation can be found, and the tumor cells adhere to the peripheral curved blood vessels. In some cases, slender blood vessels form complex networks, which are extremely similar to the structure of a myxoid liposarcoma.

3. Giant cell type: The tumor contains a large amount of osteoclast-like giant cells, mainly consisting of three kinds of cells, fibroblasts, histiocytes, and osteoclast-like giant cells. Giant cells often contain 3–5 nuclei or more than 20 nuclei in some cells, and osteoid tissue can be found in some cases.
4. Inflammatory type: A large number of xanthoma cells and acute or chronic inflammatory cells are blended in the tumor, as well as mononucleated or multinucleated tumor giant cells, or Touton giant cells distributed sporadically in the tumor, while these have not been reported in the liver.
5. Angiomatoid type: The tumor has abundant blood-containing cavities, without endothelial lining. The tumor is similar to hematoma or hemangioma grossly; however, it has not been reported in the liver.

7.4.5.5 Immunohistochemistry

Tumor cells are positive for vimentin, CD68 (Fig. 7.254), α1-AT, α1-ACT, Mac387, and lysozyme but negative for epithelial, muscular, and lymphocyte markers. The stronger the expression of ezrin protein, the poorer the prognosis the patients have.

7.4.5.6 Differential Diagnosis

Yao and Dai [158], 14.3% of the cases were misdiagnosed as hepatic cyst, liver abscess, or hepatic tumors before the surgery. The key points of differentiation of the tumor from other spindle cell tumors in the liver are shown in Table 7.15, and the differentiation of it from tumors containing cytoplasmic vacuoles are shown in Table 7.19.

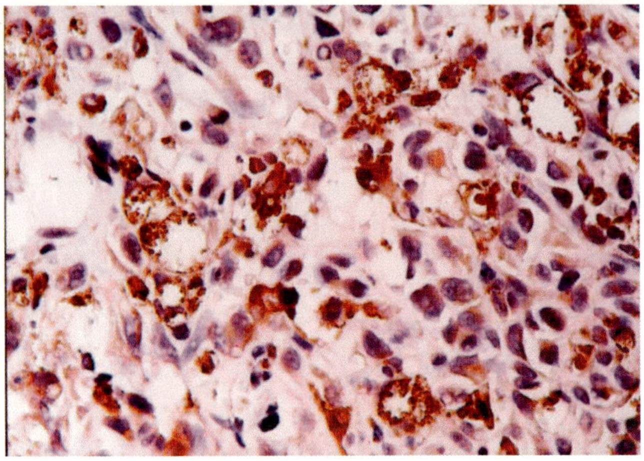

Fig. 7.254 Hepatic malignant fibrous histiocytoma. CD68 staining is positive

7.4.5.7 Treatment and Prognosis

In general, MFH is highly invasive malignant tumors, postsurgical 5-year and 10-year overall survival rate of the patients is 58% and 38%, respectively. The survival time of 33% of the patients with early radical excised hepatic MFH can reach to 2 years or even 10 years. Invasion of the diaphragm and lung is found in 32% of the cases. It has been reported that one case of MFH was resected when the tumor recur after the first surgery. The overall survival time reached over 9 years in that case. The prognostic factors include huge masses, high expression index of ezrin, and late clinical stage.

7.4.6 Undifferentiated (Embryonal) Sarcoma

Wen-Ming Cong and Zhen Zhu
Department of Pathology, Eastern Hepatobiliary Surgery Hospital, Second Military Medical University,
Shanghai, China

7.4.6.1 Pathogenesis and Mechanism

In 1978, Stocker and Ishak named the hepatic tumor found in 31 cases in American Force Institution of Pathology (AFIP) as undifferentiated (embryonal) sarcoma (UES), which mainly consists of primitive mesenchymal and myxoid stromal components and was characterized by specific PAS-positive bodies. Of all the hepatic tumors found in children at the age of 6–15 years old, UES is the third common tumor ranking after hepatoblastoma and hepatocellular carcinoma, accounting for 9–15% of all the hepatic tumors in this age group [160]. By 2013, there have been more than 200 reported cases of hepatic UES [161].

UES is a kind of embryonic mesenchymal tumor with diverse components, and the tumor cells can resemble those in various types of mesenchymal tumors in varying proportions, such as tumor cells in angiosarcoma, osteosarcoma and chondrosarcoma, lipoblasts, rhabdomyoblasts, histiocytes, or fibroblasts. The histogenesis of UES is still unknown, and UES was previously called malignant mesenchymoma. Shehata et al. [162] reported one case of an 11-month-old infant with UES and mesenchymal hamartoma (MH). Begueret et al. [163] reported one case of children tumor with UES, MH, and a transition area between the two components, finding the common mesenchymal phenotype and DNA aneuploidy among them via immunohistochemistry and DNA flow cytometry, which is supportive of the UES deriving from malignant transformation of MH. Rajaram et al. [164] applied DNA sequencing to confirm that UES originating from MH with t(11;19)(q11;q13.4) translocation contains a breakpoint of MALAT1 (metastatic adenocarcinoma of lung-associated transcript 1) gene on chromosome 11 and MHLB1 (breakpoint 1 of mesenchymal hamartoma of the liver) gene on chromosome 19 [164]. Mathews et al. [165] used the next-generation sequencing to analyze MALAT1 (metastatic adenocarcinoma of lung-associated transcript 1) gene on chromosome 11 and MHLB1 (breakpoint 1 of mesenchymal hamartoma of the liver) gene on chromosome 19 of the paraffin-embedded tissues in seven cases of hepatic mesenchymal hamartoma, demonstrating that three cases of MH had rearrangement of MHLB1 gene, suggesting that MHLB1 locus contains a CpG-rich region; thus, it may regulate C19MC miRNA gene via methylation, and genetic rearrangement may cause damage of the integrity of the region leading to malignant transformation of MH due to abnormal expression of miRNA.

In addition, Keating et al. [166] analyzed the ultrastructure and immunohistochemistry characteristics of UES in two children cases, proposing that UES may derive from malignant fibrous histiocytoma. Parham et al. [167] conducted the analysis of ultrastructure and immunohistochemistry on 13 cases of UES and 2 cases of hepatic rhabdomyosarcoma, finding a partial overlap between these two kinds of tumors in morphology and immunohistochemistry, indicating the possible origination of primitive pluripotent stem cells in the liver for UES. Recently, we conducted detection of loss of heterozygosity of microsatellite DNA to assess the clonal features of different UES cell populations, and the results showed that about 60% of the tumors are monoclonal origin, suggesting that UES may derive from pluripotent tumoral stem cells.

7.4.6.2 Clinical Features

UES is predominantly found in children and adolescents, and patients at the age of 6–15 years old account for more than 75%, and 90% of them are younger than 21 years old, with more female than male. However, the age range is from 2 months old to 86 years old, and adult patients are not rare [168]. From January 2000 to December 2011, a total of 43 cases of UES treated with surgical resection were diagnosed in Eastern Hepatobiliary Surgery Hospital, Second Military Medical University, which met the pathological diagnostic criteria of WHO and have complete clinical data. Thirty-two cases affected males (74.4%) and 11 females (35.6%) with an age ranging from 5 to 70 years (35 ± 22.49 years), while the patients younger than 14 years old and those older than 15 years old accounted for 32.6% (14/43) and 67.4% (29/43) in the present group, respectively. The main clinical manifestations include right upper abdominal discomfort and pain (74.4%), abdominal mass (55.9%), and fever (34.9%). Serum biochemical examination shows abnormalities mainly consisting of increased ALP (53.5%), AST (46.5%), and ALT (32.6%), without increased serum AFP. Half of the adult UES patients have a history of HBV infection, which may be an etiological feature of Chinese UES.

Among the 43 cases of UES diagnosed in the Department of Pathology, Eastern Hepatobiliary Surgery Hospital, Second Military Medical University, 35 cases involved the right lobe of the liver (81.4%), 3 cases the left lobe (7.0%), and 5 cases the middle lobe (11.6%). Due to the rapid growth of UES, it is often huge in volume and tends to rupture and bleed spontaneously, or directly invades the diaphragm, pleura, ribs, abdominal wall, gastrointestinal tract, and mesentery, or even involves the inferior vena cava, right atrium, and right ventricle via venous system causing pulmonary embolism. Distal metastasis to the pancreas, kidney, and adrenal gland is also found. The examinations in the lab often show increased white blood cells and abnormal liver function in 1/3–1/2 of the patients. Ultrasound type B demonstrates cystic and solid masses. While CT images show huge cystic or cystic and solid hypodensitive mass (Fig. 7.255), with multiple hyperdensitive, varying thickness septa in the center, or pseudocapsule in the surrounding of the lesions. Some cystic UES lesions are prone to be mistaken as echinococciasis of liver, while patients with fever are often misdiagnosed as liver abscess.

7.4.6.3 Gross Features

The tumors are often huge in volume. Of the 43 cases of UES diagnosed in the Department of Pathology, Eastern Hepatobiliary Surgery Hospital, Second Military Medical University, the lesions are 12.6 (3.8–25) cm in diameter and

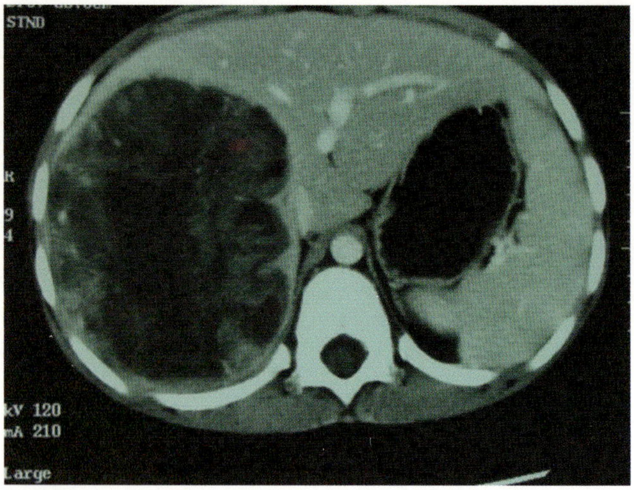

Fig. 7.255 Hepatic undifferentiated embryonal sarcoma. CT image shows huge cystic and solid tumor

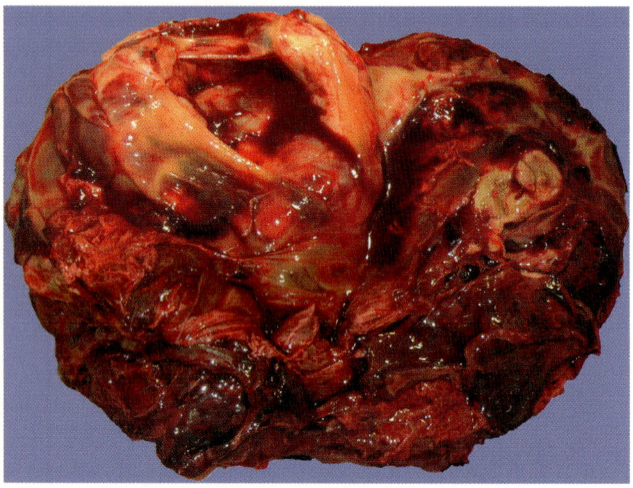

Fig. 7.256 Hepatic undifferentiated embryonal sarcoma. The tumor is deriving from MH malignant transformation, which appears cystic and solid with heamorrage and necrosis

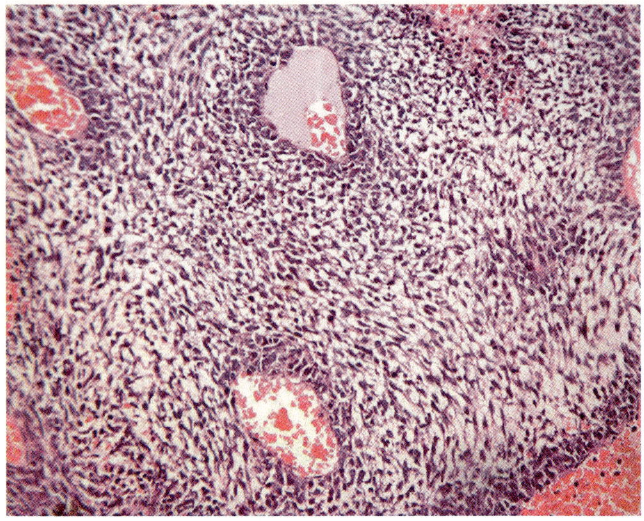

Fig. 7.257 Hepatic undifferentiated embryonal sarcoma. Spindled tumor cells are loosely distributed with poor adhesive ability

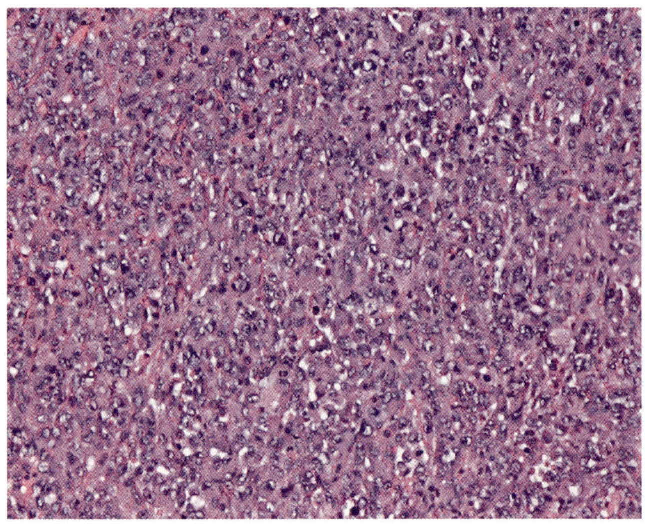

Fig. 7.258 Hepatic undifferentiated embryonal sarcoma. Densely distributed tumor cells are solid packed with active mitotic figures

1280 g in weight on average. UES lesions often have no capsules and are often soft, gelatinous, gray white, yellow or tan in color, cystic, and solid with cystic degeneration, hemorrhage, and necrosis in most cases. The diameters of the cystic cavities vary greatly, which contain brown and gelatinous contents (Fig. 7.256).

7.4.6.4 Microscopic Features

The tumor cells are spindle, stellate, or pleomorphic shaped in medium or large size, and local tumor cells are loosely distributed with poor adhesive ability (Fig. 7.257), while other areas of the tumor contain densely distributed tumor cells which are solid packed, forming cellular sheath surrounding small blood vessels (Fig. 7.258), angiosarcomatous cavity with obviously atypical cellular lining (Fig. 7.259) or loosely myxoid stromal tissue (Fig. 7.260). These tumor cells are similar to primitive embryonic mesenchymal cells which have no definite differentiation direction (Figs. 7.261 and 7.262), with bizarre or multiple nuclei, which are atypical and hyperchromatic with active nuclear mitotic figures, conspicuous nucleoli, and an increased nuclear to cytoplasmic ratio (Fig. 7.263). Both cytoplasmic eosinophilic bodies and apoptotic bodies in stroma are a key diagnostic feature for UES (Figs. 7.264 and 7.265). The eosinophilic bodies are still PAS staining positive after amylase digestion, and Masson staining shows light blue, purple, or erythrinus. Incomplete capsule can be found in the peripheral region of the tumor, and tumor cells may grow into the adjacent hepatic sinus in an invasive pattern (Fig. 7.265).

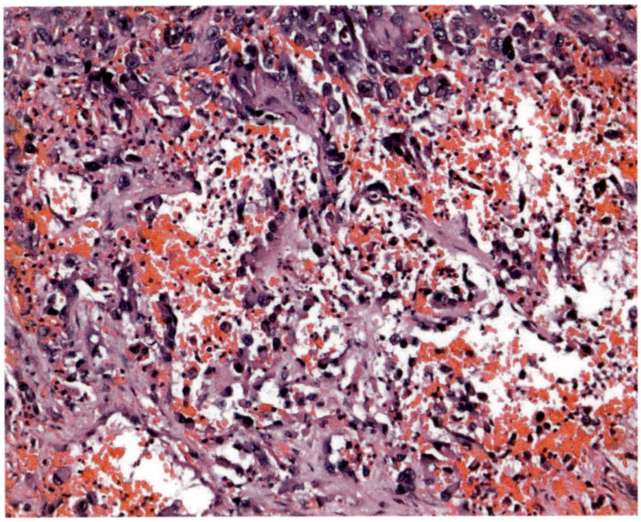

Fig. 7.259 Hepatic undifferentiated embryonal sarcoma. Angiosarcomatous cavity with obviously atypic cellular lining, focally hemorrage and necrosis

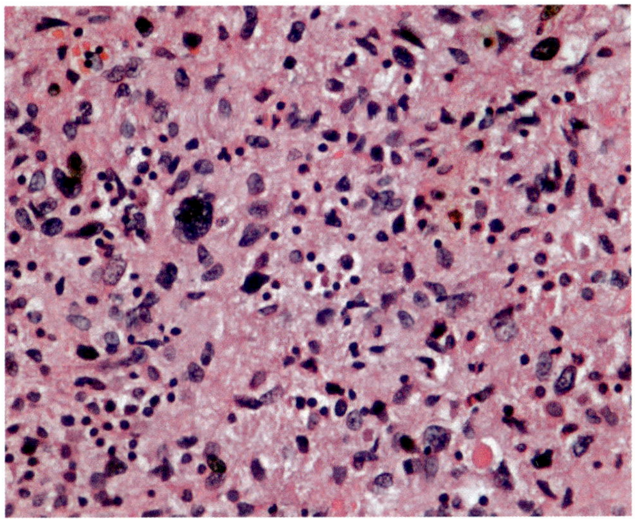

Fig. 7.261 Hepatic undifferentiated embryonal sarcoma. The tumor cells are inconsistant in size and irregular in shape, which are distributed in sheet, eosinophilic bodies kan be seen at the *lower right corner*

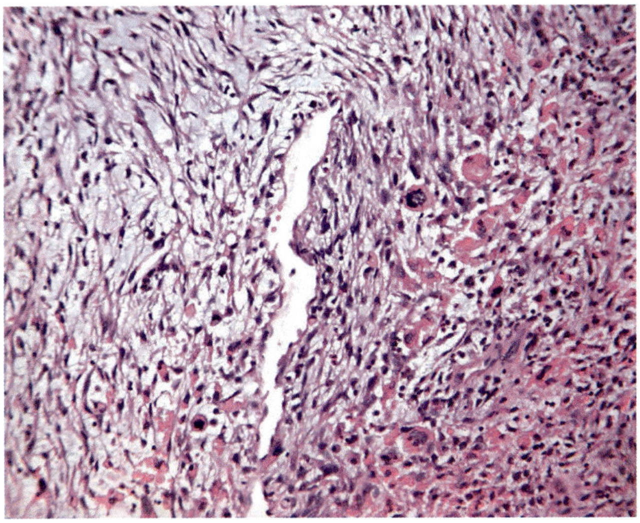

Fig. 7.260 Hepatic undifferentiated embryonal sarcoma. Stellate tumor cells if found in loosely myxoid stromal tissue

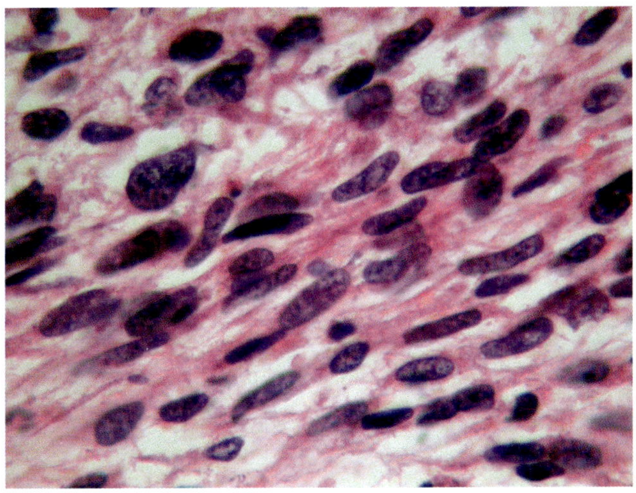

Fig. 7.262 Hepatic undifferentiated embryonal sarcoma. The tumor cells have rod-like nuclei with sparse cytoplasm

7.4.6.5 Immunohistochemistry

The tumor is composed of various mesenchymal differentiated cells; thus, the tumor cells are generally positive for vimentin (Fig. 7.266), α1-AT (Fig. 7.267), and CD68 and locally positive for BCL-2, CD10, desmin, SMA, and calponin, while they are negative for Hep Par1 (in exclusion of hepatoblastoma), myogenin (in exclusion of embryonal rhabdomyosarcoma), S-100 (in exclusion of other sarcoma), and c-kit [169, 170].

7.4.6.6 Differential Diagnosis

1. Mesenchymal hamartoma: It also contains myxoid stroma with disorderly distributed proliferated ductules, hepatocellular islets, thin-walled blood vessels, lymphatic vessels, etc.; furthermore, the cells are not highly atypical. To notice with caution, the proportion of MH cases complicated by or transforming into UES reaches as high as 45% [164]; thus, extensive sampling and careful examination of the cellular morphology are necessary.
2. Hepatoblastoma: It is mainly found in patients under the age of 3 years old and consists of immature hepatocytes, with the structure of sinus. The tumor has relatively single cellular component, which are positive for hepatocellular markers. pCEA and CD10 staining show the bile canaliculi of the tumor cells. Different from hepatoblastoma, UES shows no positive nuclear staining for β-catenin.

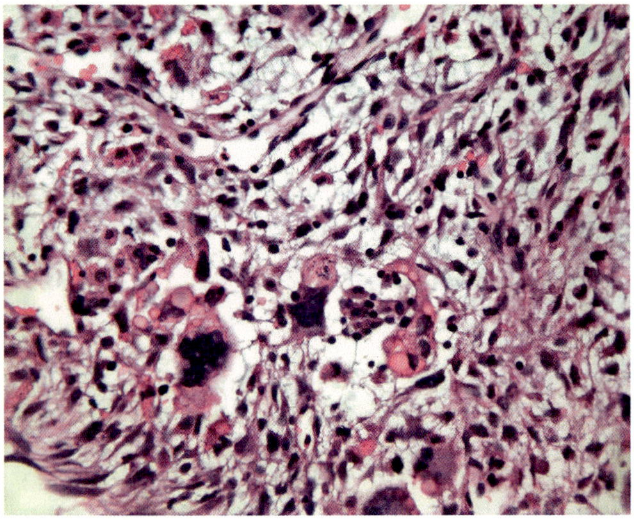

Fig. 7.263 Hepatic undifferentiated embryonal sarcoma. Giant and bizarre nucleus tumor cells with amount of eosinophilic bodies

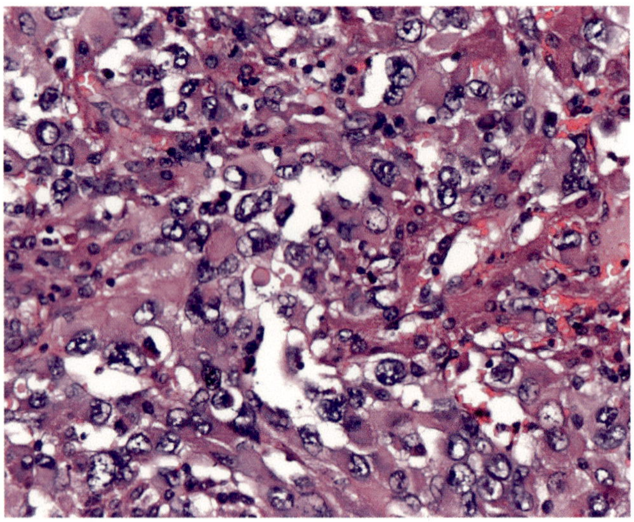

Fig. 7.264 Hepatic undifferentiated embryonal sarcoma. There is eosinophilic bodies in the center of the tumor

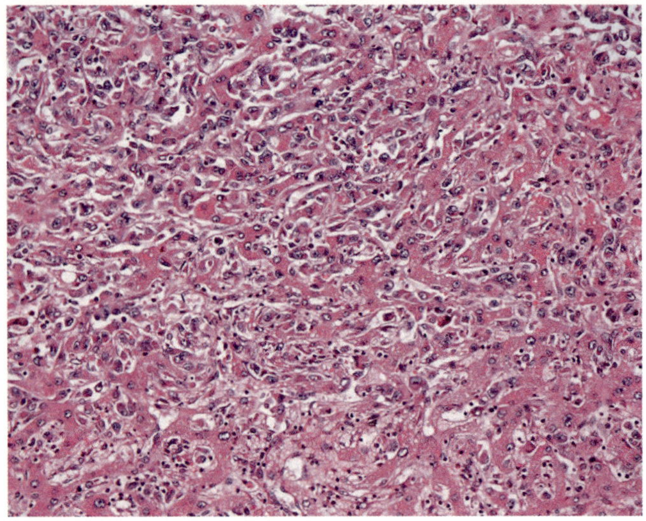

Fig. 7.265 Hepatic undifferentiated embryonal sarcoma. There is no capsule around the tumor, and the tumor cells infiltrate into the hepatic sinus and are mixed with the remnant hepatic plate

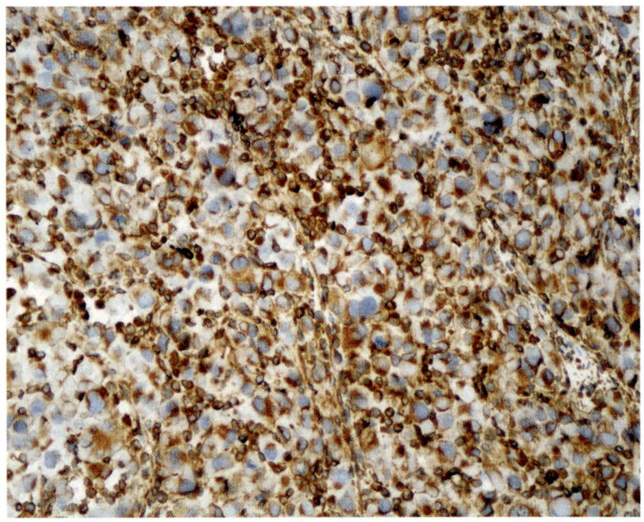

Fig. 7.266 Hepatic undifferentiated embryonal sarcoma. VI is positive

3. Malignant fibrous histiocytoma: The spindled cells are in storiform or cartwheel arrangement and are positive for CD68 and α1-AT, while the latter is negative in UES.
4. Fibrosarcoma or leiomyosarcoma: Both contain mono-component which has a defined differentiation, and no cystic or myxoid stroma is seen in the UES, without dilated bile ducts or eosinophilic bodies.

7.4.6.7 Treatment and Prognosis

UES grows rapidly with high malignancy and a poor overall prognosis. In nontreatment group, 80% of the patients survived less than 1 year after diagnosis. UES is often complicated by distal metastasis, and the lung is the most common metastatic organ. The clinical data found in Eastern Hepatobiliary Surgery Hospital, Second Military Medical University, showed that UES patients younger than 14 years old have a medium survival time of (16 ± 1.3) months, patients of 15–49 years old (11 ± 0.6) months, while those older than 50 years old (2.5 ± 1.4) months, the prognosis of the latter was significantly poorer than the former two groups ($P = 0.022$). Several studies demonstrated that UES is a type of chemotherapy-sensitive tumor, and radical resection plus comprehensive therapies is adopted in the treatment, including chemotherapy (cisplatin, doxorubicin, vincristine, and cyclophosphamide), radiotherapy, and interventional therapy, and so on. Ida et al. [171] reported one case of a patient who had a surgically excised UES which was 20 cm × 20 cm in volume and treated by systemic chemotherapy after the

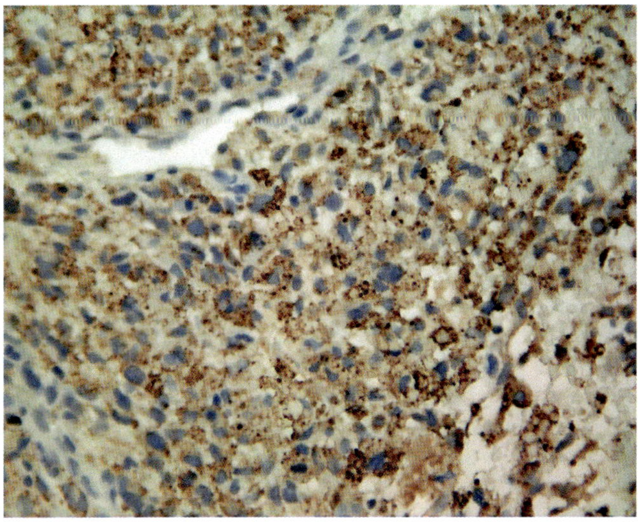

Fig. 7.267 Hepatic undifferentiated embryonal sarcoma. α_1-AT is positive

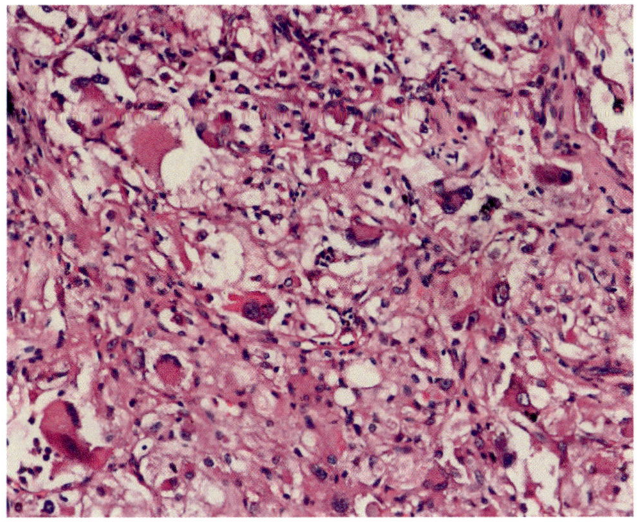

Fig. 7.268 Hepatic malignant angiomyolipoma. Tumor cells with leomorphic and bizarre nuclei are common, the cells density is increased

surgery, and we received a disease-free survival during the 52-month follow-up. Lenze et al. [168] retrospectively analyzed the prognosis in 68 cases of UES patients, older than 15 years old, of which the patients with radical resection and postsurgical chemotherapy received a median follow-up period of 28.5 (6–204) months, while those with radical resection without postsurgical chemotherapy received a median follow-up period of only 8 (2–144) months, with significant difference between the two groups. In domestic literature, Gao et al. [161] reported one case of a 7-year-old girl who was treated with surgical resection of a 17 cm in diameter UES and 3 weeks of epirubicin chemotherapy after the surgery, and no recurrence was found in the 22-month follow-up.

7.4.7 Malignant Angiomyolipoma

Ohmori et al. reported the first case of primary hepatic malignant angiomyolipoma in 1989, and there have been six cases of hepatic malignant angiomyolipoma. The patients were 54.7 years old on average with a male to female ratio of 1:2. The tumors are mainly solitary nodules or multinodules in some cases, and their average diameter was 17.2 cm. The malignant component of hepatic malignant angiomyolipoma is predominantly epithelioid cells; thus, it is actually malignant epithelioid angiomyolipoma, which was named as malignant perivascular epithelioid cell neoplasms (PEComa) by WHO. However, it is also reported that hepatic angiomyolipoma malignant transformation can occur. Nguyen et al. (2008) reported one case of hepatic malignant angiomyolipoma containing three cellular constituents, epithelioid cells, adipocytes, and blood vessels [172].

Histologically, malignant angiomyolipoma has a more obvious atypia than epithelioid cells in angiomyolipoma, which are plump spindle or polygonal cells of large sizes, with translucent and bright cytoplasm which is granular or eosinophilic, mononucleus, right-angled nucleus, or multiple nuclei, as well as Reed-Sternberg-like cells. In the nuclei, pseudo-inclusion bodies, hyperchromatin, and conspicuously nuclear atypia can be observed. Spindled tumor cells are found to protrude from the smooth muscle layer of thick-walled blood vessels, a transition between the two can be seen, or adipocytes in some cases. Epithelioid tumor giant cells may also be seen containing multiple nucleoli and center-distributed cytoplasm, as well as a translucent halo between the margin of the cytoplasm and cellular membrane (Fig. 7.268). Intracytoplasmic translucent bodies can be found, and some epithelioid cells exhibit nuclear condensation. Epithelioid tumor cells are often arranged in cord or nests, or similar to hepatocellular carcinoma, without any capsule and often invade the adjacent hepatic sinusoids (Fig. 7.269) and branches of the portal vein. As to immunohistochemistry markers, the cells mainly express melanocyte markers, including HMB-45,melan-A, and MITF, SMA may be positive, and about 10% of the tumors can focally express S-100 or strongly positive for TFE3 staining, while CD34, CD117, desmin, and h-caldesmon are rarely positive.

When making the diagnosis, it should be differentiated from benign angiomyolipoma. Folpe et al. [173] suggested to divide the perivascular tumors into benign, of uncertain malignant potential and malignant types according to seven histological features: tumor diameter>5 cm, invasive growth, high-grade nuclear, abundant cytoplasm, necrosis, mitotic figures >1/50 HPF, and invasion of blood vessels. PEComa with two or more worrisome histological features should be considered malignant. Parfitt et al. [174] reported one case of a seemingly "benign" hepatic angiomyolipoma, in which

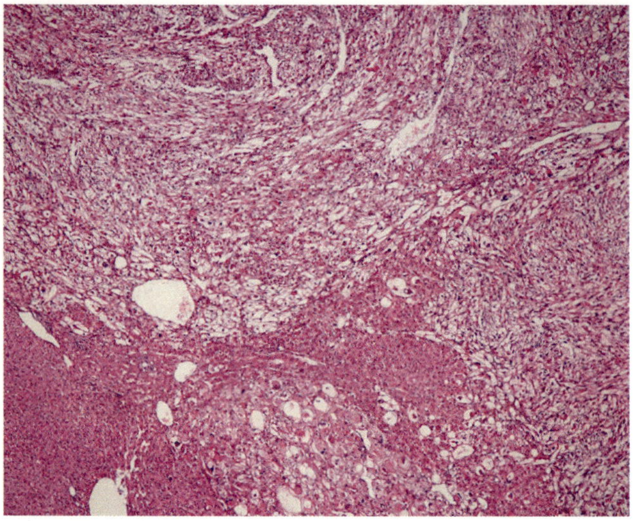

Fig. 7.269 Hepatic malignant angiomyolipoma. Epithelioid tumor cells are often arranged in multi-nodule, and often invade the adjacent hepatic sinusoids

metastasis of multiple organs was found 9 years after its primary surgical resection, including soft tissue, lung, pancreas, and urinary bladder. It was suggested that the biological behaviors of malignant hepatic angiomyolipoma are of uncertainty; thus, the diagnosis should be based on the combination of the morphology and growth features of the tumor, as well as immunohistochemistry staining of Ki-67and p53, while suspicious case should be followed up for a long period.

7.4.8 Osteosarcoma

7.4.8.1 Pathogenesis and Mechanism

Osteosarcoma is rare and primary hepatic osteosarcoma is even rarer. By 2009, only nine cases have been reported at abroad. The pathogenesis of hepatic osteosarcoma is unclear, and its histogenesis may involve the intrahepatic pluripotent stem cells which differentiate into osteoblasts and chondroblasts.

7.4.8.2 Clinical Features

Of the reported nine cases of hepatic osteosarcoma, the male to female ratio was 2:1, and the patients were 19–73 years old with an average age of 61.8 years old. The main symptoms include abdominal hard masses, pain in the hepatic zone, weight loss, etc. A few cases are complicated with HCV hepatitis-related cirrhosis. Serum AFP and CEA are often negative, and alanine aminotransferase and aspartate aminotransferase may be elevated.

7.4.8.3 Gross Features

Hepatic osteosarcoma is often large in volume with an average diameter of larger than 10 cm, and the largest lesion may reach 25 cm in diameter and 3600 g in weight. The cross section of the tumor is often gray white, tan brown or grayish yellow, and gravel, with hemorrhage and extensive necrosis or tumor thrombus in the hepatic vein and inferior vena cava, and the tumor can also directly invade into the portal area.

7.4.8.4 Microscopic Features

The histological changes are similar to those of osteosarcoma of the bone. And according to the difference in predominant cells and tumoral stroma, this type of tumor can be divided into osteoblast type, chondroblast type, fibroblast type, and mixed type. In the case of a 69-year-old female patient with primary hepatic osteosarcoma reported by Park et al. [175], the tumor is composed by polygonal or spindle-shaped tumor cells, with hyperchromatic nuclei and conspicuous atypical nuclei, which can be mingled with eosinophilic and lace-arranged osteoid stroma. Furthermore, the region of osteoblasts also contains a large number of osteoclast-like giant cells with mitotic figures. Malignant chondroblasts and fibroblasts grow in nests without any epithelial or other mesenchymal components.

7.4.8.5 Immunohistochemistry

The tumor cells are positive for vimentin, and negative for actin, desmin, SMA, CEA, AFP, and CK.

7.4.8.6 Differential Diagnosis

Metastatic osteosarcoma and hepatic tumors containing osteocomponents, such as carcinosarcoma, malignant mesenchymal adenoma, hepatoblastoma, malignant fibrous histiocytoma, undifferentiated embryonic sarcoma, etc., should be excluded. In the first place, the common feature of these tumors is that the tumoral osseous tissue is only a small part of the whole tumor.

7.4.8.7 Treatment and Prognosis

Hepatic osteosarcoma is often huge in volume and grows in invasive pattern, with tumor thrombi in the hepatic vein or portal vein, distal metastasis, and a poor prognosis. Nawabi et al. [176] reported one case of a 19-year-old female patient with primary hepatic osteosarcoma, who received postsurgical adjuvant chemotherapy (ifosfamide and mesna 14 g/m^2 for two therapeutic courses, followed by cisplatin100mg/m^2 and doxorubicin75mg/m^2) via an interval of 3 weeks. The patient survived free of tumor in 3-year postsurgical period.

7.4.9 Chondrosarcoma

Extraskeletal chondrosarcoma is rare, including myxoid chondrosarcoma and mesenchymal chondrosarcoma, and extraskeletal myxoid chondrosarcoma constitutes less than 3% of all sarcomas of soft tissue, often found in patients older than 35 years old with most frequently onset age of

50–60 years old. Male patients are two times more common than females. A total of 19 cases of extraskeletal chondrosarcoma have been reported in the literature, with an average age of 47.1 (22–62) years old and a male to female ratio of 1:2.4, of which 6 cases were classic type, 11 cases mesenchymal type, 1 case myxoid type, and the other dedifferentiated type.

Primary hepatic extraskeletal chondrosarcoma is extremely rare with one reported case of a 67-year-old male patient who had simultaneous hepatocellular carcinoma and chondrosarcoma found in different sites, while one case of a 56-year-old male patient was reported in Chinese literature with a surgically excised 15 cm × 12 cm × 10 cm mass in the right lobe of the liver, which was diagnosed as well-differentiated chondrosarcoma. One case of primary hepatic chondrosarcoma was diagnosed in Eastern Hepatobiliary Surgery Hospital, Second Military Medical University, concerning a 57-year-old male patient with positive hepatitis B surface antigen, and ultrasound type B showed a cystic and solid occupying lesion in the liver which had irregularly thickened inner wall with visible papillary protrusion. MRI demonstrated a cystic occupying lesion in the liver, and T_1-weighted images showed hypo-signal while T_2-weighted images showed hyper-signal with a little calcification. No extrahepatic tumors were found. The patient received partial hepatectomy, and the excised tumor was 18 cm × 17 cm × 11 cm in size, the cut section of which was grayish white and grayish blue with a huge cystic cavity of 13 cm × 7 cm in the center, tender tumoral tissues in the periphery, and a well-defined boundary separating it from the surrounding liver tissue. Microscopically, the tumor consisted completely of blue-stained chondroid tissue (Figs. 7.270 and 7.271) with visible pit cells and osteoclast-like giant cells, as well as large patches of mucinous degeneration and necrosis in the tumor, around which are the capsule, well-defined, adjacent liver tissue without cirrhosis. Immunohistochemically, S-100 was positive and cartilage matrix was positive in Alcian blue staining. The patient was treated with transcatheter arterial embolization 2 months after the surgery and was found in good recovery without recurrence and metastasis during the 13-month follow-up.

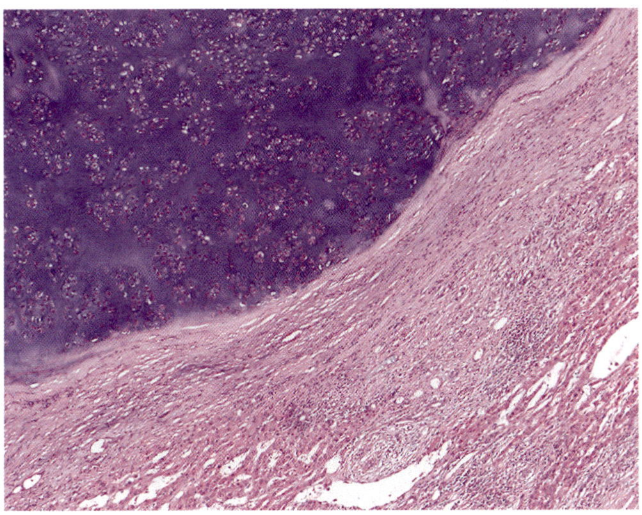

Fig. 7.270 Hepatic chondrosarcoma. There is a thick fibrous capsule around the tumor, a few hepatic cells can be seen outside the capsule

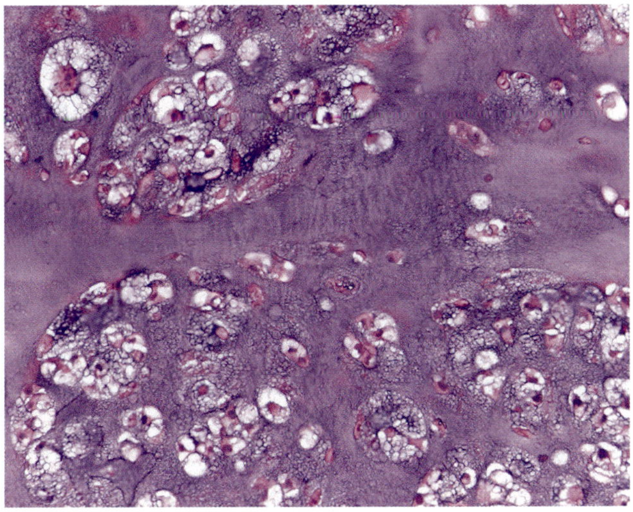

Fig. 7.271 Hepatic chondrosarcoma. The tumor consisted of osteoclast-like giant cells, as well as abundant myxoid stroma

7.5 Malignant Neurological and Endocrinic Tumors

7.5.1 Neuroendocrine Neoplasms

7.5.1.1 Pathogenesis and Mechanism

It refers to all tumors originating from peptidergic neurons and neuroendocrine cells, from inertial tumors, in slow growth with mild malignancy, to obvious malignant tumors with highly metastatic ability, etc. According to the degree of differentiation, NEN is divided into well-differentiated neuroendocrine tumor (NET) and poorly differentiated neuroendocrine carcinoma (NEC). Though the term of carcinoid tumor has been used in a history of over a century, it does not reflect the origin of NEN and the feature of hormone secretion nor does it suggest the biological behaviors of the tumor, based on which the Chinese Consensus on Pathodiagnosis of Gastrointestinal and Pancreatic neuroendocrine neoplasms (2013 version) proposed to abandon the name of carcinoid in routine pathological diagnosis, while 2010 WHO classification defined NET G1 phase as the synonym of carcinoid [4]. NEN can be found in any part of the body, including organs differentiated from foregut, midgut, and hindgut.

The pathogenesis of hepatic NEN is still not defined, which was suggested to derive from the ectopic pancreas or adrenal gland tissue in the liver or neuroendocrine cells scattered in between the biliary epithelium during embryonic development. Furthermore, chronic inflammation of biliary system can lead to intestinal metaplasia, which tends to form neuroendocrine neoplasms [177]. So far, the Chinese and English literature contains more than 100 reported cases of primary hepatic NEN. Gravante et al. [178] reviewed the English literature, summarizing the symptoms, diagnosis, and treatment of 69 cases of primary hepatic carcinoid. And Jing Zhao et al. [179] from Zhongshan Hospital, Fudan University reviewed samples of 12,600 cases with hepatectomy during 10-year period from 2000 to 2010, and 35 cases of primary hepatic NEN were diagnosed. In addition, a total of 12 cases of primary hepatic NEN have been diagnosed in the Department of Pathology, Eastern Hepatobiliary Surgery Hospital, Second Military Medical University.

7.5.1.2 Clinical Features

The patients are often aged 8–83 years old, with males accounting for 40.6%. Jing Zhao et al. reported 35 cases of primary hepatic NEN with a male to female ratio of 2.6:1. And a total of 12 cases of hepatic carcinoid have been diagnosed in the Department of Pathology, Eastern Hepatobiliary Surgery Hospital, Second Military Medical University, with a male to female ratio of 7:5, an average age of 47.3 years old. The clinical manifestations include abdominal pain or asymptomatic mass in the liver, while some tumors have gastrin-stimulating immunocompetence, and these patients may be complicated by Zollinger-Ellison syndrome, hypoglycemia, etc.

7.5.1.3 Imaging Features

Ultrasound type B shows hyper-echoes in the liver parenchyma, indicating contents of multiple microcystic tumors. And CT plain scan shows oval and solid hypodensities, while enhanced scan demonstrates patchy enhancement in arterial phase, increased enhancement in portal phase with contrast agent filling toward the center, and decreased enhancement in delayed phase. In the center of cases with high-grade malignancy, regions of liquefaction necrosis are commonly observed, and obvious heterogeneous enhancement is shown in arterial phase without significant enhancement in the central liquefaction necrosis.

7.5.1.4 Gross Features

Primary hepatic NEN is often solitary, more frequently found in the right lobe of the liver, accounting for about 49.3%, and the tumors are generally huge, solitary, and hemorrhaged well-defined masses with no capsule. The average diameter of the tumors is 9.4 (3–21.5) cm, and the cut sections are gray white with rich blood supply (Figs. 7.272 and 7.273), marked calcification, and no cirrhosis in the surrounding liver tissue. No significant difference is observed between functional and nonfunctional tumors in gross appearance.

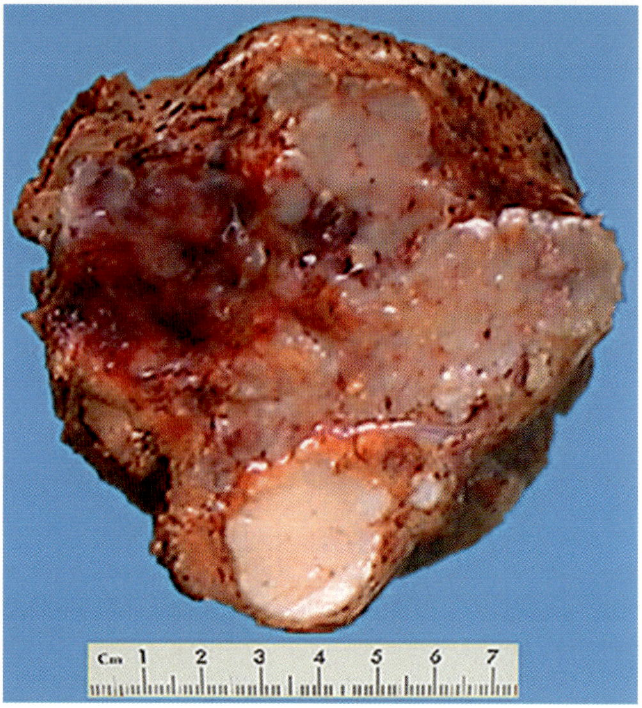

Fig. 7.272 Hepatic carcinoid. Huge *gray-white* fish-like mass with a little heamorrage

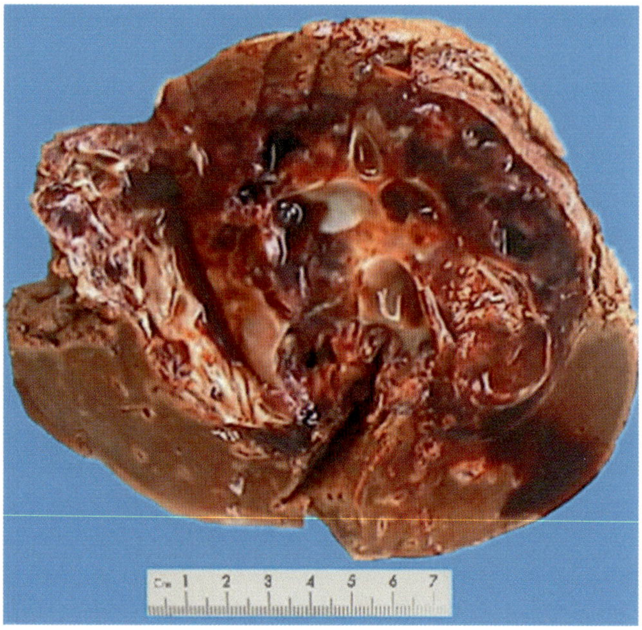

Fig. 7.273 Hepatic carcinoid. Cut surface appears as cystic and solid

7.5.1.5 Microscopic Features

It consists of tumor cells similar to neuroendocrine cells of normal digestive tract, which are consistent in size and

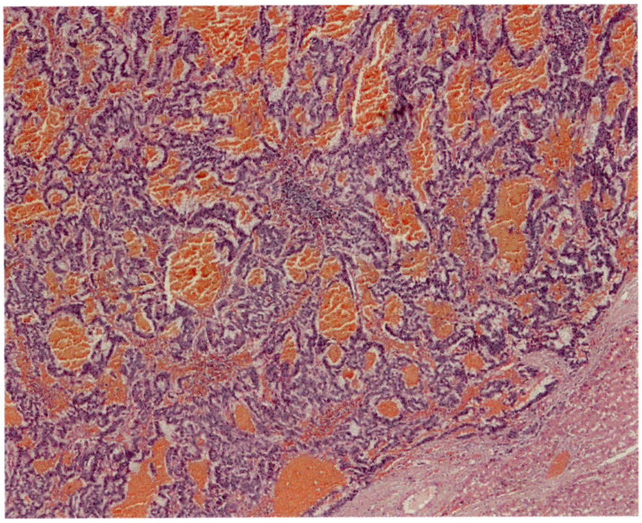

Fig. 7.274 Hepatic NET G1. Tumor cells are consistent in size, arranged in trabecular pattern and well-defined border

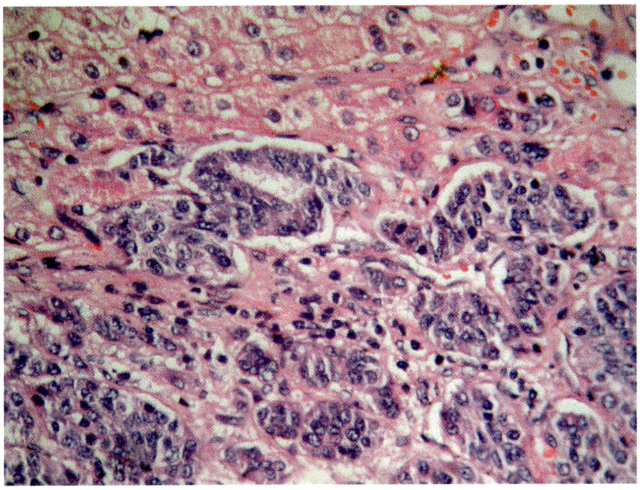

Fig. 7.275 Hepatic NET G2. There is no capsule between the tumor and the liver tissue and infiltrated into the adjacent hepatic sinus

arranged in solid nests, ribbons, lord or rosettes, etc. The tumor cells are polygonal in consistent shape and size, either small cells or medium-sized cells, containing median or abundant amount of cytoplasm, with or without nucleoli. The peri-nest fibers vary in number, with abundant small blood vessels, and no or spotty necrosis is visible. Mitotic figures are counted in 50 HPF. Ki-67 (using MIB antibody) index is estimated by 500–2000 cells of the most strongly nuclear-stained regions, and in cases of inconsistent mitotic figures and Ki-67 index, the higher grade was adopted. According to mitotic figures and Ki-67 index, NET can also be divided into G1 (Fig. 7.274) and G2 (Fig. 7.275), while NEC is classified as G3 (Table 7.20).

Neuroendocrine carcinoma (NEC) refers to poorly differentiated high-grade malignant neuroendocrine neoplasms,

Table 7.20 2010 edition WHO NEN classification [4]

NEN	Grade	Criteria
NET	G1	Mitotic figures <2/10 HPF and/or Ki-67 index ≤2%
NET	G2	Mitotic figures 2–20/10 HPF and / or Ki-67 index of 3–20%
NEC	G3	Mitotic figures >20/10 HPF and /or Ki-67 index >20%

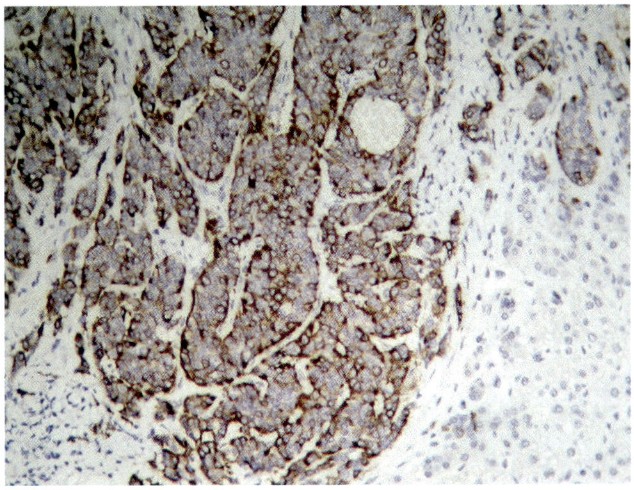

Fig. 7.276 Hepatic NET. CgA is positive in tumor cells

including small cell neuroendocrine carcinoma and large cell neuroendocrine carcinoma, the morphology of which is identical with that of corresponding tumor in the lung. The cells of small cell carcinoma are small in size, round or oval in shape, similar to lymphocyte, while some cells are elongated and fusiform, containing little cytoplasm, with obvious nuclear atypia and mitotic figures (>20/HPF). Tumor cells exhibit distributed diffusely, or arranged in nests in most cases, and multifocal necrosis can be found in the tumors. In large cell neuroendocrine carcinoma, the cells are often three times larger than lymphocytes, forming an organ-like structure, arranged in pseudorosettes or diffuse distribution, containing thick and granular chromatin, conspicuous nucleoli, abundant cytoplasm, visible mitotic figures, and obvious necrosis.

NEC includes large cell neuroendocrine carcinoma and small cell neuroendocrine carcinoma, abbreviated as large cell carcinoma and small cell carcinoma, respectively.

7.5.1.6 Immunohistochemistry

The tumor is positive for neuroendocrine markers, such as NSE, S-100 protein, CgA, Syn, CD56, etc. (Figs. 7.276 and 7.277). And CK18, CK19, and other epithelial markers can be positive, as well as focal positive CDX2. The tumor cells are argentaffin, positive in Ag-NORs, or potassium dichromate staining.

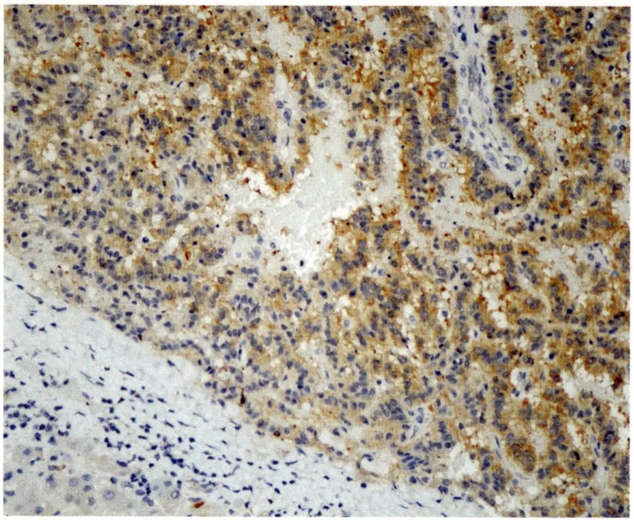

Fig. 7.277 Hepatic NET. NSE is positive in tumor cells

7.5.1.7 Electron Microscopic Observation

The cytoplasm contains dense-core-containing granules of varying sizes, the diameter of which is 200 nm.

7.5.1.8 Differential Diagnosis

Most hepatic NEN, either solitary or multiple, are metastatic, with the primary tumor in the gastrointestinal tract. In situations of undefined primary lesions after multiple examinations, the cases can be diagnosed as primary hepatic NEN with much caution. Reports in the literature also revealed the existence of finding primary lesion during the follow-up years after surgical resection of hepatic NEN; thus, the so-called "primary" hepatic NEN may be metastatic lesion with uncertain primary lesion. Hepatocellular carcinoma may show neuroendocrine differentiation; however, HCC cells are Hep Par-1 positive, pseudoglandular structures containing bile, and the trabecula is separated by endothelial cell lining sinusoids with cirrhosis in the adjacent liver tissue. Cholangiocarcinoma may contain similar small cells and fibrosis, but the former is positive for CK19 and CA19-9 staining, while it is often negative for neuroendocrine markers. Besides, a few kinds of carcinoids are concomitant lesions of multiple endocrine neoplasia type 1 (MEN-1).

7.5.1.9 Treatment and Prognosis

Surgical resection remains the mainstream for the treatment of primary hepatic NEN, and for unresectable cases, liver transplantation may receive good therapeutic effects. In the literature, three reported cases of primary hepatic NEN treated via liver transplantation, the patients gained tumor-free survival during the postsurgical periods, ranging from 38 months to 8 years [180]. In addition, the latest studies showed [181] that targeted medicines, e.g., angiogenesis inhibitor, sunitinib, immunosuppressor, everolimus, etc., can also play a role in the treatment of NET. Since NET is a potentially malignant tumor, which has risks of long-term metastasis and recurrence, poorly differentiated, grows in invasive pattern, with grade three nuclei, mitotic figures>20/10 HPF, Ki67 PI>20%, and tumoral necrosis indicates high degree of malignancy of the tumor, and the patients are suggested to have a short survival period with poor prognosis. Jing Zhao et al. [179] reported 32 cases of primary hepatic NEN with a median survival time of 37 months in postsurgical follow-up, and the average survival time was 63.4 months in NET group, while patients in NEC group survived for 17.6 months on average.

7.5.2 Malignant Peripheral Nerve Sheath Tumor

7.5.2.1 Pathogenesis and Mechanism

Malignant peripheral nerve sheath tumor (MPNST), also known as malignant schwannoma, is extremely rare, accounting for 5–10% of tumors of soft tissue. As many as 50% of the MPNST cases are found in NF1 hereditary syndrome, and about 10% of them are induced by radiation, others have no identified genetic abnormalities, or are only a concomitant lesion of neurofibromatosis. By now, only three cases of MPNST have been reported in the literature, of which only two cases are complicated with neurofibromatosis NF-1 and others are de novo. There are two cases reported in Chinese literature.

7.5.2.2 Clinical Features

The patients are aged 21–63 years old with a median onset age of 49 years old, more males than females (7/9), and early onset age is found in cases with neurofibromatosis. The clinical manifestations include abdominal pain, fever, jaundice, ascites, etc. A total of three cases of MPNST have been diagnosed in the Department of Pathology, Eastern Hepatobiliary Surgery Hospital, Second Military Medical University, and the patients are aged 46.7 years old on average (Table 7.21), with a male to female ratio of 2:1. Those with neurofibromatosis may present corresponding manifestations, such as milk-coffee spots in the skin.

7.5.2.3 Gross Features

The tumor is solid, lobulated or nodular, and large in volume with a diameter of >5 cm in most cases or even reaching 30 cm which occupies almost the whole hepatic lobe. The tumors have no or incomplete capsule, and satellite nodules of varying sizes can be visible in the surrounding liver tissue. The cross section of the tumor is dense, fleshy or jelly, with vortex and cord structures, or multicolored in cases with

Table 7.21 Clinical and pathological characteristics of three cases of hepatic malignant peripheral nerve sheath tumor

Case	Gender	Age	Location	Size (cm)	Illustration
1	Female	37	Left lobe	37 × 20 × 8	Postsurgical recurrence with peritoneal metastasis
			Left lobe	7 × 4 × 3	
2	Male	51	Left lobe	12 × 9 × 5	
			Right lobe	1 × 1 × 1	
3	Female	52	Portal area	3.5 × 2	

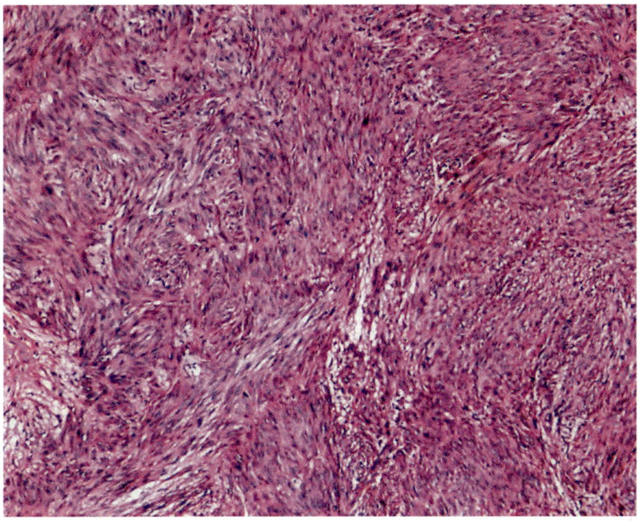

Fig. 7.278 Hepatic malignant peripheral nerve sheath tumor. The spindle cells are arranged in fascicles or storiform structures with focally myxoid degeneration

obvious hemorrhage and necrosis. In a few cases, the tumor can be white nodule protruding into intrahepatic bile ducts and large branches of the hepatic vein.

7.5.2.4 Microscopic Features

The spindle cells are arranged in fascicles or storiform structures (Fig. 7.278), and alternate cellularity regions and cell-sparse regions are found, often with myxoid stroma, paliform arranged nuclei, spiral nodules formed by a part of spindle cells, perivascular tumor cells densely arranged in eccentric structures, staghorn-like vascular lumen. The cells grow along the branches of nerve. Spindle tumor cells contain bend or curved nucleus, with perinuclear microvacuoles (Fig. 7.279), active mitosis, commonly observable necrosis, and other metaplasia tissues including the bone, cartilage, skeletal muscle, etc. Tumor cells focal degeneration, venous invasion, and satellite forming are suggestive of malignant transformation [182].

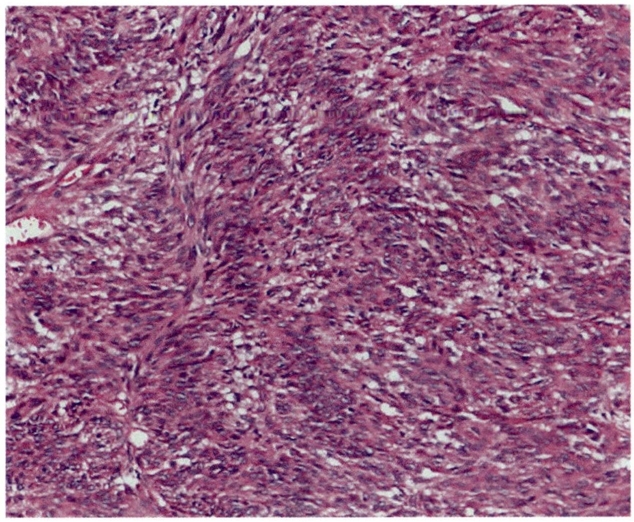

Fig. 7.279 Hepatic malignant peripheral nerve sheath tumor. Spindle tumor cells contain hyperchromatic nucleus, with peri-nuclear microvacuoles, arranging in paliform pattern

Epithelioid MPNST is a rare subtype, consisting of plump epithelioid cells with abundant eosinophilic cytoplasm and sometimes scattered in abundant extracellular matrix. The tumor cells grow in lobulated pattern, often found in malignant transformation of benign neurilemmoma, irrelevant to NF1. The diagnostic criteria of MPNST include ① tumors of the peripheral nerves; ② transitional tumors between benign tumors and other malignant peripheral nerve tumors; ③ tumors in NF1 patients, histologically similar to MPNST derived from nerves; and ④ tumors without characteristics of NF1, but with histological features of MPNST, and defined immunophenotype or ultrastructure features of Schwann cells and peripheral nerve cells differentiation [183].

7.5.2.5 Immunohistochemistry

Tumor cells are focally or weakly positive for S-100, and strongly positive for S-100 should be paid much attention to distinguish from cell-rich neurilemmoma. Vimentin is positive, and CD56 and CD57 positive rates vary greatly. Also, the tumor cells are positive for peripheral collagen IV. And epithelioid MPNST shows diffusely positive for S-100.

7.5.2.6 Differential Diagnosis

Diseases that MPNST should be distinguished from monophase synovial sarcoma, solitary fibrous tumors, undifferentiated pleomorphic sarcoma, fibrosarcoma, leiomyosarcoma, etc. The histology and immunohistochemistry features of different tumors can be referred to in related chapters and sections.

7.5.2.7 Treatment and Prognosis

Surgical resection is optimal treatment. The prognosis of MPNST is poor, and for rapid recurrence, metastasis and death are often found after surgery. Patients with NF1 have a poorer prognosis, and positive nuclear TP53 of tumor cells is suggestive of a poor prognosis.

7.6 Other Malignant Tumors

7.6.1 Carcinosarcoma

7.6.1.1 Pathogenesis and Mechanism

In 2002 version of WHO classification, hepatic carcinosarcoma was defined as hepatic epithelial malignant tumors (hepatocellular carcinoma or cholangiocarcinoma) combined with various mesenchymal sarcoma components, also known as malignant pleomorphic adenoma (malignant-mixed tumor). So far, only more than 20 cases of hepatic carcinosarcoma which meet the criteria have been reported in the literature. A total of 23 cases of carcinosarcoma have been diagnosed in the Department of Pathology, Eastern Hepatobiliary Surgery Hospital, Second Military Medical University. And in 2010 version of WHO classification, hepatic carcinosarcoma was defined as carcinoma with sarcomatoid differentiation, also known as sarcomatoid carcinoma, and suggested that sarcomatoid components were clonal evolution of differentiated tumoral components, such as hepatocellular carcinoma or cholangiocarcinoma, with varying morphology of spindled, epithelioid, or pleomorphic. It has also been proposed that carcinosarcoma is a malignant tumor consisting of epithelial and sarcomatous components. This type of tumor is generated and dedifferentiated from epithelial cells [184]. The author suggests that carcinosarcoma may differ from sarcomatoid carcinoma, for the former is a single tumor containing two definite malignant epithelial and mesenchymal cell component, such as hepatocellular carcinoma or cholangiocarcinoma complicated by leiomyosarcoma or fibrosarcoma, while the latter was previously called as metaplastic carcinoma (MC), which referred to malignant epithelial components differentiating into sarcomatoid morphology with metaplasia but possessing some of the phenotypes of epithelial tumors. Both the two types of hepatic tumors can be found in pathodiagnosis.

Goto et al. (2010) reported one case of surgically excised mass of 3 cm in size in the left lobe of the liver, consisting of the contents of hepatocellular carcinoma, cholangioadenoma, osteosarcoma, and chondrosarcoma, which was confirmed as a carcinosarcoma [185]. Lai et al. (2011) reported one case of surgically excised hepatic carcinosarcoma of 4 cm in diameter, consisting of hepatocellular carcinoma and rhabdomyosarcoma [186].

The histogenesis of epithelial and mesenchymal components in carcinosarcoma is still unclear. Thompson et al. (1996) studied the methylation status of hypoxanthine phosphoribosyltransferase gene on chromosome X, finding carcinosarcoma was monoclonal originated [187]. In 2010, Zhao et al. [188] used loss of heterozygosity of microsatellite to find that both carcinoma and sarcoma components shared the same clonal origin. In 2012, Schaefer et al. [189] conducted a comparison study on the two components in one case of hepatic carcinosarcoma using CGH and found amplification of 6p gene in both carcinoma and sarcoma components, while ten abnormal genes were found in the carcinoma part and three in the sarcoma part, indicating they might originate in monoclonal stem cell, and carcinosarcoma derives from a single cell with amplification of 6p chromosome which differentiates subsequently into two different directions of molecular progression. Luchini et al. [190] studied one case of hepatic carcinosarcoma via next-generation sequencing, finding the tumor originated from the same progenitor cell and undergoes into different clonal evolution. Simultaneous point mutations are found in TP53 gene of primary HCC, HCC satellite focus, sarcoma, and rhabdomyosarcoma components, suggesting HCC satellite foci may be the result of intrahepatic metastasis of primary carcinosarcoma. The finding that different tumoral components undergo different clonal evolution was confirmed by other molecular changes, e.g., same ABL1 mutation but different PIK3CA mutations in primary and metastatic hepatocellular carcinoma, different FGFR3 mutations in poorly differentiated sarcoma, and rhabdomyosarcoma of sarcoma component. Thus, it is believed that the term of "carcinoma with sarcomatoid differentiation" is more suitable. The author has conducted a comparison analysis on the three cases of hepatic carcinosarcoma in the Department of Pathology, Eastern Hepatobiliary Surgery Hospital, Second Military Medical University via genomic loss of heterozygosity of microsatellite, demonstrating that carcinoma and sarcoma components had different loss of heterozygosity of microsatellite loci and frequents, which suggested that they may originate in different clones and differentiate into carcinoma and sarcoma (data to be published).

7.6.1.2 Clinical Features

The patients of hepatic carcinosarcoma are aged 46–84 years old, with an average age of 60 years old and a male to female ratio of 17:7, and about 58.3% of them have a history of cirrhosis, while one-third of the patients are complicated by viral hepatitis.

7.6.1.3 Gross Features

The tumors are 11.2 (3–19) cm in diameter. And in the 23 cases of carcinosarcoma diagnosed in the Department of Pathology, Eastern Hepatobiliary Surgery Hospital, Second Military Medical University, the average age of the patients were (51.4 + 12.8) (ranged 14–70) years old, with a male to female ratio of 21:2, the rate of hepatitis B virus infection of 73.9% (17/23), of which nine cases were complicated by cirrhosis.

7.6.1.4 Microscopic Features

The epithelial component in the tumor is mainly hepatocellular carcinoma, or cholangiocarcinoma, neuroendocrine carcinoma, undifferentiated carcinoma, etc., while sarcoma component is more often osteosarcoma and chondrosarcoma, as well as rhabdomyosarcoma, leiomyosarcoma, malignant fibrous histiocytoma, fibrosarcoma, malignant peripheral nerve sheath tumor, undifferentiated spindle cell tumor, etc., with or without a transition between epithelial and mesenchymal components (Figs. 7.280 and 7.281). However, reactive stromal fibrous proliferation should not be mistaken as fibrosarcoma component. Immunohistochemistry should be done to determine the existence of both cellular components, e.g., CK (CK8, CK18 or CK7, CK19) is positive (Fig. 7.282) in carcinoma cells, S-100 is negative, chondrosarcoma tumor cells are CK negative and S-100 positive, transitional carcinoma cells can be CK and S-100 positive, leiomyosarcoma cells are SMA positive (Fig. 7.283), and fibrosarcoma components are vimentin positive (Fig. 7.284). Among the 23 cases of carcinosarcoma diagnosed in the Department of Pathology, Eastern Hepatobiliary Surgery Hospital, Second Military Medical University, 9 cases mainly contained hepatocellular carcinoma as the carcinoma component, 10 cases cholangiocarcinoma, 4 cases combined hepatocellular carcinoma-cholangiocarcinoma, and sarcoma component is more often fibrosarcoma found in 13 cases, angiosarcoma in 3 cases, leiomyosarcoma in 3 cases, MFH in 2 cases, one UES and one case of hemangio-perithelioma.

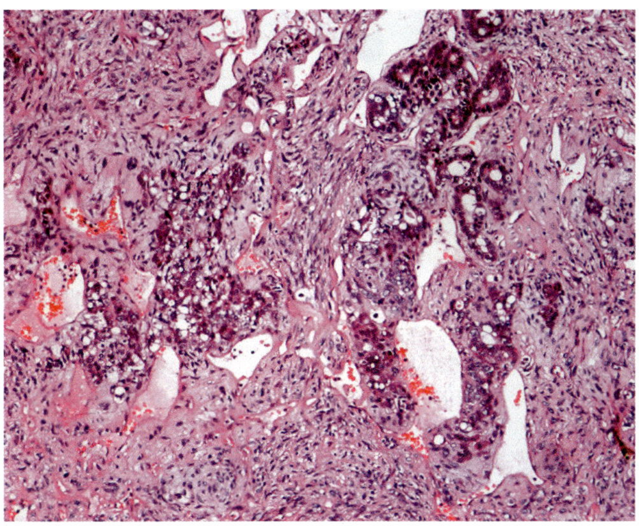

Fig. 7.280 Hepatic carcinosarcoma. The tumor consists of cholangiocarcinoma and leiomyosarcoma

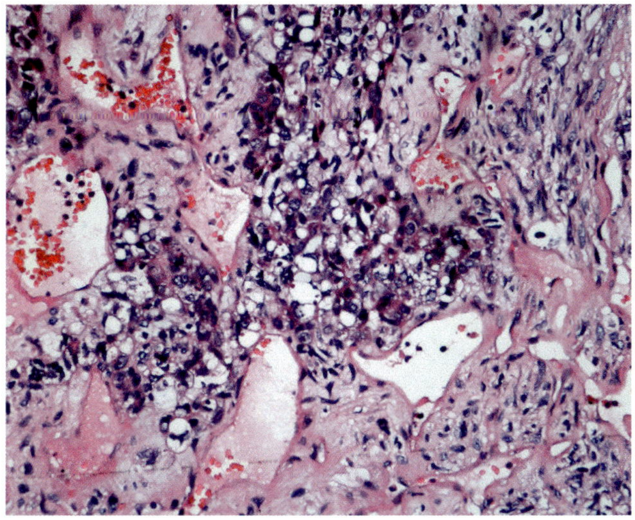

Fig. 7.281 Hepatic carcinosarcoma. Adenocarcinoma cells are mingled with leiomyosarcoma

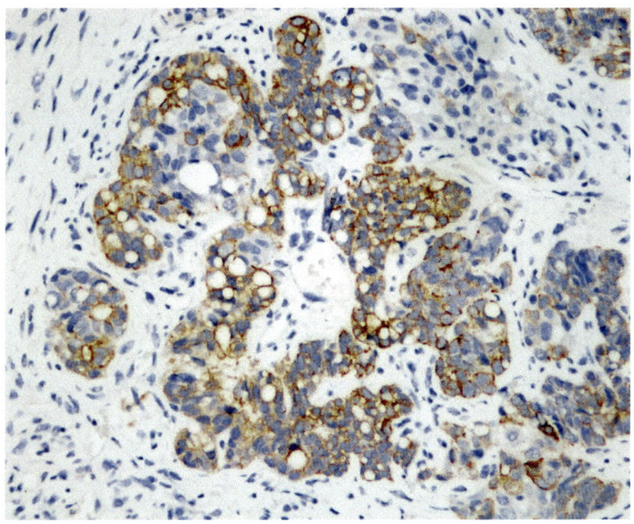

Fig. 7.282 Hepatic carcinosarcoma. Cholangiocarcinoma cells are positive for CK19

7.6.1.5 Treatment and Prognosis

Hepatic carcinosarcoma presents dual biological behaviors, with higher grade of malignancy, and most cases have metastasis of the lung and lymph nodes with a poor prognosis. Zhao (2010) found that the sarcoma component in hepatic carcinosarcoma tends to invade peritumoral hepatic sinusoid (Fig. 7.285), and postsurgically recurrent lesions also contain predominant sarcomatoid components [188]. Thus, radical surgical resection with adjuvant postsurgical comprehensive treatment is optimal. Luchini et al. [190]

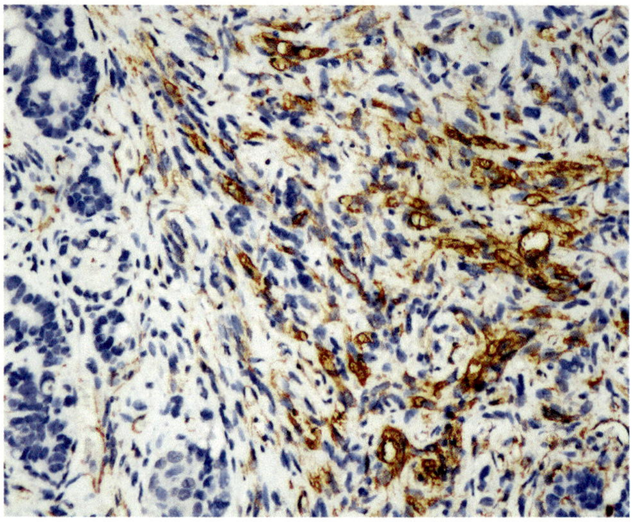

Fig. 7.283 Hepatic carcinosarcoma. Leiomyosarcoma cells are positive for SMA while cholangiocarcinoma cells are negative

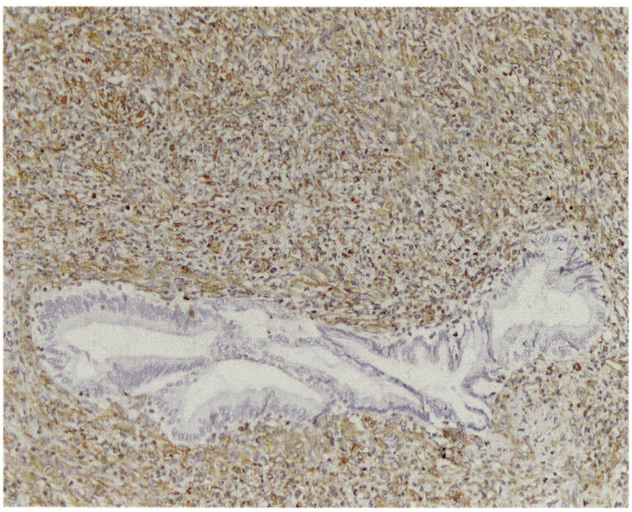

Fig. 7.284 Hepatic carcinosarcoma. Fibrosarcoma cells are positive for Vimentin while cholangiocarcinoma cells are negative

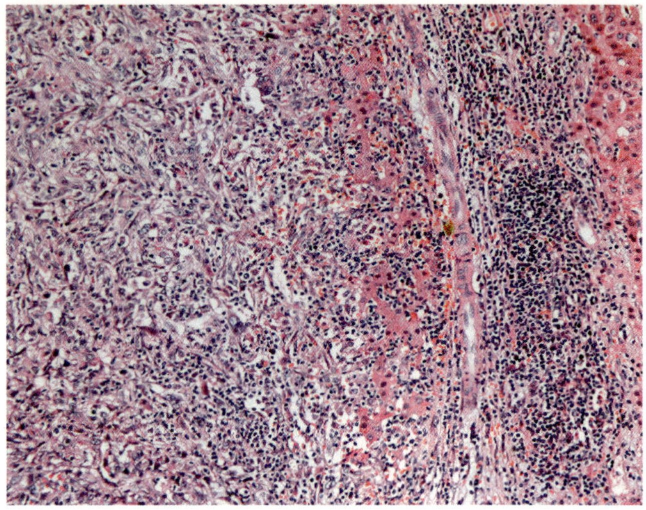

Fig. 7.285 Hepatic carcinosarcoma. Fibrosarcoma components infiltrate into the surrounding hepatic sinus

conducted sequencing and found that PIK3CA, FGFR2, FGFR3, and VEGFR2 may be the potential therapeutic molecular target of hepatic carcinosarcoma.

7.6.2 Yolk Sac Tumor

7.6.2.1 Pathogenesis and Mechanism

Primary hepatic germ cell tumors, including yolk sac tumor, choriocarcinoma, and teratoma, are relatively rare. Yolk sac tumor is a malignant germ cell tumor, mostly found in gonads, and is the most common tumor of testis in prepuberal males, accounting 70% of all germ cell tumors of the testis. Yolk sac tumor of ovary in females accounts for about 20% of female germ cell tumors. Extra-gonad germ cell tumor is rare, accounting for 1–5% of germ cell tumors, among which yolk sac tumor makes up 60%. Yolk sac tumor is common in the anterior mediastinum, posterior peritoneum, sacrococcygeum, vagina, central nervous system, and pineal gland. Primary hepatic yolk sac tumor is rare, firstly reported by Hart in 1975, and less than 20 cases have been reported in the literature. Its pathogenesis mainly involves the ectopic germ cells in the liver, or it is suggested to be originated from the abnormally differentiated pluripotent stem cells during the embryonic development. The immunohistochemistry and histological feature of yolk sac tumor are similar to those of endodermal sinus in mice, so it is also known as endodermal sinus tumor.

7.6.2.2 Clinical Features

Among the 19 cases of hepatic yolk sac tumor reported in the literature, eight patients are infants or children, with an average age of 19.9 months and a male to female ratio of 1:1, and 11 adult patients with an average age of 37.4 (24–64) years old and more females (the male to female ratio of 7:4). The main clinical manifestations include upper abdominal pain, abdominal distention, and abdominal huge mass with fever, and examination of the genital glands shows no mass. Serum AFP and β-human chorionic gonadotropin (β-HCG) significantly increase, indicating extra-gonadal yolk sac tumor.

7.6.2.3 Gross Features

The tumors are often huge masses or multiple lesions in a few cases, and the average diameter of the tumors is 12.3 (4–20) cm, with well-defined capsule. The cross section is soft and brittle, grayish tan or dark red, multinodular, or locally multicolored, with semitransparent and grayish-white myxoid regions and foci of hemorrhage and necrosis, and cystic degeneration.

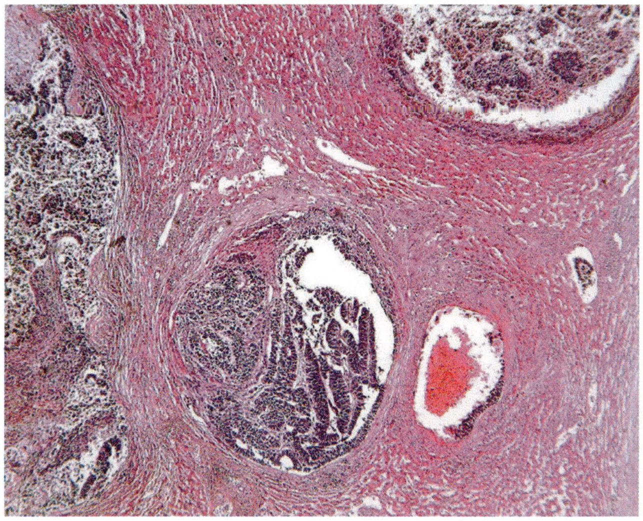

Fig. 7.286 Hepatic yolk sac tumor. Yolk sac structure with varying sizes of multi-cystic structures, lined by cubic or flat epithelium, infiltrated into the hepatic tissue

7.6.2.4 Microscopic Features

The tumor contains typical structures of yolk sac tumor similar to that in genital glands, e.g., in the background of myxoid edematous stroma, basophilic small cells form various shapes with characteristic histological figures:

① Endodermal sinus consisting of epithelial and blood vessels forming angioid structures with pseudopapilla. The cross section is similar to glomerulus (Schiller-Duval body) (Fig. 7.286).
② Yolk sac structure with varying sizes of multicystic structures, lined by cubic or flat epithelium.
③ Stellate structure which is loose and similar to a network.
④ Glandular structure, with round or irregular glands containing translucent cytoplasm, which are arranged in pushpin-like structures, with significantly increased mitotic figures and conspicuous atypia.

Abundant micro-blood vessels with tumor thrombi can be observed, which protrude the capsule, and multiple microcarcinoma foci can also be seen. Specific PAS-positive hyaline bodies can be found inside or outside the tumor cells.

7.6.2.5 Immunohistochemistry

AFP, HCG, albumin, alpha 1-AT, and transferrin staining are positive, while CD30 and CD34 are negative.

7.6.2.6 Differential Diagnosis

The diagnosis of primary hepatic yolk sac tumor should be made in exclusion of metastatic yolk sac tumors of the ovary or testis. Other tumors that should be differentiated include hepatocellular carcinoma, hepatic teratoma, hepatoblastoma, etc. Hepatoblastoma can also exhibit increased AFP, which is often found in children; however, it rarely contains Schiller-Duval bodies or cytoplasmic eosinophilic bodies histologically. Solitary and cystic tumors found in liver tissues without cirrhosis with glomerular bodies, AFP-positive hyaline bodies, stellate network structures in the background of myxoid edematous stroma, or pseudopapillary structures facilitate the diagnosis of hepatic yolk sac tumor.

7.6.2.7 Treatment and Prognosis

Surgical resection with combined adjuvant chemotherapy is reported with good therapeutic effects. Warren et al. [191] reported one case of primary hepatic yolk sac tumor treated with surgical resection combined with chemotherapy, and no recurrence was found in the 11-year follow-up after the surgery. Furthermore, AFP is not only the diagnostic indicator for yolk sac tumor but also an important index for the monitoring of therapeutic effects and recurrence of the tumor.

7.6.3 Chorioepithelioma

7.6.3.1 Pathogenesis and Mechanism

Chorioepithelioma, also known as choriocarcinoma, is commonly found in the genital gianas and uterus; extra-gonadal chorioepithelioma is rare. And the diagnosis of extra-gonadal primary choriocarcinoma in male patients should be made after exclusion of testicular tumors via consecutive section. For female patients, primary choriocarcinoma of the ovary and uterus should also be excluded before the diagnosis of primary extra-gonadal chorioepithelioma. It is multiple masses consisting of trophoblast cells similar to those in placenta, which can cause severe hemorrhage, and is extremely rare. Seven cases have been reported in the literature by now. It shares the possible pathogenesis of ectopic germ cells in other extra-gonadal chorioepithelioma. Elevated levels of serum β-HCG are found in some patients with hepatoblastoma and hepatocellular carcinoma, indirectly suggesting the potential origin of epithelial metaplasia in the liver for hepatic chorioepithelioma, which is not supported by the finding of no hepatocellular carcinoma components in the tumor based on the reported cases.

7.6.3.2 Clinical Features

Shi [192] reported five cases of hepatic chorioepithelioma, all affecting male adults, and the patients were aged 41.6 years old (36–48 years old) on average and clinically manifested as right upper abdominal pain and abdominal distention. Two cases of metastasizing to the lung and brain with symptoms such as headache, nausea, cough, hemoptysis, shortness of breath, and their serum β-HCG were elevated with average level of 5300 mIU/ml (560–16 500mIU/ml), while serum AFP, CEA, and CA19-9 were normal. All these five patients received histological examination of serial sections of the testis, finding no scars or germ cell tumor degeneration-related pathological evidence.

7.6.3.3 Gross Features

The tumor is often a huge mass with hemorrhage and 11 (9–13) cm in diameter, soft, with necrosis, or multiple hemorrhaged nodules.

7.6.3.4 Microscopic Features

The tumor is similar to uterine chorioepithelioma, consisting of two cellular components forming dual morphology, polygonal trophoblasts and syncytiotrophoblasts. Mononuclear trophoblasts have clear intercellular borders, with round or irregular nuclei, conspicuous nucleoli and mitotic figures [192], translucent cytoplasm, mingled with large and multinucleated syncytiotrophoblasts, which have abundant eosinophilic or basophilic cytoplasm, with moderate to severe nuclear atypia, hyperchromatic nuclei, and rare nucleoli. The tumor cells are arranged in micropapillary or cluster structures. Hemorrhage and necrosis are extensive inside the tumor, often with tumor thrombi in micro-blood vessels, diffuse hemorrhage, and well-defined slender fibrous capsule separated the tumor from the normal liver tissue.

Theegarten D et al. [193] reported one case of huge mixed malignant germ cell tumor located in the left lobe of the liver, in a size of 14 cm × 9 cm × 8 cm, serum detection: AFP: 1391 μg/ml, β-HCG: 6565 U/ml. Biopsy revealed that the tumor consisted of embryonic sarcoma (AFP, PLAP, and CD30 positive) and choriocarcinoma (β-HCG positive), with tumor thrombus in the portal vein and lymphatic metastasis.

7.6.3.5 Immunohistochemistry

Identical to embryonic chorioepithelioma, the tumor cells are positive for β-HCG, human placental lactogen, and P63, and Ki67 positive rate can reach higher than 70%, while AFP, CK7, and CK20 are negative [192].

7.6.3.6 Differential Diagnosis

Primary hepatic chorioepithelioma is rare, so careful examination of primary tumors in sites of the body in the patients such as genitals (uterus, ovary, or testis) should be conducted, mediastinum and posterior retroperitoneum, and the diagnosis of primary hepatic chorioepithelioma can only be made after exclusion of metastatic choriocarcinoma. In addition, it should also be distinguished from metastatic undifferentiated carcinoma.

7.6.3.7 Treatment and Prognosis

Primary hepatic chorioepithelioma has a poor prognosis. Shi et al. [192] reported five cases of primary hepatic chorioepithelioma, two cases of which were localized in the liver and received surgical resection plus postsurgical chemotherapy, while three cases had metastasis in other organs at the time of diagnosis who received poorly differentiated carcinoma-targeted chemotherapy with unsatisfactory effects. The five patients died of the tumor in 2–8 months after diagnosis, and it was noted that the levels of serum HCG decreased significantly when treatment was effective.

7.6.4 Malignant Teratoma

7.6.4.1 Pathogenesis and Mechanism

Teratoma contains the tissues of two or more embryonic layers and can be divided into mature teratoma (benign teratoma) and immature teratoma (malignant teratoma). Embryologically, teratoma originates from the primitive immature germ cells, which was hindered during the migration from hindgut of allantois to gonads in the first week of embryonic development. Willis theory suggests it originates from the pluripotent stem cells of invaginated planula, which avoid the primitive commands in embryonic development. The tumor is often found in the ovary, testis, anterior mediastin, posterior peritoneum, sacrococcygeum, and cranium or occasionally discovered in the gastrointestinal tract, while hepatic cases are rare. In current literature, more than 40 cases of hepatic teratoma have been reported, with only a few containing malignant components. The disease may derive from malignant transformation of benign teratoma or directly generated malignant teratoma.

7.6.4.2 Clinical Features

Jian-guo Zhao et al. [194] reported one case of hepatic immature teratoma, and the patients were all females, aged 19 years old on average. CT images show a mass in the segments VI and VII of the right lobe of the liver, which was 20 cm long and 16 cm in diameter, with partial cystic degeneration, and compression of the right kidney, head of the pancreas, and descending duodenum was also found. Serum tests: AFP 154.1 ng/ml, CA 19–9238.4 IU/ml, CA 125301.8 IU/ml. During the operation, the tumor was seen to occupy most of the right lobe of the liver, sized 20 cm × 15 cm × 15 cm, and the cut section was cystic and solid, mainly solid, with mucus in the cyst, and no cirrhosis in the liver tissue. Xu et al. (2010) reported one case of a 34-year-old male with a 16 cm × 12 cm × 8 cm tumor in the right lobe of the liver, and it was composed of mixed yolk sac tumor and immature teratoma components histologically, which was treated with surgical resection combined with postsurgical chemotherapy. The patient died from recurrence of the tumor 5 months later [195].

7.6.4.3 Gross Feature

The tumor is huge with a capsule as teratoma in other parts of the body, and the cross section is solid or multilobular. Cystic lesions are often spherical, while solid lesions are often multilobular. The cysts contain serum, mucus or blood, and few hairs. The parenchyma is soft, fish-like, grayish white or pink, and often with hemorrhage and necrosis.

7.6.4.4 Microscopic Features

The tumors contain mature and immature tissues derived from all the three embryonic layers, the former of which include the bone, cartilage, hair, skin, fat, primitive kidney tissue, pancreas and other endocrine tissues, squamous epithelium, and nerve tissue, while the latter mainly include squamous cell carcinoma and sarcomatoid stroma, without yolk sac tumor components, and partial cells contain obviously increased mitotic figures with significant atypia.

7.6.4.5 Differential Diagnosis

Yolk sac tumor: completely consisting of malignant tumor components without any components of benign germ cell tumor, and metastasis should first be excluded in the diagnosis.

7.6.4.6 Treatment and Prognosis

The optimal treatment is surgical resection for the disease; however, the prognosis is poor. The patients often die from systemic metastasis. For patients with growing teratoma syndrome, liver transplantation can improve their prognosis. Eghtesad et al. [196] reported one case of hepatic multiple teratomas with metastasis in posterior peritoneum, in vivo liver transplantation, and resection of the tumor in the posterior peritoneum was operated contributing to the patient's tumor-free survival in the postsurgical 15-month period.

7.6.5 Malignant Rhabdoid Tumor

7.6.5.1 Pathogenesis and Mechanism

Malignant rhabdoid tumor (MRT) is a type of malignant tumors with uncertain histogenesis or differentiation, which was first reported as a kind of primary malignant tumors of the kidney by Bechwith and Palmer in 1978. The tumor can also be found in extrarenal organs, namely, extrarenal rhabdoid tumor, as well as tumors in the central nervous system, posterior peritoneum, the liver, and other organs. But primary hepatic MRT is rare, and the literature only reported 30 cases so far. Molecular biological study shows that homozygous loss of the SMARCB1 gene (in chromosome22q11.2) exists in as many as 35% of the patients, often caused by translocation of chromosome 22q11.2 and the other chromosome arms. All newly diagnosed MRT cases are required to be undergone genetic tests to exclude deletion or mutation of SMARCB1 gene. In addition, the risk of developing neurofibromatosis in familial members with mutations in the SMARCB1 gene is high. Other studies show that tumor suppressor genes, e.g., hSNF5/INI1/BAF47 on the chromosome 22q11.2 are related with MRT [197].

7.6.5.2 Clinical Features

The age of the patients with hepatic MRT is often 2 months to 9 years old. Most patients are younger than 2 years old, with a median onset age of 8 months. The main clinical manifestations include vomiting, anorexia, hepatic or abdominal mass, or tumor rupture as the first symptom. Serum AFP is normal; however, Martelli et al. (2013) reported one case of hepatic MRT in children, with serum AFP level of 197 ng/ml [197]. In a few cases, vasoactive intestinal polypeptide (VIP) increases. CT images show enormous occupying hypodensities in the liver, accompanied by necrosis and irregular calcification, or cystic degeneration in a few cases [198]. It is common to find pulmonary and lymphatic metastasis in patients with this disease.

7.6.5.3 Gross Features

Huge tumor is found which tends to occupy the whole lobe of the liver, and the cut section is soft, fleshy, and grayish white or grayish brown, with foci of hemorrhage and necrosis or partial cystic degeneration. Martelli et al. (2013) reported one case of a 7-month-old baby girl with recurrence and pulmonary metastasis 3 months after surgical resection of a 3 cm × 10 cm × 5 cm MRT in the right lobe of the liver [197].

7.6.5.4 Microscopic Features

Similar to the morphology of renal MRT, the tumor is composed of loosely arranged, large and oval or polygonal cells, which are like "RT" or rhabdomyoblasts. The tumor cells contain large and vacuolated nuclei, with obvious nucleoli, nuclear deviation, as well as abundant eosinophilic cytoplasm. PAS-positive hyaline inclusion bodies or hyaline bodies can be observed in the perinuclear cytoplasm, with clear outlines [199], and their ultrastructure shows that hyaline inclusion bodies are densely arranged in swirl intermediate filaments in a length of about 10 nm. PTAH staining shows no cross striation in the cytoplasm.

7.6.5.5 Immunohistochemistry

The tumor is CK, CK18, CK7, CK19, CD99, EMA, and vimentin positive, and NSE and S-100 can also be positive, suggesting a neuroectodermal differentiation, but myogenic markers, e.g., desmin, SMA, and myoglobin are negative. The absence of INI protein expression indicating hSNF5/INI1/BAF47 gene mutation is of diagnosis significance [197].

7.6.5.6 Electron Microscopic Observation

Perinuclear intermediate filaments are characteristic, 10 nm in diameter, and arranged in swirl and dense structures, without Z zone or sarcomere [200].

7.6.5.7 Differential Diagnosis

It should be primarily differentiated from hepatic malignant tumors in children, including hepatocellular carcinoma, hepatoblastoma, angiosarcoma, epithelioid hemangioendothelioma, leiomyosarcoma, carcinosarcoma, undifferentiated embryonic sarcoma, etc. Main key points in the diagnosis of MRT are infant; patches of the large polygonal tumor cells, vacuolar nucleus, clear nucleoli, eosinophilic cytoplasm, hyaline inclusion bodies; the immunohistochemistry shows a biphasic differentiation of vimentin and epithelial antigen; and the ultrastructural cytoplasmic intermediate filaments. Accordingly, it can be identified with the embryonic rhabdomyosarcoma, which shows positive staining of desmin and myoglobin and negative of CK staining. And hepatoblastoma should be excluded in infant cases, which shows the hepatocellular differentiation. In addition, malignant melanoma and poorly differentiated carcinoma contain visible rhabdoid cells, as well as many other tumor components which are visible in multiregional sampling, while MRT consists completely of tumor rhabdoid cells.

7.6.5.8 Treatment and Prognosis

MRT is a highly aggressive malignancy. The treatment includes surgical resection and chemotherapy, but it is not sensitive to chemotherapy. Due to the huge volume of the tumor, surgical treatment receives poor prognosis. And among the 25 cases with follow-up data reported in the literature, the median survival time was 2 months (from 5 days to more than 6 years), and the mortalities at 3, 6, and 12 months were 60%, 76%, and 84%, respectively. Even patients with metastasis can receive long-term survival if the treatment is effective.

7.6.6 Gastrointestinal Stromal Tumors

7.6.6.1 Pathogenesis and Mechanism

Gastrointestinal stromal tumor (GIST) is the most common gastrointestinal mesenchymal tumors which is specific in histology with KIT (CD117) positive. The most common involved sites are the stomach (60%), followed by jejunoileum (30%), duodenum (4–5%), the rectum (4%), colon and appendix (1–2%), esophagus (< 1%), or other organs in the gastrointestinal tract, such as the mesentery, omentum majus, retroperitoneum, pancreas, urethra, urinary bladder, and the liver. By 2014, a total of six cases of primary hepatic GIST have been reported in the English literature [201–206], and the patients are aged 46.2 years on average (ranged 17–79 years), with a male to female ratio of 5:1. Gastrointestinal stromal tumors originate from Cajal cells, and primary hepatic GIST may originate from intrahepatic-undifferentiated stem cells which can differentiate into Cajal cells, due to the hepatic origination of ventral bud in foregut from the perspective of embryogenesis.

7.6.6.2 Gross Features

The average diameter of the tumor is 12.9 (5.1–20) cm, and the cut section was cystic or solid and white grayish with a well-defined border, tenderness in solid parts, visible necrosis and hemorrhage.

7.6.6.3 Microscopic Features

Similar to the histomorphology of gastrointestinal GIST, hepatic GIST cell can be spindle cell type or epithelioid cell type. Of the six cases of reported primary hepatic GIST, four cases concerned spindle cell type, one case epithelioid cell type, and one mixed type. Spindle cell-type GIST consists of spindled tumor cells arranged in short fascicles or interwoven structures, with short stab nuclei, perinuclear vacuoles in some tumor cells, varying degrees of nuclear atypia, mitotic figures of 0/50–75/50 HPF, well-defined border between the tumor and the surrounding liver tissue, and thin capsules (Fig. 7.287). A few cases show tumor cells around blood vessels (Fig. 7.288), with hyperplasia of the fibrous stroma, infiltration of inflammatory cells, and little necrosis.

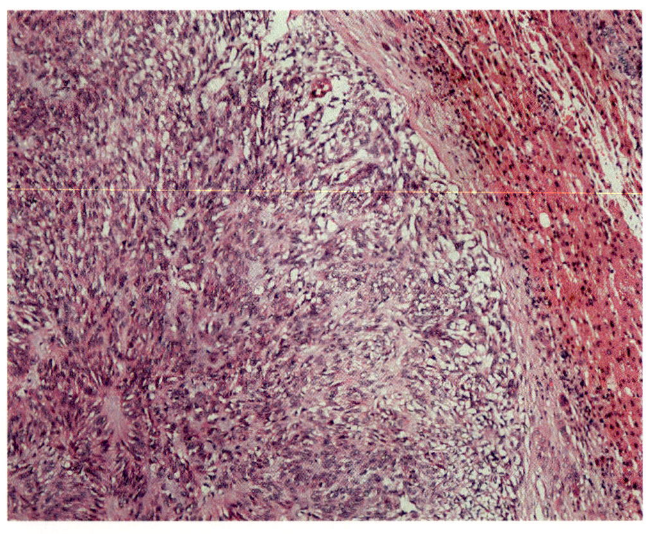

Fig. 7.287 Hepatic GIST. Thin capsule between the tumor and the surrounding liver tissue, and obvious myxoid background

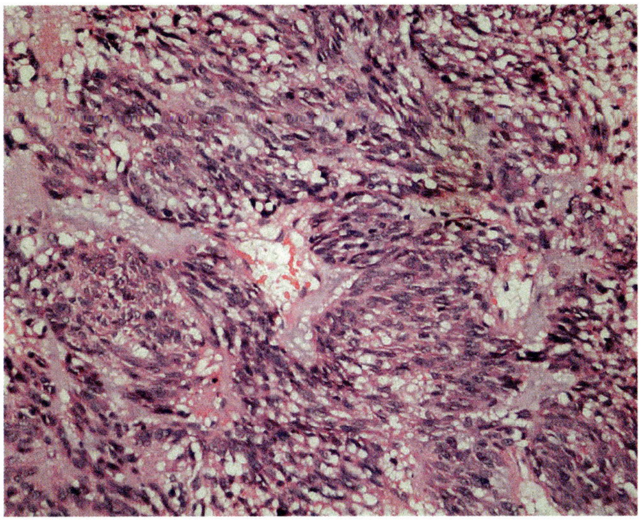

Fig. 7.288 Hepatic GIST. There are abundant blood vessels in the tumor and around which are tumor cells

Epithelioid cell-type GIST contains round or polygonal tumor cells, with translucent cytoplasm, clear intercellular borders, obvious nuclear atypia, and common mitotic figures.

7.6.6.4 Immunohistochemistry

More than 95% of GIST lesions are CD117 positive, and other related markers include CD34, nestin, PKC theta, DOG-1, and SMA, while they are negative for desmin, S100, and GFAP.

7.6.6.5 Molecular Detection

Mutation testing is helpful in the diagnosis and differential diagnosis of some difficult cases of GIST to predict the effects of molecular-targeted therapy and guide clinical treatment. Currently, recommended polymerase chain reaction (PCR) amplification sequencing can ensure the accuracy and consistency of testing results. Based on variation of gene point mutations, selection of testing genes should be demonstrated, and the genes include exons of number 9 (11%), 11 (67.5%), 13 (0.9%), and 17 (< 0.5%) in c-kit gene, and exons of number 12 (0.9%), 18 (6.3%) and 14 (0.3%) in PDGFRA gene. Most of the GIST (65–85%) gene mutations are located in c-kit gene exon 11 or 9 [207–209]; thus, priority of these two exons can be given in testing, with corresponding addition of tests on c-kit gene for exon 14 and 18 [210]. C-kit gene mutation types include frameshift deletion, mononucleotide substitutions, and copy and insertion, and deletion mutations often involve codon 557 and 558, with the most common mononucleotide substitutions of V559A, V559D, V560D, W557R, and L576P.

GIST with mutations of exon 11 in c-kit gene is sensitive to treatment of imatinib (Gleevec), and cases with exon 9 mutation have an early resistance for imatinib showing poor efficacy. Cases with PDGFRA gene mutation are sensitive to imatinib, but those with substitution mutation D842V of codon 18 are not; thus, tumors with these kinds of mutation types are resistant to imatinib. Those with c kit and PDGFRA gene mutations belong to primary resistance groups, and imatinib shows ineffectiveness in most of these cases.

7.6.6.6 Treatment and Prognosis

In pathodiagnosis, malignant evaluation can be made referring to relevant risk classifications of gastrointestinal GIST. But on the whole, GIST is a highly malignant tumor, and cases of GIST with small lesions and metastasis are not rare. Primary hepatic GIST should be surgically removed, and for patients with unresectable lesions or with metastasis and recurrence, molecular-targeted treatment using tyrosine kinase inhibitor, e.g., imatinib, would significantly control the disease development, especially for cases with c-kit gene exon 11 mutations suggested by gene sequencing, the effects of which are reported to be the best. De Chiara et al. [205] reported one case of primary hepatic GIST with multiple metastases in the lung 14 months after surgery, and the pulmonary lesions disappeared shortly after oral imatinib of 400 mg/d. Furthermore, the patient received tumor-free survival during the 2-year follow-up [211].

7.6.7 Malignant Melanoma

Primary hepatic malignant melanoma is rare with unknown origin. It was found that primary hepatic melanoma weakly expressed Hep Par-1, which may be transformed by the liver cells. At present, there are 14 reported cases of hepatic melanoma in Chinese and 8 cases in foreign literature. Domestic patients are 35.2 years old on average (ranged 27–64 age old years) with a male to female ratio of 4:3, including four cases with multiple lesions, and solitary tumors are 11.4 (4–16) cm in diameter. No current diagnostic criteria for primary malignant melanoma are conclusive. Willis et al. proposed the following reference index for primary malignant melanoma, including three necessary conditions: pathological diagnosis of malignant melanoma, especially meeting the morphological characteristics of primary malignant melanoma; no present and previous malignant melanoma in other parts of the body; and no unknown type of skin disease or a history of eye surgery, and three secondary conditions: solitary; at least one large lesion, especially >5 cm in diameter; and biopsy to exclude occult primary foci. And it was put forward that primary malignant melanoma can be diagnosed when the tumor meets the three necessary conditions and one of the secondary conditions; thus, the diagnosis of primary hepatic malignant melanoma can be referred to this criteria.

The cut sections of the tumors are grayish yellow or grayish white, with clear boundaries, partial cystic or solid components, visible hemorrhage and necrosis, cirrhosis in the surrounding liver tissue in some cases. Microscopically, epithelioid tumor cells contain melanin granules, and the tumor cells are spindle, round, or irregular shaped and arranged in acini, nests, or cords, with round or oval nuclei, large nucleoli, obvious nuclear atypia, and diffuse infiltrative growth in the surrounding area, fibrous separation between the peripheral region and the surrounding liver tissue tumor. And cases with cells containing less melanin granules should be identified from hepatocellular carcinoma via immunohistochemistry. Malignant melanoma is strongly positive for HMB45, a broad-spectrum melanoma, and S-100, but negative for high molecular weight CK, CK18, CK19, LCA, NSE, EMA, Hep-1, desmin, etc. Electron microscopy shows cytoplasmic melanin bodies. Complete resection plus systemic chemotherapy is a commonly used method for treatment.

7.6.8 Malignant Mesothelioma

7.6.8.1 Pathogenesis and Mechanism

Malignant mesothelioma is reported to originate in the pleura (70%), peritoneum (20–25%), pericardium, or testis, which has a serous cellular lining, and 80–90% of the cases have close relationship with inhaled asbestos fibers. The process from the initial exposure to airborne asbestos fibers to generation of malignant mesothelioma may be 25–40 years. Occasionally, cases of malignant mesothelioma in the falciform ligament of the liver and liver duodenum ligament are reported, while those primarily found in the liver parenchyma are rare and may derive from mesothelial cells of Glisson's sheath and subsequently invade into the hepatic parenchyma [212]. By 2013, only seven cases of hepatic malignant mesothelioma have been reported in the literature [213].

7.6.8.2 Clinical Features

Of all the seven cases of defined primary hepatic malignant mesothelioma, the median age of the patients was 62 (53–68) years old, with a male to female ratio of 2.5:1, and one patient had a determined history of asbestos exposure. The clinical manifestations of primary hepatic malignant mesothelioma are similar to those of a nonoccupational case, and some patients had significantly increased serum γ-glutamyl and alkaline phosphatase [213]. All the tumors are located in the right lobe of the liver. A total of three cases of primary hepatic malignant mesothelioma have been diagnosed in the Department of Pathology Eastern Hepatobiliary, Surgery Hospital, Second Military Medical University, and the average age of the patients was 50 (41–58) years old, with a male to female ratio of 1:2. DeStephano et al. (1985) reported one case of malignant cystic tumor in the liver, affecting a 6-month-old infant, and showed a skin differentiation lesion which was similar to peritoneal mesothelioma with postsurgical recurrence by immunohistochemistry and electron microscopy, and this case may be the youngest one among all the patients with primary hepatic malignant mesothelioma [214].

7.6.8.3 Gross Features

The tumors are often solitary nodules, located under the liver capsule, in an average diameter of 7.8 (3.2–16) cm, and most of the lesions are larger than 10 cm. The cut sections are often yellow or brown, and solid ones often contain polycystic cavities and hemorrhage.

7.6.8.4 Microscopic Features

Either histologically or immunohistochemistrically, hepatic malignant mesothelioma and classic malignant mesothelioma are similar. In the seven cases of primary hepatic mesothelioma reported in the literature, five cases (71.4%) were epithelioid type, and two cases (28.6%) were dual-phase type [epithelioid with spindle cells (sarcomatoid type)]. Microscopically, the epithelioid tumor cell-type mesothelioma are cellularity, which are round or polygonal, with abundant and pale eosinophilic cytoplasm, irregular nuclei with atypia, obvious nucleoli and active mitosis figures, arranged in cords, tubular, papillary, or adenoid patterns, and cystic dilatation of multiple lumen can be found (Fig. 7.289). The cystic walls are coated by cubic or columnar epithelial cells, and a part of them contain translucent cytoplasm (Fig. 7.290); sarcomatoid-type cells show trabecular arrangement, abundant eosinophilic cytoplasm, unclear cellular boundaries, obvious nuclei and nucleoli, while some tumor cells are similar to signet ring cells or microcystic cavities in epithelioid hemangioendothelioma. The tumors often contain hemorrhage and necrosis foci with no capsule and invade into the surrounding hepatic sinusoid (Fig. 7.291). And the boundaries between the lesions and the surrounding liver tissue are clear, while no fibrous capsules are formed and residual small hepatocyte islands and bile ducts can be found in the tumors.

7.6.8.5 Immunohistochemistry

Mesotheliomas were positive for calretinin, D2–40, WT-1, vimentin (Fig. 7.292), mesothelin (MC) (Fig. 7.293), thrombomodulin, and p53, and Ki-67 positive rate can be as high as 20%. CK7 can also be positive (Fig. 7.294), while they are negative for adenocarcinoma markers (CEA, CD15 and berep4, bg8, MOC31), as well as CD34 and CD31.

7.6.8.6 Differential Diagnosis

The biggest difference or differential point between mesotheliomas and sarcomas lies in the biphasic differentiation

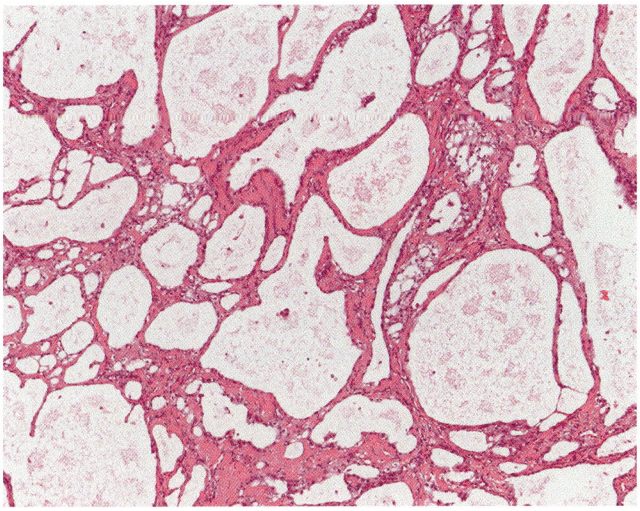

Fig. 7.289 Hepatic malignant epithelioid mesothelioma. Cystic dilatation of multiple lumen can be found

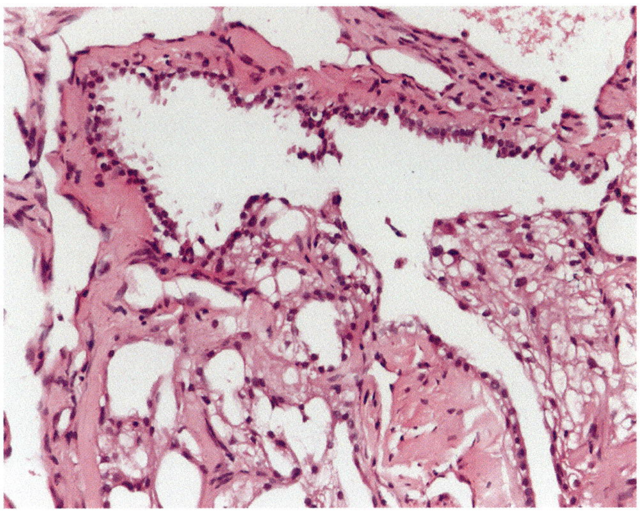

Fig. 7.290 Hepatic malignant epithelioid mesothelioma. The cystic walls are coated by cubic or columnar epithelial cells, and a part of them contain translucent cytoplasm

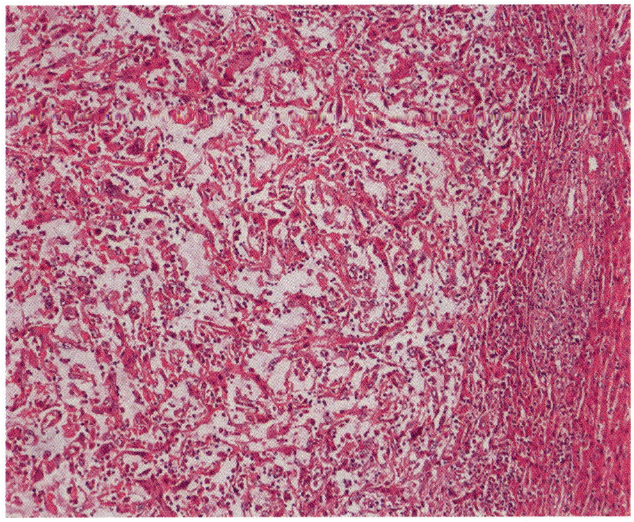

Fig. 7.291 Hepatic malignant mesothelioma. The epithelioid tumor cells are arranged as glandular pattern and invade into the surrounding hepatic sinusoid

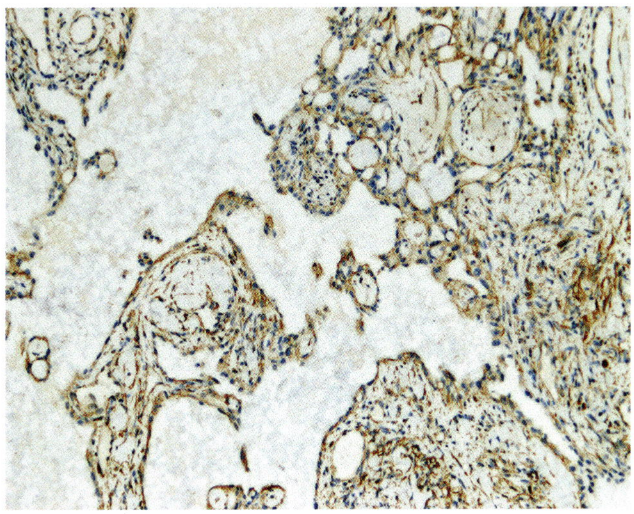

Fig. 7.292 Hepatic malignant mesothelioma. Vimentin stain is positive

characteristics in histology and immunohistochemistry of the former, as well as positive mesothelial cell markers. Also, attention needs to be paid to the exclusion of metastasis of pleural, peritoneal, and other stromal tumors into the liver.

7.6.8.7 Treatment and Prognosis

In the reported seven cases of primary hepatic malignant mesothelioma, six cases were treated with surgical resection including three cases with postsurgical recurrence, two cases of epithelioid type, and one case of dual phase type. The postsurgical serum γ-glutamine transfer peptide and alkaline phosphatase decreased to normal [213].

7.6.9 Synovial Sarcoma

Hui Dong and Wen-Ming Cong
Department of Pathology, Eastern Hepatobiliary Surgery Hospital, Second Military Medical University, Shanghai, China

7.6.9.1 Pathogenesis and Mechanism

Synovial sarcoma is the fourth soft tissue tumor, often found in the extremities, with the most common site of the knee, and other sites include the heart, kidney, prostate, pleura, mediastinum, liver, gastrointestinal tract, posterior perito-

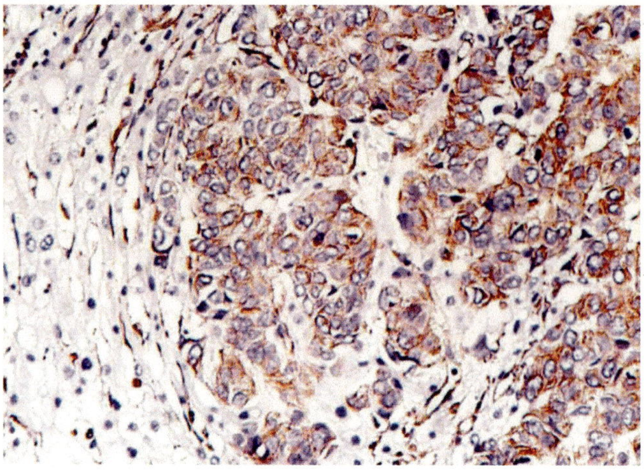

Fig. 7.293 Hepatic malignant mesothelioma. MC stain is positive

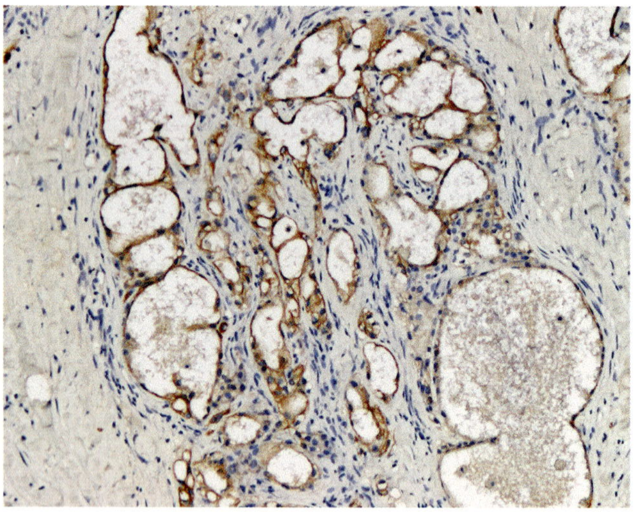

Fig. 7.294 Hepatic malignant mesothelioma. CK7 stain is positive

neum, and peripheral nerve. The histological origin of synovial sarcoma is not clear, and it has been proposed to derive from the synovial cells or pluripotent mesenchymal cells which can differentiate into synovial cells. Holla et al. (2006) reported the first case of primary hepatic synovial sarcoma in the English literature, and so far, only three cases have been reported [215–217]. Ninety percent of the synovial sarcoma contains translocation of chromosome (X; 18) (p11.2; q11.2), and DNA sequencing confirmed the presence of SYT-SSX1 fusion gene. All the three cases of primary hepatic synovial sarcoma reported in the literature contained this molecular genetic abnormality.

7.6.9.2 Clinical Features

The tumors are often found in young adults or teenagers. The three cases of primary hepatic synovial sarcoma reported in the literature affected one 18-year-old female, one 13-year-old boy, and one 60-year-old female. General clinical symptoms include fatigue, nausea, vomiting, abdominal distention, and right upper abdominal pain. Imaging displays massive hepatic space occupying lesions.

7.6.9.3 Gross Features

The tumors are large in an average diameter of 15(2.1–21) cm, with or without multinodules, and no or incomplete capsule is found.

7.6.9.4 Microscopic Features

Synovial sarcoma is a kind of malignant tumors with biphasic differentiation, composed of fibrous and epithelial cell types. Dual-phasic synovial sarcoma contains both components, and monophasic type contains one component, while poorly differentiated type is rare. In the literature, the reported three cases of hepatic synovial sarcoma are all monophasic fibrous type.

Monophasic fibrous synovial sarcoma consists of only plump spindle tumor cells, with oval or elongated nuclei, hyperchromatin nuclear, small nucleoli, and obvious mitotic figures in areas with hyperplasia (can be >20/10 HPF). The cellular boundaries are not obvious. And the tumor cells are arranged in a fascicular or storiform pattern, while cell-sparse areas show myxoid stroma degeneration, and some parts of the tumor contain expansive and staghorn blood vessels, similar to hemangio-perithelioma, with visible vascular invasion and local hemorrhage and necrosis and no epithelial component. The surrounding liver tissue may be compressed to form pseudocapsule or a slim capsule.

7.6.9.5 Immunohistochemistry

Monophasic cells are positive for vimentin, Bcl-2, and TLE-1 and may be focal positive for SMA, CK7, and EMA, while they are negative for DOG1, CD117, CD34, Syn, desmin, CD99, Hep Par-1, HMB45, and S-100.

7.6.9.6 Molecular Pathology

RT-PCR can be used to detect expression of SYT-SSX fusion gene in paraffin-embedded tissue of synovial sarcoma (SYT-SSX type 1 accounts for 66.7% and SYT-SSX type II 33.3%), and cytogenetics confirms the existence of translocation of t(x;18)(p11.2;q11.2) and breakpoints on short arm of chromosome X and long arm of chromosome 18, which are of diagnostic value.

7.6.9.7 Differential Diagnosis

The diagnosis of primary hepatic synovial sarcoma metastatic tumors should first be excluded before the diagnosis of primary hepatic synovial sarcoma. Immunohistochemistry is necessary to differentiate it from fibrosarcoma, leiomyosarcoma, hemangio-perithelioma, and spindle-cell carcinoma, and cytogenetic tests should be used to confirm the diagnosis when necessary.

7.6.9.8 Treatment and Prognosis

Monophasic synovial sarcoma has a low degree of malignancy. Surgery is still the preferred method of treatment, and postsurgical chemotherapy is required. Even so, cases with recurrence or metastasis a few months after surgery are also frequently discovered.

7.6.10 Osteoclast-Like Giant Cell Tumors

7.6.10.1 Pathogenesis and Mechanism

Osteoclast-like giant cell tumors (OCGT) are common in the skeletal system, but primary cases in the liver are rare, and the first case of hepatic OCGT was reported by Munoz et al. [218] who suggested that it might originate from Kupffer cells in the liver. To date, 14 cases of hepatic OCGT (Table 7.22) have been reported in the English literature. It was supported that OCGT derives from mono-histiocytes according to the expression of histiocytic and mesenchymal markers, e.g., CD68 and vimentin [219], while other suggestions of OCGT origination have also been proposed such as precursor of bile duct epithelial cells [220] or the situations in which tumor cells release chemokines that attract histiocyte/mononuclear macrophage in the bone marrow resulting in fusion and formation of osteoclast-like giant cells which can express epithelial markers. Bauditz et al. [221] suggested OCGT with osteoclast-like giant cells should be referred to as undifferentiated carcinoma which is more appropriate, indicating the origin and invasive growth of the tumor. Noteworthy is that Tanahashi et al. (2009) reported one case of hepatic tumor containing HCC and OCGT components, between which observed a transitional region, suggesting that the tumor originated from HCC and underwent sarcomatoid change and generate reactive osteoclast-like giant cells [222].

7.6.10.2 Clinical Features

The 14 cases of hepatic OCGT affected 11 males and the male to female ratio was 3.7:1. The age of the patients ranged 28–87 years old, with an average of 56.6 years old. The most common symptom is abdominal pain, which may be accompanied by lethargy, fever, and so on. About half of the patients have extrahepatic metastasis when they started medical examination or treatment, and lymphatic metastasis is common with the lung as the most frequently metastatic organ. Laboratory examination shows normal levels of serum AFP, CEA, and CA19-9. About half of the patients have hepatocellular carcinoma, who also have a history of hepatitis B, and a few have cirrhosis.

7.6.10.3 Gross Features

Cauliflower-like masses are found, which are large in size, often 5–12 cm in diameter, with cystic liquefaction, hemorrhage and necrosis, a number of small calcification foci and central scars.

7.6.10.4 Microscopic Features

The tumor tissue is a mixture of three kinds of cells: (1) pleomorphic mononuclear cells, the most cell type which is widely distributed in the tumor, mostly fusiform or oval shaped with varying degrees of nuclear atypia and observable mitotic figures; (2) osteoclast-like giant cells, the morphology of which is similar to that of osteoclast in bone tissues, containing 10–20 small irregular nuclei; and (3) multinucleated cells, containing multiple oval or polygonal bizarre nuclei, with mitotic figures. In addition, hepatic OCGT can also contain adenocarcinoma components (Fig. 7.295).

7.6.10.5 Immunohistochemical Characteristics

All the three types of cells express α1-AT, α1-chymotrypsin, vimentin, and CD68 but do not express AFP, CEA, AE1/3, HMW, CK7, and CK20.

7.6.10.6 Differential Diagnosis

The pancreas is the most common site to find OCGT in the digestive system, and metastatic pancreatic OCGT should be first excluded in the diagnosis of hepatic OCGT, as well as HCC with osteoclast-like giant cells.

7.6.10.7 Treatment and Prognosis

The main biological behaviors of OCGT are undefined, and the prognosis of this type of tumors in the digestive tract is generally poor. The tumors usually have strong invasiveness; thus, complete surgical resection is difficult, with the postsurgical survival time of less than 1 year [219]. It has been reported that OCGT is often accompanied by metastasis before or during the surgery, and the operation effect is not satisfactory. There is no experience in radiotherapy or chemotherapy for the treatment of the tumor; however, Rudloff et al. (2005) pointed out that tumor embolization may be a palliative treatment option. Bauditz et al. [221] reported a case treated with surgical resection combined with postsurgical chemotherapy of carboplatin, etoposide, and paclitaxel, plus local burning, and the patient survived without recurrence or metastasis during the postsurgical 15-month follow-up till now.

Table 7.22 Fourteen cases of OCGT reported in the English literature

Reference	Gender	Age (years)	Symptoms	Complications	Treatment	Diameter	Follow-up
Munoz [218]	Male	87	Somnolence, weight loss	Metastasis to the lymph nodes surrounding the lung, adrenal gland, omentum, and pancreas	None	11 cm	Death from hepatic failure 32 days later
Kuwano [223]	Male	54	Fatigue, weight loss	Metastasis to the lung, hepatocellular carcinoma	Surgery	12 cm	Death 42 days later
Horie [224]	Male	66	Abdominal pain, hematemesis	Invasion of the duodenum	Local chemotherapy	Huge	Death 42 days later
Hood [225]	Female	37	Abdominal and right shoulder pain	Invasion of anterior abdominal wall, hepatocellular carcinoma	Surgery plus radiotherapy and chemotherapy	Huge	Death 8 months later
Rudloff [219]	Female	61	Abdominal pain	–	Surgery	10 cm	Death from peritoneal and pulmonary metastasis 3 months later
Ahaouche [226]	Male	57	Abdominal pain	–	Surgery	6 cm	Death 3 months later
Andreola [227]	Male	71	–	–	–	–	Death 20 days later
Haratake [228]	Male	59	Persistent fever	–	–	Fist	Death 1 month later
McClugage [229]	Male	71	–	Hepatocellular carcinoma	–	–	Death 30 days later
Sasaki [230]	Male	42	–	Hepatocellular carcinoma	Surgery	–	Death 28 days later
Ikeda [231]	Male	76	Chronic hepatitis C for several years	Metastasis to the vertebral body and both lungs	Surgery	–	Death 5 months later
Chetty [232]	Male	28	Chronic hepatitis B for several years	Hepatocellular carcinoma	–	–	Death 7 days later
Bauditz [221]	Male	45	Symptomless	Hepatocellular carcinoma	Surgery plus radiotherapy and chemotherapy	7 cm	No recurrence or metastasis during the following 15 days
Zhang [233]	Female	38	Recurrence 15 months after surgery	Metastasis to abdominal and thoracic cavities	Surgery		Rapidly worsen healthy condition

7.6.11 Desmoplastic Small Round Cell Tumor

Wen-Ming Cong and Yu-Yao Zhu
Department of Pathology, Eastern Hepatobiliary Surgery Hospital, Second Military Medical University, Shanghai, China

7.6.11.1 Pathogenesis and Mechanism

Desmoplastic small round cell tumor (DSRCT) is a rare soft tissue tumor and was named by Gerald et al. for the first time in 1991. Only about 300 cases of DSRCT with a few primary hepatic cases are reported in the current literature. About 12 cases of hepatic DSRCT have been reported in the literature, either primary or direct involvement of the liver in DSRCT of other organs, and the liver is the most common site for the metastasis of DSRCT [234]. Whether the disease involves metastasis in the liver is also an evaluation index for the grading of DSRCT [235]. The pathogenesis of DSRCT is unknown. And due to the expression of epithelial, mesenchymal, neuroendocrine, and other immunohistochemistry markers, it may be derived from pluripotent stem cells with multiple differentiation [236], and characteristic

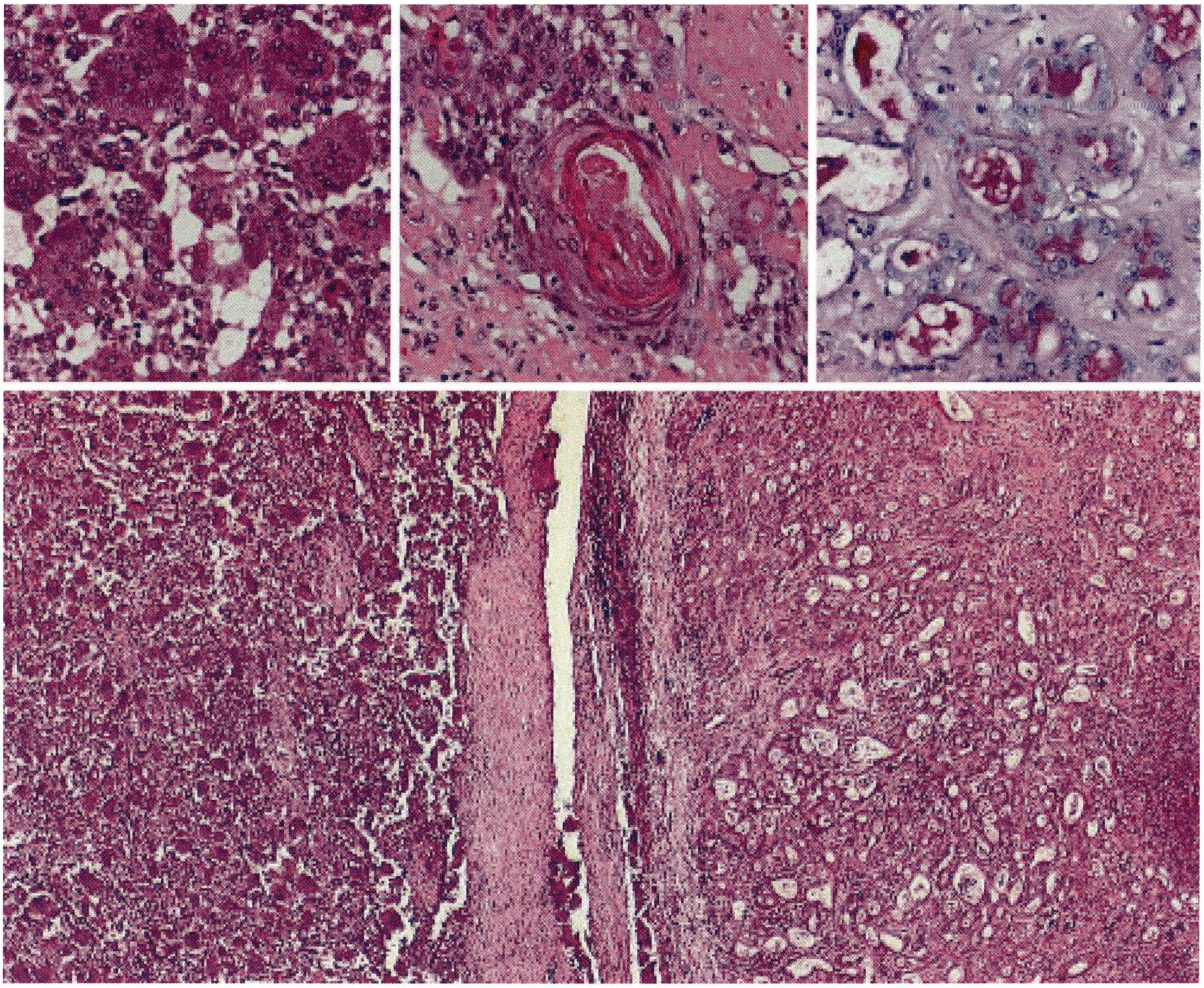

Fig. 7.295 Hepatic osteoclast-like giant cell tumors. Histology (HE, × 20–40) of OGCT of the liver with a mixed cell population of osteoclastic giant cells and pleomorphic mononuclear cells (*left*), adenocarcinomatous component with mucinous inclusions (PAS, *upper right*) and squamous cell differentiation (*middle*) (Quote from: Bauditz J)

break and translocation of t(11; 22)(p13;q12) on chromosome 11 and 22 to form EWS-WT1 fusion gene are of diagnostic value.

7.6.11.2 Clinical Features

DSRCT is often found in children and young or middle-aged males, and the average age of the patients is 25.44 years old (2–66 years old) based on the reports of 132 cases in China and abroad, with a male to female ratio of 4:1. More than half of the cases are found in the abdominal cavity, followed by pelvic cavity, para-testis regions in males, liver, groin, iliac fossa, ankle joint, neck, arm, leg, calve, etc. The clinical manifestations include abdominal distention, abdominal pain and abdominal mass, and so on. A domestic report made by Chen Xi-gang et al. described a case of a 66-year-old female with a huge mass in the right lobe of the liver, with intrahepatic volume of 8 cm × 6 cm × 5 cm and extrahepatic volume of 16 cm × 12 cm × 10 cm, which was surgically excised and diagnosed as DSRCT, with invasion of gastric antrum, descending duodenum, and hepatic flexure of the colon. Combined organ resection was conducted and post-surgical chemotherapy was administrated. The patient survived in good condition during the 12-month follow-up [237].

Plain scan CT shows abdominal or pelvic soft tissue mass. Laboratory examination often reveals normal tumor markers, while serum CA125 can be elevated to 200 U/ml in 80% of the cases with abdomen-located lesions.

7.6.11.3 Gross Features

Grossly, the mass is poorly defined, rounded, similar rounded or irregular nodular with central necrosis and ranges from 3 to 24 cm (average 10.7 cm). On cut section, it is hard and tough with unconspicuous capsule and adhesion of the tumor

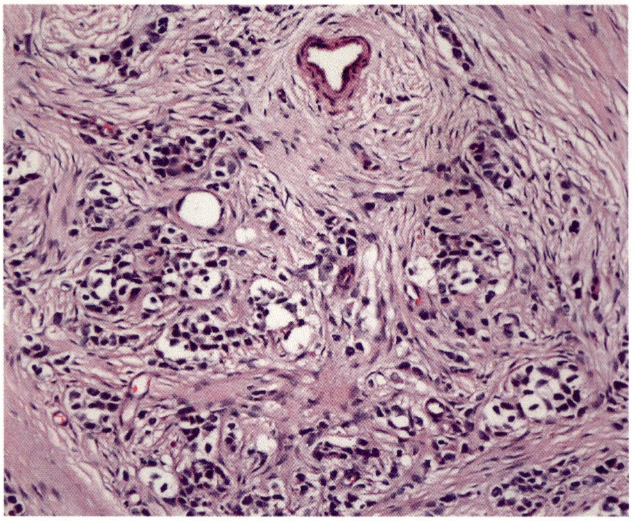

Fig. 7.296 Desmoplastic small round cell tumor. Tumor cells are arranged in irregular small nests or solid cords, surrounded by dense and collagen-rich connective tissue

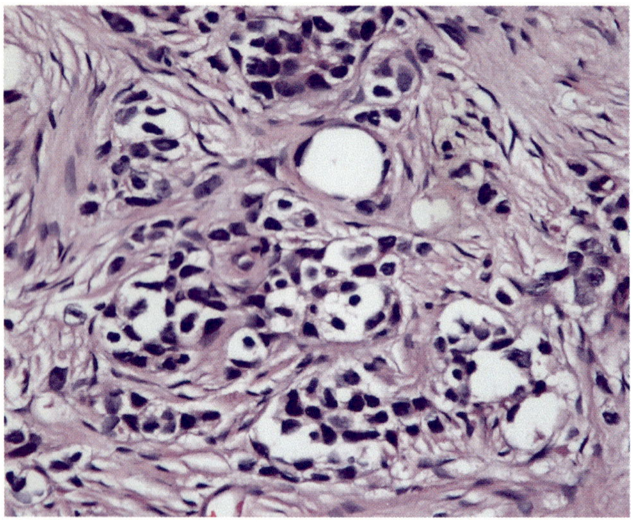

Fig. 7.297 Desmoplastic small round cell tumor. The tumor cells are small and round in consistent shape and size with round or oval nuclear and unclerar nucleoli, little translucent cytoplasm

surface to the surrounding tissue. One case of abdominal DSRCT have been diagnosed in the Department of Pathology, Eastern Hepatobiliary, Surgery Hospital, Second Military Medical University, which was 5.2 cm in diameter with hepatic metastatic lesion of 0.2 cm in diameter, hard, and adhesive to the gastric tissue on the surface of the tumor.

7.6.11.4 Microscopic Features

No clear originating tissue or origin of the tumor is found; thus, it is not easy to determine its origin. The tumor is composed of small tumor cells and surrounding fibrous stroma. Tumor cells are arranged in irregular small nests or solid cords, surrounded by dense and collagen-rich connective tissue. The tumor cells are small and round in consistent shape and size, with stromal infiltration, hyperchromatic round or oval nuclei, unclear nucleoli, visible mitotic figures, and little translucent cytoplasm (Figs. 7.296 and 7.297). Metastasis foci can infiltrate into hepatic sinusoid and a few residual hepatocytes in between the tumor cells. In the case of the tumor diagnosed in the Department of Pathology, Eastern Hepatobiliary, Surgery Hospital, Second Military Medical University, the lesion contains a small amount of residual tumor tissue, and the tumor cell to interstitial tissue ratio was 1:3. The tumor grows in infiltrative pattern with invasion of muscular layer of the stomach, accompanied by multiple intra-abdominal metastasis including the liver, omentum, and transverse mesocolon. Wang et al. [238] reported four cases of primary renal DSRCT in children accompanied by calcification foci, suggesting that calcification is the pathological feature of this tumor.

7.6.11.5 Immunohistochemistry

The tumor cells have the feature of multi-differentiation; thus, they show multiple immunophenotypes, and different proportions of staining of the following immunohistochemistry markers are found: EMA (80.5–90.6%), CK (69–88.1%) (Fig. 7.298a), vimentin (95.56–100%) (Fig. 7.298b), desmin (86.6–97.8%), WT1 (81.4%), NSE (75–84.4%) (Fig. 7.298c), MIC2 (51.3%), INI-1 (100%), and SMA (76.9%) [239, 240]. In addition, partial staining of CD99 (30%), Syn (13.3%), chromogranin (21%), S-100 (12.5%), etc. has also been reported [240], as well as increased proliferation index by PCNA (Fig. 7.298d).

7.6.11.6 Molecular Pathology

Cytogenetics shows translocation of chromosome 11 and 12, namely, t(11;12)(p13;q12), and fusion gene EWS-WT1 can be detected by PCR.

7.6.11.7 Differential Diagnosis

1. EWS/PNET: Similar to DSRCT, EWS/PNET also consists of small round cells forming patches or nests. Generally, EWS/PNET lesions are positive for CD99 and vimentin in immunohistochemistry staining and negative for CK and myogenic marker. Different from chromosome translocation of DSRCT, the characteristic chromosomal translocation of EWS/PNET is t(11;22)(q24;q12) [241].
2. Neuroblastoma: It is common in children, with negative staining for CK, WT1, and desmin in immunohistochemistry, containing rich nerve fibers in the stroma and usually visible ganglion cells. And neural immunohistochemistry markers are positive in this type of tumor [242].
3. Advanced lymphoma: Its histological behaviors are similar to those of DSRCT to some degrees; however, lymphoma often grows diffusely with positive lymphocytic

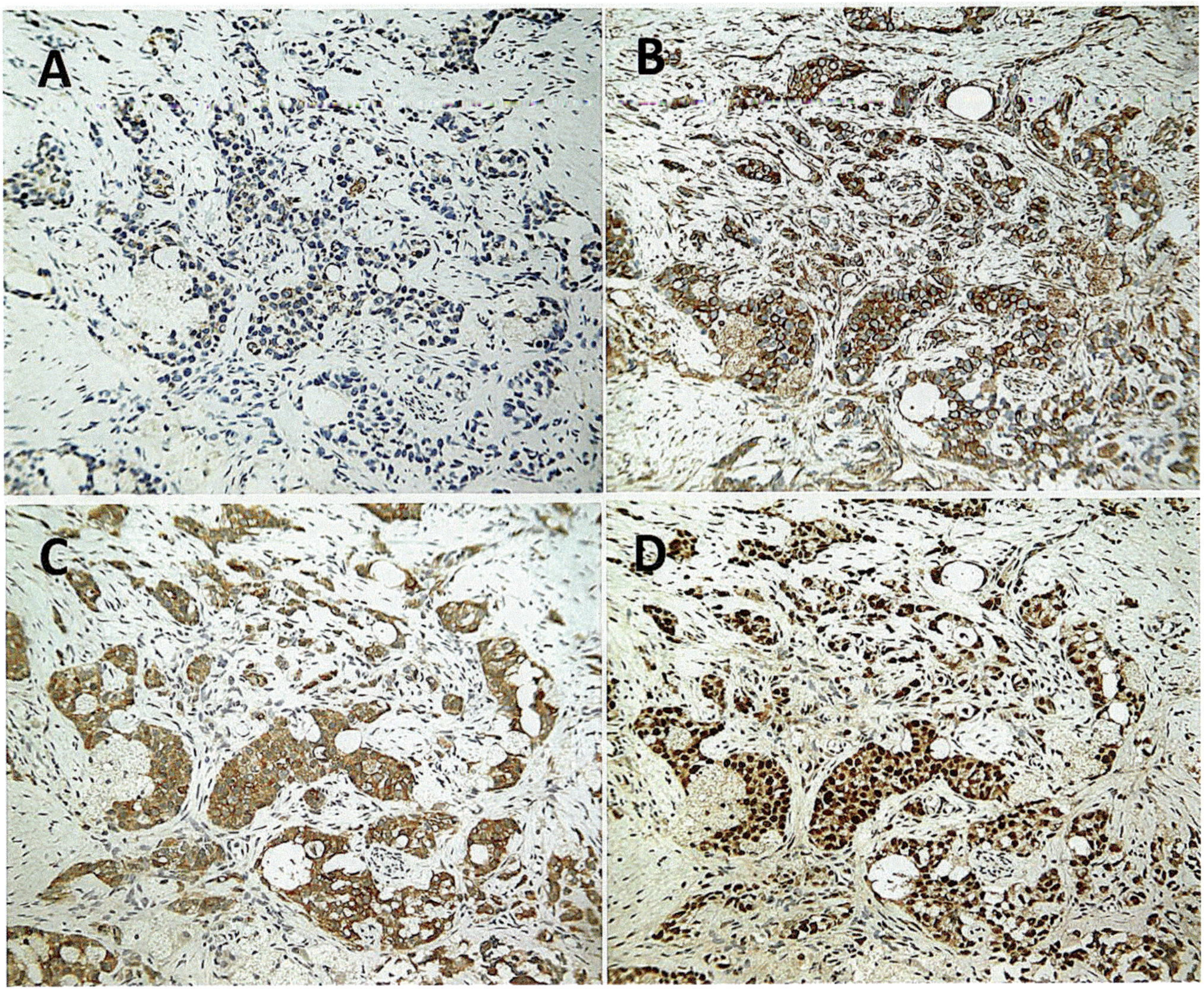

Fig. 7.298 Desmoplastic small round cell tumor. The characteristic of the immunohistochemical stain: (**a**) CK; (**b**) Vimentin; (**c**) NSE; (**d**) PCNA

markers and negative epithelial, neurogenic, and myogenic markers.

7.6.11.8 Treatment and Prognosis

The principles of treatment for hepatic DSRCT are similar to those of DSRCT in other organs. The prognosis of the tumor is poor with a 5-year survival rate of only 15%. And the therapeutic strategy of this tumor remains controversial, due to its low incidence and high invasiveness. Despite of multiple treatment plans suggested, no reliable criteria or definite and effective therapy can be found. But generally speaking, the treatment should include effective surgical resection and postsurgical chemotherapy. Al Balushi et al. [243] conducted autologous bone marrow transplantation in three patients who were sensitive to chemotherapy, followed by partial tumor resection, which achieved good therapeutic effects, and two patients have already survived 6 years and 2 years, respectively. Lal et al. [244] summarized the treating experience in 66 cases of DSRCT and found higher postsurgical survival rate in patients with extensive resection than that of cases with no resection. Modak et al. [245] proposed that GD2 and 8H9 antibodies can be used as potential targets for immunotherapy of DSRCT.

References

1. Jemal A, Bray F, Center MM, et al. Global cancer statistics. CA Cancer J Clin. 2011;61(2):69–90.
2. El-Serag HB, Rudolph KL. Hepatocellular carcinoma: epidemiology and molecular carcinogenesis. Gastroenterology. 2007;132(7):2557–76.
3. Siegel R, Naishadham D, Jemal A. Cancer statistics, 2012. CA Cancer J Clin. 2012;62(1):10–29.
4. Theise ND, Park YN, Curado MP, et al. Tumours of the liver and intrahepatic bile ducts. In: Bosman FT, Carneiro F, Hruban RH, et al., editors. WHO classification of tumours of the digestive system. Geneva: WHO Press; 2010. p. 195–261.

5. Cong WM, Dong H, Tan L, et al. Surgicopathological classification of hepatic space-occupying lesions: a single-center experience with literature review. World J Gastroenterol. 2011;17(19):2372–8.
6. Zhang T, Zhang J, You X, et al. Hepatitis B virus X protein modulates oncogene Yes-associated protein by CREB to promote growth of hepatoma cells. Hepatology. 2012;56(6):2051–9.
7. Liu H, Xu L, He H, et al. Hepatitis B virus X protein promotes hepatoma cell invasion and metastasis by stabilizing Snail protein. Cancer Sci. 2012;103(12):2072–81.
8. Jiang YF, He B, Li NP, et al. The oncogenic role of NS5A of hepatitis C virus is mediated by up-regulation of survivin gene expression in the hepatocellular cell through p53 and NF-kappa B pathways. Cell Biol Int. 2011;35(12):1225–32.
9. Wurmbach E, Chen YB, Khitrov G, et al. Genome-wide molecular profiles of HCV-induced dysplasia and hepatocellular carcinoma. Hepatology. 2007;45(4):938–47.
10. Cheng D, Zhao L, Zhang L, et al. p53 controls hepatitis C virus non-structural protein 5A-mediated downregulation of GADD45 alpha expression via the NF-kappa B and PI3K-Akt pathways. J Gen Virol. 2013;94(Pt 2):326–35.
11. Wang J, Liu XM. Assessment of dietary aflatoxins exposure in chinese residents. Chin J Food Hyg. 2007;19(3):238–40.
12. Baffy G, Brunt EM, Caldwell SH. Hepatocellular carcinoma in non-alcoholic fatty liver disease: an emerging menace. J Hepatol. 2012;56(6):1384–91.
13. Jia D, Wei L, Guo W, et al. Genome-wide copy number analyses identified novel cancer genes in hepatocellular carcinoma. Hepatology. 2011;54(4):1227–36.
14. Li M, Zhao H, Zhang X, et al. Inactivating mutations of the chromatin remodeling gene ARID2 in hepatocellular carcinoma. Nat Genet. 2011;43(9):828–9.
15. Kan Z, Zheng H, Liu X, et al. Whole-genome sequencing identifies recurrent mutations in hepatocellular carcinoma. Genome Res. 2013;23(9):1422–33.
16. Liu L, Dai Y, Chen J, et al. Maelstrom promotes hepatocellular carcinoma metastasis by inducing epithelial-mesenchymal transition by way of Akt/GSK-3beta/Snail signaling. Hepatology. 2014;59(2):531–43.
17. Kanai T, Hirohashi S, Upton MP, et al. Pathology of small hepatocellular carcinoma. A proposal for a new gross classification. Cancer. 1987;60(4):810–9.
18. Jakate S, Yabes A, Giusto D, et al. Diffuse cirrhosis-like hepatocellular carcinoma: a clinically and radiographically undetected variant mimicking cirrhosis. Am J Surg Pathol. 2010;34(7):935–41.
19. Rodriguez-Peralvarez M, Luong TV, Andreana L, et al. A systematic review of microvascular invasion in hepatocellular carcinoma: diagnostic and prognostic variability. Ann Surg Oncol. 2013;20(1):325–39.
20. Greaves M, Maley CC. Clonal evolution in cancer. Nature. 2012;481(7381):306–13.
21. Del Rosario AD, Bui HX, Singh J, et al. Intracytoplasmic eosinophilic hyaline globules in cartilaginous neoplasms: a surgical, pathological, ultrastructural, and electron probe x-ray microanalytic study. Hum Pathol. 1994;25(12):1283–9.
22. Stumptner C, Heid H, Fuchsbichler A, et al. Analysis of intracytoplasmic hyaline bodies in a hepatocellular carcinoma. Demonstration of p62 as major constituent. Am J Pathol. 1999;154(6):1701–10.
23. International Consensus Group for Hepatocellular Neoplasia, The International Consensus Group for Hepatocellular Neoplasia. Pathologic diagnosis of early hepatocellular carcinoma: a report of the international consensus group for hepatocellular neoplasia. Hepatology. 2009;49(2):658–64.
24. Yong KJ, Gao C, Lim JS, et al. Oncofetal gene SALL4 in aggressive hepatocellular carcinoma. N Engl J Med. 2013;368(24):2266–76.
25. Kee KM, Wang JH, Lin CY, et al. Validation of the 7th edition TNM staging system for hepatocellular carcinoma: an analysis of 8,828 patients in a single medical center. Dig Dis Sci. 2013;58(9):2721–8.
26. Nault JC, De Reynies A, Villanueva A, et al. A hepatocellular carcinoma 5-gene score associated with survival of patients after liver resection. Gastroenterology. 2013;145(1):176–87.
27. Shirabe K, Toshima T, Kimura K, et al. New scoring system for prediction of microvascular invasion in patients with hepatocellular carcinoma. Liver Int. 2014;34(6):937–41.
28. Tsujita E, Yamashita Y, Takeishi K, et al. Poor prognostic factors after repeat hepatectomy for recurrent hepatocellular carcinoma in the modern era. Am Surg. 2012;78(4):419–25.
29. Kadalayil L, Benini R, Pallan L, et al. A simple prognostic scoring system for patients receiving transarterial embolisation for hepatocellular cancer. Ann Oncol. 2013;24(10):2565–70.
30. Okuda K, Nakashima T, Obata H, et al. Clinicopathological studies of minute hepatocellular carcinoma. Analysis of 20 cases, including 4 with hepatic resection. Gastroenterology. 1977;73(1):109–15.
31. Moribe T, Iizuka N, Miura T, et al. Methylation of multiple genes as molecular markers for diagnosis of a small, well-differentiated hepatocellular carcinoma. Int J Cancer. 2009;125(2):388–97.
32. Llovet JM, Chen Y, Wurmbach E, et al. A molecular signature to discriminate dysplastic nodules from early hepatocellular carcinoma in HCV cirrhosis. Gastroenterology. 2006;131(6):1758–67.
33. Lu XY, Xi T, Lau WY, et al. Pathobiological features of small hepatocellular carcinoma: correlation between tumor size and biological behavior. J Cancer Res Clin Oncol. 2011;137(4):567–75.
34. Cong Wm WM. Small hepatocellular carcinoma - current and future approaches. Hepatol Int. 2013;7(3):805–12.
35. Tremosini S, Forner A, Boix L, et al. Prospective validation of an immunohistochemical panel (glypican 3, heat shock protein 70 and glutamine synthetase) in liver biopsies for diagnosis of very early hepatocellular carcinoma. Gut. 2012;61(10):1481–7.
36. Eggert T, Mcglynn KA, Duffy A, et al. Epidemiology of fibrolamellar hepatocellular carcinoma in the USA, 2000-10. Gut. 2013;62(11):1667–8.
37. Honeyman JN, Simon EP, Robine N, et al. Detection of a recurrent DNAJB1-PRKACA chimeric transcript in fibrolamellar hepatocellular carcinoma. Science. 2014;343(6174):1010–4.
38. Malouf GG, Job S, Paradis V, et al. Transcriptional profiling of pure fibrolamellar hepatocellular carcinoma reveals an endocrine signature. Hepatology. 2014;59(6):2228–37.
39. Kaseb AO, Shama M, Sahin IH, et al. Prognostic indicators and treatment outcome in 94 cases of fibrolamellar hepatocellular carcinoma. Oncology. 2013;85(4):197–203.
40. Weeda VB, Murawski M, Mccabe AJ, et al. Fibrolamellar variant of hepatocellular carcinoma does not have a better survival than conventional hepatocellular carcinoma–results and treatment recommendations from the Childhood Liver Tumour Strategy Group (SIOPEL) experience. Eur J Cancer. 2013;49(12):2698–704.
41. Garancini M, Goffredo P, Pagni F, et al. Combined hepatocellular-cholangiocarcinoma: a population-level analysis of an uncommon primary liver tumor. Liver Transpl. 2014;20(8):952–9.
42. Wakasa T, Wakasa K, Shutou T, et al. A histopathological study on combined hepatocellular and cholangiocarcinoma: cholangiocarcinoma component is originated from hepatocellular carcinoma. Hepato-Gastroenterology. 2007;54(74):508–13.
43. Coulouarn C, Cavard C, Rubbia-Brandt L, et al. Combined hepatocellular-cholangiocarcinomas exhibit progenitor features and activation of Wnt and TGF beta signaling pathways. Carcinogenesis. 2012;33(9):1791–6.

44. Cai X, Zhai J, Kaplan DE, et al. Background progenitor activation is associated with recurrence after hepatectomy of combined hepatocellular-cholangiocarcinoma. Hepatology. 2012;56(5):1804–16.
45. Yamaguchi R, Nakashima O, Ogata T, et al. Hepatocellular carcinoma with an unusual neuroendocrine component. Pathol Int. 2004;54(11):861–5.
46. Garcia MT, Bejarano PA, Yssa M, et al. Tumor of the liver (hepatocellular and high grade neuroendocrine carcinoma): a case report and review of the literature. Virchows Arch. 2006;449(3):376–81.
47. Akiba J, Nakashima O, Hattori S, et al. Clinicopathologic analysis of combined hepatocellular-cholangiocarcinoma according to the latest WHO classification. Am J Surg Pathol. 2013;37(4):496–505.
48. Yeh MM. Pathology of combined hepatocellular-cholangiocarcinoma. J Gastroenterol Hepatol. 2010;25(9):1485–92.
49. Komuta M, Spee B, Vander Borght S, et al. Clinicopathological study on cholangiolocellular carcinoma suggesting hepatic progenitor cell origin. Hepatology. 2008;47(5):1544–56.
50. Woo HG, Lee JH, Yoon JH, et al. Identification of a cholangiocarcinoma-like gene expression trait in hepatocellular carcinoma. Cancer Res. 2010;70(8):3034–41.
51. Yin X, Zhang BH, Qiu SJ, et al. Combined hepatocellular carcinoma and cholangiocarcinoma: clinical features, treatment modalities, and prognosis. Ann Surg Oncol. 2012;19(9):2869–76.
52. Park YH, Hwang S, Ahn CS, et al. Long-term outcome of liver transplantation for combined hepatocellular carcinoma and cholangiocarcinoma. Transplant Proc. 2013;45(8):3038–40.
53. Groeschl RT, Turaga KK, Gamblin TC. Transplantation versus resection for patients with combined hepatocellular carcinoma-cholangiocarcinoma. J Surg Oncol. 2013;107(6):608–12.
54. Lu XY, Xi T, Lau WY, et al. Hepatocellular carcinoma expressing cholangiocyte phenotype is a novel subtype with highly aggressive behavior. Ann Surg Oncol. 2011;18(8):2210–7.
55. Govaere O, Komuta M, Berkers J, et al. Keratin 19: a key role player in the invasion of human hepatocellular carcinomas. Gut. 2014;63(4):674–85.
56. Bridgewater J, Galle PR, Khan SA, et al. Guidelines for the diagnosis and management of intrahepatic cholangiocarcinoma. J Hepatol. 2014;60(6):1268–89.
57. Aishima S, Kuroda Y, Nishihara Y, et al. Proposal of progression model for intrahepatic cholangiocarcinoma: clinicopathologic differences between hilar type and peripheral type. Am J Surg Pathol. 2007;31(7):1059–67.
58. Nakanuma Y, Xu J, Harada K, et al. Pathological spectrum of intrahepatic cholangiocarcinoma arising in non-biliary chronic advanced liver diseases. Pathol Int. 2011;61(5):298–305.
59. Palmer WC, Patel T. Are common factors involved in the pathogenesis of primary liver cancers? A meta-analysis of risk factors for intrahepatic cholangiocarcinoma. J Hepatol. 2012;57(1):69–76.
60. Li M, Li J, Li P, et al. Hepatitis B virus infection increases the risk of cholangiocarcinoma: a meta-analysis and systematic review. J Gastroenterol Hepatol. 2012;27(10):1561–8.
61. Razumilava N, Gores GJ. Classification, diagnosis, and management of cholangiocarcinoma. Clin Gastroenterol Hepatol. 2013;11(1):13–21.. e11; quiz e13-14
62. Cong WM, Bakker A, Swalsky PA, et al. Multiple genetic alterations involved in the tumorigenesis of human cholangiocarcinoma: a molecular genetic and clinicopathological study. J Cancer Res Clin Oncol. 2001;127(3):187–92.
63. Sia D, Tovar V, Moeini A, et al. Intrahepatic cholangiocarcinoma: pathogenesis and rationale for molecular therapies. Oncogene. 2013;32(41):4861–70.
64. Rizvi S, Gores GJ. Pathogenesis, diagnosis, and management of cholangiocarcinoma. Gastroenterology. 2013;145(6):1215–29.
65. Blechacz B, Gores GJ. Cholangiocarcinoma: advances in pathogenesis, diagnosis, and treatment. Hepatology. 2008,48(1):308–21.
66. Francis H, Alpini G, Demorrow S. Recent advances in the regulation of cholangiocarcinoma growth. Am J Physiol Gastrointest Liver Physiol. 2010;299(1):G1–9.
67. Fan B, Malato Y, Calvisi DF, et al. Cholangiocarcinomas can originate from hepatocytes in mice. J Clin Invest. 2012;122(8):2911–5.
68. Zender S, Nickeleit I, Wuestefeld T, et al. A critical role for notch signaling in the formation of cholangiocellular carcinomas. Cancer Cell. 2013;23(6):784–95.
69. Andersen JB, Spee B, Blechacz BR, et al. Genomic and genetic characterization of cholangiocarcinoma identifies therapeutic targets for tyrosine kinase inhibitors. Gastroenterology. 2012;142(4):1021–31.. e1015
70. Oishi N, Kumar MR, Roessler S, et al. Transcriptomic profiling reveals hepatic stem-like gene signatures and interplay of miR-200c and epithelial-mesenchymal transition in intrahepatic cholangiocarcinoma. Hepatology. 2012;56(5):1792–803.
71. Karakatsanis A, Papaconstantinou I, Gazouli M, et al. Expression of microRNAs, miR-21, miR-31, miR-122, miR-145, miR-146a, miR-200c, miR-221, miR-222, and miR-223 in patients with hepatocellular carcinoma or intrahepatic cholangiocarcinoma and its prognostic significance. Mol Carcinog. 2013;52(4):297–303.
72. Edge SB, Compton CC. The American Joint Committee on Cancer: the 7th edition of the AJCC cancer staging manual and the future of TNM. Ann Surg Oncol. 2010;17(6):1471–4.
73. Nathan H, Aloia TA, Vauthey JN, et al. A proposed staging system for intrahepatic cholangiocarcinoma. Ann Surg Oncol. 2009;16(1):14–22.
74. Yamasaki S. Intrahepatic cholangiocarcinoma: macroscopic type and stage classification. J Hepato-Biliary-Pancreat Surg. 2003;10(4):288–91.
75. Jiang W, Zeng ZC, Tang ZY, et al. A prognostic scoring system based on clinical features of intrahepatic cholangiocarcinoma: the Fudan score. Ann Oncol. 2011;22(7):1644–52.
76. Wang Y, Li J, Xia Y, et al. Prognostic nomogram for intrahepatic cholangiocarcinoma after partial hepatectomy. J Clin Oncol. 2013;31(9):1188–95.
77. Zhou YM, Yang JM, Wang XF, et al. Characteristics of extrahepatic lymph node metastases in intrahepatic cholangiocarcinoma. Chin J Dig Surg. 2007;6(2):96–8.
78. Rimola J, Forner A, Reig M, et al. Cholangiocarcinoma in cirrhosis: absence of contrast washout in delayed phases by magnetic resonance imaging avoids misdiagnosis of hepatocellular carcinoma. Hepatology. 2009;50(3):791–8.
79. Nakanuma Y, Sato Y, Harada K, et al. Pathological classification of intrahepatic cholangiocarcinoma based on a new concept. World J Hepatol. 2010;2(12):419–27.
80. Spolverato G, Ejaz A, Kim Y, et al. Tumor size predicts vascular invasion and histologic grade among patients undergoing resection of intrahepatic cholangiocarcinoma. J Gastrointest Surg. 2014;18(7):1284–91.
81. Liau JY, Tsai JH, Yuan RH, et al. Morphological subclassification of intrahepatic cholangiocarcinoma: etiological, clinicopathological, and molecular features. Mod Pathol. 2014;27(8):1163–73.
82. Ji LH, Zhao G, Wu ZY. Typing and staging and treatment of intrahepatic cholangiocarcinoma. Chin. J. Dig. Surg. 2010;3:193–6.
83. Aishima S, Nishihara Y, Iguchi T, et al. Lymphatic spread is related to VEGF-C expression and D2-40-positive myofibroblasts in intrahepatic cholangiocarcinoma. Mod Pathol. 2008;21(3):256–64.

84. Dong H, Cong WL, Zhu ZZ, et al. Evaluation of immunohistochemical markers for differential diagnosis of hepatocellular carcinoma from intrahepatic cholangiocarcinoma. Chin J Oncol. 2008;30(9):702–5.
85. Aishima S, Fujita N, Mano Y, et al. Different roles of S100P overexpression in intrahepatic cholangiocarcinoma: carcinogenesis of perihilar type and aggressive behavior of peripheral type. Am J Surg Pathol. 2011;35(4):590–8.
86. Ruys AT, Groot Koerkamp B, Wiggers JK, et al. Prognostic biomarkers in patients with resected cholangiocarcinoma: a systematic review and meta-analysis. Ann Surg Oncol. 2014;21(2):487–500.
87. Kloppel G, Adsay V, Konukiewitz B, et al. Precancerous lesions of the biliary tree. Best Pract Res Clin Gastroenterol. 2013;27(2):285–97.
88. Nakanuma Y, Sato Y, Ojima H, et al. Clinicopathological characterization of so-called "cholangiocarcinoma with intraductal papillary growth" with respect to "intraductal papillary neoplasm of bile duct (IPNB)". Int J Clin Exp Pathol. 2014;7(6):3112–22.
89. Nishino R, Honda M, Yamashita T, et al. Identification of novel candidate tumour marker genes for intrahepatic cholangiocarcinoma. J Hepatol. 2008;49(2):207–16.
90. Becker NS, Rodriguez JA, Barshes NR, et al. Outcomes analysis for 280 patients with cholangiocarcinoma treated with liver transplantation over an 18-year period. J Gastrointest Surg. 2008;12(1):117–22.
91. Arnaoutakis DJ, Kim Y, Pulitano C, et al. Management of biliary cystic tumors: a multi-institutional analysis of a rare liver tumor. Ann Surg. 2014;261(2):361–7.
92. Vogt DP, Henderson JM, Chmielewski E. Cystadenoma and cystadenocarcinoma of the liver: a single center experience. J Am Coll Surg. 2005;200(5):727–33.
93. Dai YH, Yeo YH, Li YF, et al. Hepatobiliary cystadenocarcinoma without mesenchymal stroma in a female patient: a case report. BMC Gastroenterol. 2014;14:109.
94. Shibahara H, Tamada S, Goto M, et al. Pathologic features of mucin-producing bile duct tumors: two histopathologic categories as counterparts of pancreatic intraductal papillary-mucinous neoplasms. Am J Surg Pathol. 2004;28(3):327–38.
95. Yang XW, Yang J, Li L, et al. The outcome of ipsilateral hemihepatectomy in mucin-producing bile duct tumors. PLoS One. 2014;9(4):e92010.
96. Sasaki M, Matsubara T, Kakuda Y, et al. Immunostaining for polycomb group protein EZH2 and senescent marker p16INK4a may be useful to differentiate cholangiolocellular carcinoma from ductular reaction and bile duct adenoma. Am J Surg Pathol. 2014;38(3):364–9.
97. Kanamoto M, Yoshizumi T, Ikegami T, et al. Cholangiolocellular carcinoma containing hepatocellular carcinoma and cholangiocellular carcinoma, extremely rare tumor of the liver: a case report. J Med Investig. 2008;55(1–2):161–5.
98. Lee W. Intrahepatic lymphoepithelioma-like cholangiocarcinoma not associated with epstein-barr virus: a case report. Case Rep Oncol. 2011;4(1):68–73.
99. Shinoda M, Kadota Y, Tsujikawa H, et al. Lymphoepithelioma-like hepatocellular carcinoma: a case report and a review of the literature. World J. Surg. Oncol. 2013;11:97.
100. Nemolato S, Fanni D, Naccarato AG, et al. Lymphoepithelioma-like hepatocellular carcinoma: a case report and a review of the literature. World J Gastroenterol. 2008;14(29):4694–6.
101. Arakawa Y, Shimada M, Ikegami T, et al. Mucoepidermoid carcinoma of the liver: report of a rare case and review of the literature. Hepatol Res. 2008;38(7):736–42.
102. Guo XQ, Li B, Li Y, et al. Unusual mucoepidermoid carcinoma of the liver misdiagnosed as squamous cell carcinoma by intraoperative histological examination. Diagn Pathol. 2014;9:24.
103. Iimuro Y, Asano Y, Suzumura K, et al. Primary squamous cell carcinoma of the liver: an uncommon finding in contrast-enhanced ultrasonography imaging. Case Rep Gastroenterol. 2011;5(3):628–35.
104. Avezbadalov A, Aksenov S, Kaplan B, et al. Asymptomatic primary squamous cell carcinoma of the liver. J Commun Support Oncol. 2014;12(2):75–6.
105. Liu J. Y HY, He J. Primary squamous cell carcinoma of the liver: report of a case. Acad J Second Mil Med Uni. 2009;30(1):108–10.
106. Shimizu S, Oshita A, Tashiro H, et al. Synchronous double cancers of primary hepatic adenosquamous carcinoma and hepatocellular carcinoma: report of a case. Surg Today. 2013;43(4):418–23.
107. Park SY, Cha EJ, Moon WS. Adenosquamous carcinoma of the liver. Clin Mol Hepatol. 2012;18(3):326–9.
108. Liu Y, Sang XT, Gao WS, et al. The first case of primary epithelial-myoepithelial carcinoma in the liver. Chin J Surg. 2006;44(21):1477–9.
109. Tsuneyama K, Hoso M, Kono N, et al. An unusual case of epithelial-myoepithelial carcinoma of the liver. Am J Surg Pathol. 1999;23(3):349–53.
110. Haas S, Gutgemann I, Wolff M, et al. Intrahepatic clear cell cholangiocarcinoma: immunohistochemical aspects in a very rare type of cholangiocarcinoma. Am J Surg Pathol. 2007;31(6):902–6.
111. Khera R, Uppin SG, Uppin MS, et al. Clear cell papillary cholangiocarcinoma: a case report with review of literature. Indian J Pathol Microbiol. 2014;57(1):105–8.
112. Kim YI, Kim ST, Lee GK, et al. Papillary cystic tumor of the liver. A case report with ultrastructural observation. Cancer. 1990;65(12):2740–6.
113. Ishak Kg GZ, Stocker J. Tumors of the liver and intrahepatic bile ducts, vol. 276. Washington, DC: American Registry of Pathology; 2001.
114. Montell Garcia M, Romero Cabello R, Romero Feregrino R, et al. Angiosarcoma of the liver as a cause of fulminant liver failure. BMJ Case Rep. 2012.
115. Poggi Machuca L, Ibarra Chirinos O, Lopez Del Aguila J, et al. Hepatic angiosarcoma: case report and review of literature. Rev Gastroenterol Peru. 2012;32(3):317–22.
116. Dimashkieh HH, Mo JQ, Wyatt-Ashmead J, et al. Pediatric hepatic angiosarcoma: case report and review of the literature. Pediatr Dev Pathol. 2004;7(5):527–32.
117. Yang KF, Leow VM, Hasnan MN, et al. Primary hepatic angiosarcoma: difficulty in clinical, radiological, and pathological diagnosis. Med J Malays. 2012;67(1):127–8.
118. Mehrabi A, Kashfi A, Fonouni H, et al. Primary malignant hepatic epithelioid hemangioendothelioma: a comprehensive review of the literature with emphasis on the surgical therapy. Cancer. 2006;107(9):2108–21.
119. Tsarouha H, Kyriazoglou AI, Ribeiro FR, et al. Chromosome analysis and molecular cytogenetic investigations of an epithelioid hemangioendothelioma. Cancer Genet Cytogenet. 2006;169(2):164–8.
120. Cao Y, Zou XM, Feng L, et al. Cytogenetic alterations in lung epithelioid hemangioendothelioma. Carcinog Teratog Mutagen. 2009;21(3):185–8.
121. Simonelli C, Tedeschi R, Gloghini A, et al. Plasma HHV-8 viral load in HHV-8-related lymphoproliferative disorders associated with HIV infection. J Med Virol. 2009;81(5):888–96.
122. Wang XD, Hui Y. Advances in the genotyping of human herpesvirus 8. Int J Dermatol Venereol. 2009;35(2):3.
123. Bronowicki JP, Bineau C, Feugier P, et al. Primary lymphoma of the liver: clinical-pathological features and relationship with HCV infection in French patients. Hepatology. 2003;37(4):781–7.

124. Sekiguchi Y, Yoshikawa H, Shimada A, et al. Primary hepatic circumscribed Burkitt's lymphoma that developed after acute hepatitis B: report of a case with a review of the literature. J Clin Exp Hematop. 2013;53(2):167–73.
125. Haider FS, Smith R, Khan S. Primary hepatic lymphoma presenting as fulminant hepatic failure with hyperferritinemia: a case report. J Med Case Rep. 2008;2:279.
126. Lei KI. Primary non-Hodgkin's lymphoma of the liver. Leuk Lymphoma. 1998;29(3–4):293–9.
127. Li XQ, Cheuk W, Lam PW, et al. Inflammatory pseudotumor-like follicular dendritic cell tumor of liver and spleen: granulomatous and eosinophil-rich variants mimicking inflammatory or infective lesions. Am J Surg Pathol. 2014;38(5):646–53.
128. Ge R, Liu C, Yin X, et al. Clinicopathologic characteristics of inflammatory pseudotumor-like follicular dendritic cell sarcoma. Int. J. Clin. Exp. Pathol. 2014;7(5):2421–9.
129. Chao MW, Gibbs P, Wirth A, et al. Radiotherapy in the management of solitary extramedullary plasmacytoma. Intern Med J. 2005;35(4):211–5.
130. Soutar R, Lucraft H, Jackson G, et al. Guidelines on the diagnosis and management of solitary plasmacytoma of bone and solitary extramedullary plasmacytoma. Br J Haematol. 2004;124(6):717–26.
131. Palumbo A, Rajkumar SV, San Miguel JF, et al. International Myeloma Working Group consensus statement for the management, treatment, and supportive care of patients with myeloma not eligible for standard autologous stem-cell transplantation. J Clin Oncol. 2014;32(6):587–600.
132. Lee JY, Won JH, Kim HJ, et al. Solitary extramedullary plasmacytoma of the liver without systemic monoclonal gammopathy. J Korean Med Sci. 2007;22(4):754–7.
133. Straetmans J, Stokroos R. Extramedullary plasmacytomas in the head and neck region. Eur Arch Otorhinolaryngol. 2008;265(11):1417–23.
134. Miyabe K, Masaki A, Nakazawa T, et al. Histiocytic sarcoma of the bile duct. Intern Med. 2014;53(7):707–12.
135. Llamas-Velasco M, Cannata J, Dominguez I, et al. Coexistence of Langerhans cell histiocytosis, Rosai-Dorfman disease and splenic lymphoma with fatal outcome after rapid development of histiocytic sarcoma of the liver. J Cutan Pathol. 2012;39(12):1125–30.
136. Wang E, Hutchinson CB, Huang Q, et al. Histiocytic sarcoma arising in indolent small B-cell lymphoma: report of two cases with molecular/genetic evidence suggestive of a 'transdifferentiation' during the clonal evolution. Leuk Lymphoma. 2010;51(5):802–12.
137. Feldman AL, Arber DA, Pittaluga S, et al. Clonally related follicular lymphomas and histiocytic/dendritic cell sarcomas: evidence for transdifferentiation of the follicular lymphoma clone. Blood. 2008;111(12):5433–9.
138. Vos JA, Abbondanzo SL, Barekman CL, et al. Histiocytic sarcoma: a study of five cases including the histiocyte marker CD163. Mod Pathol. 2005;18(5):693–704.
139. Zhang X, Kryston JJ, Michalak WA, et al. Histiocytic sarcoma in the small intestine: a case report with flow cytometry study and review of the literature. Pathol Res Pract. 2008;204(10):763–70.
140. Purgina B, Rao UN, Miettinen M, et al. AIDS-related EBV-associated smooth muscle tumors: a review of 64 published cases. Pathol Res Int. 2011;2011:561548.
141. Villella JA, Bogner PN, Jani-Sait SN, et al. Rhabdomyosarcoma of the cervix in sisters with review of the literature. Gynecol Oncol. 2005;99(3):742–8.
142. Corapcioglu F, Memet Ozek M, Sav A, et al. Congenital pineoblastoma and parameningeal rhabdomyosarcoma: concurrent two embryonal tumors in a young infant. Childs Nerv Syst. 2006;22(5):533–8.
143. Barr FG, Smith LM, Lynch JC, et al. Examination of gene fusion status in archival samples of alveolar rhabdomyosarcoma entered on the Intergroup Rhabdomyosarcoma Study-III trial: a report from the Children's Oncology Group. J Mol Diagn. 2006;8(2):202–8.
144. Rudzinski ER, Anderson JR, Lyden ER, et al. Myogenin, AP2beta, NOS-1, and HMGA2 are surrogate markers of fusion status in rhabdomyosarcoma: a report from the soft tissue sarcoma committee of the children's oncology group. Am J Surg Pathol. 2014;38(5):654–9.
145. Besnard-Guerin C, Newsham I, Winqvist R, et al. A common region of loss of heterozygosity in Wilms' tumor and embryonal rhabdomyosarcoma distal to the D11S988 locus on chromosome 11p15.5. Hum Genet. 1996;97(2):163–70.
146. Besnard-Guerin C, Cavenee WK, Newsham I. A new highly polymorphic DNA restriction site marker in the 5′ region of the human tyrosine hydroxylase gene (TH) detecting loss of heterozygosity in human embryonal rhabdomyosarcoma. Hum Genet. 1994;93(3):349–50.
147. Sabbioni S, Barbanti-Brodano G, Croce CM, et al. GOK: a gene at 11p15 involved in rhabdomyosarcoma and rhabdoid tumor development. Cancer Res. 1997;57(20):4493–7.
148. Afify A, Mark HF. Trisomy 8 in embryonal rhabdomyosarcoma detected by fluorescence in situ hybridization. Cancer Genet Cytogenet. 1999;108(2):127–32.
149. Barr FG, Chatten J, D'cruz CM, et al. Molecular assays for chromosomal translocations in the diagnosis of pediatric soft tissue sarcomas. JAMA. 1995;273(7):553–7.
150. De Alava E, Ladanyi M, Rosai J, et al. Detection of chimeric transcripts in desmoplastic small round cell tumor and related developmental tumors by reverse transcriptase polymerase chain reaction. A specific diagnostic assay. Am J Pathol. 1995;147(6):1584–91.
151. Downing JR, Khandekar A, Shurtleff SA, et al. Multiplex RT-PCR assay for the differential diagnosis of alveolar rhabdomyosarcoma and Ewing's sarcoma. Am J Pathol. 1995;146(3):626–34.
152. Arden KC, Anderson MJ, Finckenstein FG, et al. Detection of the t(2;13) chromosomal translocation in alveolar rhabdomyosarcoma using the reverse transcriptase-polymerase chain reaction. Genes Chromosom Cancer. 1996;16(4):254–60.
153. Schoofs G, Braeye L, Vanheste R, et al. Hepatic rhabdomyosarcoma in an adult: a rare primary malignant liver tumor. Case report and literature review. Acta Gastroenterol Belg. 2011;74(4):576–81.
154. Heerema-Mckenney A, Wijnaendts LC, Pulliam JF, et al. Diffuse myogenin expression by immunohistochemistry is an independent marker of poor survival in pediatric rhabdomyosarcoma: a tissue microarray study of 71 primary tumors including correlation with molecular phenotype. Am J Surg Pathol. 2008;32(10):1513–22.
155. Neville HL, Andrassy RJ, Lobe TE, et al. Preoperative staging, prognostic factors, and outcome for extremity rhabdomyosarcoma: a preliminary report from the Intergroup Rhabdomyosarcoma Study IV (1991–1997). J Pediatr Surg. 2000;35(2):317–21.
156. Tomimaru Y, Nagano H, Marubashi S, et al. Sclerosing epithelioid fibrosarcoma of the liver infiltrating the inferior vena cava. World J Gastroenterol. 2009;15(33):4204–8.
157. Coindre JM, Mariani O, Chibon F, et al. Most malignant fibrous histiocytomas developed in the retroperitoneum are dedifferentiated liposarcomas: a review of 25 cases initially diagnosed as malignant fibrous histiocytoma. Mod Pathol. 2003;16(3):256–62.
158. Yao D, Dai C. Clinical characteristics of the primary hepatic malignant fibrous histiocytoma in China: case report and review of the literature. World J Surg Oncol. 2012;10(2)
159. Li YR, Akbari E, Tretiakova MS, et al. Primary hepatic malignant fibrous histiocytoma: clinicopathologic characteristics and prog-

nostic value of ezrin expression. Am J Surg Pathol. 2008;32(8):1144–58.
160. Wei ZG, Tang LF, Chen ZM, et al. Childhood undifferentiated embryonal liver sarcoma: clinical features and immunohistochemistry analysis. J Pediatr Surg. 2008;43(10):1912–9.
161. Gao J, Fei L, Li S, et al. Undifferentiated embryonal sarcoma of the liver in a child: a case report and review of the literature. Oncol Lett. 2013;5(3):739–42.
162. Shehata BM, Gupta NA, Katzenstein HM, et al. Undifferentiated embryonal sarcoma of the liver is associated with mesenchymal hamartoma and multiple chromosomal abnormalities: a review of eleven cases. Pediatr Dev Pathol. 2011;14(2):111–6.
163. Begueret H, Trouette H, Vielh P, et al. Hepatic undifferentiated embryonal sarcoma: malignant evolution of mesenchymal hamartoma? Study of one case with immunohistochemical and flow cytometric emphasis. J Hepatol. 2001;34(1):178–9.
164. Rajaram V, Knezevich S, Bove KE, et al. DNA sequence of the translocation breakpoints in undifferentiated embryonal sarcoma arising in mesenchymal hamartoma of the liver harboring the t(11;19)(q11;q13.4) translocation. Genes Chromosom Cancer. 2007;46(5):508–13.
165. Mathews J, Duncavage EJ, Pfeifer JD. Characterization of translocations in mesenchymal hamartoma and undifferentiated embryonal sarcoma of the liver. Exp Mol Pathol. 2013;95(3):319–24.
166. Keating S, Taylor GP. Undifferentiated (embryonal) sarcoma of the liver: ultrastructural and immunohistochemical similarities with malignant fibrous histiocytoma. Hum Pathol. 1985;16(7):693–9.
167. Parham DM, Kelly DR, Donnelly WH, et al. Immunohistochemical and ultrastructural spectrum of hepatic sarcomas of childhood: evidence for a common histogenesis. Mod Pathol. 1991;4(5):648–53.
168. Lenze F, Birkfellner T, Lenz P, et al. Undifferentiated embryonal sarcoma of the liver in adults. Cancer. 2008;112(10):2274–82.
169. Kiani B, Ferrell LD, Qualman S, et al. Immunohistochemical analysis of embryonal sarcoma of the liver. Appl Immunohistochem Mol Morphol. 2006;14(2):193–7.
170. Nishio J, Iwasaki H, Sakashita N, et al. Undifferentiated (embryonal) sarcoma of the liver in middle-aged adults: smooth muscle differentiation determined by immunohistochemistry and electron microscopy. Hum Pathol. 2003;34(3):246–52.
171. Ida S, Okajima H, Hayashida S, et al. Undifferentiated sarcoma of the liver. Am J Surg. 2009;198(1):e7–9.
172. Nguyen TT, Gorman B, Shields D, et al. Malignant hepatic angiomyolipoma: report of a case and review of literature. Am J Surg Pathol. 2008;32(5):793–8.
173. Folpe AL, Mentzel T, Lehr HA, et al. Perivascular epithelioid cell neoplasms of soft tissue and gynecologic origin: a clinicopathologic study of 26 cases and review of the literature. Am J Surg Pathol. 2005;29(12):1558–75.
174. Parfitt JR, Bella AJ, Izawa JI, et al. Malignant neoplasm of perivascular epithelioid cells of the liver. Arch Pathol Lab Med. 2006;130(8):1219–22.
175. Park SH, Choi SB, Kim WB, et al. Huge primary osteosarcoma of the liver presenting an aggressive recurrent pattern following surgical resection. J Dig Dis. 2009;10(3):231–5.
176. Nawabi A, Rath S, Nissen N, et al. Primary hepatic osteosarcoma. J Gastrointest Surg. 2009;13(8):1550–3.
177. Experts Group of Chinese pancreatic neuroendocrine tumors of gastrointestinal pathology Consensus in 2013. Consensus on pathological diagnosis of gastrointestinal pancreatic neuroendocrine tumors in China (2013Edition). Chin. J. Pathol. 2013;42(10):691–4.
178. Gravante G, De Liguori CN, Overton J, et al. Primary carcinoids of the liver: a review of symptoms, diagnosis and treatments. Dig Surg. 2008;25(5):364–8.
179. Zhao J, Yang B, Xu C, et al. Study on clinicopathologic grading system and prognosis of primary hepatic neuroendocrine neoplasms. Chin. J. Pathol. 2012;41(2):102–6.
180. Fenwick SW, Wyatt JI, Toogood GJ, et al. Hepatic resection and transplantation for primary carcinoid tumors of the liver. Ann Surg. 2004;239(2):210–9.
181. Karampelas IN, Syrigos KN, Saif MW. Targeted agents in treatment of neuroendocrine tumors of pancreas. JOP. 2014;15(4):351–3.
182. Fiel MI, Schwartz M, Min AD, et al. Malignant schwannoma of the liver in a patient without neurofibromatosis: a case report and review of the literature. Arch Pathol Lab Med. 1996;120(12):1145–7.
183. Kobori L, Nagy P, Mathe Z, et al. Malignant peripheral nerve sheath tumor of the liver: a case report. Pathol Oncol Res. 2008;14(3):329–32.
184. Heywood G, Burgart LJ, Nagorney DM. Ossifying malignant mixed epithelial and stromal tumor of the liver: a case report of a previously undescribed tumor. Cancer. 2002;94(4):1018–22.
185. Goto H, Tanaka A, Kondo F, et al. Carcinosarcoma of the liver. Intern Med. 2010;49(23):2577–82.
186. Lai Q, Levi Sandri GB, Melandro F, et al. An unusual case of hepatic carcinosarcoma. G Chir. 2011;32(8–9):372–3.
187. Thompson L, Chang B, Barsky SH. Monoclonal origins of malignant mixed tumors (carcinosarcomas). Evidence for a divergent histogenesis. Am J Surg Pathol. 1996;20(3):277–85.
188. Zhao Q, Su CQ, Dong H, et al. Hepatocellular carcinoma and hepatic adenocarcinosarcoma in a patient with hepatitis B virus-related cirrhosis. Semin Liver Dis. 2010;30(1):107–12.
189. Schaefer IM, Schweyer S, Kuhlgatz J. Chromosomal imbalances in primary hepatic carcinosarcoma. Hum Pathol. 2012;43(8):1328–33.
190. Luchini C, Capelli P, Fassan M, et al. Next-generation histopathologic diagnosis: a lesson from a hepatic carcinosarcoma. J Clin Oncol. 2014;32(17):e63–6.
191. Warren M, Thompson KS. Two cases of primary yolk sac tumor of the liver in childhood: case reports and literature review. Pediatr Dev Pathol. 2009;12(5):410–6.
192. Shi H, Cao D, Wei L, et al. Primary choriocarcinoma of the liver: a clinicopathological study of five cases in males. Virchows Arch. 2010;456(1):65–70.
193. Theegarten D, Reinacher A, Graeven U, et al. Mixed malignant germ cell tumour of the liver. Virchows Arch. 1998;433(1):93–6.
194. Zhao JG, Cai B, Qiu B, et al. A case report of immature hepatic teratoma. Chin J Hepatol. 2010;18(1):72–72.
195. Xu AM, Gong SJ, Song WH, et al. Primary mixed germ cell tumor of the liver with sarcomatous components. World J Gastroenterol. 2010;16(5):652–6.
196. Eghtesad B, Marsh WJ, Cacciarelli T, et al. Liver transplantation for growing teratoma syndrome: report of a case. Liver Transpl. 2003;9(11):1222–4.
197. Martelli MG, Liu C. Malignant rhabdoid tumour of the liver in a seven-month-old female infant: a case report and literature review. Afr J Paediatr Surg. 2013;10(1):50–4.
198. Abe T, Oguma E, Nozawa K, et al. Malignant rhabdoid tumor of the liver: a case report with US and CT manifestation. Jpn J Radiol. 2009;27(10):462–5.
199. Yuri T, Danbara N, Shikata N, et al. Malignant rhabdoid tumor of the liver: case report and literature review. Pathol Int. 2004;54(8):623–9.
200. Hsueh C, Kuo TT. Congenital malignant rhabdoid tumor presenting as a cutaneous nodule: report of 2 cases with review of the literature. Arch Pathol Lab Med. 1998;122(12):1099–102.
201. Zhou B, Zhang M, Yan S, et al. Primary gastrointestinal stromal tumor of the liver: report of a case. Surg Today. 2014;44(6):1142–6.

202. Kim HO, Kim JE, Bae KS, et al. Imaging findings of primary malignant gastrointestinal stromal tumor of the liver. Jpn J Radiol. 2014;32(6):365–70.
203. Ochiai T, Sonoyama T, Kikuchi S, et al. Primary large gastrointestinal stromal tumor of the liver: report of a case. Surg Today. 2009;39(7):633–6.
204. Luo XL, Liu D, Yang JJ, et al. Primary gastrointestinal stromal tumor of the liver: a case report. World J Gastroenterol. 2009;15(29):3704–7.
205. De Chiara A, De Rosa V, Lastoria S, et al. Primary gastrointestinal stromal tumor of the liver with lung metastases successfully treated with STI-571 (imatinib mesylate). Front Biosci. 2006;11:498–501.
206. Hu X, Forster J, Damjanov I. Primary malignant gastrointestinal stromal tumor of the liver. Arch Pathol Lab Med. 2003;127(12):1606–8.
207. Corless CL, Fletcher JA, Heinrich MC. Biology of gastrointestinal stromal tumors. J Clin Oncol. 2004;22(18):3813–25.
208. Dang YZ, Gao J, Li J, et al. The clinicopathologic features and gene mutation status of gastrointestinal stromal tumor (with the analysis of 660 cases of patients). Chin J Pract Surg. 2013;33(1):61–5.
209. He HY, Fang WG, Zhong HH, et al. Status and clinical implication of c-kit and PDGFRA mutations in 165 cases of gastrointestinal stromal tumor (GIST). Chin J Pathol. 2006;35(5):262–6.
210. Expert Committee of Csco on Gastrointestinal Stromal Tumor. Consensus on diagnosis and treatment of gastrointestinal stromal tumor in China (2013 Edition). Chin Clin Oncol. 2013;18(11):1025–32.
211. Agaimy A. Gastrointestinal stromal tumors (GIST) from risk stratification systems to the new TNM proposal: more questions than answers? A review emphasizing the need for a standardized GIST reporting. Int. J. Clin. Exp. Pathol. 2010;3(5):461–71.
212. Leonardou P, Semelka RC, Kanematsu M, et al. Primary malignant mesothelioma of the liver: MR imaging findings. Magn Reson Imaging. 2003;21(9):1091–3.
213. Inagaki N, Kibata K, Tamaki T, et al. Primary intrahepatic malignant mesothelioma with multiple lymphadenopathies due to non-tuberculous mycobacteria: a case report and review of the literature. Oncol Lett. 2013;6(3):676–80.
214. Destephano DB, Wesley JR, Heidelberger KP, et al. Primitive cystic hepatic neoplasm of infancy with mesothelial differentiation: report of a case. Pediatr Pathol. 1985;4(3–4):291–302.
215. Holla P, Hafez GR, Slukvin I, et al. Synovial sarcoma, a primary liver tumor--a case report. Pathol Res Pract. 2006;202(5):385–7.
216. Srivastava A, Nielsen PG, Dal Cin P, et al. Monophasic synovial sarcoma of the liver. Arch Pathol Lab Med. 2005;129(8):1047–9.
217. Xiong B, Chen M, Ye F, et al. Primary monophasic synovial sarcoma of the liver in a 13-year-old boy. Pediatr Dev Pathol. 2013;16(5):353–6.
218. Munoz PA, Rao MS, Reddy JK. Osteoclastoma-like giant cell tumor of the liver. Cancer. 1980;46(4):771–9.
219. Rudloff U, Gao ZQ, Fields S, et al. Osteoclast-like giant cell tumor of the liver: a rare neoplasm with an aggressive clinical course. J Gastrointest Surg. 2005;9(2):207–14.
220. Westra WH, Sturm P, Drillenburg P, et al. K-ras oncogene mutations in osteoclast-like giant cell tumors of the pancreas and liver: genetic evidence to support origin from the duct epithelium. Am J Surg Pathol. 1998;22(10):1247–54.
221. Bauditz J, Rudolph B, Wermke W. Osteoclast-like giant cell tumors of the pancreas and liver. World J Gastroenterol. 2006;12(48):7878–83.
222. Tanahashi C, Nagae H, Nukaya T, et al. Combined hepatocellular carcinoma and osteoclast-like giant cell tumor of the liver: possible clue to histogenesis. Pathol Int. 2009;59(11):813–6.
223. Kuwano H, Sonoda T, Hashimoto H, et al. Hepatocellular carcinoma with osteoclast-like giant cells. Cancer. 1984;54(5):837–42.
224. Horie Y, Hori T, Hirayama C, et al. Osteoclast-like giant cell tumor of the liver. Acta Pathol Jpn. 1987;37(8):1327–35.
225. Hood DL, Bauer TW, Leibel SA, et al. Hepatic giant cell carcinoma. An ultrastructural and immunohistochemical study. Am J Clin Pathol. 1990;93(1):111–6.
226. Ahaouche M, Cazals-Hatem D, Sommacale D, et al. A malignant hepatic tumour with osteoclast-like giant cells. Histopathology. 2005;46(5):590–2.
227. Andreola S, Lombardi L, Scurelli A, et al. Osteoclastoma-like giant-cell tumor of the liver. Case Rep Tumori. 1985;71(6):615–20.
228. Haratake J, Yamada H, Horie A, et al. Giant cell tumor-like cholangiocarcinoma associated with systemic cholelithiasis. Cancer. 1992;69(10):2444–8.
229. Mccluggage WG, Toner PG. Hepatocellular carcinoma with osteoclast-like giant cells. Histopathology. 1993;23(2):187–9.
230. Sasaki A, Yokoyama S, Nakayama I, et al. Sarcomatoid hepatocellular carcinoma with osteoclast-like giant cells: case report and immunohistochemical observations. Pathol Int. 1997;47(5):318–24.
231. Ikeda T, Seki S, Maki M, et al. Hepatocellular carcinoma with osteoclast-like giant cells: possibility of osteoclastogenesis by hepatocyte-derived cells. Pathol Int. 2003;53(7):450–6.
232. Chetty R, Learmonth GM, Taylor DA. Giant cell hepatocellular carcinoma. Cytopathology. 1990;1(4):233–7.
233. Zhang J, Chen L, Li F, et al. Recurrent and metastatic osteoclast-like giant cell tumor of the liver revealed by FDG PET/CT. Clin Nucl Med. 2012;37(10):1016–7.
234. Jordan AH,Pappo A. Management of desmoplastic small round-cell tumors in children and young adults. J Pediatr Hematol Oncol. 2012;34(Suppl 2): S73–5.
235. Dufresne A, Cassier P, Couraud L, et al. Desmoplastic small round cell tumor: current management and recent findings. Sarcoma. 2012;2012:714986.
236. Feng ZZ, Li DC, Liu DC, et al. Desmoplastic small round cell tumor: a report of 2 cases and literature review. Chin J Clin Exp Pathol. 2008;24(1):83–5.
237. Chen XG, Peng MH, Luo RZ, et al. Desmoplastic small round cell tumor in liver (A case report and review of the literature). J Pract Oncol. 2002;17(1):61–3.
238. Wang LL, Perlman EJ, Vujanic GM, et al. Desmoplastic small round cell tumor of the kidney in childhood. Am J Surg Pathol. 2007;31(4):576–84.
239. Rekhi B, Ahmed S, Basak R, et al. Desmoplastic small round cell tumor-clinicopathological spectrum, including unusual features and immunohistochemical analysis of 45 tumors diagnosed at a tertiary cancer referral centre, with molecular results t(11; 22)(p13; q12) (EWS-WT1) in select cases. Pathol Oncol Res. 2012;18(4):917–27.
240. Zhang J, Xu H, Ren F, et al. Analysis of clinicopathological features and prognostic factors of desmoplastic small round cell tumor. Pathol Oncol Res. 2014;20(1):161–8.
241. Chang F. Desmoplastic small round cell tumors: cytologic, histologic, and immunohistochemical features. Arch Pathol Lab Med. 2006;130(5):728–32.
242. Li M, Cai MY, Lu JB, et al. Clinicopathological investigation of four cases of desmoplastic small round cell tumor. Oncol Lett. 2012;4(3):423–8.
243. Al Balushi Z, Bulduc S, Mulleur C, et al. Desmoplastic small round cell tumor in children: a new therapeutic approach. J Pediatr Surg. 2009;44(5):949–52.
244. Lal DR, Su WT, Wolden SL, et al. Results of multimodal treatment for desmoplastic small round cell tumors. J Pediatr Surg. 2005;40(1):251–5.
245. Modak S, Gerald W, Cheung NK. Disialoganglioside GD2 and a novel tumor antigen: potential targets for immunotherapy of desmoplastic small round cell tumor. Med Pediatr Oncol. 2002;39(6):547–51.

Hepatic Tumors in Children

8

Xiang-Ru Wu

8.1 Introduction

8.1.1 New Classification of Hepatic Tumors in Children

Hepatic tumors are extremely rare in children, and the overall incidence is estimated to be only 1.5/1000, 000 in under 18-year-old population, accounting for 1% of all children solid tumors. In children population, two thirds of the hepatic tumors are malignant, with hepatoblastoma (43%) and hepatocellular carcinoma (23%) as the most common [1, 2]. Other hepatic tumors are even rarer in children, among which benign angioma ranks the third (10%), followed by sarcoma (6%), hepatic mesenchymal hamartoma (6%), benign hepatocellular proliferated tumors (adenoma and focal nodular hyperplasia (7%), and a few rare tumors (5%). In 2011, classification of hepatic tumors in children (consensus) was formulated by international institutes for researches on hepatic tumors in children (Table 8.1).

8.1.2 Requirements of Tissue Sampling and Delivery for Diagnosing Hepatic Tumors in Children

Diagnostic biopsy must be provided with the age, serum AFP, imaging data, and clinical information of the children, aiming at obtaining adequate tumor tissue for histological diagnosis and classification and obtaining fresh juncture tissue between the tumor and normal liver tissue for cytogenetics and of molecular biology.

Biopsy must be conducted before the start of chemotherapy, because chemotherapy of hepatic tumors in children may have impacts on the differentiation and induction which is still not clear. The international institutions are endeavoring to collect large quantities of pre- and post-chemotherapy data for these tumors for comparison, study, and analysis; thus, the present histological classifications are applied only to the pathodiagnosis of pre-chemotherapy specimens.

At present, the guidelines of children's oncology group (COG) recommend sampling methods to obtain the liver tumors which are as follows: percutaneous needle aspiration, laparoscopic or open needle biopsy, or wedge biopsy. According to the condition of pediatric patient, the tumor size, and the location, different choices can be made. Because of the heterogeneity commonly found in hepatic tumors in children, the adequacy of the biopsy specimens is crucial for accurate pathodiagnosis and typing. And uncertainties exist in aspects of sampling, including how much tissue can reflect the whole tumor in biopsy and how representative of the biopsy is. Thus, the guidelines require ultrasound or imaging-guided sampling according to the different regions of the tumor tissue via coarse needle biopsy, obtaining no less than ten strips, and each strip of tissue should be not less than 1 cm × 0.3 cm in size. If possible, take a small amount of adjacent nontumor liver tissue for inspection. And in order to avoid dissemination of the tumor inside the needle tract, it is recommended to use coaxial needle, which achieves removal of tumor tissue and tissue in the needle at the same time. Intraoperative frozen pathodiagnosis should be avoided, for frozen sections are generally used only for margin assessment. Fine needle aspiration is not suitable for tumor diagnosis, since the obtained cells or tissues are far from enough for the assessment of the tumor.

Biopsy or resected specimens should be sent to the Department of Pathology freshly, and if tumor specimens are sufficient in amount, molecular biology of cytogenetics and tests can be done when necessary, which is important in the study of the mechanisms and the improvement of the treatment of tumors. Hopefully, in the future study, some prognostic index in molecular biology can be beneficial in deciding whether to reduce the drug in the treatment to avoid toxicity or to reduce the intensity of treatment to improve prognosis. According to the experience of COG, the

X.-R. Wu (✉)
Xin Hua Hospital, Shanghai Jiao Tong University School of Medicine, Shanghai, China
e-mail: xiangruwu6@hotmail.com

W.-M. Cong (ed.), *Surgical Pathology of Hepatobiliary Tumors*, DOI 10.1007/978-981-10-3536-4_8

Table 8.1 Consensus on the classification of hepatic tumors in children (2011)

Epithelial tumors
Hepatocellular[a]
Benign and tumorlike lesions
Hepatocellular adenoma (adenomatosis)
Focal nodular hyperplasia
Macroregenerative nodule
Precancerous lesion
Dysplastic nodules
Malignant lesion
Hepatoblastoma
Epithelial subtypes
Pure fetal with low mitotic activity
Fetal, mitotically active
Pleomorphic, poorly differentiated
Embryonal
Small-cell undifferentiated
INI1 negative
INI1 positive
Epithelial mixed (any/all above)
Cholangioblastic
Epithelial macrotrabecular pattern
Mixed epithelial and mesenchymal
Without teratoid features
With teratoid features
Hepatocellular carcinoma
Classic HCC
Fibrolamellar HCC
Hepatocellular neoplasm, NOS[b]
Bile duct
Benign
Bile duct adenoma/hamartoma, others
Malignant
Cholangiocarcinoma
Combined (hepatocellular cholangiocarcinoma)
Mesenchymal tumor
Benign
Vascular
Infantile hemangioma
Mesenchymal hamartoma
PEComas
Malignant
Embryonal sarcoma
Rhabdomyosarcoma
Vascular
Epithelioid hemangioendothelioma
Angiosarcoma
Other malignant tumors
Undefined tumors
Malignant rhabdoid tumor
INI1 (*INI1* mutation)
INI1+
Nested stromal-epithelial tumor
Others
Germ cell tumors
Teratoma
Yolk sac tumor
Desmoplastic small round cell tumor (DSRCT)
Peripheral primitive neuroectodermal tumor (pPNET)
Metastatic(and secondary)
Solid tumors (neuroblastoma, Wilms' tumor, others)
Acute myeloid leukemia (M7)

Reprint with permission from Dolores, et al. Modern Pathology 2013, Vol 27(3), Towards and international pediatric liver tumor consensus classification

[a]Only for pre-chemotherapy lesions

[b]Tentative classification, possibly containing previously called transition hepatocellular tumors

diagnosis of simple fetal-type HB with low mitotic activity in the resected specimen is very important in the prognosis and treatment, which can prevent these children from chemotherapy. Total removal of the tumors can cure the children, so first-stage operations should be increased as possible, not only to reduce unnecessary chemotherapy but also for a better understanding of small-cell undifferentiated composition in the tumor and evidence and experience on deciding the lowest proportion of tumor components to have an impact on the prognosis.

In order to ensure the access to poorly differentiated areas (such as small-cell undifferentiated type) in resected tumor, sampling should be conducted in each different regions of the tumor. The total number of samples should be at least equal to or larger than the number of centimeters of the maximum diameter of the tumor on the tumor resection specimens. These sampling parts should include ink-marked margins and involved large blood vessels (such as the portal vein, hepatic vein, and inferior vena cava), and both the sampling position and the infiltration degree of large blood vessels are required to be recorded in detail. While tumor size and location of certain hepatic segment should be recorded in cases with multifocal tumors, the conditions of tumor cells growing in small blood vessels, which are either in or outside the tumor, are required to be reported.

For post-chemotherapy resected specimens, pathological examination is mainly aimed at accurately describing and comparing the changes before and after chemotherapy (such as the ratio of tumor necrosis and the type of residual viable tumor) and molecular biological characteristics related to the survival tumor cells (such as expression of drug-resistant genes).

8.2 Malignant Hepatic Tumors in Children

8.2.1 Epithelial Tumors

8.2.1.1 Hepatoblastoma (HB)

Pathogenesis and Mechanism

HB is the most common pediatric hepatic malignant tumor, accounting for 1% of all malignant tumors found in children under 15 years old, and nearly 90% of them are discovered in young patients under the age of 5, 70% in patients under 2 years old, and 4% at birth. Most of hepatic tumors in children are sporadic, and the male-to-female ratio is 1.4–2: 1, and some cases are related to familial tumor syndrome (Table 8.2), metabolic diseases, individual susceptibility, and so on, while the exact etiology is still unknown. In recent years, the incidence of HB has been rising, possibly related to the increased survival rate of low birth weight infants, as it has been reported that the lower the birth weight, the higher the risk of developing HB, and the risk values of developing HB in patients with birth weight of <1000 g, 1000–1500 g, and 2000–2500 g are 15.64, 2.53, and 1.21, respectively [3]. Other hereditary syndromes (Beckwith-Wiedemann syndrome, Li-Fraumeni syndrome, familial adenomatous polyposis, Edward's syndrome, etc.), chromosome abnormalities (2, 8, 13, 18, 21 trisomy, etc.), environmental factors (parents with exposure to metal, petroleum products, paint, acetaminophen, tobacco, etc.), and some of the common chromosome recessive hereditary metabolic diseases (such as glycogen storage disease type I) can increase the risk of HB. The molecular mechanism and tumor signal transduction pathway activation play a role in the genesis of HB, mainly involving pathways such as Wnt pathway, hepatocyte growth factor/C-Met (PI3K/AKT and MAPK) pathway, insulin-like growth factor (IGF) pathway, sonic hedgehog (SHH) pathway [12], Notch pathway [13], and so on.

Clinical Features

Among the 50 cases of HB treated by surgical resection and pathodiagnosis in Eastern Hepatobiliary Surgery Hospital, Second Military Medical University during the period from January 1983 to December 2013, the patients were under the age of 18 years with a male-to-female ratio of 2.57: 1 (36:14) and an average age of 43.6 (6–210, median 27.5) months, of which patients under 4 years old account for 64%, while 74% of the patients go to the hospital because of abdominal pain or accidentally found abdominal mass, and 24% are found in physical examination. In a case affecting a Chinese female infant who developed jaundice 3 days after birth, abdominal huge mass was found and resected 40 days after birth, which was located in the left lobe of the liver and was mixed type with a size of 10 cm × 8 cm. HB patients often manifest abdominal swelling, secondary hepatomegaly, weight loss or gain, abdominal pain, and digestive tract symptoms, such as nausea, vomiting, and decreased appetite, and jaundice is found in only 5% of the patients. The tumors are located in deep parts and the child cannot express itself, resulting in huge or dissemination of the tumor at primary diagnosis; irregular mass can be palpated in the right upper abdomen in physical examination, which is hard even exceeding midline and pelvic brim in some cases. Some cases are associated with some clinical syndrome associated with developmental malformations, and a few have sexual

Table 8.2 Common hepatic tumor-related hereditary diseases in children

Disease	Classification	Chromosome	Gene
Trisomy 18	Hepatoblastoma	18	
Beckwith-Wiedemann syndrome	Hepatoblastoma	11p15.5	p57KIP2
	Hemangioendothelioma		
Familial adenomatous polyposis	Hepatoblastoma, adenoma, hepatocellular carcinoma, cholangioadenoma	5q21,22	APC
Li-Fraumeni syndrome	Hepatoblastoma, undifferentiated sarcoma	17p13	P53
Glycogen storage disease type I	Hepatoblastoma, adenoma, hepatocellular carcinoma	17	Glucose-6-phosphatase
Hereditary tyrosinemia	Hepatocellular carcinoma	15q23–25	Fumaryl acetoacetic acid lyase
Alagille syndrome	Hepatocellular carcinoma	20p12	Jagged-1
Other familial cholestasis syndromes	Hepatocellular carcinoma, cholangiocarcinoma	18q21–22, 2q24	FIC-1, BSEP (ABCB11)
Neurofibromatosis	Hepatocellular carcinoma, malignant neurinoma, hemangiosarcoma	17q11.2	
Ataxia telangiectasia	Hepatocellular carcinoma	11q22–23	ATM
Fanconi anemia	Hepatocellular carcinoma, hepatic adenoma, fibrolamellar carcinoma of the liver	20q13.2–13.3	FAA, FAC\BRCA2
		1q42, 3p, others	
Tuberous sclerosis	Angiomyolipoma	9q34, 16p13	TSC1, TSC2

precocity or androphany due to secretion of gonadotropins by the tumor, e.g., increased levels of serum chorionic gonadotrophin and testosterone. Seventy percent of the HB patients may be associated with anemia, 50% with thrombocytosis, and 80–90% with significantly increased serum alpha-fetoprotein (AFP), while undifferentiated small-cell HB and few fetal HB have normal or slightly increased serum AFP. The AFP level shows parallel changes with the disease course and can be used to evaluate and assess the residual of the tumor and reaction of postsurgical chemotherapy and monitor tumor recurrence. Since AFP is produced by the fetal liver, neonatal serum AFP level can be extremely high, and the AFP concentration in normal full-term infants can be up to more than 100,000 ng/ml which gradually decreases months after birth to <10 ng/ml at 1 year old. So for infants <1 year old, careful evaluation and assessment should be made. All the 50 cases of HB diagnosed in Eastern Hepatobiliary Surgery Hospital, Second Military Medical University, had no previous history of viral hepatitis, 78% of which have serum AFP of ≥1000 μg/L. And distal metastasis at the time of diagnosis was found in 20% of HB cases, with the lung as the most common metastatic site, and other metastatic sites include the bone, brain, eye, ovary, and so on.

Controversy remains in whether adults can develop HB, and 2010 WHO classification of hepatic and intrahepatic bile duct tumors did not describe adult HB, but there have been 50 cases of adult HB in the literature. Compared to pediatric HB, both adult and pediatric HB contain similar numbers of tumor nodules, but pediatric type tends to involve the right lobe of the liver (55–60%), while adult cases often involve both the left and right lobe in a similar proportion. About 90% of pediatric cases have significantly increased serum AFP level, while adult HB displays normal serum AFP levels, and cases with AFP > 200 μ g/l only account for 25%. Pulmonary metastasis can be found in pediatric HB, while adult HB may present metastasis in the lymph nodes and visceral organs including the lung. The prognosis of adult HB aged older than 45 years old is markedly poorer than that of patients under 45 years old.

Pathological Staging

1. Pre-/posttreatment tumor extension (PRETTEXT/POSTTEXT) staging by the International Childhood Liver Tumors Strategy (SIOPEL). This system is based on the segmental anatomy of the liver, with the basic index, e.g., the number and extension of tumors involving four hepatic lobes (left lateral lobe, left internal lobe, right anterior lobe, and right posterior lobe), without any involvement of histopathology. It is widely used in the formulation of therapeutic strategy and evaluation of the prognosis (Table 8.3), and the 2005 edition added the annotation of invasion extension. The recommendations made by COG suggested surgical guidelines which include the following: (1) PRETEXT stages I and II at diagnosis, lobular or segmental resection of the liver can be conducted; (2) POSTTEXT stage II or III, without vascular invasion grossly (V−, P−), lobular or tri-segmental resection of the liver after neoadjuvant chemotherapy is suitable; (3) POSTTEXT stage III, with vascular invasion grossly (V+, P+); or POSTTEXT stage IV, extremely complex surgical resection or liver transplantation after neoadjuvant chemotherapy can be adopted [4–7].

Table 8.3 PRETTEXT/POSTTEXT staging of hepatoblastoma

Stage	Characteristics
Stage I	Tumors are confined in one hepatic lobe (segments 2 and 3 in the left lateral lobe, or segments 6 and 7 in the right posterior lobe), with no invasion of three adjacent lobes
Stage II	Solitary or multiple nodules involving one or two hepatic lobes, with no invasion of two adjacent lobes
Stage III	Huge tumors with involvement of three hepatic lobes except one adjacent lobe with several subtypes, including right anterior tumor involving left internal lobe or multinodular tumor with exemption of involvement of the right anterior and/or left lateral lobe or left internal and right anterior lobes
Stage IV	Huge tumors or multinodular tumors involving all four hepatic lobes
Annotation	
V	Involvement of the inferior vena cava or all three major hepatic veins (right, middle, and left)
P	Left and right branches of portal vein
E	Extrahepatic involvement, such as the diaphragm, abdominal wall, stomach, colon, etc.
M	Distal metastasis (commonly seen in the lung, barely seen in the bone and brain)
C	Caudate lobe
F	Multinodular tumors
N	Involvement of lymph nodes

Of the 50 cases of pediatric HB diagnosed and excised in Eastern Hepatobiliary Surgery Hospital, Second Military Medical University, cases at PRETEXT stages I, II, III, and IV account for 34%, 52%, 12%, and 2%, respectively. All these 14 cases affecting female patients (100%) were stage I–II, while of the 36 cases affecting male patients, 29 cases were (81.6%) stage I–II, with worse PRETEXT staging in male HB patients than females.

2. North American children's oncology association risk stratification for HB. This system grades the risk of HB into four stages from low risk to high risk, involving multiple index related to surgery and pathology (Table 8.4) and can be referred to and applied in the clinical practice [4].

Table 8.4 North American children's oncology association risk stratification for hepatoblastoma

Stage	Features
Stage I	Extremely low risk: simple fetal type, tumors resected at diagnosis, PRETEXT stage I or II, hepatic segmental resection, or standard lobular resection
Stage II	Low risk: all histology status, tumors resected at diagnosis, PRETEXT stage I or II
Stage III	Moderately low risk: PRETEXT stage III or IV; extrahepatic tumors (invasion of hepatic vein/portal vein/extrahepatic tissues); undifferentiated small-cell type
Stage IV	High risk: metastasis at diagnosis, serum AFP < 100 ng/ml

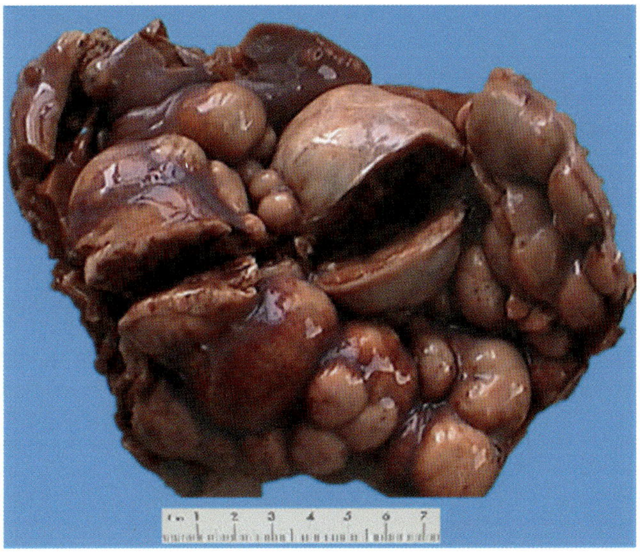

Fig. 8.1 Hepatoblastoma. The tumor presents multi-nodular in shape

3. Maibach et al. [8] (2012) included serum AFP concentration, metastasis, PRETEXT staging, age, and pathological parameters to form a stratification diagram of influencing factors for PRETEXT staging and prognosis of HB, dividing the disease-free survival (DFS) of HB patients into three groups: PRETEXT stage I/II/III, without any other risk factors, 3-year DFS reaches 90%; PRETEXT stage IV, and/or multinodular tumors, and/or >5 years old, and/or AFP ≥ 1.2 × 10^6 ng/ml, 3-year EFS reaches 70%; and undifferentiated small-cell tumor, and/or AFP<100 ng/ml, and/or metastasis, 3-year DFS is 49%.

Gross Features

About 80% of HB lesions are solitary masses, and 58% are located in the right lobe and 15% located in the left lobe, and 27% of the cases involve the left and right lobe. Single huge lesion across the midline or bilobular multifocal lesion can also be found. The tumors are 5–20 cm in diameter, slightly lobulated, or protrude on the surface of the liver. The cut sections show well-defined borders between the tumor and the surrounding liver tissue with a pseudocapsule separating the two, and the tumors are grayish white, brown, or green, commonly seen with hemorrhage and necrosis. Of the 50 cases of surgically resected HB diagnosed in Pathology, Eastern Hepatobiliary Surgery Hospital, Second Military Medical University, the average diameter was 11.2 (2.5–20) cm (Figs. 8.1 and 8.2).

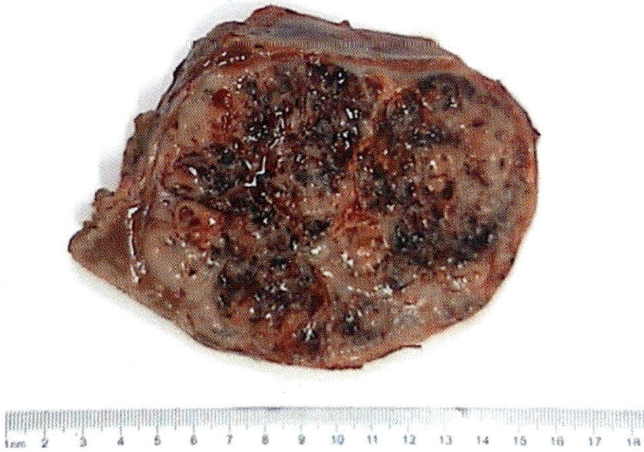

Fig. 8.2 Hepatoblastoma. The cut section shows well defined borders, and the tumors are *gray-white* with extensive hemorrhage and necrosis

Histological Classification

In 2011 Los Angeles COG Liver Tumor Forum edited the classification of HB, mainly including the following types (Table 8.5):

1. Well-differentiated fetal type (WDF). Also known as pure fetal HB with low mitotic activity, this type accounts for 7% of all epithelial HB. The tumor cells are smaller than nonneoplastic hepatocytes and similar to the size of fetal hepatocytes, with a diameter of 10–20 μm, and are consistently round and cubic in shape. The nuclei are small, round, and center located, with thin chromatin, clear cell membrane, and nonobvious nucleolus. Some cells contain varying amounts of glycogen or lipid resulting in eosinophilic or translucent cytoplasm, which are called as "DAR cells" and "bright cells" (Fig. 8.3). The tumor cells are arranged in cords or thin trabecules, with 2–3 cellular layers and mitotic figures <2个/10HPF (Fig. 8.4). Extramedullary hematopoiesis (EMH) can be easily found. The diagnosis of WDF is only for pre-chemotherapy completely resected specimens, and according to the treatment guidelines of COG, this type of HB does not need postsurgical chemotherapy after complete resection, with tumor-free survival rate of 100%.
2. Crowded fetal type (CF). Also known as mitotically active fetal type, the cells of the tumor are morphologically

Table 8.5 Histological classification and characteristics of hepatoblastoma

Epithelial type	Features
Fetal type	Well differentiated: consistent cellular size (10–20 μm), bright or dark cells, round nucleus, trabecular arrangement, mitotic figures <2/HPF, EMH
	Cell-rich: mitotic figures >2/HPF, obvious nucleolus, litter cytoplasmic glycogen
Polymorphic/poorly differentiated	Cellular anaplasia, significant nuclear atypia, increased karyoplasmic ratio, marked nucleoli
Embryonal	Cellular diameter ranged 10–15 μm, increased karyoplasmic ratio, irregular nucleus, primitive tubular structure, EMH
Macrotrabecular pattern	Epithelial (fetal or embryonal type) type, trabecular arrangement, intersinusoidal trabecules are thicker than five cells
Small-cell undifferentiated type	Cellular diameter ranged 5–10 μm, clusters or diffuse distribution, little amphophilic cytoplasm, round or oval nucleus, exquisite chromatin, nonobvious nucleolus, mitotic figures+/−, necrosis, common apoptosis, INI1+/−
Cholangioblastic type	Tumoral cholangial or tubular structures, often found at the margin of epithelial islets, or as the main component
Mixed type	
Without teratomatoid features	Epithelial and mesenchymal components: spindle cells, osteoid, fibrous, chondro
With teratomatoid features	Epithelium and mesenchyma, primitive nerve epithelium, primitive endoderm, melanoma, squamous and epithelial components

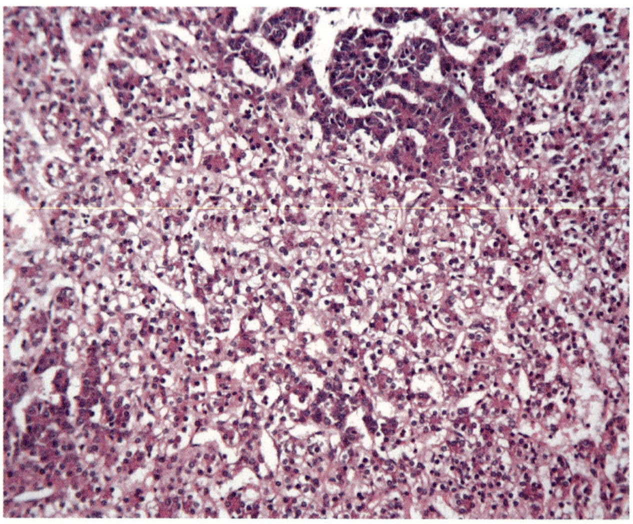

Fig. 8.3 Fetal hepatoblastoma, Some cells contain varying amounts of glycogen or lipid resulting in eosinophilic or translucent cytoplasm, which are called as "dark cells" and "bright cells"

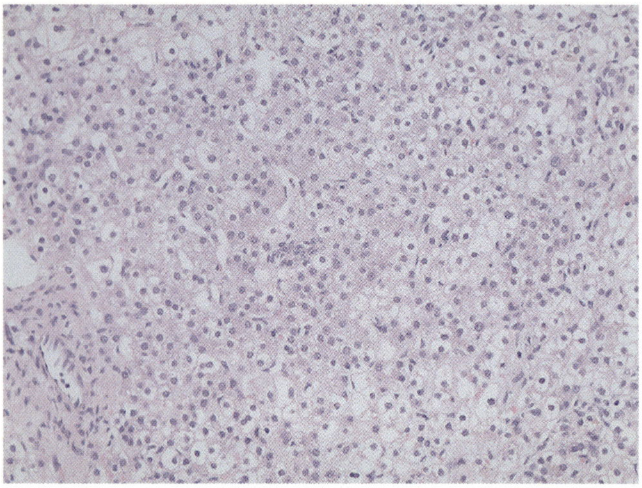

Fig. 8.4 Fetal hepatoblastoma. Well-differentiated neoplastic cells are consistent in size

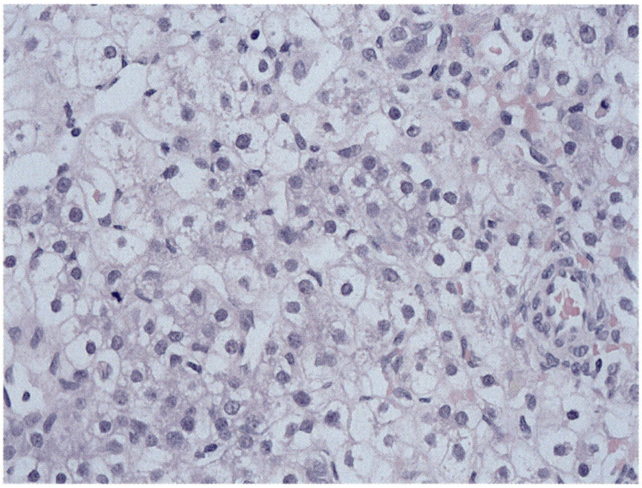

Fig. 8.5 Crowded fetal type hepatoblastoma. Tumor cellular density is increased and the cells have clear boundaries

similar to WDF but with more cellular density, clear boundaries, increased karyoplasmic ratio, visible nucleolus, and increased mitotic figures >2个/10HPF (Fig. 8.5). This type is often found in a mixture with WDF, and these tumors with defined CF regions should be treated with postsurgical adjuvant chemotherapy. Glypican-3 staining is beneficial in the differential diagnosis of the two types.

3. Embryonal type. This type of tumors is morphologically similar to the cells in the embryonic liver tissue during sixth to eighth weeks of gestation, which are 10–15 μm in diameter, round or angular, scant cytoplasm, increased karyoplasmic ratio, a little eosinophilic cytoplasm, and unclear cellular membrane. They are arranged in flaky and trabecular, acinar, or rosette-shaped clusters (Fig. 8.6) or papilla similar to yolk sac tumor (Fig. 8.7). Visible primitive tubular structures are formed with accidental

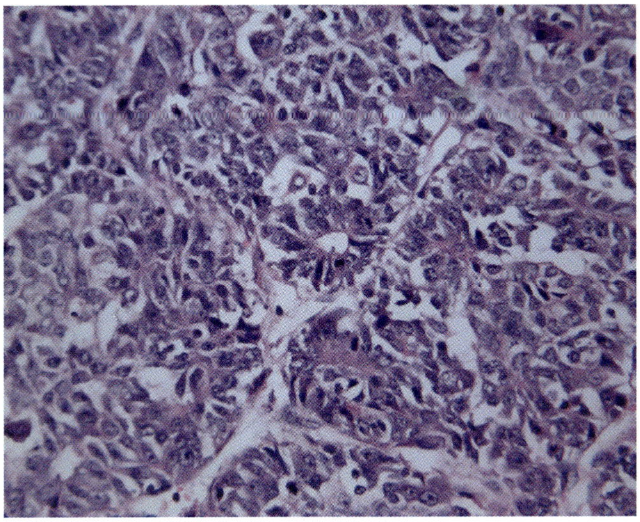

Fig. 8.6 Embryona type hepatoblastoma. The tumor cells are arranged in rosettes shaped clusters with active nuclear mitotic figures

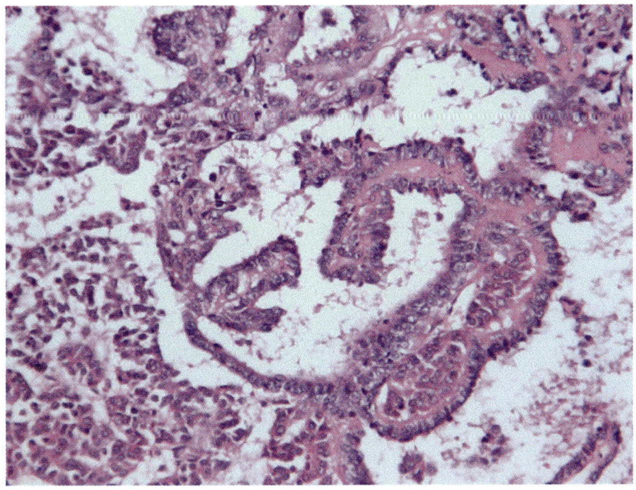

Fig. 8.7 Embryona type hepatoblastoma. The tumor cells are arranged in papillary glandular structure

tumor cells in the loose myxoid background distributed in microcystic arrangement; tumor cells are densely distributed with obvious nuclear overlap. Extramedullary hematopoiesis (EMH) can also be observed (Fig. 8.8).

4. Pleomorphic/poorly differentiated. Previously known as "anaplastic fetal type" and "hepatocellular carcinoma type," it is a rare type of HB, seen in post-chemotherapy metastatic specimens, the morphology of which is similar to pleomorphic tumor cells containing rich eosinophilic cytoplasm in fetal or embryonal HB, increased karyoplasmic ratio, obvious nuclear atypia, thick chromatin, conspicuous nucleolus, visible mitotic figures, or even anaplastic features, including large cells (3–4 times the size of the adjacent cells) and pathological mitotic figures (Fig. 8.9). If these pleomorphic tumor cells grow in huge trabecular pattern, it is difficult to differentiate it from hepatocellular carcinoma, and typical HB regions found in the tumor may facilitate the diagnosis. Rare cases contain simultaneously the components of HB and HCC; however, the relationship between the prognosis and the type of tumor is still not determined.
5. Cholangioblastic type. This type of HB is rare with some tumor cells undergoing cholangiolar differentiation [9], with or without cholangiolar structures which can be located inside or surrounding the tumor. The cholangioblasts are often cubic rather than columnar, with round nuclei and thick chromatin (Fig. 8.10), which express cholangioepithelial immunophenotypes (CK7, CK19 positive).

Differential Diagnosis

(1) Cholangioblasts and tubular or acinar structures in embryonal HB cells in the latter are smaller with less cytoplasm and obvious mitotic figures and express glypican-3, while the former are often negative for glypican-3 (Table 8.2).

(2) Cholangiolar ducts formed by cholangioblasts and reactive proliferated bile ducts β-catenin staining facilitate the differentiation of these two compositions, and the former show positive expression in the nuclei, while the latter are positive on the cell membrane.

(3) Other pediatric cholangioblastic tumors
  (a) Ductal plate tumor: It is rare, with visible ductal platelike structures which are densely distributed.
  (b) Intrahepatic cholangiocarcinoma in children: It contains diffuse desmoplastic features, which cannot be observed in cholangioblastic HB.
  (c) Hepatic nested stromal-epithelial tumor (see contents below).

6. Small-cell undifferentiated type (SCU). Tumor cells are larger than lymphocytes (7–8 μm), and the nuclei are round or oval, with little amphophilic cytoplasm, fine chromatin, inconspicuous nucleoli, rare mitotic figures, and obvious necrosis and apoptosis, in clusters or diffuse distribution or arranged in nests or organ structures (Fig. 8.11). It is often mixed with other types of HB. These small cells can express simultaneously epithelial and mesenchymal markers. HB consisting of single SCU component is rare, accounting only for less than 5% of all HB cases, and is mainly found in infants. Generally, the diagnosis of this type of HB can be made when the tumor contains at least 75% of SCU components.

Recently, it has been reported that some SCU have the biological features of MRT, such as loss of expression of nuclear integrase interactor 1 (INI1) in tumor cells, and molecular biological tests confirmed the same change as in

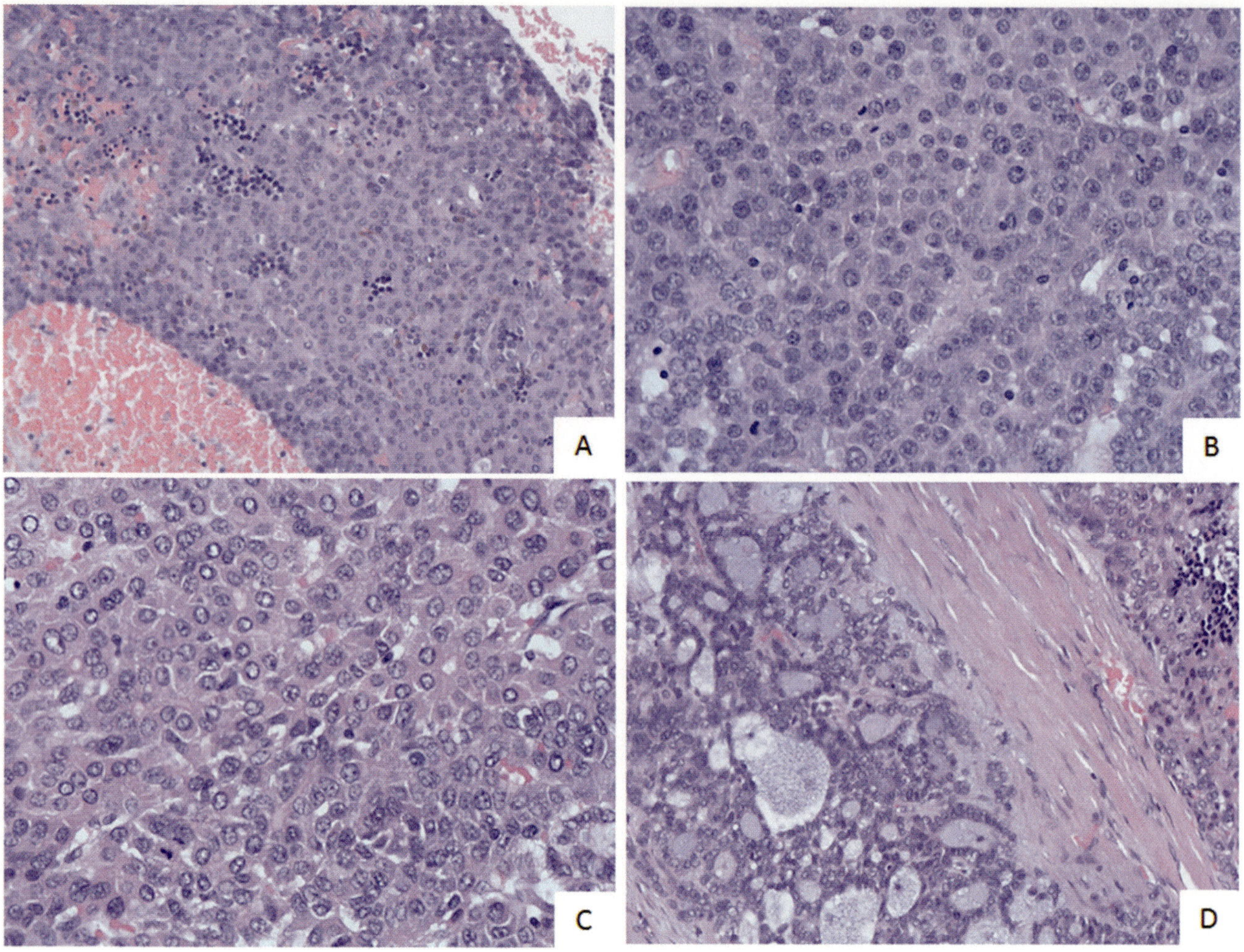

Fig. 8.8 Embryona type hepatoblastoma. (**a**) Tumor cells are high-density with overlapping nuclear; (**b**) Tumor cells has scant cytoplasm and the higher karyoplasmic ratio with unclear cellular memberane; (**c**) Tumor cells are round or angular with eosinophilic cytoplasm and visible nucleoli; (**d**) Tumor cells are arranged in glandular or micro-cystic shape

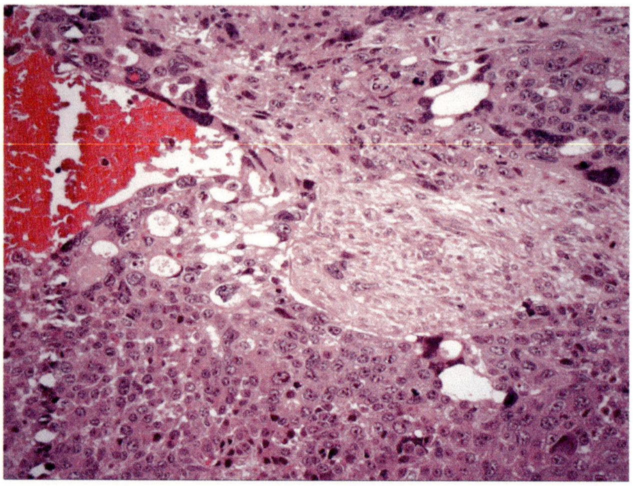

Fig. 8.9 Pleomorphic hepatoblastoma. Pleomorphic and anaplastic tumor giant cells with abundant eosinophilic cytoplasm

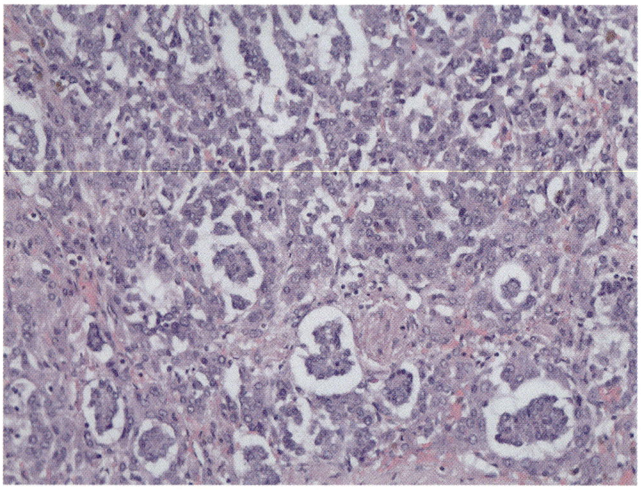

Fig. 8.10 Cholangioblastic type hepatoblastoma, tumor cells undergone cholangio-differentiation with focal cholangiolar structures can be seen

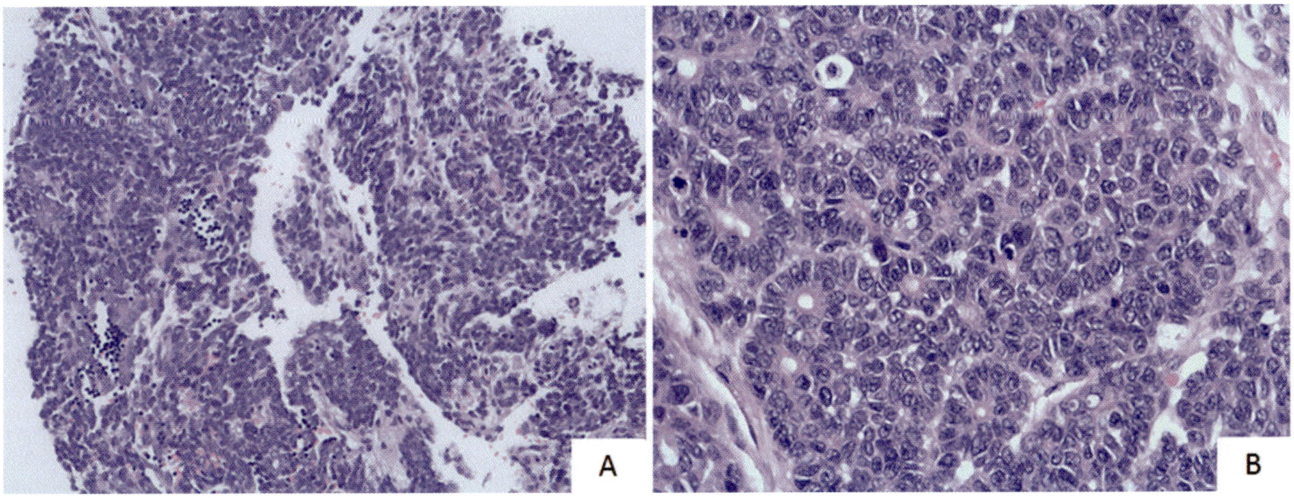

Fig. 8.11 Small-cell undifferentiated type hepatoblastoma. (**a**) Small tumor cells are distributed diffusely, or arranged in nests or organ structures; (**b**) Focal rosette structure can be seen

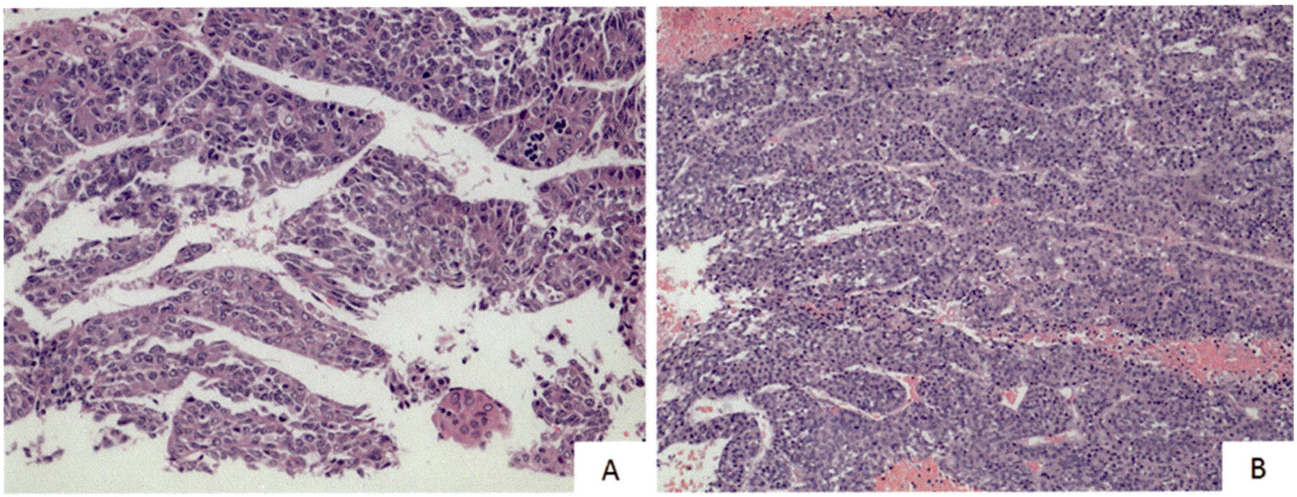

Fig. 8.12 Macrotrabecular pattern hepatoblastoma. (**a**) tumor cells forming macrotrabecules are embryonal; (**b**) thickness of hepatocellular plates ≥5 cells

MRT; thus, it has been suggested that SCU with loss of expression of INI1 may belong to MRT lineage. Clinical studies have shown that the prognosis in INI1 expression group of small-cell component in HB is better than that in loss of expression of INI1 group; thus, distinguishing the difference is crucial for evaluation of prognosis and selection of adjuvant chemotherapy. For SCU with loss of expression of INI1, further tests of INI1 mutation/deletion should be conducted, and cases with morphological rhabdoid features (loss of adhesiveness, eccentric nucleus, clear nucleolus, eosinophilic cytoplasm, perinuclear inclusion bodies) are recommended to be diagnosed as MRT. In addition to INI1 gene mutation, the typical histomorphological features are still the important basis for the diagnosis of MRT in children.

7. Macrotrabecular pattern. It accounts for less than 5% of HB, which was first reported by Gonzalez-Crussi et al. and characterized by the following features, including thickness of neoplastic cell plates ≥5 cells; tumor cells forming macrotrabecules are fetal, embryonal, polymorphic, or similar to tumor cells of HCC (Fig. 8.12); the macrotrabecular growth of the cells can be the single pattern or coexistent with other growth patterns in the same tumor. It is not an easy task to differentiate macrotrabecular HB and macrotrabecular HCC, which needs to combine the clinical, morphological, immunophenotypic, and even molecular biological examinations.

Current clinical data has not adequately established the relationship between the type and prognosis. For more observational details and targeted researches, it is suggested to divide macrotrabecular HB into two subtypes: hepatocytic/HCC cell-like and fetal/embryonic cell-like, and if a report contains the term of focal macrotrabecular type, the cell type which forms the macrotrabecules should be included.

8. Mixed epithelial and mesenchymal type without teratoid features. This type of tumor accounts for 20–30% of HB, and the tumor consists of embryo/fetal, primitive mesenchymal components and multiple differentiated mesenchymal tissues. Primitive mesenchymal components showed increased cell density, spindle, less cytoplasm, and fibroblasts/myofibroblasts (Fig. 8.13); mild myxoid stromal degeneration is locally parallel arranged, within which are visible collagen indicating the origin of fibroblasts; differentiated mesenchymal tissues show that mature fibrous tissues form septa, osteoid tissue, and chondroid tissue (Fig. 8.14), and the cells in osteoid stroma are irregular and angular with short processes, which are difficult to distinguish from osteoblasts according to its morphology, while immunohistochemistry shows that these osteoid stroma-generating cells contain the features of epithelial differentiation, as well as visible mixture and transition of them and adjacent embryonic/fetal components in some regions which also suggests their epithelial origin. It has been reported in the literature that osteoid stroma can be more marked in post-chemotherapy tumor samples.

9. Mixed epithelial and mesenchymal type with teratoid features. Various teratoid components can be seen in 20% of mixed HB, such as squamous epithelium, mucinous epithelium, melanin, the bone, cartilage, striated muscle, primitive neuroepithelium, and primitive endoderm, which can be scattered or mixed with other ingredients in

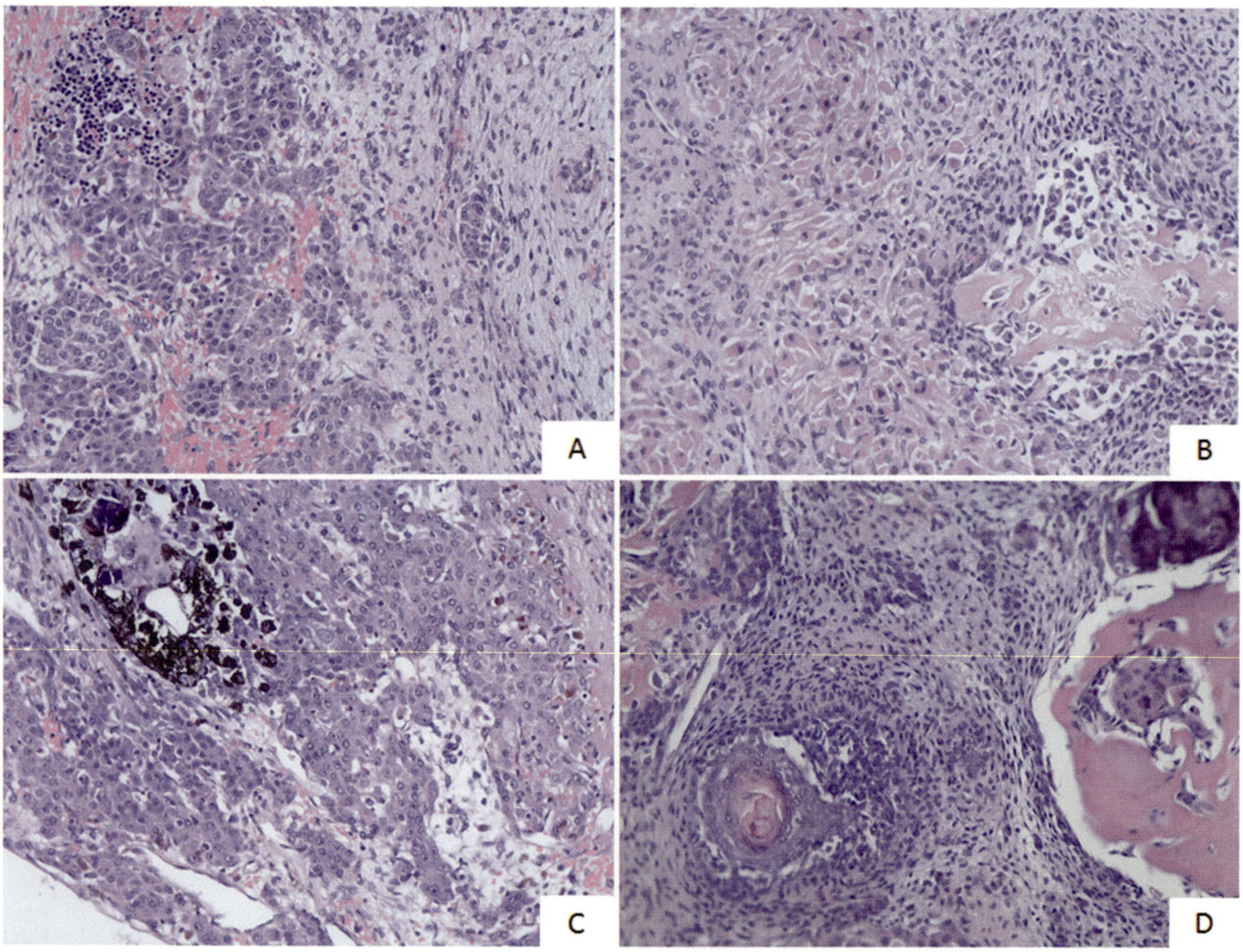

Fig. 8.13 Mixed epithelial and mesenchymal type hepatoblastoma. (**a**) Embryo epithelial components (*left*) are mixed with primitive mesenchymal components (*right*); (**b**) osteoid and striated muscle components; (**c**) Embryo epithelial components and melanin components; (**d**) osseous and squamous epithelium components

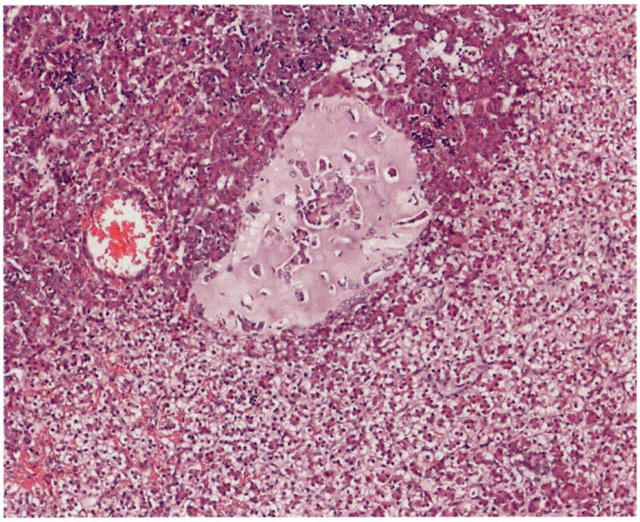

Fig. 8.14 Mixed epithelial and mesenchymal type hepatoblastoma. Osteoid tissue occur in the fetal HB

the tumor. Primitive adenoepithelial cells were columnar, mucus-generating cytoplasm, darkly stained chromatin, crowded and overlapping nuclei, easily found mitotic figures and apoptosis, and arranged in irregular glandular or tubular structures, with desmoplastic reaction in the surroundings. This type of HB should be differentiated from true teratoma, for the latter contains no regions of fetal or embryonal HB and rare reports of coexistence of teratoma and HB in the same tumor.

Immunohistochemistry

Currently, common antibodies used in diagnosis and classification of HB mainly include AFP, glypican-3 (GPC-3), β-catenin, vimentin, panCK, CK7, CK19, HepPar1, INI1, GS (glutamine synthetase), etc.

Cellular and Molecular Genetics

The most common cytogenetic abnormalities of HB include chromosomes 2, 8, 18, and 20 and trisomy 22; genetic rearrangement of 1q,4q on chromosomes 2 and 22; as well as formation of double minutes. And acquisition of chromosome may be associated with poor prognosis [10, 11].

Treatment and Prognosis

During the recent four decades, the overall survival rate of HB patients has been raised from 30% to higher than 80%, due to improvement in surgery and combined chemotherapy. Surgical resection remains the key therapy for HB, and chemotherapy helps in the transformation of unresectable tumors into resectable ones, as well as postsurgical adjuvant therapies. Radiotherapy does not play any role in the treatment of HB; thus, it is not recommended in routine therapeutic plans. Liver transplantation is suitable for pediatric patients receiving total hepatectomy, and the posttransplantation 5-year survival rate reaches 83% [6].

It is generally believed that the WDF HB receives a good prognosis [14], which needs no chemotherapy after complete resection in stage I, and the disease-free survival rate reaches 100%, while the CF type needs postsurgical adjuvant chemotherapy. For pleomorphic and poorly differentiated ones, the association between macrotrabecular type and the prognosis is still uncertain. SCU possesses strongly invasive biological behaviors which relate to low survival rate, and this histological type is an important prognostic index indicating a higher risk of death; thus, more intensive chemotherapy is recommended in cases with SCU components in biopsy specimens. However, due to the limited number of cases, it is not clear whether the correlation between this type and the prognosis significantly depends on the existence or proportion of SCU, and COG recommended that the pathological report should include the proportion of SCU component in order to facilitate retrospectively analysis of these data in the future.

For pediatric patients with unresectable tumors who receive chemotherapy, the prognosis is related to the post-chemotherapy decreased level of AFP. It has been reported that the patients in whom the AFP level decreases by two logarithmic grades after four courses of chemotherapy received a survival rate of 75%, while those, who have AFP level decreased by less than two logarithmic grades before their second surgery, show an extremely low survival rate.

8.2.1.2 Hepatocellular Carcinoma (HCC)

Pathogenesis and Mechanism

In children, HCC accounts for about one fourth of all the malignant tumors in the liver, ranking the second. Infection of hepatitis B virus (HBV) is the key pathogenic factor for typical hepatocellular carcinoma in the Far East. It generally takes 10–20 years for HBV to exert its carcinogenic effect after infection of HBV after birth; however, pre-birth or perinatal infection of HBV can cause rapid integration of the viral genome into the host DNA to generate chromosomal abnormalities (e.g., acquisition, deletion), activating some of the oncogenes (e.g., P53, cyclin A, D1, etc.), due to the rapid growth of the liver, resulting in hepatocellular carcinoma (HCC) in infants. And because of the high carrying rate of HBV, the incidence of pediatric HCC had been once raised markedly, which has decreased significantly in recent two decades, due to the wide vaccination with HBV vaccine in children. Infection of hepatitis C virus has a smaller impact on children than adults. Fibrolamellar HCC (FL-HCC) is more common in children and teenagers, without viral infection, and is irrelevant with cirrhosis, the pathogenesis of which remains unknown.

Pediatric HCC is also associated with some hereditary syndromes, autosomal recessive inheritance-related metabolic diseases (such as α1-antitrypsin deficiency, Gaucher disease, Alagille syndrome, glycogen storage disease type I, genetic tyrosine syndrome type I, etc.), and chronic cholestatic syndromes (congenital extrahepatic biliary atresia, Byler syndrome, long-term use of intestinal nutrition, familial cholestatic syndrome) (Table 8.2). And children with occult genetic and metabolic disorders present onset of the disease before the age of 10 years, the manifestations of which are similar to those in adult cases.

Clinical Features

Over 80% of the patients manifest abdominal pain or mass, with or without a number of other symptoms, such as anorexia, fever, nausea, vomiting, and jaundice, and the gastrointestinal symptoms usually indicate tumor progression, while rupture and hemoperitoneum are rare. It has been found that 60–70% of the pediatric patients show significantly elevated serum AFP, which is normal or mildly elevated in cases of FL-HCC without relationship with cirrhosis, mild anemia, polycythemia, and thrombocytosis which are common. And only a small part of pediatric patients present elevated serum levels of transaminase (ALT and AST), lactate dehydrogenase (LDH), alkaline phosphatase (ALP), and bilirubin, which are different from adult HCC.

Gross Features

The tumors are solitary or multiple, and more than 70% of the cases involve both the left and right hepatic lobes, which are 2–25 cm in diameter. The sections are grayish white or grayish red and soft or hard, with common hemorrhage and necrosis. More than 60% of the patients have micro- or macronodular cirrhosis in the surrounding liver tissue, which is related with complicated liver diseases, such as biliary atresia and hereditary tyrosine disease. FL-type lesions are often solitary, with grayish white, hard, and rare cirrhosis.

Histological Classification

Typical HCC and FL-HCC are similar to those in adults. See details in related chapters.

Differential Diagnosis

1. Macrotrabecular HB and typical HCC. These two tumors have overlapping morphological features; thus, it is difficult to differentiate one from the other, histologically. Comprehensive analysis of factors, such as clinical data, imaging, and sensitivity to chemotherapy, should be considered. For example, HBV infection is more common in the latter, and multiple nodules or vascular invasions are rare in the former, even in cases with progressive tumors, while the former is sensitive to chemotherapy.
2. Transitional hepatocellular tumor (tentative classification). Malignant hepatocellular tumors, non-special type (hepatocellular malignant neoplasm, NOS), also known as transitional liver cell tumor (TLCT), are a kind of tumor with features between hepatoblastoma and hepatocellular carcinoma.

In 2002, Prokurat reported the first groups of cases of malignant hepatic epithelial tumors in children at older ages and adolescent patients, which were primarily diagnosed as HB according to the histological morphology of the biopsy, but they all manifested some extraordinary features: onset age >5 years, significantly increased AFP, high aggression in clinical course, and deficient reaction to chemotherapy which can be observed in HB. Most of the tumors are located in the right lobe of the liver forming huge solitary masses, which are shown on CT as inhomogeneous lesions with hypodensity, and the expansive masses compress the surrounding liver tissue, with diffuse necrosis in the center. The tumors are pleomorphic, consisting of various kinds of tumor cells of epithelioid (fetal, embryonic, pleomorphic), atypical mature hepatocyte-like cells, HCC-like cells, hepatocyte-like multinucleated giant cells, and poorly differentiated median large-sized undefined tumor cells. Different from the trabecular arrangement of HCC, NOS is often solid and grows invasively in flakes or diffuse, with alveolar or adenoid structures in a rare case (express CK7, CK19), absent of typical sinus blood vessel networks with little and immature stroma. Immunohistochemistry shows diffuse expression of AFP in tumor cells and combined expression of β-catenin on the membrane, the nuclei, or the cytoplasm (Fig. 8.15).

For this group of tumors with component of HB and HCC in the same tumor but different features in clinical, imaging, and biological behaviors compared with HB and HCC, it is difficult to make the accurate diagnosis, even according to the combined examinations of immunohistochemistry and other adjuvant molecular biological tests. Thus, it is supposed that these tumor cells may be tentative cells between HB and HCC cells and a new subtype of pediatric hepatic tumor, which needs to be supported by more data of cases and molecular studies. To better investigate this undefined class of tumors, in 2011 Los Angeles COG Consensus proposed to tentatively classify them as "hepatocytic malignant tumors, non-special type (HMN, NOS)."

Cellular and Molecular Genetics

Cases of pediatric HCC are rare, and the knowledge and researches on their biological features are limited. Different from molecular biological changes of adult HCC, the existence of overlapping between the two is still not defined. It has been found that some cases of FL-HCC contain abnormal chromosomes 7 and 8, but the invasiveness of tumors

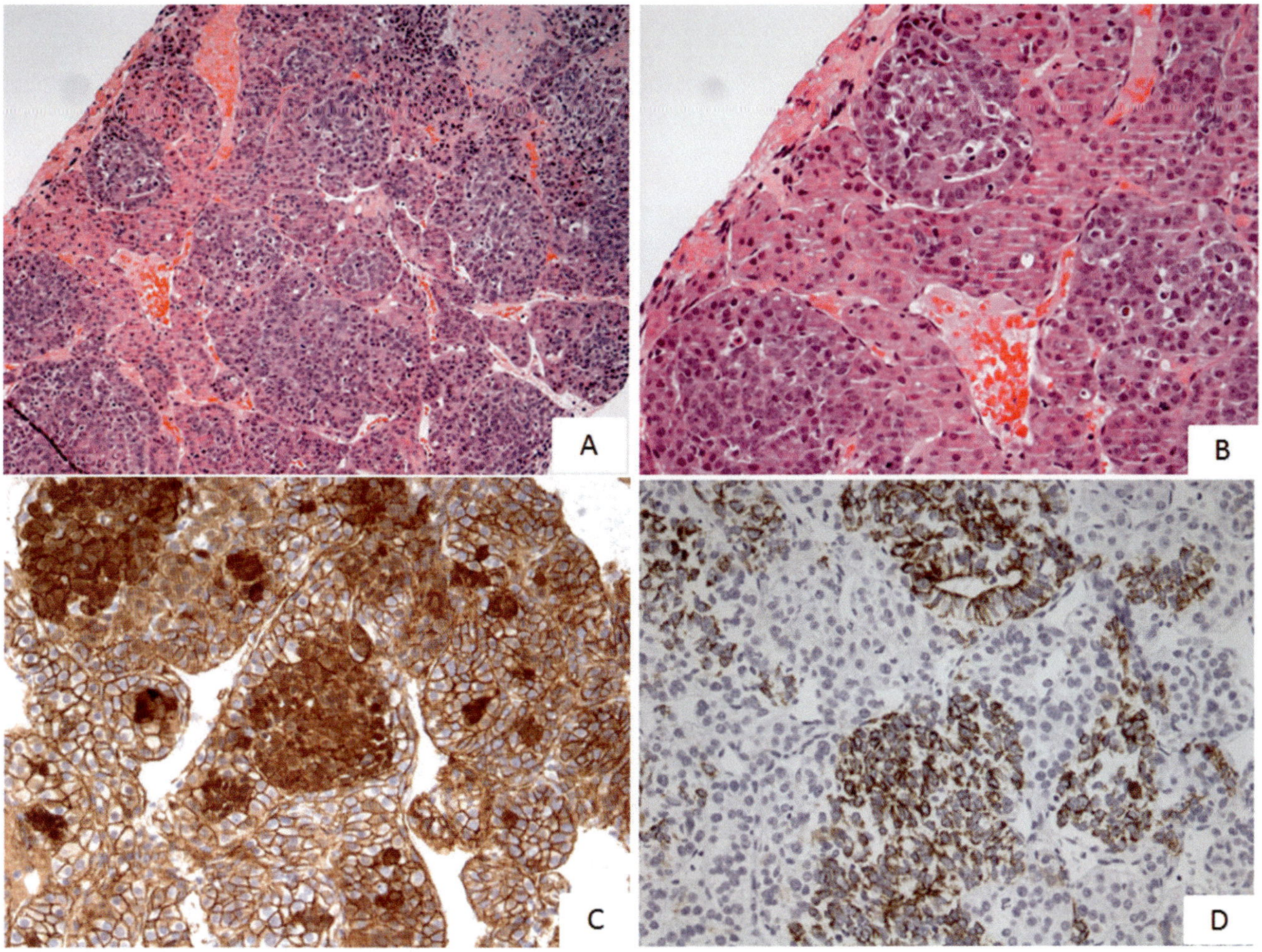

Fig. 8.15 Hepatocytic malignant tumors, non-special type. (**a**) Tumor cells are arranged in sheet, nests or nodular pattern; (**b**) The tumor cells resemble embryonic HB cells in the center while HCC-like cells are distributed in the peripheral area; (**c**) Immunohistochemistry shows diffuse membrane expression of β-catenin in HCC-like cells while expression of β-catenin on in the nuclei or cytoplasm in the embryonic HB like cells; (**d**) Some tumor cells express CK19

with abnormal chromosomes is much stronger than those without these abnormalities, irrelevant with age, gender, or tumor size. Typical HCC has a pathogenesis with molecular mechanism possibly related to genetic mutations induced by activation of tumor signal transduction pathways, such as AFP, TP53 mutation, β-catenin mutation, etc.; however, no evidence on the correlation of this phenomenon with FL-HCC has been reported.

Treatment and Prognosis

Pediatric HCC should be treated by combined surgery and neoadjuvant chemotherapy, and for unresectable cases even at the time of diagnosis, chemotherapy can reduce the volume of the tumor to increase the resection rate. Local ablation and transcatheter arterial chemoembolization are suitable for post-chemotherapy unresectable tumors. Liver transplantation should be conducted in patients with unresectable tumors; however, extrahepatic involvement, lymphatic metastasis, grossly visible vascular invasion, and distal metastasis are contraindications for liver transplantation.

Prognosis of pediatric HCC is poor with the 5-year overall survival rate of only around 25%, and the main factors for evaluation of prognosis include the chance of complete resection, presurgical tumor size, PRETEXT stage, metastasis, etc. Though FL-HCC was previously regarded to have a slightly better prognosis compared to typical HCC probably due to more common FL-type young cases and absence of cirrhosis, the biological behaviors of pediatric FL-HCC and typical HCC are similar in children, while the median survival time of patients with the former is longer than that of the latter, and no significant difference has been found in 5-year survival rates between the two groups.

8.2.2 Mesenchymal Tumors

8.2.2.1 Embryonal Sarcoma (ES)

Also known as undifferentiated (embryonal) sarcoma (UES)

Pathogenesis and Mechanism

The incidence of UES ranked the third of the pediatric hepatic malignant tumors, without significant gender and racial differences, partly associated with the Li-Fraumeni syndrome (Table 8.2). The histogenesis of UES is unclear, and studies have found that some UES and hepatic mesenchymal hamartoma share the same chromosomal abnormalities and genetic changes, suggesting that it may derive from malignant transformation of the latter [15], while the hypothesis of origination from pluripotent stem cells in the hepatic mesenchymal is mostly accepted.

Clinical Features

Sixty-three percent of the cases are found in patients aged 6–10 years and 88% under the age of 15 years, while adult cases are rare. The main symptoms include abdominal pain, abdominal mass, jaundice, poor appetite, vomiting, lethargy, fever, etc. Dyspnea and cardiac souffle can be found in a few cases with tumor thrombi involving the inferior vena cava and right cardiac atrium or ventricle. Acute abdomen caused by tumor rupture is rare. Serum AFP is generally normal, and abnormal liver function is found in one third to one half of the cases. The most common finding in lab examination is elevated serum level of alkaline phosphatase, while bilirubin generally shows no obvious abnormality. Since the tumor can produce erythropoietin, it can lead to secondary erythrocytosis. The lesions are more common in the right lobe of the liver, and ultrasound showed that the tumors are cystic or solid, isoechoic, or hyperechoic compared with the surrounding liver parenchyma, and CT or MRI demonstrates hypodensities of the occupying lesions with hyperdense septa. Hepatic arteriography shows few blood vessels inside the tumors.

Gross Features

The tumors are large in volume, and range from 10–30 cm. On the cut section, they are grayish white or grayish yellow, jelly, and often with hemorrhage, necrosis, or cystic degeneration, intracystic brown colloid substance, clear boundaries, and pseudocapsules formation around tumors. These lesions grow outward from the tumor or with a pedicle, and no obvious cirrhosis is visible in the surrounding liver tissue.

Microscopic Features

The tumor was composed of significantly atypical stellate, spindle, or polygonal cells with diversity in histomorphology due to various myxoid stromal proportions and cell densities. The myxoid regions contain fewer cells, while cell-rich regions contain abundant tumor cells with marked atypia, abundant eosinophilic cytoplasm, PAS- and PAS-D-positive eosinophilic bodies, common mitotic figures, as well as pathological mitotic figures, inconspicuous nucleolus, a proliferation index of above 30%, and scattered multinucleated tumor giant cells. Hyperplastic and atypical cholangiolar structures can be found around the tumor cell nests without epithelial components found in the metastatic lesions; thus, these are considered to be cholangiolar invagination or residue, rather than tumor components. Reticular fiber proliferated around tumor cell nest, with collagen, hyaline, and extramedullary hematopoiesis in the stroma. It has been reported that a small amount of osteoid stroma, fibroblasts, smooth muscle blast cells, or fat blast cell-like composition can be found in the tumors, as well as mesenchymal hamartoma-like structures in rare cases. Necrosis, fibrosis, and calcification can be visible in tumors after chemotherapy.

Immunohistochemistry

Tumor cells show epithelial and mesenchymal immunophenotypes with multiple directions of differentiation which are mild in specificity and need groups of antibodies to exclude other tumors. These tumor cells express vimentin, Bcl2, panCK (punctiform expression in the cytoplasm), CD10, calponin, desmin, SMA, P53, α1-AT, α1-ACT, CD56 (expression on the membrane), and CD68. They generally do not express myoglobin, myogenin, h-caldesmon, S100, ALK, NSE, CEA, FVII, and AFP.

Ultrastructure

Within the cytoplasm of tumor cells are visible dilated rough endoplasmic reticulum and densely deposited lysosomes, related to eosinophilic bodies observed under the light microscope. Dilated mitochondria and mitochondria-rough endoplasmic reticulum complex can also be found, as well as intracellular lipid droplets in the cytoplasm, scattered actin microfilaments, and glycogen granules.

Molecular Genetics

Various chromosomal variations can be found; the more common type is ploidy abnormalities (such as sub-diploid, aneuploid, near triploid, near hexaploid), acquisition of chromosome (1q, 5p, 6q, 8p, 12q), and chromosomal deletion (9p, 11p, 14). Part of the UES contains the same translocation of chromosomes 11 and 19 as in mesenchymal hamartoma.

Treatment and Prognosis

UES is highly malignant with an extremely poor prognosis, and local metastasis is more common than distal metastasis and dissemination, which is reported to involve the lung, bone, pleura, and peritoneum. The mortality rate of the tumor reaches 80%, and the median post-diagnostic survival time is 11 months. A small number of children receiving comprehensive treatment with neoadjuvant chemotherapy have a survival time reaching 5 years. The treatment should include radical surgery and intensive combined chemotherapy, while radiotherapy is not a part of the standard treatment for UES, for effective dosage of radiotherapy is more than the liver can tolerate. Due to high rate of local recurrence, local radiotherapy can only be adopted as an adjunct treatment for surgery and chemotherapy and is suitable for high-risk patients with intraoperative tumorous overflow, spontaneous rupture, etc., and cases with positive margin can be treated by radiotherapy; however, the minimum dosage of effective radiotherapy has not been determined. For unresectable or recurrent cases, liver transplantation can be an option.

8.2.2.2 Embryonal Rhabdomyosarcoma (ERMS)

Pathogenesis and Mechanism

ERMS is the most common type of pediatric hepatic rhabdomyosarcoma, accounting for 1% of all hepatic neoplasms, mainly deriving from intrahepatic and biliary system. Since it derives from the biliary system lined with mucosa and looks like grapes, it is also known as botryoid rhabdomyosarcoma. The etiology is still unknown, and the tumor cells may originate from multipotent stem cells in the portal area and muscle containing tissues such as intra- and extrahepatic biliary systems. It has been reported that estrogen may stimulate the primitive stem cells to differentiate into striated muscle and undergo malignancy.

Clinical Features

The tumor is more common in children under the age of 5 years, and patients older than 15 years old are rare. The most common symptom is obstructive jaundice, which is often accompanied by cholemia, clay-colored stools, hepatomegaly, fever, abdominal distention, nausea, and vomiting, which makes it easy to misdiagnose the lesions as hepatitis and common bile duct cyst. Imaging (including CT, MRI, ultrasonography, and cholangiography) shows the locations of the obstruction clearly, and serum AFP is generally normal.

Gross Features

The tumors are solitary or multiple botryoid or polypoid lesions, located in the lumen of the bile ducts without capsules. The diameter of the lesions is often 0.2–14 cm, and the cut sections are fish- or jellylike with superficial inflammations, hemorrhage, ulcer, or necrosis. Dilatation of proximal obstructive bile ducts is often found, with significantly thickened wall and narrowed lumen of the involving bile ducts.

Microscopic Features

The tumor is often located in the submucosal regions, which are covered by a layer of cubic biliary epithelium, which may contain hyperplasia, inflammation, ulcer, or squamous metaplasia. The characteristic feature of the tumor is the aggregation of undifferentiated cells close to the inferior of the epithelium, forming a wide band parallel with the mucosa, known as cambium layer. The tumor cells are rhabdomyoblasts in various degrees of differentiation, which are round, spindle, or strip shaped, containing less eosinophilic cytoplasm, hyperchromatin, common mitotic figures, or even cross striation in some cases. The tumor cells are distributed in loose myxoid matrix (Fig. 8.16a, b). In cases with infection, a large number of acute or chronic inflammatory cells infiltrate into the stroma, which may cover up the tumor cells leading to misdiagnosis.

Immunohistochemistry

The tumor cells express myogenic antibodies, such as desmin (Fig. 8.16c), myoglobin, myoD1, and myogenin (Fig. 8.16d). The latter two are highly sensible and specific to tumors deriving from striated muscle; thus, their positive expression is of much diagnostic value. Some of these tumor cells can express CD99.

Treatment and Prognosis

The treatment is often surgical resection, and since the tumors extend along the biliary system into the liver, complete resection of the tumors can be achieved in only 20–40% of the cases involving lymphatic metastasis and local dissemination into the duodenum, stomach, pancreas, etc. Recently, preoperative standard chemotherapy surgical resection has elevated the resection rate, which significantly improves the therapeutic effects, and the 5-year survival rate can reach up to 66%.

8.2.2.3 Angiosarcoma

Pathogenesis and Mechanism

In children, hepatic angiosarcoma accounts less than 2.5% of all hepatic tumors, the etiology of which is unknown. And the related factors found in the pathogenesis of adult angiosarcoma (such as exposure to thorium and vinyl chloride, oral administration of androgen, anabolic steroids, diethylstilbestrol, etc.), definite genetic changes, or hereditary syndromes have not been reported to be associated with children's cases. Rare reports concern pediatric cases of infantile-type hepatic angiosarcoma which was transformed into angiosarcoma via malignancy.

Clinical Features

The onset age of the tumor is 1.5–18 years, and it can be rarely seen in newborns. The median age is 4 years, which is

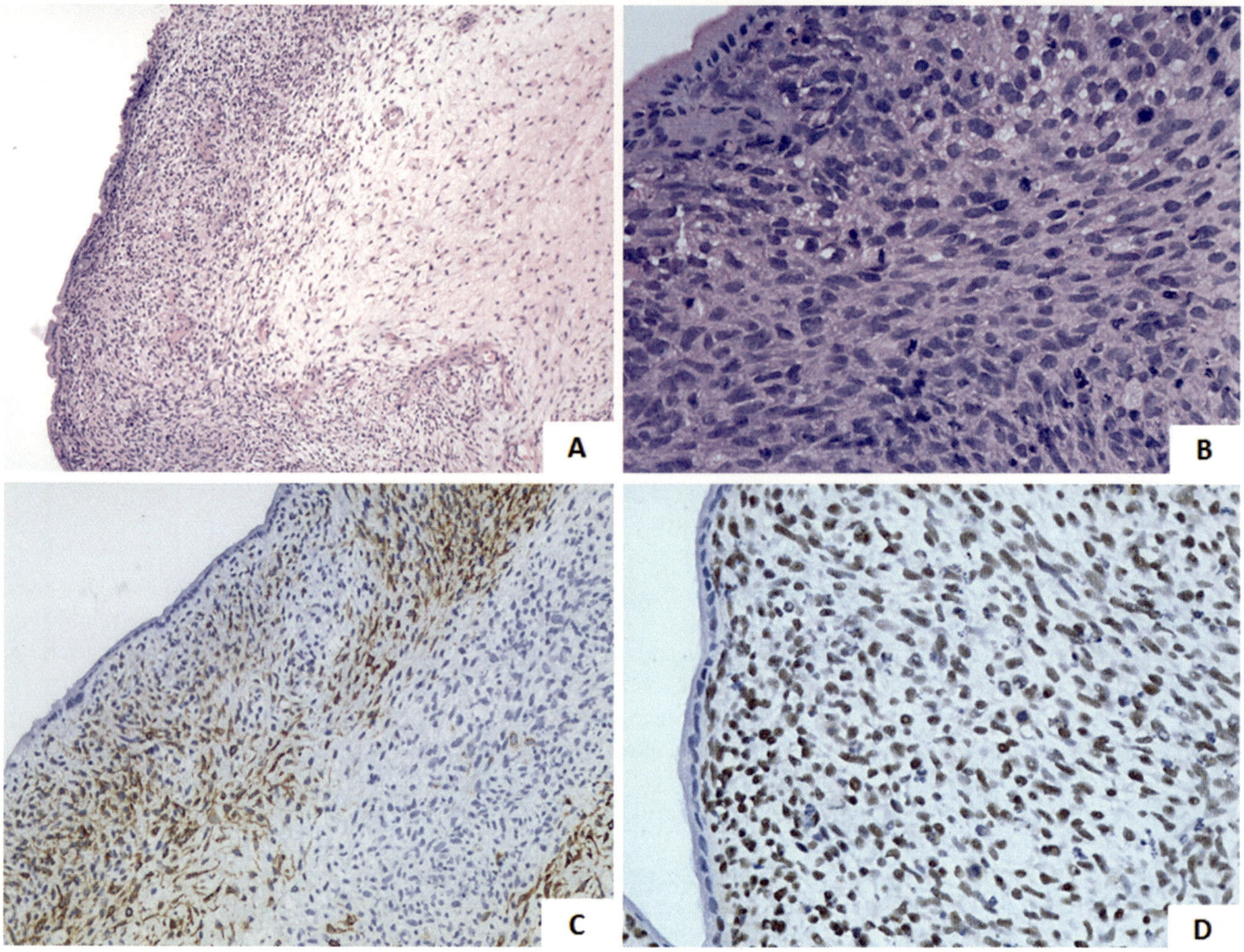

Fig. 8.16 Embryonal rhabdomyosarcoma. (**a**) The aggregation of undifferentiated cells are close to the inferior of the epithelium; (**b**) rhabdomyoblasts with common mitotic figures; (**c**): The tumor cells express desmin; (**d**) The tumor cells express myogenin

older than the predilection age of infantile-type angioma under the age of 1 year. Female patients are more common with a male-to-female ratio of about 1:2, and the most common symptom is rapidly enlarging abdominal masses, with or without jaundice, diarrhea, abdominal pain, and vomiting. Manifestations caused by congestive heart failure, commonly seen in infantile-type hepatic angioma, are rare in angiosarcoma. Some pediatric patients have a history of hepatic multiple infantile-type angiomas, which transform into angiosarcoma after recurrence.

Gross Features

Hepatic angiosarcoma has often multiple nodules, with single nodule bounded clearly, the diameter of 7–10 cm, and the cut section is often dark red, solid, or honeycomb-like, with marked hemorrhage and necrosis.

Microscopic Features

The tumors show the morphology of infantile angioma in some cases, or solid cell masses with Kaposi's features, such as whirlpool arrangement of spindle cells in the tumor, with visible vascular cavities, or forming spongy angioma-like or sprout structure. The angioendothelial cells in the tumor are often atypical with multilayer and papillary hyperplasia, hyperchromatin, and common mitotic figures. PAS-positive eosinophilic bodies can be found inside or outside the tumor cells. Atypical vascular infiltration and permeation of endothelial cells can be found in adjacent hepatic sinusoids. Pediatric hepatic angiosarcoma differs from adult angiosarcoma, for the former contains the whirlpool arrangement of sarcomatoid cells apart from general feature of angioma, which are called as Kaposi's spindle cells.

Immunohistochemistry

Tumor cells express vascular markers, including CD34, CD31, F8, vimentin, and α1-ACT, but do not express CK, AFP, CEA, and desmin.

Treatment and Prognosis

Generally, the tumors are mainly treated by surgery plus postsurgical combined adjuvant chemotherapy. Hepatic angiosarcoma is insensitive for radiotherapy; thus, radiotherapy does not belong to conventional treatment. For tumors with unresectable or recurrent lesions, liver transplantation can be an option. However, the overall therapeutic effects are poor, and metastasis to the lung, bone, kidney, adrenal gland, spleen, pleura, peritoneum, mesenterium, etc. is often found. The survival time was generally less than 2 years.

8.2.2.4 Malignant Rhabdoid Tumor (MRT)

Pathogenesis and Mechanism

Primary extrarenal MRT in the liver is rare, and less than 60 cases have been reported so far. It is a group of highly malignant tumors with unknown origin and differentiation direction, mainly found in infants and young children [16]. Current studies have confirmed the inactivation of INI1 gene (located on chromosome 22q11.2) in the tumor.

Clinical Features

The onset age for the tumor is under 2 years and slightly more in male than female patients, with a median age of 8 months. The clinical manifestations are fever, vomiting, loss of appetite, lethargy, abdominal distention, and right upper abdominal masses, and spontaneous tumor rupture is found in a few cases. Serum AFP is generally normal. Since a part of the tumors can secrete parathyroid hormone and vasculointestinal peptide-like substance, it can cause hypercalcemia and watery diarrhea.

Gross Features

The tumors are often huge in volume, and the sections are inhomogeneous in texture and grayish white in color, with common hemorrhage and necrosis.

Microscopic Features

The tumors are polymorphic, e.g., flask-like arrangement without obvious trabecular or hepatic sinusoid structures surrounding the blood vessels and forming papillary or epithelioid structures. The tumor cells are round or polygonal, containing median to large amounts of eosinophilic cytoplasm, with perinuclear PAS-positive inclusion bodies, and the nuclei are vacular with dissymmetric conspicuous nucleoli (Fig. 8.17a, b).

Immunohistochemistry

The tumor cells show multidirectional differentiation, with diffuse strongly positive vimentin and focal-positive CK, EMA, S100, neuroendocrine markers (CD99, NSE, SYN), and myogenic markers (SMA, MSA) (Fig. 8.17c), while they do not express desmin, myoglobin, CGA, AFP, cyclin, D1, and HepPar1. Loss of nuclear expression of INI1 is of diagnostic value (Fig. 8.17d).

Molecular Genetics

Deletion of chromosome 22q11.21-q12.1

Differential Diagnosis

Cases with cellular components of primitive differentiation should be distinguished from Ewing sarcoma/PNET, small-cell undifferentiated HB, and other small round cell malignant tumors [17]. And loss of expression of INI1 in immunohistochemistry staining, FISH, and INI1 mutation tests is helpful in the diagnosis of this type of tumor [18].

Treatment and Prognosis

There is no standard effective treatment for the tumor, and the therapeutic results are unsatisfactory. Surgery plus chemotherapy is considered to be optimal therapy; however, most of the tumors are too large at diagnosis to be surgically resected, and even the intensive combined chemotherapy cannot improve the prognosis. The lung is the most common site for the metastasis of the tumor. The average survival time for the patients with the tumor is less than 6 months, and the overall mortality reaches 89%. A few cases of MRT treated by a comprehensive treatment including liver transplantation are reported to have a long-term survival period [19].

8.2.2.5 Nested Stromal-Epithelial Tumor (NSET)

According to the differences in histological composition, the disease is also known as desmoplastic nested spindle cell tumor, ossifying stromal-epithelial tumor and calcifying nested stromal-epithelial tumors [20, 21].

Pathogenesis and Mechanism

Recently, a new described pediatric primary hepatic tumor refers to a rare mixed tumor with epithelial and mesenchymal components, and only 30 cases of the tumor have been reported by now. Neither histogenesis of the tumor nor the relationship of the tumor with other infantile embryonic hepatic tumors is clear. And it has been proposed that it may derive from hepatic mesenchymal stem cells with primitive biliary differentiation without definite causes. Calcification is found in the tumor which can lead to ossification.

Clinical Features

The onset age of the disease is 2–33 years, and most of the reported cases affect patients under the age of 10 years with

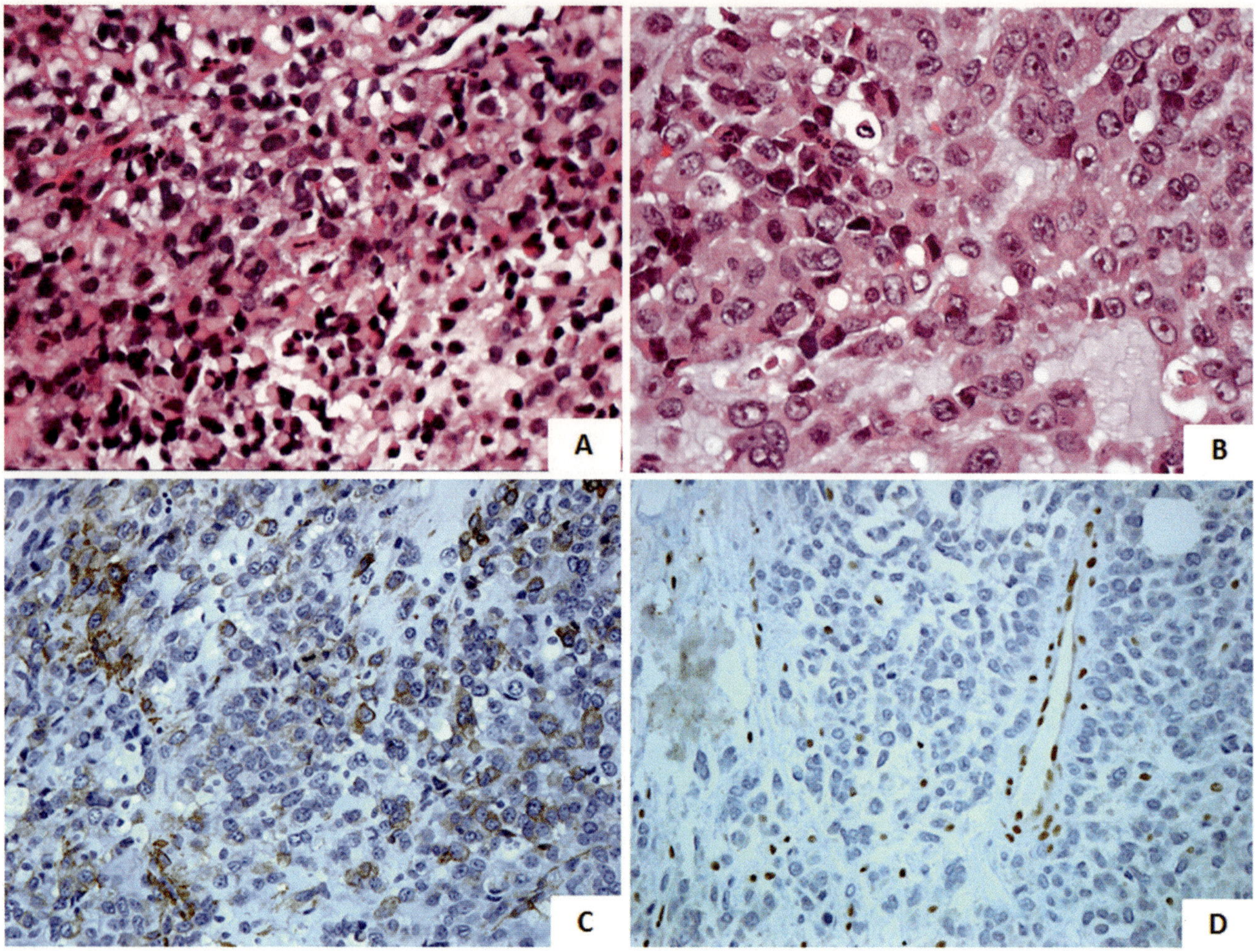

Fig. 8.17 Malignant rhabdoid tumor. (**a**) The tumor cells are arranged in sheets, containing abundant eosinophilic cytoplasm; (**b**) the large nuclei are vacuolar with conspicuous nucleoli; (**c**) Tumor cells express SMA; (**d**) Loss of nuclear expression of INI1 while it is positive in vascular endothelium and lymphocytes

more female patients. A case of a 33-year-old male has also been reported. Mostly, the tumor was detected incidentally, and cases involving hormone-related syndromes (such as Cushing's syndrome) have also been reported, with or without a history of childhood liver calcification nodules, hydronephrosis and nephroblastoma (disease), renal dysplasia, growth retardation, omphalocele, etc. Most of the pediatric patients have no clinical symptoms or a history of hepatitis. The serum alkaline phosphatase and γ-glutamyl transferase may be mildly elevated.

Gross Features

The tumor, mostly in the liver, has a well-defined border, without obvious capsule, and the diameter is 4–30 cm. The cut sections are multinodular, grayish brown, and fine granular in appearance with varying sizes of soft zones, with or without visible focal necrosis, cystic degeneration, and calcification, and gravel parts are mostly located in the liver.

Microscopic Features

It is a non-hepatocellular and non-bile duct tumor with nested epithelial and spindle cells. The tumor cells include spindle cells and (or) epithelioid cells, which are arranged in nests with plump spindle or polygonal epithelioid cells in the center. The nests are surrounded by dense fibrous tissue and varying amounts of myofibroblasts. And a small number of bile duct components are found in or surround the nests, either invaginated or remained cholangioles. Psammoma bodies, focal calcification, and ossification can be found in the stroma in varying amounts. Tumor cells are bounded clearly, with round or oval nuclei, little atypia, clear nuclear membrane, fine chromatin, or small nucleoli, and mitotic figures are rare (1–2/10HPF). The cytoplasm is eosinophilic or pale and transparent. The epithelioid cells have marked membrane. No dysplasia bile duct plates can be found in the tumor. Pseudorosette structures can be found in nests of recurrent tumors with mucus secretion, vascular infiltration, and mitotic figures.

Immunohistochemistry

Tumor cells diffusely or focally express vimentin and CK, and WT1 gene C and N terminal antibodies show diffuse strong expression in the cytoplasm or punctate expression near the nucleus. They express EMA, CD56, CK8, CK18, CK19, CK5/CK6, NSE, S100, CD117, PR, and some mesenchymal antibodies to different degrees, but do not express SYN, CHG-A, CD57, HepPar1, CEA, CK7, CK20, Bcl2, HMB45, inhibin, calretinin and desmin, CD34, α1-ACT, ER, TTF1, and CD99. The proliferated fibrous stroma expresses collagen IV and SMA, while ACTH can be expressed in patients with Cushing's syndrome.

Ultrastructure

Spindle and epithelioid tumor cells have visible local basement membrane and well-developed cell junctions, and intracytoplasmic mitochondria and rough endoplasmic reticulum are scarce, with local accumulation of intermediate filaments and no neuroendocrine particles. It is reported that a few cases containing abundant mitochondria and rough endoplasmic reticulum have strongly invasive clinical course, intrahepatic recurrence, and lymphatic metastasis.

Differential Diagnosis

1. Desmoplastic small round cell tumor (DSRCT). The histological features are similar to NEST, but DSRCT is more often found in young males with highly invasive clinical course, no formation of tubular structure and diffuse calcification, and perinuclear punctuate-positive desmin in immunohistochemistry. The detection of EWS1-WT1 fusion gene is the "gold standard" for the diagnosis of DSRCT.
2. Ewing/PNET with or without glandular and pseudochrysanthemum structures, it is positive for CD99, and EWS/PNET fusion gene can be detected.
3. Mixed epithelial and mesenchymal teratoid HB. It is more common in infants and young children, with elevation of serum AFP level and expression of HepPar1.
4. Synovial sarcoma. Fusion gene of SYT-SSX can be found.
5. Primary or metastatic spindle cell sarcomatoid carcinoma. It contains obvious carcinoma components.
6. Metastatic KIT-negative gastrointestinal stromal tumor (GIST). It often contains visible perinuclear vacuoles which are arranged in paliform structures. Part of GIST lesions can express epithelial marker (CK18, CK8) to varying degrees, and it is of much difficulty in the differentiation from NSET which does not express CD34.
7. Metastatic primitive sex cord stromal tumor. This tumor is inhibin and ER positive and EMA negative, which can be an evidence in differential diagnosis from NSET.

Treatment and Prognosis

Complete resection of the tumor can cure the patients, though local recurrence can be found in a few cases, which can be treated by re-surgery or local ablation. Chemotherapy regimens have not been defined, and it has been found that chemotherapy regimens for HB and soft tissue sarcoma can decrease the tumor size for patients with local recurrence which cannot be resected without obvious necrosis. And multiple recurrence and lymphatic metastasis indicate poor prognosis. For patients with unresectable tumors and no extrahepatic lesions, liver transplantation is a suitable option. At present, it is believed that the tumor is of low malignancy and unpredictable biological behaviors, which needs long-term follow-up.

8.2.2.6 Metastatic Tumors of the Liver

The most common metastatic tumors of the liver in children include neuroblastoma, Wilms' tumor, yolk sac tumor, lymphatic and hematopoietic tumors, and others reported in the literature, such as EBV-related leiomyosarcoma after liver transplantation.

8.3 Section Three Benign Hepatic Tumors and Tumorlike Lesions in Children

8.3.1 Epithelial Tumors and Tumorlike Lesions

8.3.1.1 Hepatocellular Adenoma (HCA)

Pathogenesis and Mechanism

HCA is a rare benign tumor in children, mostly found in adolescents, and related to oral contraceptives or overexposure to hormones or some genetic diseases, such as glycogen deposition disease types I, III, and IV; galactosemia; severe immunodeficiency; familial adenomatous polyposis; Hurler syndrome (mucopolysaccharidosis) and familial diabetes; β-Mediterranean anemia and androgen-treated Fanconi anemia; etc. Recently, obesity is considered to be a risk factor for HCA subtype.

Clinical Features

The patients manifest as no or mild symptoms, such as abdominal pain, nausea, vomiting, and acute abdomen due to intratumoral hemorrhage or intraperitoneal hemorrhage. Laboratory examination shows normal or only slightly elevated serum transaminase, alkaline phosphatase, and bilirubin. Imaging examination is helpful in the detection of the masses. And angiography shows vascular tumor with decreased amounts of blood vessels in some parts of the tumors. Current imaging technology is still unable to diagnose the HCA; either can it distinguish early malignant transforming.

Pathological Characteristics

Pathological characteristics of HCA in children are similar to those in adults which have been described previously.

(2) Focal nodular hyperplasia (FNH)

Pathogenesis and Mechanism

FNH is rare in children, accounting for only 0.045% in the whole pediatric population. The pathogenesis of FNH is still undetermined and may involve congenital (hereditary telangiectasia, congenital absent portal vein, Budd-Chiari syndrome, etc.) or acquired hepatic vascular abnormalities, leading to secondary liver parenchyma hyperplasia. It may also associate with vascular injuries resulting in thrombosis and hepatocellular hyperplasia due to revascularization. It has been reported that the genesis of pediatric FNH may be related to previous treatment for malignant tumors, such as some chemotherapeutic drugs for neuroblastoma. And the incidence of FNH is 5.1% in pediatric patients with malignant tumors who survive more than 2 years, more than 100 times the total incidence of all the pediatric population, which also suggests the latter theory that severe venous occlusive lesion is a risk factor for FNH. There is still controversy about the relationship of the incidence of FNH in older children and adolescents and oral contraceptives.

Clinical Features

Pediatric FNH is mainly found in young people under the age of 15 years, with the predilection age of 6–10 years and more female patients, and the incidence in females is three times than that in males. Ninety percent of the patients have no clinical symptoms, and the tumor is found only in routine physical examination via imaging methods. Patients with huge lesions may manifest as abdominal pain, weight loss, vomiting, diarrhea, and other symptoms. Laboratory examination demonstrates normal results, with generally normal serum AFP. Imaging identification of various benign and malignant or metastatic tumors, which are rich in blood vessels, e.g., HCA and HCC, is critical. CT plain scan shows FNH as hypodense lesions, while enhanced scan demonstrates homogeneous densities, with enhancement in the center indicative of central scar. The typical performance in MRI includes iso- or hypo-signals on T_1-weighted images and iso- or hyper-signals on T_2-weighted images showing central scars as hyper-signals. Angiography shows that the lesions have one or multiple nourishing vessels, with centrifugal perfusion, i.e., the blood flows from the nutrient artery to the periphery of the lesion. The imaging often shows no typical features in pediatric FNH, and the central scars may be insignificant in cases with small lesions, while rare FNH with central scars can be found in tumor patients.

Pathological Characteristics

Gross and microscopic characteristics of FNH in children are similar to those in adults which have been described previously.

8.3.2 Mesenchymal Tumors

8.3.2.1 Infantile hemangioma (IH)

Pathogenesis and Mechanism

Also known as hemangioendotheliomas, infantile hemangiomas are the most common benign hepatic tumor in children, which are more often found in infants under the age of 1 year, are sporadic, and share the same clinical course with cases found in the skin, including proliferation and spontaneous degeneration after maturation. The etiology is unclear, and it may involve some congenital diseases, such as congenital heart diseases, trisomy 21 syndrome, ectopic liver in the thoracic cavity, etc. [22, 23].

Clinical Features

About 33% of IH lesions are developed in neonatal phase, and cases with onset within 6 months after birth account for 86%. IH is rare in children older than 3 years old, and the male-to-female ratio in pediatric patients is about 1:1.7. Hepatomegaly, congestive heart failure, and anemia are typical clinical triad. Most of the patients manifest as abdominal masses, and 10–15% of them have symptoms associated with congestive heart failure, including increased cardiac output, elevated end-diastolic blood pressure of left and right ventricles, decreased systolic pressure gradient of pulmonary arterial outflow, and slightly increased pulmonary artery pressure. Thirty percent of the patients have accompanied solitary or multiple extrahepatic lesions, which are mostly found in the skin, and other sites include the brain, lung, eye, lymph nodes, pancreas, posterior peritoneum, adrenal gland, bone, placenta, and so on. Other clinical manifestations include jaundice (20%), fever, dysplasia, hemolytic anemia, thrombocytopenia, etc, while a few cases show hepatic failure or tumor rupture resulting in death. Elevation of serum AFP can be detected in some patients, while neonatal AFP level can reach as high as 2500 ng/ml which will gradually decline to normal and thus still belongs to normal level considering the age of these patients. It has been reported that the patients may have severe hypothyroidism [24]. Imaging performance is helpful in the diagnosis of IH, as CT shows clearly bounded hypodensities, with or without punctuate calcification, with faster marginal enhancement compared to central enhancement, while MRI can present the flow characteristics and the structure of the surrounding blood vessels.

Gross Features

The tumors often contain multiple lesions, with single lesion of 0.5–15 cm in diameter, involving the left or the right lobe, or even both in rare cases. Lesions located near the liver surface may contain an umbilication pit in the center. The sections show that the lesions are clearly bounded, brownish red or light brown in color, soft, and cavernous, and infarction, hemorrhage, fibrosis, and gravel calcification can be visible in the central region of huge lesions. Cases treated with preoperative hepatic artery ligation or embolization may show infarction involving the whole tumor.

Microscopic Features

The natural course of IH includes proliferation phase and degradation phase, with different tumor morphology in different phases. The proliferation phase shows lobulated and cell-rich tumor nodules in the liver parenchyma, consisting of densely distributed plump vascular endothelial cells and perivascular cells, forming small or tiny capillary cavities, in between, which slender fibrous stromata and residue bile duct cells or liver cells can be found in it. Endothelial cells and perivascular cells contain enlarged nuclei, abundant pale cytoplasm, easily found mitotic figures which are often no more than 5/HPF, or large and irregularly thick-walled output veins in a few cases. For patients without preoperative interventional therapies, intravascular thrombosis, hemosiderin deposition, and necrosis are rare. Degradation phase contains decreased capillaries in the lesions, with obviously thickened basement membrane and hyalinization. The increased apoptosis bodies and perivascular mast cells can be seen in the thickened basement membrane, without marked inflammation or thrombosis. During the terminal stage of degradation phase, only a few residues of normal-sized capillaries and small veins can be observed; however, the obviously thickened basement membrane and hyalinization can also be seen, as well as a few vascular signs without epithelial lining.

Immunohistochemistry

The tumors express vascular markers such as CD31, CD34, and F8, while perivascular cells express SMA, and both do not express desmin. The vascular basement membrane shows diffusely and strongly positive expression of merosin. Since the vascular endothelium in IH shares the same immunophenotype as capillaries in placental villi, it expresses GLUT1 [25], Lewis Y antigen (LeY), FcγRII, CD15, CCR6, and indoleamine 2,3-dioxygenase (IDO), of which GLUT1 is the most important marker to identify IH from other vascular lesions.

Differential Diagnosis

Solitary congenital hepatic angioma is currently considered as congenital vascular malformation with capillary proliferation, which is formed before birth and rapidly degrades after birth. Its morphology is similar to that of skin-type congenital nonprogressive hemangiomas (RICH) with rapidly involuting course, and large patches of central necrosis and calcification can be found in the recession course. Negative expression of GLUT1 is of diagnostic value.

Treatment and Prognosis

IH is a benign tumor with rapid growth after birth in its natural course, and it shows slow degradation in childhood phase, despite infant deaths are not rare, and the overall survival rate is about 70%. The main leading causes for death include congestive heart failure, jaundice, hepatic failure due to diffuse multiple lesions, and disseminated intravascular coagulation (DIC). The treatment should be based on the degree of spontaneous degradation and relevant complications, and medication is optimal. For cases with insignificant effects on decrease of tumor size, surgical resection, hepatic artery ligation, and transcatheter arterial embolization are options. Liver transplantation is the terminal method for the treatment.

8.3.2.2 Mesenchymal Hamartoma (MH)

Pathogenesis and Mechanism

The incidence of MH ranks the second in benign hepatic tumors in children, and patients under the age of 2 years account for 85%. About 15% of the cases affect newborns, and less than 5% are found in children older than 5 years old, with a higher incidence in boys compared to girls. Its genesis may involve the embryonic ductal plate dysplasia and mesoderm developmental abnormalities; thus, intestinal malrotation, Beckwith-Wiedemann syndrome, biliary atresia, congenital heart disease, and other diseases can be seen in these patients [26].

Clinical Features

It generally manifests as abdominal distention due to progressive enlargement of the painless mass, with or without dyspnea, loss of appetite, vomiting, weight loss, or less commonly seen thrombocytopenia, pulmonary artery hypertension, obstructive jaundice, ascites, congestive heart failure, etc. Lab examinations show generally normal hepatic functions with slightly elevation of serum AFP due to regeneration of liver cells surrounding the tumor, and rare cases present significant increase in AFP level, which may be difficult to identify from HB clinically. Imaging shows marked macrocysts, polycysts, or cystic and solid masses, often hypodense, with a few blood vessels and thin mobile fibrous septa inside the cysts or intracystic hyperdense wall-attaching nodules with calcification in the surroundings.

Gross Features

In general, 75% of the MH cases are located in the right lobe of the liver, 22% involve the left lobe, and only 3% are found in both the left and right hepatic lobes. A few cases show lesions grown with protrusion on the surface of the liver and a pedicle. And the cut sections show that the tumor grows in extensive pattern, and the maximum diameter reaches up to 30 cm without any capsule, but the boundary can be well defined. There are varying sizes and numbers of cysts of the tumor, and the younger the patient is, the fewer and smaller the cysts are. Tumors contain a majority of solid regions, indicating the genesis of cysts is consistent with the enlargement of the tumor. Clear, light-yellow, or jelly contents can be found in the cysts. Irregularly compressed liver parenchyma is visible in the surroundings of the tumor, as well as bile ducts and blood vessels.

Microscopic Features

The tumor consists of varying amounts of loose connective tissue, angiolymphoid cystic cavities, bile ducts, and cholangiolar ducts. The bile ducts can be branches or rarely cystic, containing no bile in the cavities; stellate cells are scattered in the loose stroma with mucinous degeneration or concentrically distributed around the bile ducts with collagenization. In the stroma, proliferated and disorderly arranged small blood vessels, lymphatic ducts, and hepatocellular islets can be observed. The cystic walls consist of loose/dense mesenchymal tissues without epithelial linings (Fig. 8.18), covered by cubic epithelium in older pediatric patients (>1 year old). The solid regions may contain fat, smooth muscle and bone, or focal extramedullary hematopoiesis in 5% of MH cases, scattered plasma cells, or lymphocytes. Generally, there is no mitotic figure or invasion of the adjacent liver tissue.

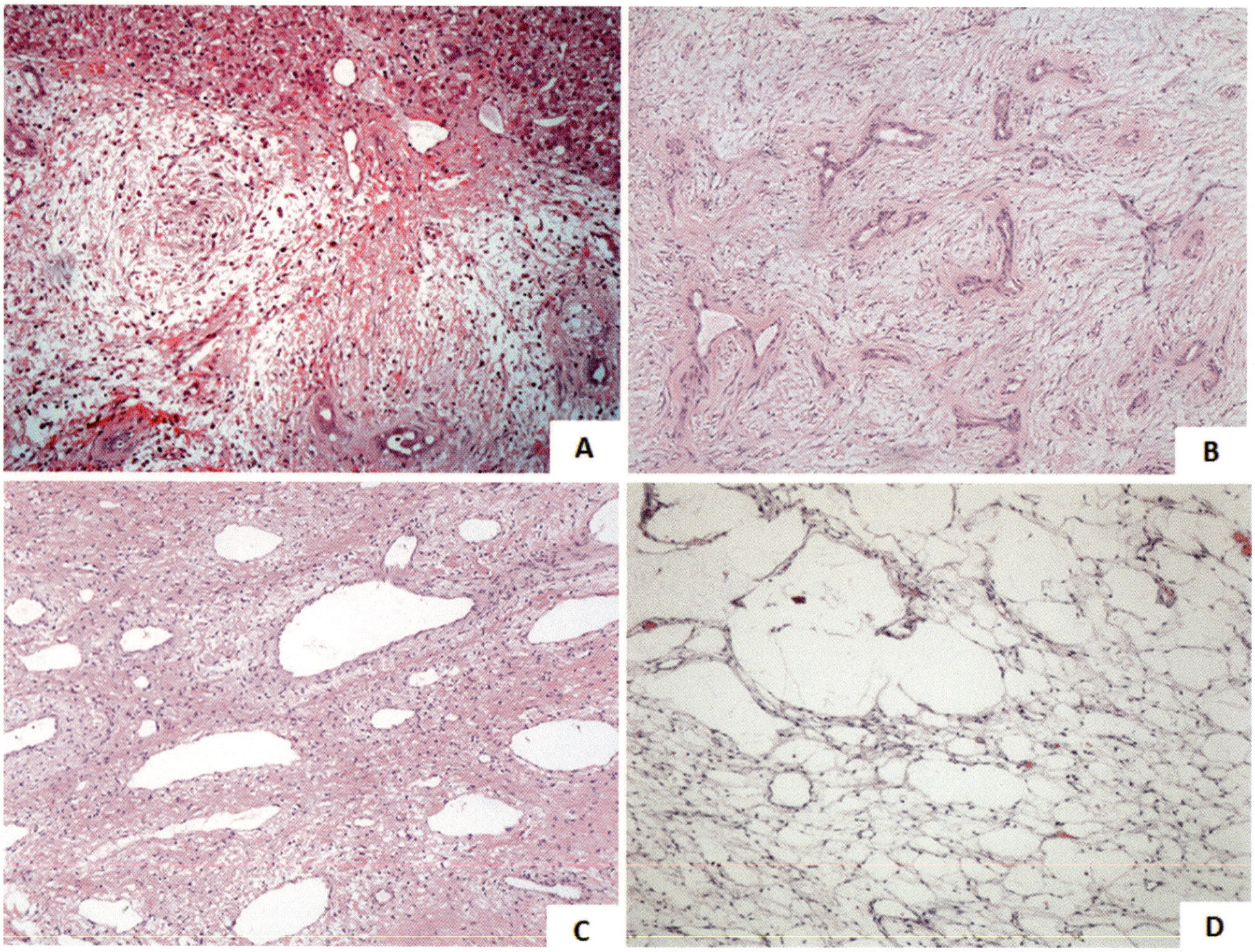

Fig. 8.18 Mesenchymal hamartoma. (**a**) stellate cells scattered in the loose stroma with mucinous degeneration; (**b**) concentrically distributed around the bile ducts with collagenzation and the bile ducts can be branches; (**c**) angiolymphoid cystic cavities can be seen focally; (**d**) dilated cystic area

Immunohistochemistry

Mesenchymal cells express vimentin, desmin, and SMA, which can be focal or diffuse positive, and cholangioepithelial cells express CK7 and CK19, while blood vessels and lymphatic vessels express CD34, CD31, F8, and D2–D40, respectively.

Molecular Genetics

The chromosomal abnormalities of MH include balanced translocation of chromosomes 15 and 19, translocation of chromosomes 11 and 19, rearrangement of chromosome 19q13.4, and complicated translocation of chromosomes 11, 17, and 19, which confirm the tumoral nature of MH, rather than hamartomatous lesions. Moreover, some of these abnormalities of chromosomal loci are identical to those in UES, which is indicative of the potential relation between them.

Differential Diagnosis

The patients have elevated AFP, which is easily misdiagnosed as HB; however, histomorphological differential diagnosis is relatively easy. Cystic MH should be distinguished from cholangiocystadenoma, angioma, and lymphoma.

Treatment and Prognosis

The currently known MH contains the same chromosomal change as UES, and it has been reported that MH could develop UES; thus, local and radial resection has been recommended. Patients without any complications have a general good prognosis during the long-term clinical follow-up, while those with severe cardiopulmonary complications have a poor prognosis.

Acknowledgment Professor C.W. Chow from Royal Children Hospital, Melbourne, Australia, for providing related pathological figures

References

1. Litten JB, Tomlinson GE. Liver tumors in children. Oncologist. 2008;13(7):812–20.
2. Finegold MJ, Egler RA, Goss JA, et al. Liver tumors: pediatric population. Liver Transpl. 2008;14(11):1545–56.
3. Tanimura M, Matsui I, Abe J, et al. Increased risk of hepatoblastoma among immature children with a lower birth weight. Cancer Res. 1998;58(14):3032–5.
4. Eichenmuller M, Gruner I, Hagl B, et al. Blocking the hedgehog pathway inhibits hepatoblastoma growth. Hepatology. 2009;49(2):482–90.
5. Lopez-Terrada D, Gunaratne PH, Adesina AM, et al. Histologic subtypes of hepatoblastoma are characterized by differential canonical Wnt and Notch pathway activation in DLK+ precursors. Hum Pathol. 2009;40(6):783–94.
6. Meyers RL, Czauderna P, Otte JB. Surgical treatment of hepatoblastoma. Pediatr Blood Cancer. 2012;59(5):800–8.
7. Lopez-Terrada D, Alaggio R, De Davila MT, et al. Towards an international pediatric liver tumor consensus classification: proceedings of the Los Angeles COG liver tumors symposium. Mod Pathol. 2014;27(3):472–91.
8. Meyers RL, Tiao G, Ville De Goyet J, et al. Hepatoblastoma state of the art: pre-treatment extent of disease, surgical resection guidelines and the role of liver transplantation. Curr Opin Pediatr. 2014;26(1):29–36.
9. Roebuck DJ, Aronson D, Clapuyt P, et al. 2005 PRETEXT: a revised staging system for primary malignant liver tumours of childhood developed by the SIOPEL group. Pediatr Radiol. 2007;37(2):123–32.. quiz 249-150
10. Maibach R, Roebuck D, Brugieres L, et al. Prognostic stratification for children with hepatoblastoma: the SIOPEL experience. Eur J Cancer. 2012;48(10):1543–9.
11. Zimmermann A. Hepatoblastoma with cholangioblastic features ('cholangioblastic hepatoblastoma') and other liver tumors with bimodal differentiation in young patients. Med Pediatr Oncol. 2002;39(5):487–91.
12. Sainati L, Leszl A, Stella M, et al. Cytogenetic analysis of hepatoblastoma: hypothesis of cytogenetic evolution in such tumors and results of a multicentric study. Cancer Genet Cytogenet. 1998;104(1):39–44.
13. Tomlinson GE, Douglass EC, Pollock BH, et al. Cytogenetic evaluation of a large series of hepatoblastomas: numerical abnormalities with recurring aberrations involving 1q12-q21. Genes Chromosom Cancer. 2005;44(2):177–84.
14. Malogolowkin MH, Katzenstein HM, Meyers RL, et al. Complete surgical resection is curative for children with hepatoblastoma with pure fetal histology: a report from the Children's Oncology Group. J Clin Oncol. 2011;29(24):3301–6.
15. Lauwers GY, Grant LD, Donnelly WH, et al. Hepatic undifferentiated (embryonal) sarcoma arising in a mesenchymal hamartoma. Am J Surg Pathol. 1997;21(10):1248–54.
16. Martelli MG, Liu C. Malignant rhabdoid tumour of the liver in a seven-month-old female infant: a case report and literature review. Afr J Paediatr Surg. 2013;10(1):50–4.
17. Wagner LM, Garrett JK, Ballard ET, et al. Malignant rhabdoid tumor mimicking hepatoblastoma: a case report and literature review. Pediatr Dev Pathol. 2007;10(5):409–15.
18. Alaggio R, Boldrini R, Di Venosa B, et al. Pediatric extra-renal rhabdoid tumors with unusual morphology: a diagnostic pitfall for small biopsies. Pathol Res Pract. 2009;205(7):451–7.
19. Ravindra KV, Cullinane C, Lewis IJ, et al. Long-term survival after spontaneous rupture of a malignant rhabdoid tumor of the liver. J Pediatr Surg. 2002;37(10):1488–90.
20. Makhlouf HR, Abdul-Al HM, Wang G, et al. Calcifying nested stromal-epithelial tumors of the liver: a clinicopathologic, immunohistochemical, and molecular genetic study of 9 cases with a long-term follow-up. Am J Surg Pathol. 2009;33(7):976–83.
21. Meir K, Maly A, Doviner V, et al. Nested (ossifying) stromal epithelial tumor of the liver: case report. Pediatr Dev Pathol. 2009;12(3):233–6.
22. Selby DM, Stocker JT, Waclawiw MA, et al. Infantile hemangioendothelioma of the liver. Hepatology. 1994;20(1 Pt 1):39–45.
23. North PE. Pediatric vascular tumors and malformations. Surg Pathol Clin. 2010;3(3):455–94.
24. Christison-Lagay ER, Burrows PE, Alomari A, et al. Hepatic hemangiomas: subtype classification and development of a clinical practice algorithm and registry. J Pediatr Surg. 2007;42(1):62–7.. discussion 67-68
25. Mo JQ, Dimashkieh HH, Bove KE. GLUT1 endothelial reactivity distinguishes hepatic infantile hemangioma from congenital hepatic vascular malformation with associated capillary proliferation. Hum Pathol. 2004;35(2):200–9.
26. Stringer MD, Alizai NK. Mesenchymal hamartoma of the liver: a systematic review. J Pediatr Surg. 2005;40(11):1681–90.

9 Tumors of the Gallbladder

Wen-Ming Cong and You-Wen Qian

9.1 Benign Tumors of the Gallbladder

9.1.1 Benign Epithelial Tumors and Precancerous Lesion of the Gallbladder

9.1.1.1 Gallbladder Adenoma

Pathogenesis and Mechanism

Generalized polypoid lesions of the gallbladder (PLG) refer to all the protruding lesions on the mucosal surface of the gallbladder, the incidence of which is 3–7% in a healthy population and 2–12% in cholecystectomy specimens [1]. GP can be divided into two major categories, pseudo and true GP. Pseudo-polyps include cholesterol polyps, adenomatoid polys, etc., and true polyps include adenoma and adenocarcinoma [2] or polypoid gallbladder lymphoma in some cases [3].

Gallbladder adenoma is the most common and most important benign neoplastic polyp in PLG, and the vast majority of cases are related to chronic cholecystitis, cholelithiasis, liver schistosomiasis, and other factors [4]. The long-term stimulation of chronic inflammation and stones promote the initiation and development of gallbladder adenoma, while adenoma can also develop from adenomyomatous hyperplasia of the gallbladder. Malformation of the distal end of the common bile duct leads to pancreatic juice regurgitation causing chronic inflammation and metaplasia, which may relate to the development of gallbladder adenoma. Furthermore, the process of hyperplasia/metaplasia → dysplasia/adenoma → carcinoma may be a sequential development pattern, and gallbladder polyps in patients at an age of >50 years old, with lesions of >1 cm in diameter and without pedicles, have a markedly increased risk of canceration [2].

W.-M. Cong (✉) • Y.-W. Qian
Department of Pathology, Eastern Hepatobiliary Surgery Hospital, Second Military Medical University, Shanghai, China
e-mail: wmcong@smmu.edu.cn

Clinical Features

The incidence of gallbladder adenoma in surgically resected specimens is 0.3–0.5%, and more female patients are found with a male to female ratio of about 3:7. It can be found in patients at any age with a median age of 58 years old. About 50% of the cases are accompanied by gallbladder stones, and Gardner syndrome or Peutz-Jegher syndrome can be found in a few cases. Cases with abnormal junction of pancreaticobiliary duct are discovered occasionally. The patients often manifest as no clinical symptoms, and enlargement of the gallbladder can be presented when the tumor is located in the neck of the gallbladder causing disruption of bile discharge.

Gross Features

Gallbladder adenoma is often solitary, with or without pedicles. As to the size of the lesion, Koga et al. conducted a study showing that 94% of benign PLG are sized in a diameter<1 cm, while 88% of the malignant lesions are sized in a diameter>1 cm. Around 50% of the adenoma are located in the body of the gallbladder, 35% at the bottom, and the rest of cases are found in the neck of the gallbladder. Multiple adenoma account for less than 10%, and rare cases involve adenoma occupying the majority of the gallbladder or located in the whole gallbladder wall. Based on the histological features, it can be classified into tubular adenoma, papillary adenoma, and tubulopapillary adenoma, among which tubular adenoma is the most common type, often presented as clearly bounded nodules with smooth surface. Papillary adenoma is slender, papillary, and lobulated (Fig. 9.1). One case of huge papillary adenoma was reported in China (1999), which was 5 cm × 4 cm × 3 cm in size and filling the whole gallbladder. Tubulopapillary adenoma contains both tubular and papillary parts.

Microscopic Features

According to histological morphology, gallbladder adenoma can be divided into tubular, papillary, and tubulopapillary types, while based on the cellular morphology, it can be divided into pyloric gland type, intestinal type, biliary type,

W.-M. Cong (ed.), *Surgical Pathology of Hepatobiliary Tumors*, DOI 10.1007/978-981-10-3536-4_9

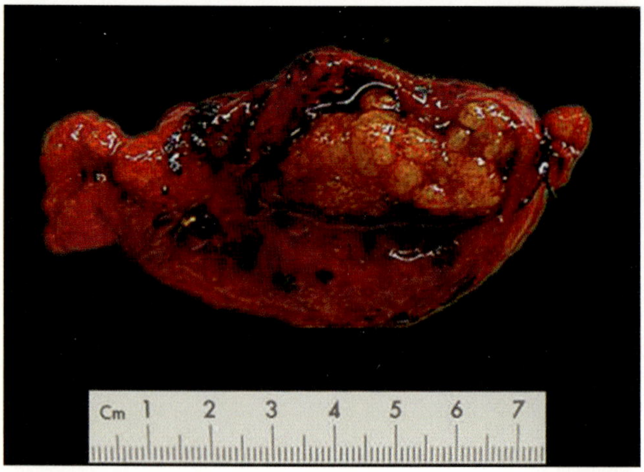

Fig. 9.1 Papillary adenoma: the tumor is lobulated, with slender papillae on the surface

and foveolar type (Fig. 9.2a–d). Each type has relatively specific immunohistochemistry markers, such as pyloric gland type (92% $MUC6^+$), intestinal type (100% $CK20^+$; 75% $CDX2^+$; 50% $MUC2^+$), biliary type (66% $MUC1^+$), and foveolar type (100% $MUC5AC^+$).

1. Tubular adenoma: The tumor consists of tubular glands which are lined by cubic or columnar epithelium and often located in the lamina propria, with clear boundary and a covering of normal gallbladder epithelium (Fig. 9.3a, b). Pyloric gland type accounts for 90% and intestinal type accounts for 10%. Pyloric gland type tubular adenoma consists of densely arranged pyloric glands, some of which are dilated into microcysts, and the glands are lined with mucus-secreting cubic or columnar epithelium. The cells contain lightly stained or vacuolar nuclei, and goblet cells and Paneth cells can be found between columnar epithelial cells, while squamous metaplasia can be visible in rare cases. 5-serotonin, somatostatin, pancreas polypeptides, or gastrin staining in immunohistochemistry can show the endocrine cells in small clusters. Large or intestinal-type tubular adenoma contains atypical hyperplasia in the epithelium, and 63% of the cases exhibit pseudopyloric gland proliferation in the nearby gallbladder epithelium, while Rokitansky-Aschoff sinuses (hyperplasia, subsidence and extension of normal gallbladder mucosa into the muscle layer) can be found in the adenoma tissues (Fig. 9.4a–b), which should be differentiated from adenocarcinoma.

2. Papillary adenoma: The tumor is divided into intestinal type and bile duct type. The former is composed of papillary glands lined with cubic or columnar epithelium, and there are more goblet cells, Paneth cells, and endocrine cells mixed between the epithelial cells. The pseudostratified epithelial cells contain little or rare cytoplasmic mucus secretion. The nuclei are round or long spindle and darkly stained, with a few mitotic figures (Fig. 9.5a–b). Sometimes it shows villous protrusions on the cell surface which can be diagnosed as villous adenoma, similar to the same kind of colon lesions. Tubular and villous structures can be found in a few cases named as villioustublar adenoma with varying degrees of epithelial dysplasia. Bile duct type is rare, which is coated with bile duct cuboidal epithelium on the papilla, and rare malignant transformation can be found [5].

3. Tubulopapillary adenoma: The tumor is composed of tubular glands and papillary structures, and each component at least accounts for more than 20% (Fig. 9.6a–b). The tubular glands can be pyloric gland type or intestinal type, with papillary structures lined with columnar epithelial cells containing mucous. Paneth cells and endocrine cells can be found in a few cases or with hyperplasia of pseudopyloric gland.

9.1.1.2 Cystadenoma

Cystadenoma is often found in extrahepatic biliary system, while gallbladder cystadenoma is rare and more common in middle-aged females. Grossly, the tumor can be lobulated, polycystic, or monocystic, containing mucus, serum, or hemorrhage, with calcification in the cystic wall. Cases with huge lesions may be accompanied by symptoms due to obstructive jaundice or cholecystitis. Under the microscope, the inner layer of the cyst wall is composed of columnar or cubic mucus-secreting epithelium, and the stroma is abundant and similar to ovarian stroma, with expression of estrogen and progesterone receptors. The interstitial tissues often contain varying degrees of fibrosis, and its outer layer is hyalinized fibrous tissue. It should be differentiated from gallbladder echinococcosis, abscess, adenomyomatosis, and septum gallbladder, and around 13% of the gallbladder adenoma may undergo malignant transforming into cystadenocarcinoma [6, 7].

According to the statistics in foreign literature, the canceration rate of gallbladder adenoma is 6–36%, while a group of domestic data shows the rate is 1.7%. In general, the gallbladder adenoma is not an important precancerous lesion for gallbladder carcinoma, because the incidence rate of gallbladder adenoma is very low and only 3% of early gallbladder carcinoma contain adenoma in the paracancerous adjacent mucosa [8]. In addition, gallbladder adenoma often has a β-catenin mutation which is rare in gallbladder carcinoma, and those genetic changes, often found in gallbladder carcinoma such as TP53, P16, and KRAS, cannot be found in gallbladder adenoma [9–11]. It is worth noticing that gallbladder adenoma or hyperplastic polyps with the following conditions should be closely followed up or treated by

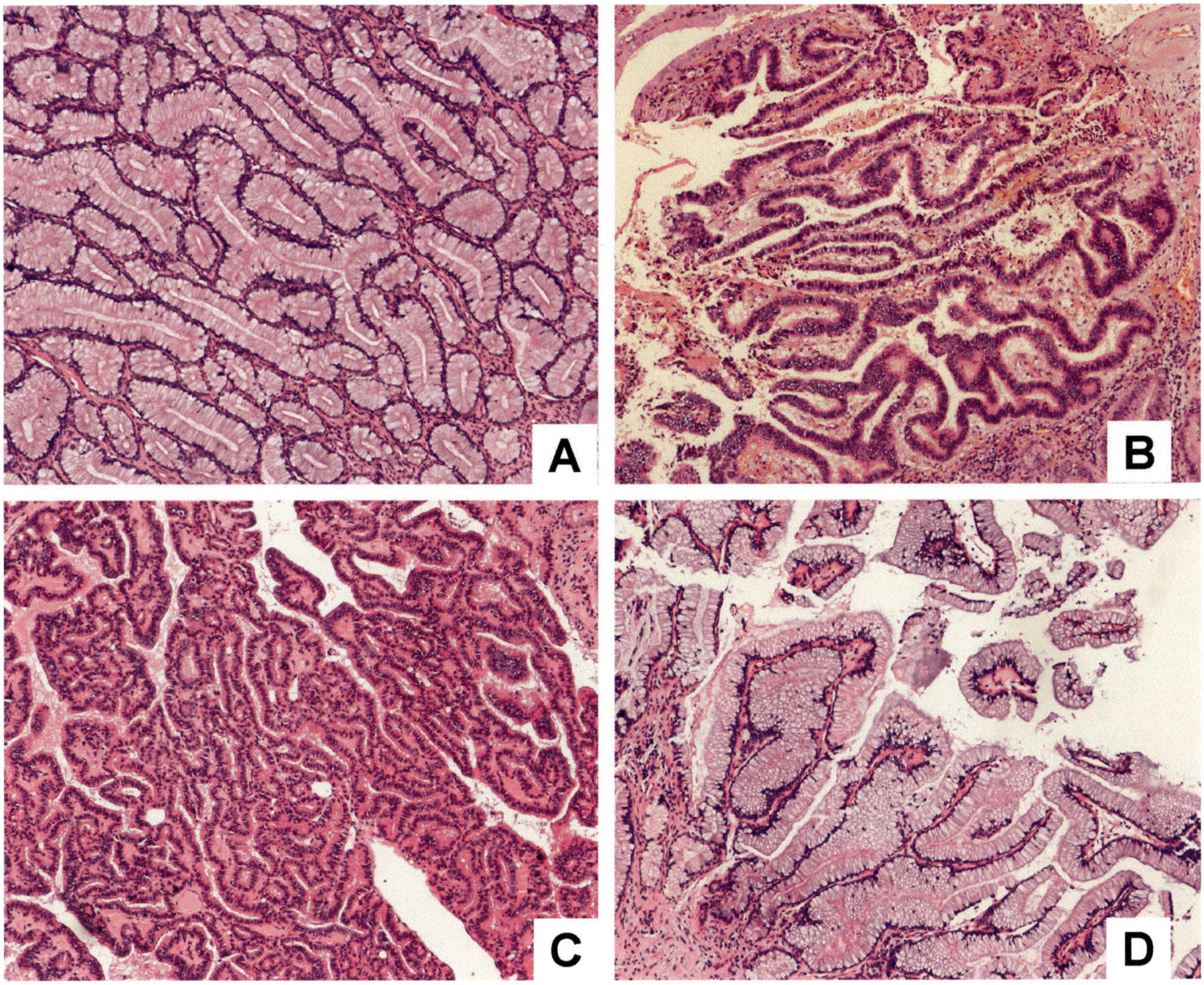

Fig. 9.2 Gallbladder adenoma: (**a**) pyloric gland type, (**b**) intestinal type, (**c**) biliary type, (**d**) foveolar type

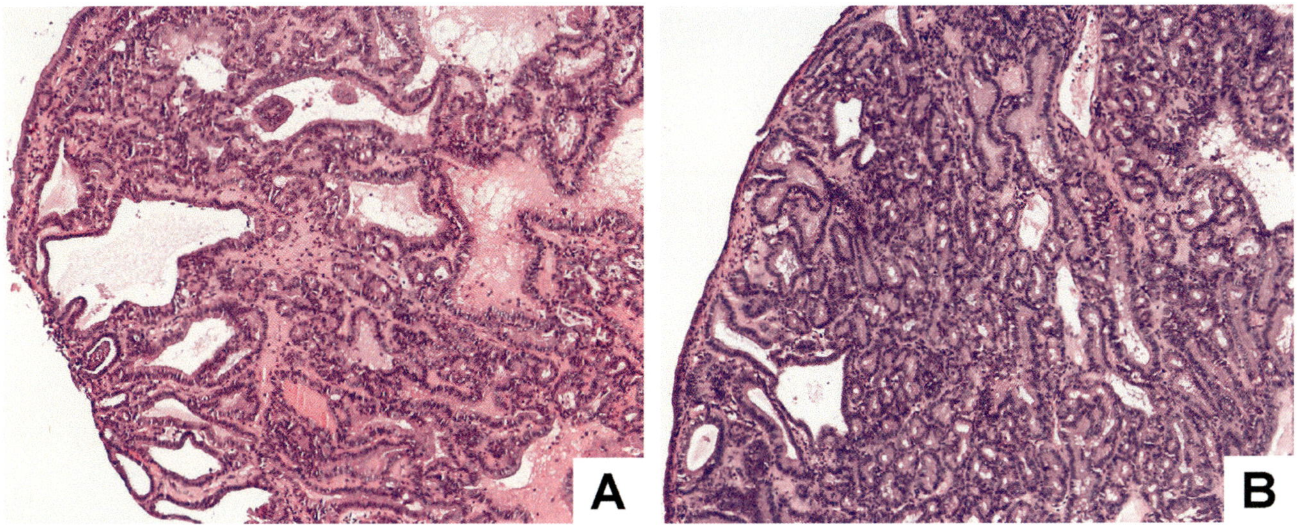

Fig. 9.3 Tubular adenoma: the tubular glands are lined with well-differentiated columnar epithelium (**a** & **b**)

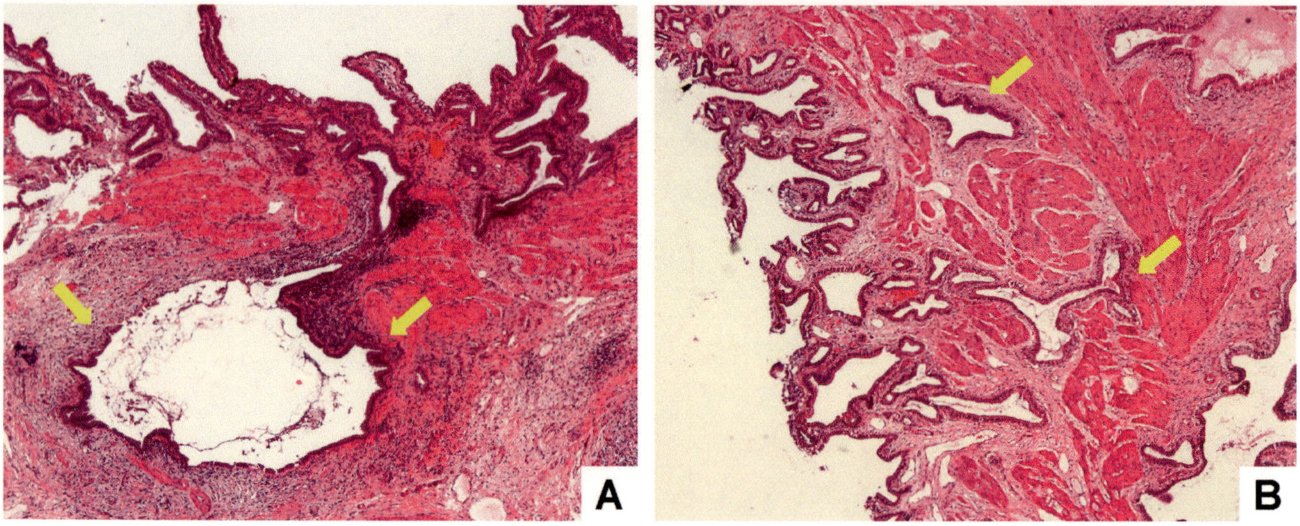

Fig. 9.4 Rokitansky-Aschoff sinuses: (**a**) Rokitansky-Aschoff sinuses refer to the hyperplasia, subsidence, and extension of normal gallbladder mucosa into the muscle layer (*arrows*); (**b**) *arrows* show the dilated Rokitansky-Aschoff sinuses among smooth muscle bundles

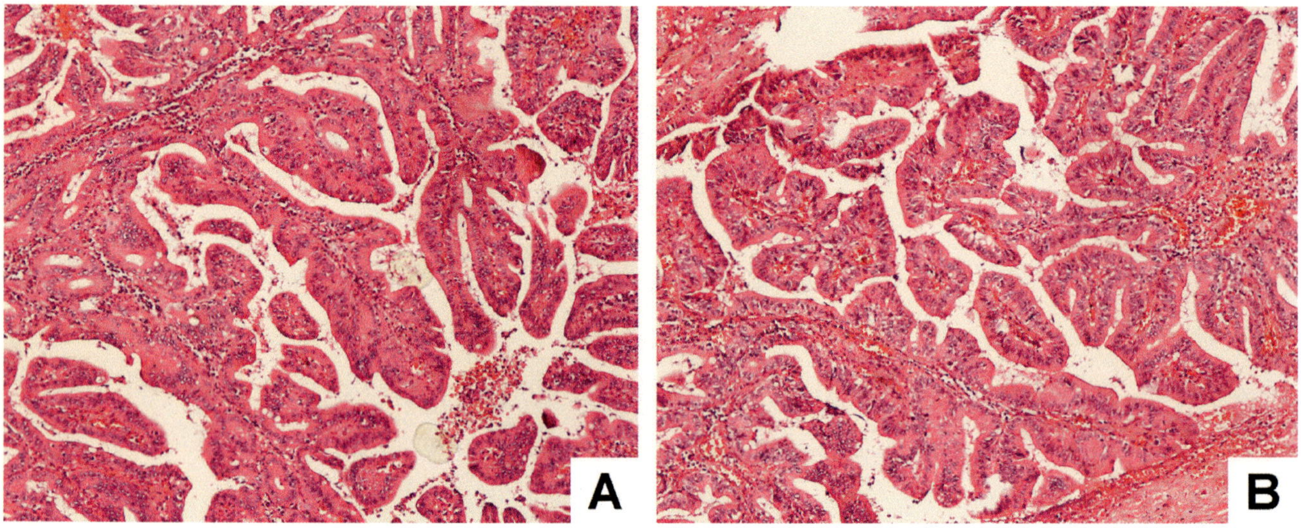

Fig. 9.5 Papillary adenoma: (**a**) papillary glands lined with cubic or columnar epithelium; (**b**) fibrovascular cores of the papilla

surgical resection as soon as possible: ① diameter of the lesions >1 cm,② diameter of the lesions <1 cm with rapid increase in volume (it has been reported that adenoma which was only 0.4 cm in diameter had already undergone malignancy), ③ multiple adenoma, ④complication with gallbladder stones, ⑤ wide base of the lesions with locally thickened gallbladder mucosa, and ⑥ older than 50 years old.

9.1.1.3 Biliary Intraductal Neoplasia (BilIN) and Carcinoma In Situ (CIS) of the Gallbladder

Biliary intraductal neoplasia in the gallbladder is often difficult to be identified due to complication with chronic cholecystitis, and the mucosal surface may be flat, papillary, granular, or nodular, with flat mucosa as the most common type. The main evaluation index includes ① cellular and nuclear atypia (cellular and nuclear pleomorphism, increased karyoplasmic ratio, thickened or irregular nuclear membrane, darkly stained chromatin), ② cellular and nuclear polarity, and ③ structural atypia (multilayered cellular and nuclear arrangement, micro-papillar or pseudo-papilla structure). And WHO classified gallbladder BilIN into the following three grades [12]:

BilIN-1 (low grade): The epithelium shows flat or low/micro-papillary structure, and the nuclei are almost in situ, with focal pseudostratified nuclei in rare cases which are still located in the lower two thirds of the epithelium.

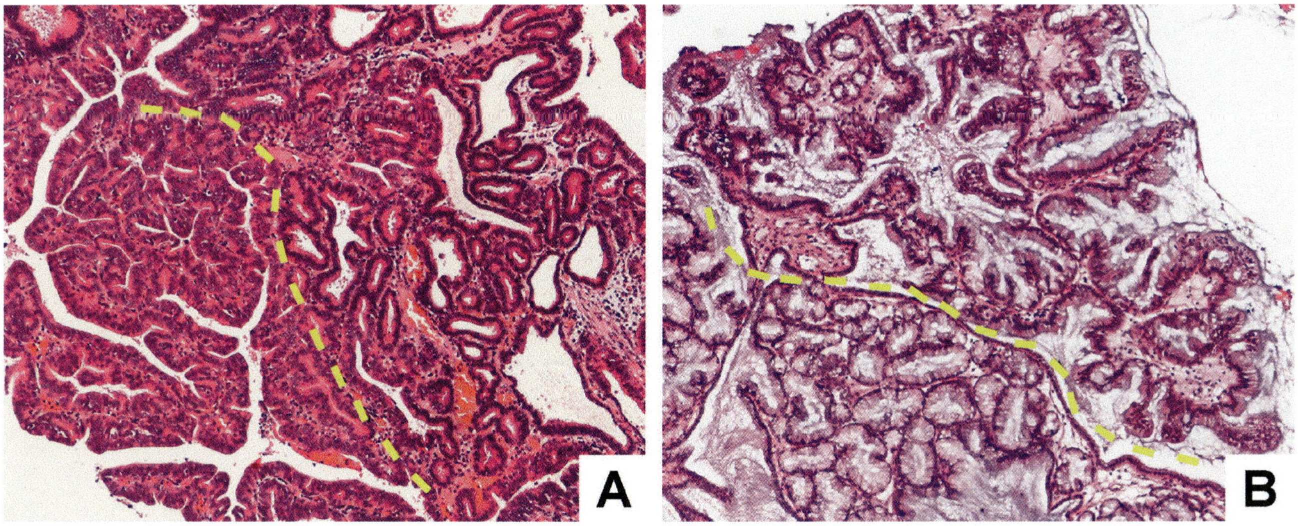

Fig. 9.6 Tubulopapillary adenoma: the tumor is composed of tubular glands and papillary structures (**a** & **b**) (the *dotted line* shows the boundary)

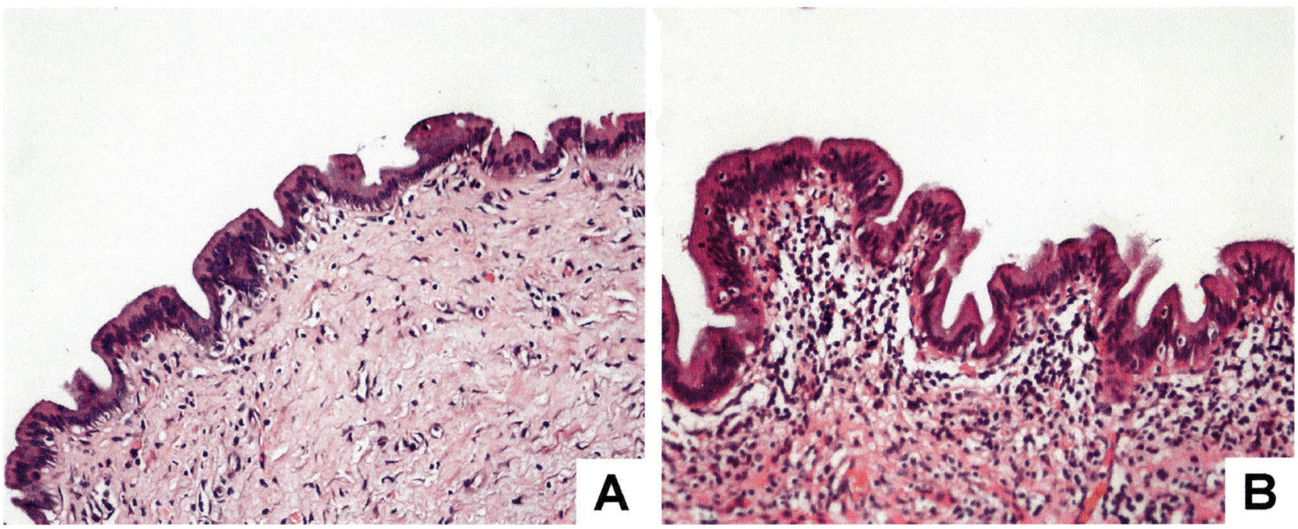

Fig. 9.7 BilIN-1 (**a** & **b**)

Cytology shows mildly abnormal nuclei, which have slight irregular nuclear membrane, increased karyoplasmic ratio, and elongated nuclei consistent in size and shape (Fig. 9.7a, b).

BilIN-2 (moderate grade): It can be flat or pseudo- or micropapillary, often with absence of non-diffused cellular polarity, pseudostratified nuclei reaching the luminal surface, which are still located in the lower two thirds of the epithelium. Cytology shows obvious nuclear dysplasia and enlargement, darkly stained chromatin, irregular nuclear membrane, varying degrees of inconsistency in the size and shape of the nuclei, and rare mitotic figures (Fig. 9.8a, b).

BilIN-3 (high grade): It often contains visible pseudo-papilla or micro-papilla, and cytology shows that it is similar to carcinoma without invasion throughout the base membrane. Diffuse and severe disappearance of cellular polarity can be found with nuclei located on the luminal surface. The epithelial cells protrude into the luminal surface in small bud clusters, forming cribriform structures. Malignant features can be observed in cytological examination, including markedly irregular nuclear membrane, darkly stained chromatin, and abnormally increased nuclei with visible mitotic figures (Fig. 9.9a, b).

BilIN-3 has a incidence of 0.5–3% in patients with gallbladder stones, which is often accompanied by pyloric gland and intestinal metaplasia, and shares similar clinical features

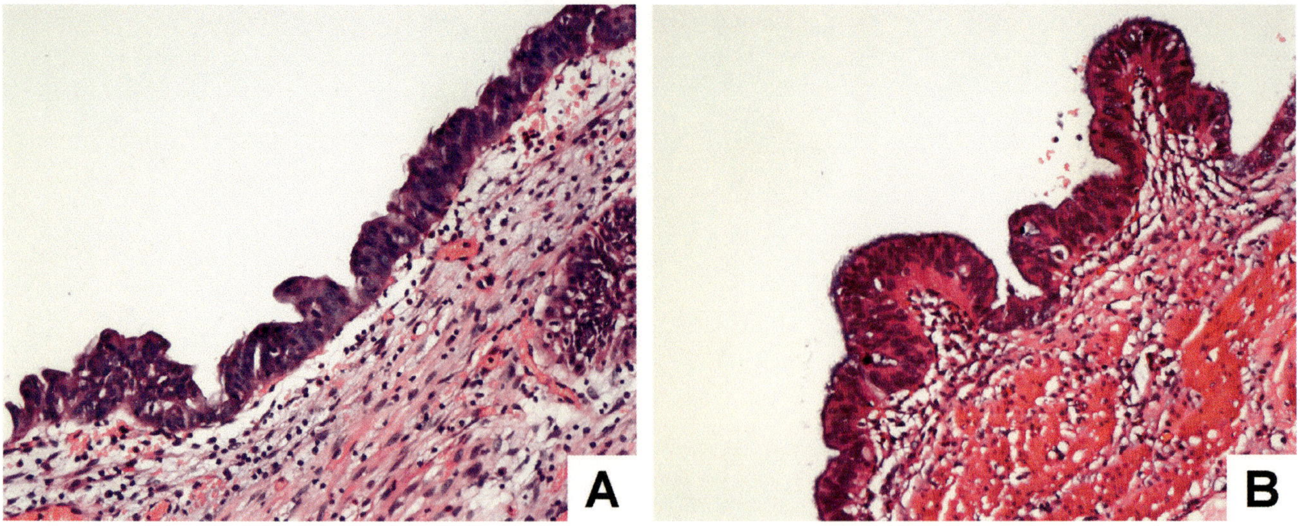

Fig. 9.8 BilIN-2 (**a** & **b**)

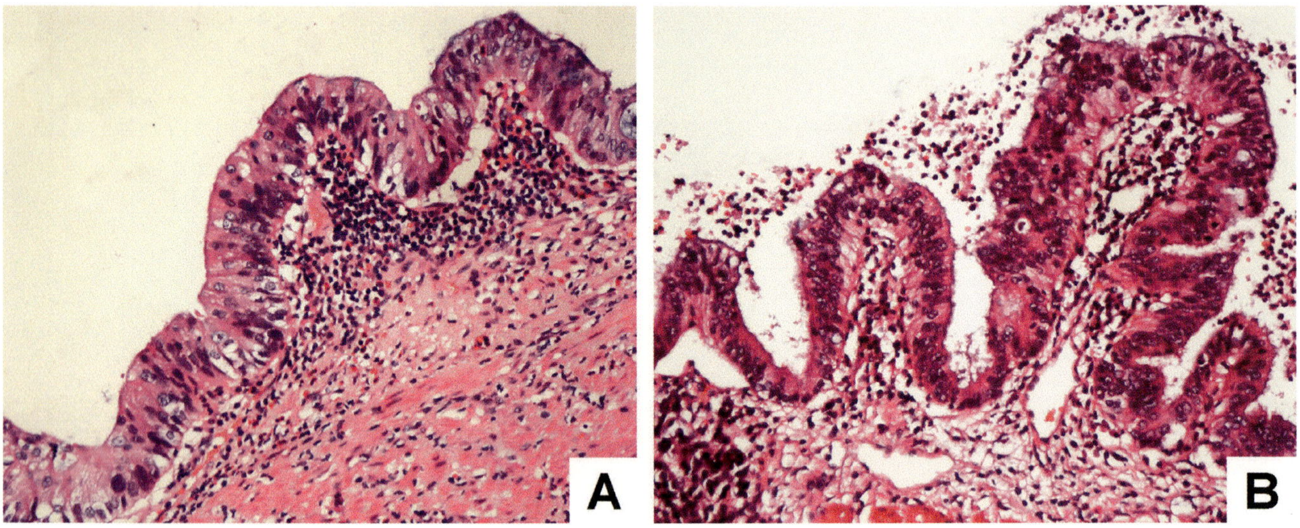

Fig. 9.9 BilIN-3 (**a** & **b**)

with gallbladder carcinoma, such as onset age, high-prevalence areas, predilection sites and molecular biological changes, etc. BilIN-3 is often a complication of gallbladder carcinoma and considered to be a precancerous lesion for gallbladder carcinoma, induced by cholelithiasis, familial adenomatous polyposis, sclerosing cholangitis and pancreatic-biliary reflux, and so forth [13]. The area of dysplasia is clearly separated from the surrounding normal epithelium. However, high-grade intraepithelial neoplasia in Rokitansky-Aschoff sinus should be identified from interstitial infiltration in gallbladder carcinoma [12]. And if the microscopic examination shows a lesion as BilIN-3, more samples should be examined to exclude gallbladder carcinoma. The morphological type of BilIN-3 can be the same with or different from the concomitant invasive cholangiocarcinoma in cases with both tumors. Immunohistochemistry demonstrates that the cells in intraepithelial neoplasia are positive for CEA, CA19-9, p53, and S100 A4 [14]. Different from dysplasia, reactive hyperplasia often contains flat epithelium, with no papillary structure or metaplasia and little changes in cellular polarity, slightly enlarged cell, round or oval and slightly enlarged nuclei, smooth nuclear membrane, and fine and uniformly distributed chromatin. Unlike dysplasia which contains monotype of cells, its cellular components are diverse, including columnar mucus-secreting cells, low cuboidal cells, and atrophic epithelioid and pencil-like cells, and the transition between it and normal epithelium is also gradual without clear boundaries.

Carcinoma in situ (CIS) shares the morphological characteristics with BilIN-3, but the lesions are confined to the mucosa and can be divided into micro-papillary type and flat type grossly. Dysplastic cells with obvious features of malignant tumors can be identified as CIS, such as frequent mitotic figures (2–10/HPF), crowded nuclei, enlarged glands, lessened stroma, close or back-to-back arrangement of the glands, lining of pseudostratified epithelium, and disappearance of cellular polarity, with intestinal metaplasia (Fig. 9.10). Albores-Saavedra et al. (2004) suggested that Rokitansky-Aschoff sinus with CIS is different from invasive glands in tubular tumors in that the former contain superficial epithelium connected to the invaginated epithelium with mixture of recognizable normal and tumorous epithelium, condensed bile content in the elongated and extended glandular cavities, and no invasion of smooth muscles. In addition, CIS extends along the Rokitansky-Aschoff sinus showing long glandular cavities through intramuscular connective tissues, while tumorous glands are often small- and medium-sized glands invading smooth muscle bundles or intramuscular connective tissues [15]. Furthermore, gallbladder stones can also result in multiple forms of mucosal changes of the gallbladder. Martinez-Guzman et al. (1998) analyzed 1096 cases of gallbladder stones, finding that mucosal epithelium with pseudopyloric gland metaplasia accounted for 50%, intestinal metaplasia 16%, low-grade atypical hyperplasia 40%, high-grade atypical hyperplasia 16%, carcinoma in situ 1.5%, and infiltrative carcinoma 2.6%, and the average age of patients with the latter four types of lesions was 42, 48, 53, and 61 years old separately. Segovia Lohse HA et al. (2013) conducted an analysis on the statistics of 1514 cases of cholecystitis, showing that pseudopyloric gland metaplasia accounted for 22.6%, intestinal metaplasia 2.1%, atypical hyperplasia 0.2%, and gallbladder carcinoma 0.6%, and the average age of the patients was 47, 46, 54, and 63 years old [16]. Both aforementioned data suggest that carcinogenesis is a gradually developmental process. As to the treatment for cases with BilIN-3 and invasive carcinoma confined to the lamina propria, surgical resection is the mainstream.

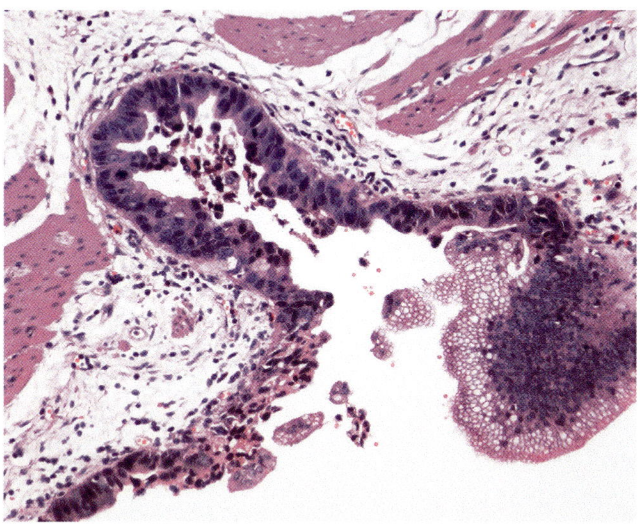

Fig. 9.10 CIS: the lesion involves the whole mucous layer but confined to the lamina propria

9.1.2 Benign Mesenchymal Tumors of the Gallbladder

Benign mesenchymal tumors of the gallbladder are rare, with a total incidence of less than 0.1% of all the specimens obtained in cholecystectomy. And the gross and microscopic morphology of these tumors are similar to the same kind of lesions at other sites.

9.1.2.1 Fibroma

Fibroma is often located in the bottom of the gallbladder, and the diameter of the lesions is often 0.8–1.2 cm, consisting of fibrous tumor cells or ganglion cells in rare cases [17].

9.1.2.2 Leiomyoma

Leiomyoma can be nodules in the gallbladder wall protruding into the cystic cavities, and leiomyoma of the gallbladder duct may cause obstruction. The lesions are often about 1 cm or even 4 cm in diameter. The microscopic observation shows the tumor consists of interdigitated bundles of leiomyomatous cells [18].

9.1.2.3 Hemangioma

Hemangioma is often cavernous angioma, and eight cases have been reported in the English literature [19], while three domestic cases have also been reported. Macroscopically, it is often lobulated, purple, and spongy, with a diameter of up to 6–8 cm, and can be connected to other intrahepatic blood vessels causing corresponding symptoms due to rupture, hemorrhage, and compression on the surrounding tissues. The patients may sometimes manifest as heart failure. Preoperative diagnosis of hemangioma is difficult, and it should be differentiated from malignant tumors of the gallbladder and hepatic tumors. Microscopically, the tumor consists of vascular cavities lined with vascular endothelium.

9.1.2.4 Lipoma

Lipoma consists of mature adipose tumor cells, and one domestic case of primary huge lipoma was reported by Nianxin Xia et al. (2008), which was located in the subserosa of the gallbladder and 8 cm × 7 cm in size, and the patient manifested it as discomfort in the right shoulder, who was treated by surgical resection with a good prognosis [20].

9.1.2.5 Neurofibroma

Similar incidences are found in male and female patients, and the average onset age is 57.9 (32–77) years old. Approximately 50% of the patients are complicated by gallbladder stones. The tumors are small and located frequently in the neck of the gallbladder in a diameter of 0.4–1.5 cm. A case with the diameter up to 8.6 cm has also been reported. Under the microscope, they are composed of wavy slender spindle cells (Schwann cells), and their morphology and histogenesis are the same as those in other organs. Furthermore, they are related to NF-1 gene [21].

9.1.2.6 Paraganglioma

The tumors are located in the subserosa, usually well circumscribed as small round nodules, which can be up to 4.5 cm in diameter, protruding to the serosa. There have been eight cases reported in the foreign literature [22]. Microscopically principal cells are arranged in typical nest or acinar structures. Endocrine markers, e.g., CgA, Syn, etc., are positive, which needs to be identified from clear cell carcinoma.

9.1.2.7 Granular Cell Tumor (GCT)

GCT is rare, often found in young or middle-aged female patients. Clinically, cases with involvement of bile duct show cholecystalgia or abdominal pain or occasional obstructive jaundice, while those with involvement of the gallbladder may be asymptomatic. Involvement of cystic duct can result in complications, such as cholecystitis or gallbladder mucous cyst or hydrocholecystis, and gallbladder stones occasionally. Grossly, the tumors are light yellow, solid, and nodular, with unclear boundaries, and often protrude into the cavity of the gallbladder. The microscopic morphology of GCT in the gallbladder is similar to the same kind of lesions in skin and other organs [23].

9.1.2.8 Cystic Lymphangioma

So far, only 11 cases of cystic lymphangioma have been reported in the foreign literature, with a male to female ratio of 5:6, and the average onset age is 36 (17–66) years old. The maximum diameter can be up to 20 cm, and clinical symptoms due to compression by the lesions can be found in half patients, possibly complicated by acute Inflammation, rupture of the cyst, and intracystic hemorrhage. Symptomatic or huge lesions should be surgically resected. Microscopic examination shows the tumor consists of lymphatic tissues, lined with monolayer of endothelial cells, and the walls of varying thicknesses contain discontinuous smooth muscle inside. The morphology of the tumor is the same to the kind of lesions in other parts [24] (Fig. 9.12).

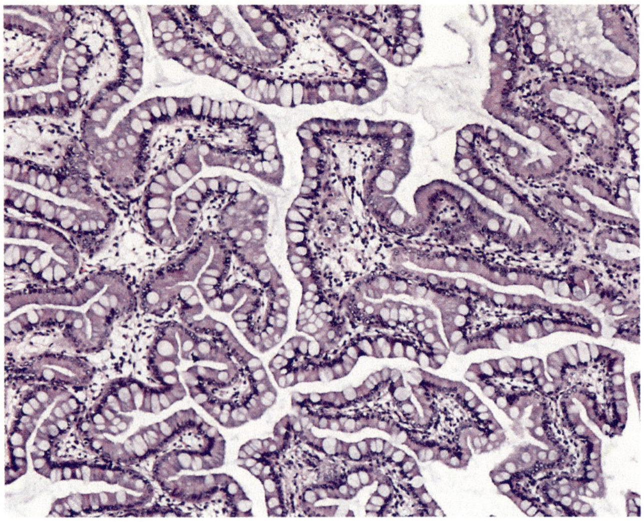

Fig. 9.11 Intestinal metaplasia: columnar epitheliums of the gallbladder adenoma mixed with many metaplastic goblet cells

9.2 Malignant Tumors of the Gallbladder

9.2.1 Carcinoma of the Gallbladder

9.2.1.1 Pathogenesis and Mechanism

The incidence of carcinoma of the gallbladder ranks the sixth in gastrointestinal carcinomas and the first in malignant biliary tumors accounting for 85–90%, with <two cases per 100,000 people in low incidence area of the world. The incidence of gallbladder carcinoma in China is reported to be 2–5%. However, the pathogenesis of gallbladder carcinoma is still unclear, and 60–90% of the patients are complicated by gallbladder stones, suggesting the close relationship between cholelithiasis and gallbladder carcinoma. In addition, infection such as chronic cholecystitis and carcinogenic derivatives of cholic acid in the bile may also play a role in the pathogenesis of gallbladder carcinoma. Other risk factors include genetic susceptibility, geographical region, race and gender, obesity, smoking, *Salmonella* or *Helicobacter pylori* and other infectious factors, abnormal junction of pancreaticobillary duct, ulcerative colitis, familial polyposis, porcelain gallbladder, primary sclerosing cholangitis, etc. [25]. Recent studies found that the pathogenesis of gallbladder carcinoma involves accumulated mutations of multiple genes, such as activation of oncogene *K-ras* and telomerase; mutation and inactivation of anti-oncogene *p53*, *p16, and FHIT*; loss of heterozygosity of 3p and 8p alleles; and microsatellite instability of *Rb gene* [26], and its carcinogenic mechanism follows the sequential pattern of hyperplasia/metaplasia→dysplasia→carcinoma, which takes 5–15 years [27].

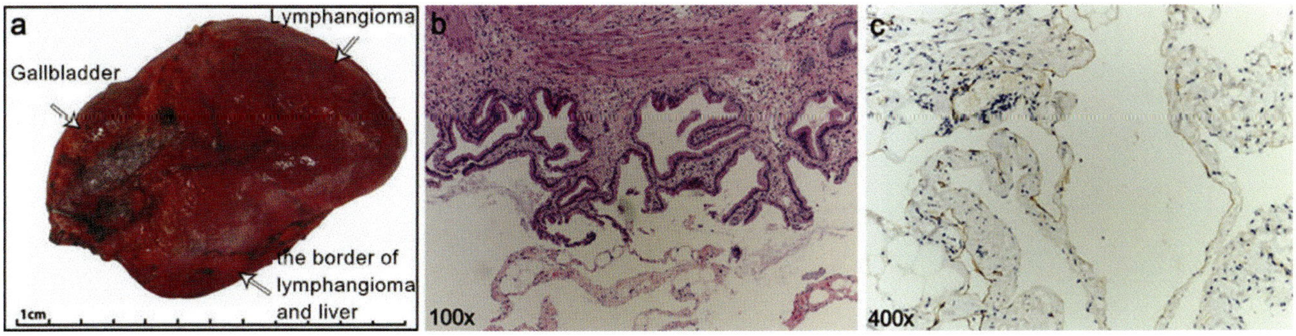

Fig. 9.12 Lymphangioma of the gallbladder: (**a**) gross specimen; (**b**) the tumor consists of lymphatic tissues, lined with monolayer of endothelial cells; (**c**) positive staining of endothelial cells with lymphatic marker D2–40

9.2.1.2 Clinical Features

It is mainly found in the elderly, and 90% of the patients are older than 50 years old with an average age of 67 years old. More female patients are involved with a male to female ratio of 1:(3, 4). Recent studies show that this gender difference may be related to estrogen and its receptors [28, 29] A total of 1089 cases of adenocarcinoma of the gallbladder have been diagnosed in the Department of Pathology, Eastern Hepatobiliary Surgery Hospital, Second Military Medical University from 2007 to August 2014, the average age of the patients was 59.9 (29–83) years old, including 433 males and 656 females, and the male to female ratio was 1:1.52. The clinical symptoms for gallbladder carcinoma include abdominal pain, jaundice, nausea and vomiting, etc., which are general gastrointestinal symptoms and difficult to identify from manifestations in patients with cholelithiasis; thus, it is difficult to make early diagnosis. Resectable lesions account for less than 20%. Some patients have enlarged gallbladder due to obstruction of cystic duct caused by the tumor. Serum CEA and CA19-9 levels are often increased, and hypercalcemia, leukocytosis, and elevation of serum HCG or AFP levels can be found in a few cases.

9.2.1.3 Gross Features

Carcinoma of the gallbladder can be grossly divided into three basic types, named massive type, nodular type, and invasive type, and the latter is the most common one, presenting diffuse thickening and hardening of the gallbladder wall, involving an area of up to 5 cm^2 of the whole gallbladder. The sections are solid, firm, and hard in texture. The tumors can also be huge polypoid masses or nodules filling the whole cystic cavity. Occasionally, dumbbell-shaped gallbladder can also be observed due to cyclic infiltration. Generally, papillary adenoma has no pedicle and is polypoid or cauliflower shaped, while mucinous adenocarcinoma and signet ring cell carcinoma are superficially coated with myxoid jelly. Carcinoma of the gallbladder is most commonly found at the bottom of the gallbladder (60%), followed by the cystic body (30%), and rarely in the neck (10%); however, most cases involve the majority of the gallbladder when discovered, and it is difficult to identify the initiation site of the tumor. Direct invasion of the adjacent liver parenchyma is often found due to penetration throughout the gallbladder wall (Fig. 9.13).

9.2.1.4 Microscopic Features

Adenocarcinoma

Adenocarcinoma is the most common histological type of gallbladder carcinoma, accounting for around 80% of all gallbladder carcinoma. According to the cellular morphology, gallbladder carcinoma can be divided into biliary type, intestinal type, and foveolar pattern. Biliary type is the most common type, in which the glands are lined with biliary epithelial cubic or columnar cells. Intestinal type contains tumor cells forming tubular or papillary structures, similar to colonic epithelium, containing a large number of goblet cells, and varying amounts of endocrine and Paneth cells. Foveolar type is the rarest and characterized by cells with basal location of the nuclei and large amounts of mucus contents in the cytoplasm.

Based on the degree of differentiation, gallbladder carcinoma can also be divided into well-differentiated, moderately differentiated, and poorly differentiated adenocarcinoma. Well-differentiated adenoma is mainly composed by well-differentiated tubular adenocarcinoma (Fig. 9.14), and the glands are lined with cubic or columnar epithelial cells, containing atypia nuclei with darkly stained chromatin and obvious nucleoli. These cells are multilayered or pseudostratified in arrangement, absent in polarity. About one third the tumors contain focal intestinal gland differentiation with varying number of endocrine cells, while Paneth cells are rare. The stroma of the carcinoma tissues contains marked fibrous hyperplasia. Poorly differentiated adenocarcinoma shows glandular differentiation to a certain degree, but most of the tumor cells are displayed in solid masses or cords (Fig. 9.15), with obvious fibrous hyperplasia. Some of the poorly differentiated adenocarcinoma cells are mainly

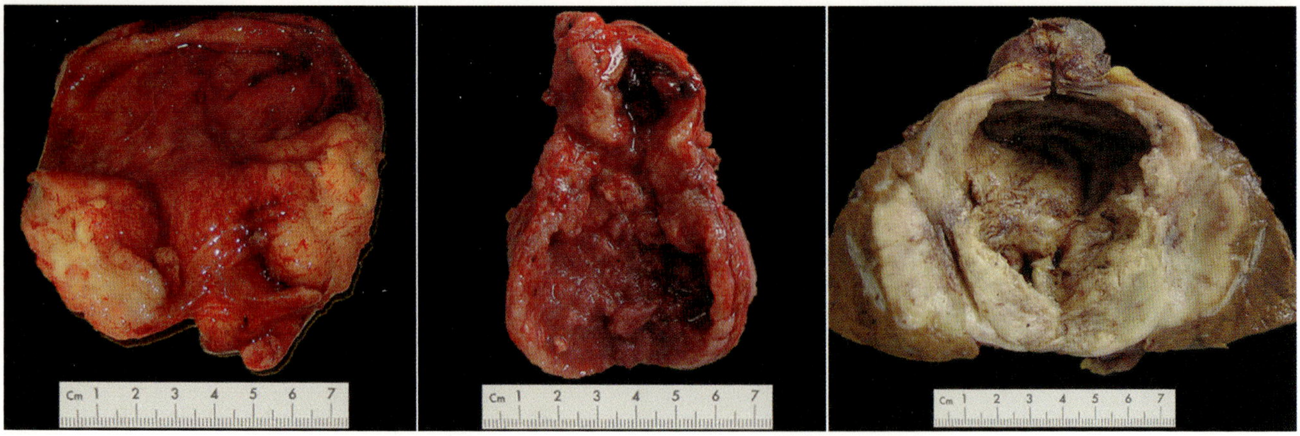

Fig. 9.13 Gross types: *left* massive type, *middle* nodular type, *right* invasive type

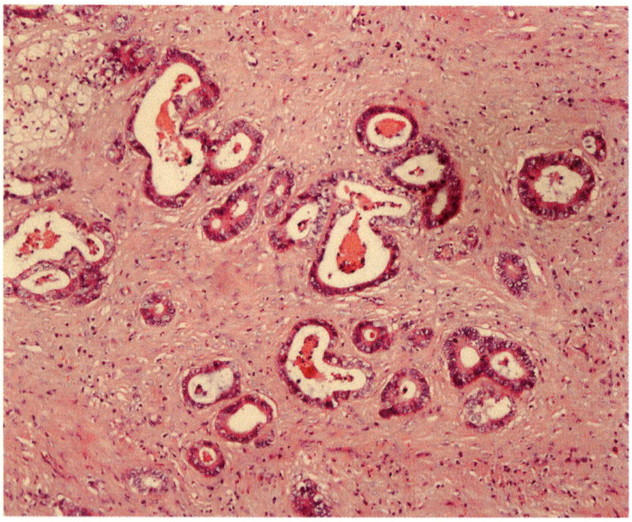

Fig. 9.14 Well-differentiated gallbladder adenocarcinoma: the glands are lined with cubic or columnar epithelial cells

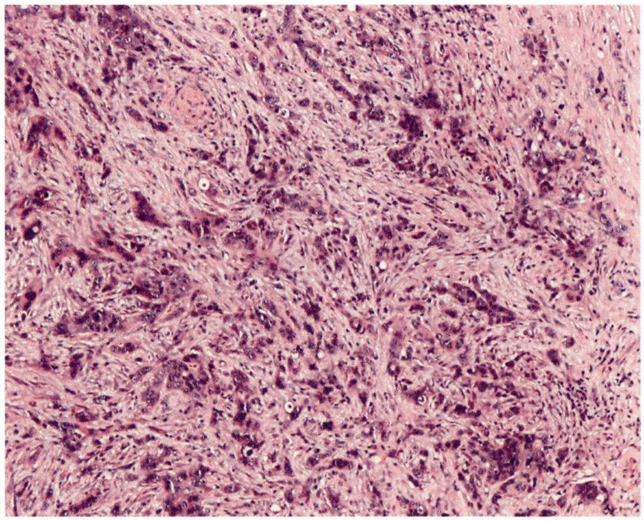

Fig. 9.15 Poorly differentiated gallbladder adenocarcinoma: the tumor cells are arranged in nest-like distribution or irregular glandular structures, with obvious atypia

small and round cells, distributed in patches, nodules, or cords, with vesicular nuclei, marked nucleoli, and little cytoplasm, and they should be differentiated from large cell lymphoma. Moderately differentiated adenocarcinoma is a tumor between well- and poorly differentiated adenocarcinomas (Fig. 9.16). Infiltration of the perineural tissues can always be observed in the adenocarcinoma of the gallbladder, with vascular tumor thrombus and invasion of the adjacent liver tissue (Fig. 9.17a–d). And the glands may contain varying amounts of mucus in the cavities, which is often salivary mucus, different from that in normal gallbladder and cholycystitis. The tumors can be cribriform or angiosarcomatoid, as well as osteoclast-like giant cells and trophoblast cells. Okada et al. classified the growth pattern of gallbladder carcinoma in the cystic wall into two groups, infiltrative growth type (IG type) and destructive growth type (DG type). Tumors in DG group have a poorer differentiation with lymphatic metastasis and vascular and perineural invasion, and their prognosis is poor [30] (Fig. 9.18).

9.2.1.5 Immunohistochemistry

Biliary type is often positive for CEA, MUC1, MUC2, p53, and CK7, intestinal type is often positive for CDX2, MUC2, CEA, and CK20, while foveolar type is positive for MUC5AC.

Cystadenocarcinoma

Cystadenocarcinoma of the gallbladder may derive from malignancy of cystadenoma, showing mono- or polycystic masses. The glands of the tumors are lined with epithelium which is similar to well-differentiated carcinoma, with or without varying number of endocrine cells [31]. Radical resection should be conducted with much caution via soft and gender operations to prevent rupture of the cysts and out-

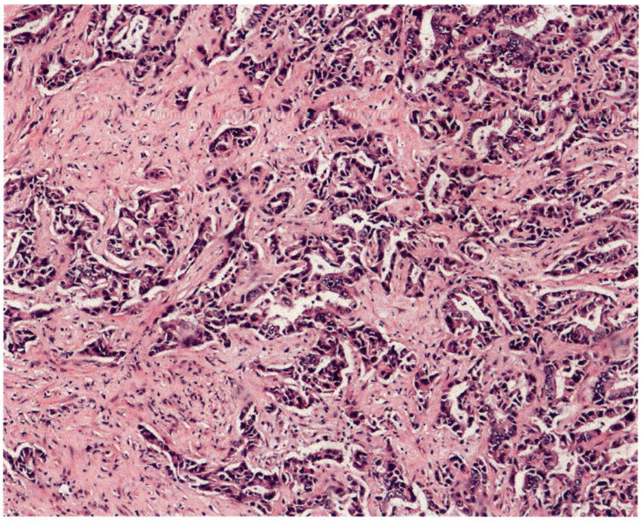

Fig. 9.16 Moderately differentiated gallbladder adenocarcinoma: moderately differentiated adenocarcinoma is a tumor between well- and poorly differentiated adenocarcinomas

flow of the cystic fluid, which can cause implantation and metastasis in the abdominal cavity [5].

Papillary Adenocarcinoma

The tumors are mainly papillary, lined with cubic or columnar epithelium, and they often contain varying amounts of mucus, while the degree of differentiation of the carcinoma cells is also inconsistent (Figs. 9.19 and 9.20). The tumors often show focal intestinal epithelial differentiation, with a large number of goblet cells, endocrine cells, and Paneth cells. Papillary adenocarcinoma grows primarily in the cavities and may fill the cystic cavity before the invasion of the cystic wall.

Intestinal-Type Adenocarcinoma

The tumors form tubular or papillary structures, similar to colonic epithelium, with many goblet cells (Fig. 9.21) and different numbers of endocrine cell and Paneth cells [32].

Mucinous Adenocarcinoma

This type accounts for about 2.5% of gallbladder carcinoma, more common in middle-aged or elderly females. The lesions are large in size with an average diameter of 4.8 cm and are jelly on gross appearance which are similar to colloid carcinoma of the colon. The tumor contains extracellular mucus, which occupies more than 50% of the surface of the tumor. Microscopic observations show three growth patterns: tumorous glands lined with columnar cells, filled with mucus (Fig. 9.22); small clumps or long cords of carcinoma cells, containing abundant mucus, similar to signet ring cells; and mucus lake containing floating carcinoma cell masses. Well-differentiated cases should be differentiated from myxoid cysts or rupture of benign tubular or papillary R-A sinus which is filled with mucus. The prognosis is poor, since diffuse infiltration of cystic wall is often found, resulting in ulceration, perforation, and peritoneal metastasis, and the 3-year survival rate is only 1%. MUC2 can be used as a marker in the differential diagnosis from other gallbladder carcinomas [33].

Clear Cell Carcinoma

Clear cell carcinoma is rare, and the diagnosis could be made after the exclusion of metastasis of renal clear cell carcinoma. The tumors mainly consist of glycogen-containing clear cells, some of which have eosinophilic cytoplasm. The carcinoma cells have clear boundaries and darkly stained nuclei and are arranged in nests, sheets, cords, trabeculaes, tubules, or papilla (Fig. 9.23). Some of these carcinoma cells contain subnuclear vaculoes, similar to secretory phase endometrium, and careful observation helps to find the classic or mucinous adenocarcinoma region, with cells infiltrating the submucosa with partial invasion of adjacent liver tissue. The tumorous stroma contains abundant sinusoids, and obviously hyalinized fibrous septa can be found in deep infiltration area, as well as focal infiltration of lymphocytes. Most of the cases are positive for PAS, CK7, CK20, CEA, and EMA, and a few cases are positive for AFP [34].

Signet Ring Cell Carcinoma

More than 90% of the tumors consist of mucus containing carcinoma cells, and the nuclei are deviated to one side of the cytoplasm forming a signet ring shape, due to the pushing of mucus (Fig. 9.24a–d). The carcinoma cells often arrange in diffuse sheets or nests [35]. A small amount of foam like histocytes may be observed in a few cases, which should be carefully differentiated from signet ring cells.

Adenosquamous Carcinoma

Adenosquamous carcinoma accounts for about 2% of gallbladder carcinomas, which consist of two components, adenocarcinoma and squamous carcinoma, in a varying proportion of different degrees of differentiation. It is generally believed that these two components occupy identical proportion; however, more than 30% of each component should be confirmed based on the consideration of deviation in distribution of tumor cells and sample drawing. Tumors with a certain component accounting for 15–30% can be described as adenosquamous carcinoma, with adenocarcinoma or squamaous carcinoma as predominant component; while those with components accounting for less than 15% should be defined as adenocarcinoma or squamaous carcinoma with other tumorous components. There is a transition between the two components. Squamous carcinoma is nest-like, containing cells of varying sizes with obvious atypia, rich cytoplasm, clear boundaries, marked nucleoli, and visible mitotic figures, with or without keratin

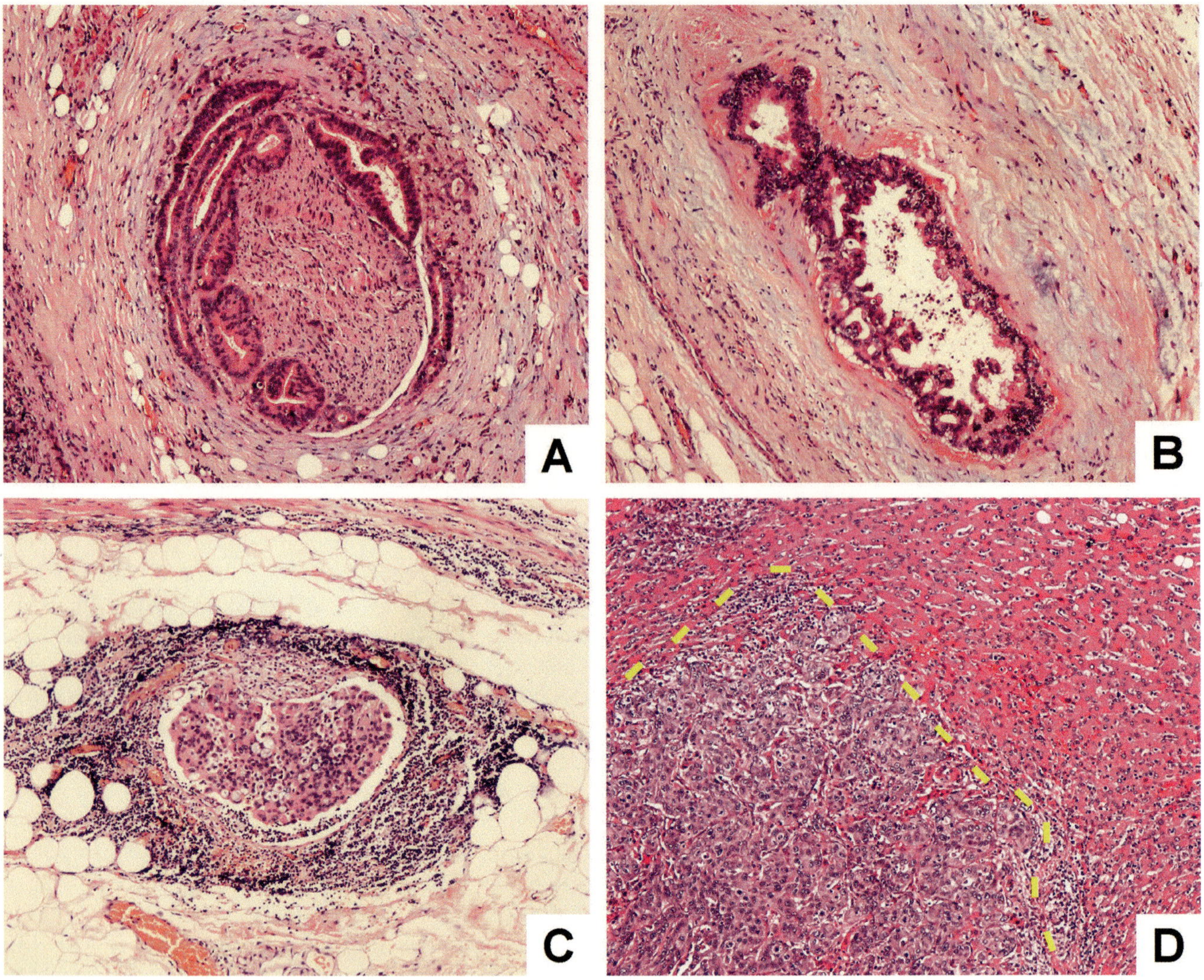

Fig. 9.17 Gallbladder adenocarcinoma: (**a**) perineural infiltration; (**b**) vascular tumor thrombus; (**c**) lymphatic tumor thrombus; (**d**) invasion of the adjacent liver tissue (the *dotted line* shows the boundary)

pearl, keratinization in a single cell and intercellular bridges. Adenocarcinoma component contains tumor cells distributed in irregular glands containing mucus, and the cells are obviously atypic [36] (Fig. 9.25a–b). A few adenosquamous carcinoma may contain endocrine cells. And immunohistochemistry shows that squamous carcinoma component is positive for CK5/6 and CK34βE12, while adenocarcinoma component is positive for CK7 and CEA. Generally, the malignant degree of adenosquamous carcinoma of the gallbladder is much higher than that of common adenocarcinoma, and the prognosis is poor.

Squamous Cell Carcinoma

Squamous cell carcinoma accounts for about 4% of gallbladder carcinomas and is grossly a grayish white, widely invasive mass, often deriving from squamous metaplasia of gallbladder mucosal epithelium. The tumors consist of squamous carcinoma cells [36] (Figs. 9.26 and 9.27) and can be divided into keratinizing and nonkeratinizing type. Generally, the tumor cells are positive for keratin and p63, while some poorly differentiated squamous cell carcinomas are mainly composed of spindle cells, which should be differentiated from some sarcomas, such as malignant fibrous histiocytoma or fibrosarcoma. Pure squamous cell carcinoma should be diagnosed based on careful examination of the specimens and multiple wide sampling, in order to exclude focal and small adenocarcinoma component. Its prognosis is poorer than common adenocarcinoma; however, lymphatic metastasis is rare.

Neuroendocrine Neoplasms (NEN)

The 2010 edition of WHO classification of neuroendocrine tumors of the gallbladder includes neuroendocrine tumor (NET), neuroendocrine carcinoma (NEC), and mixed adeno-

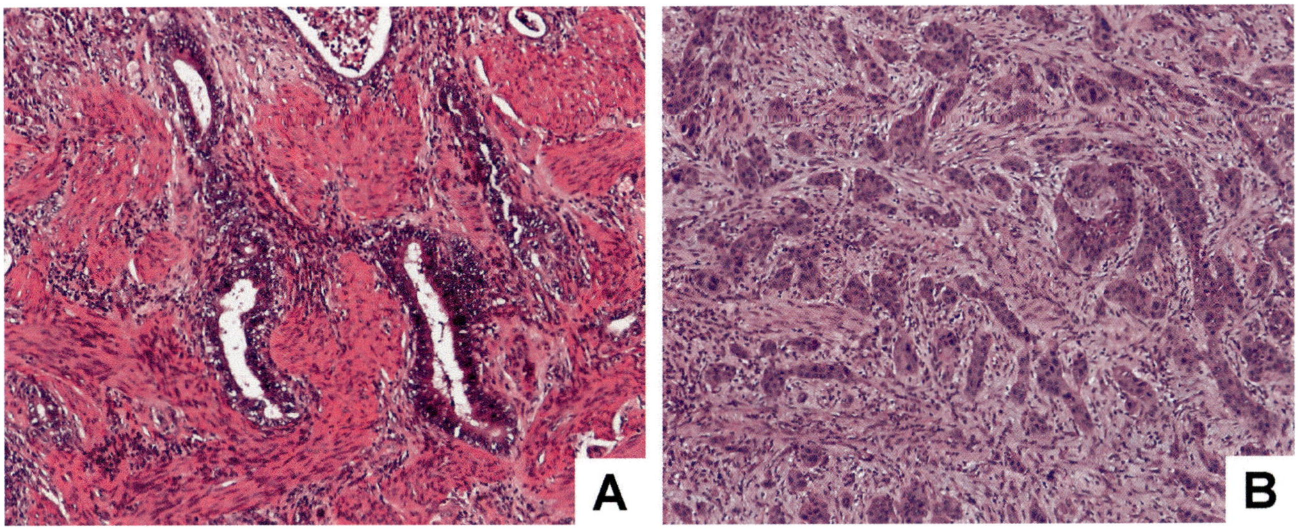

Fig. 9.18 Gallbladder adenocarcinoma: (**a**) cancer cells of IG type show infiltrative growth in the muscle layer (through the intermuscular space) without muscle layer destruction; (**b**) cancer cells of DG type invade the subserosal layer with destruction of the muscle layer. The DG type was accompanied by a stromal desmoplastic reaction which is active and irregular fibrosis due to the tumor invasion

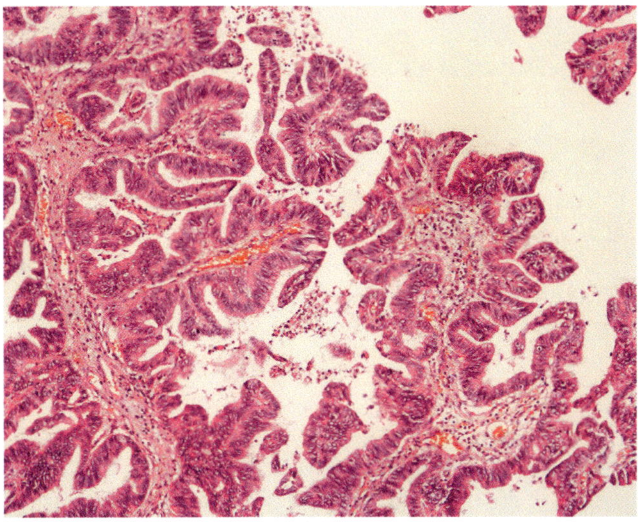

Fig. 9.19 Well-differentiated papillary adenocarcinoma

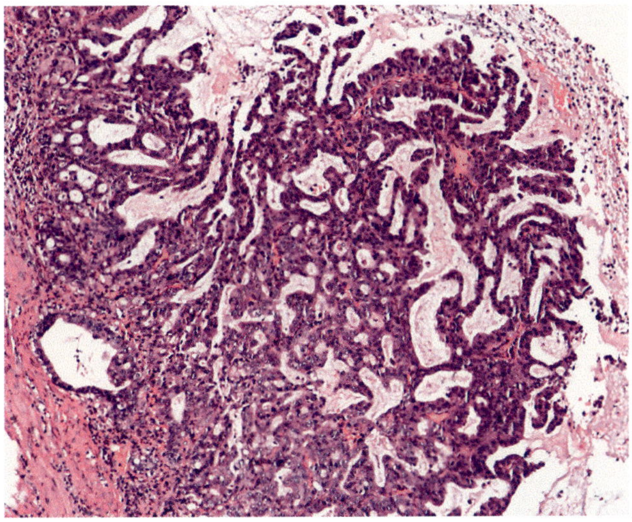

Fig. 9.20 Moderately differentiated papillary adenocarcinoma

neuroendocrine carcinoma (MANEC). Synonyms for NET include carcinoid tumor and well-differentiated endocrine tumors/carcinoma. And NET can also be divided into NET G1 (carcinoid) and NET G2. Synonyms for NEC include poorly differentiated endocrine carcinoma, high-grade neuroendocrine carcinoma, and small- and large cell endocrine carcinoma [12].

Carcinoid was first described by Joel (1929), and about 50 cases of gallbladder carcinoid have been reported in the current literature, considered to be rare tumors accounting for 0.2% of all carcinoids. Carcinoid is often solitary and 0.3–0.5 cm in size, often <2 cm in diameter, grayish white or grayish yellow, and polypoid or nodular in the submucosa. The microscopic images show that the tumor is solid and arranged in nests, cords, and glands. It occasionally grows penetrating the muscular layer. The cells are consistent in size, containing round or oval nuclei, nonobvious nucleoli, and red-stained cytoplasm. And immunohistochemistry shows that it is positive for neuroendocrine markers (Fig. 9.28). Cases of clear cell carcinoid of the gallbladder are rare, and only four cases have been reported in the literature, which were all found in middle-aged males, characterized by a large number of micro-lipid vacuoles in the cytoplasm. Ishida et al. (2012) reported one case of clear cell carcinoid of the gallbladder without VHL (Von Hippel-Lindau disease, an autosomal dominant inherited disease, characterized by clear cell tumors of multiple organs), and the Ki-67 index was only 0.8%. Immunohistochemistry showed that the

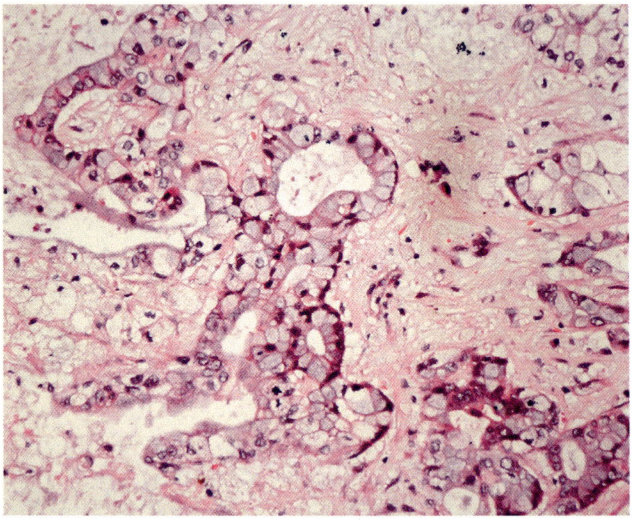

Fig. 9.21 The tumourous glands abound with goblet cells (similar to colonic epithelium)

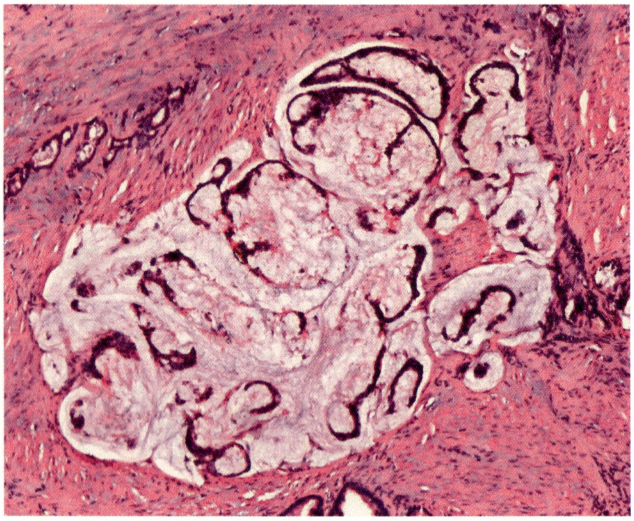

Fig. 9.22 The ruptured tumourous glands are full of mucus

tumor was positive for CgA and Syn, while it was negative for somatostatin and S-100. Furthermore, focal expression of CgA and Syn can be detected in the paratumorous regions with gastric gland metaplasia, while clear cell carcinoid with VHL is positive for somatostatin [37].

Neuroendocrine Carcinoma (NEC)

Neuroendocrine carcinoma is a kind of tumor with strong invasiveness, high degree of malignancy, and poor clinical prognosis. The tumor can be found to invade the liver with lymphatic metastasis even when it is small; however, its clinical manifestations and imaging features show no specificity compared to adenocarcinoma of the gallbladder, and sometimes these two tumors are difficult to distinguish from each other even in histology. Immunohistochemistry shows specific neuroendocrine expression, which is the key point of diagnosis. Surgical resection or systemic chemotherapy is commonly used in the treatment.

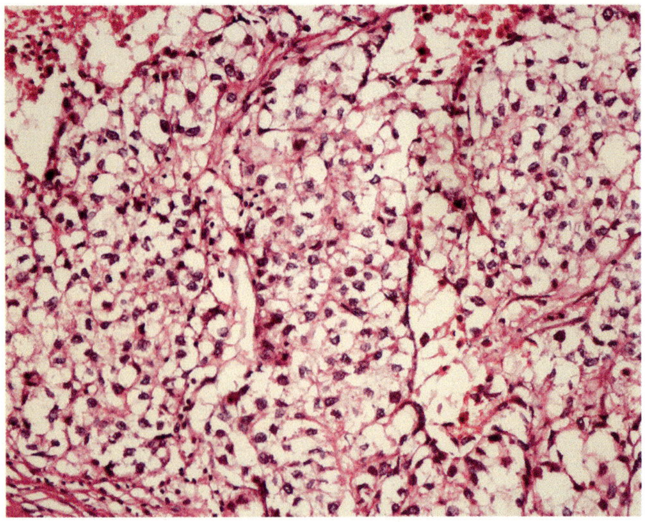

Fig. 9.23 Clear cell carcinoma is arranged in nests, with hyaline cytoplasmic inclusions

1. Small cell neuroendocrine carcinoma (SCNEC) accounts for 0.5–3.5% of malignant tumors of the gallbladder, and less than 100 cases have been reported in the literature, with the onset age of 25–86 years old which is averaged at 67 years old and female patients accounting for 66% [38]. The histomorphology of SCNEC is similar to that of small cell carcinoma of the lung, with poorly differentiated carcinoma cells, which are small round or short spindle cells, arranged in nests, sheets, cords, or ribbons, occasionally with Homer Wright rosettes and tubular structures. Diffuse necrosis and subepithelial invasive growth are the main characteristics. The nuclei are round or oval and darkly stained, with nonobvious nucleoli and common mitotic figures (15–20/10HPF) (Fig. 9.29a, b). Immunohistochemistry shows diffusely positive results for NSE and Syn and scattered positive images for CgA. In addition, tumor cells can also express epithelial markers, such as CK, CEA, AE1/AE3, etc., often with overexpression of p53 gene and loss of expression of pRb. Under electron microscope, the tumor cells contain round and dense core particles surrounded by capsules. And about 22% of the cases contain focal carcinoma areas, with 10% containing squamous cell carcinoma or carcinosarcoma areas, while half the SCNEC of the gallbladder may be complicated by other tumors. SCNEC of the gallbladder is highly malignant, and about 75% of the patients are found to have tumors with invasion of the serosa or metastasis during the operation, of which 90% are with muscular involvement. The average postsurgical

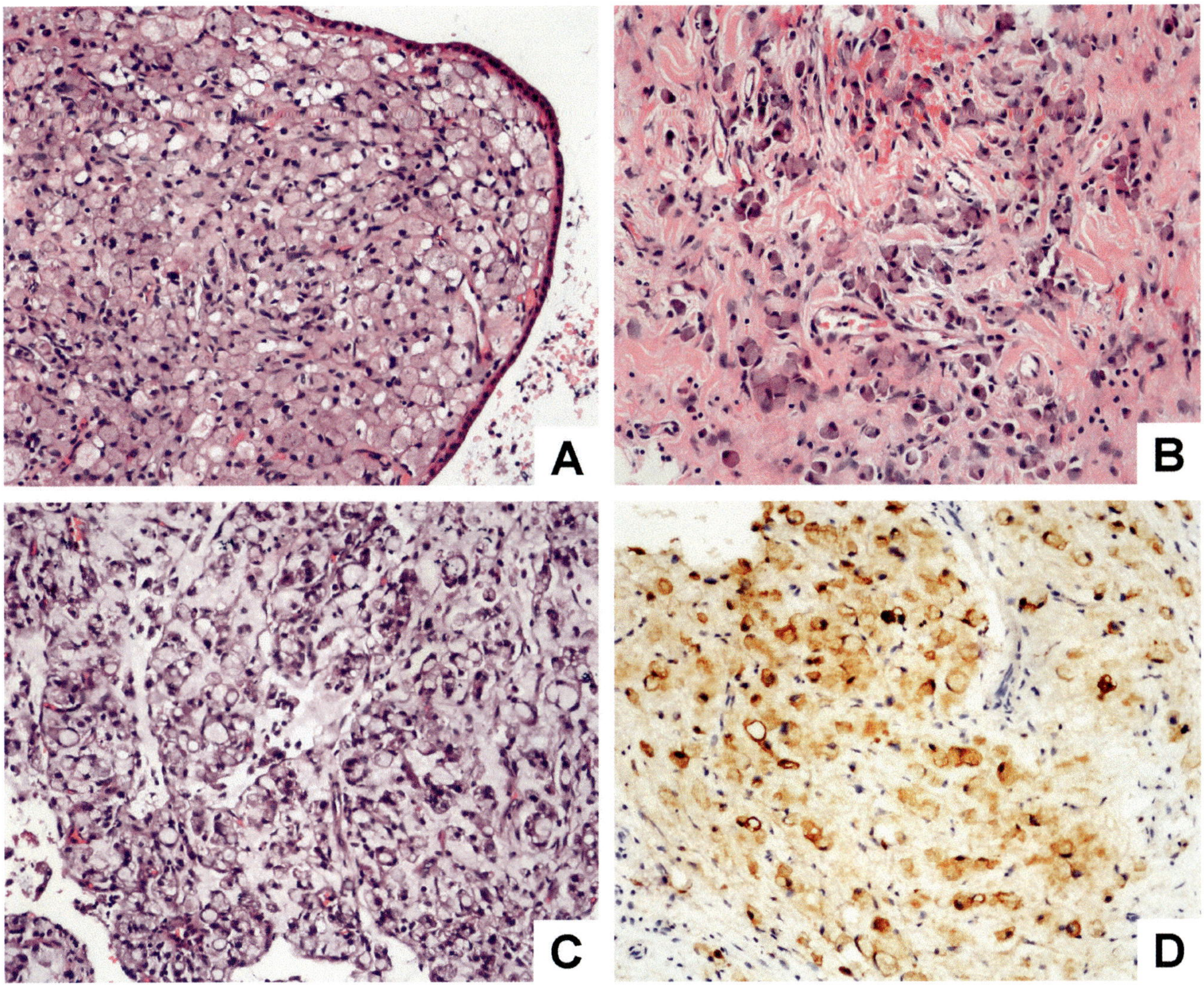

Fig. 9.24 (**a**) The tumor consists of mucus-containing carcinoma cells, arranged in nests under the mucosa; (**b**) muscular invasion; (**c**) the nuclei are deviated to one side of the cytoplasm forming a *signet ring* shape; (**d**) positive staining of *signet-ring-like* cells with epithelial marker CK

survival time for cases with simple surgical resection is 4 months, 1-year survival rate is 21%, and 5-year survival rate is 0 [39].

2. Large cell neuroendocrine carcinoma (LCNEC): LCNEC of the gallbladder was first reported by Papotti et al. in 2000, which accounts for 0.5% of all neuroendocrine neoplasms and 2.1% of all malignant tumors of the gallbladder [39]. The tumor is often organ-like or solid and nest-like, arranged in ribbons, and the tumor cells are often large, polygonal, with abundant eosinophilic cytoplasm, containing large, round or oval nuclei with obvious atypia and vacuoles and obvious nucleoli. Immunohistochemistry shows that it is positive for CD56, Syn, CgA, and CK, with a Ki-67 index>50%. Diffuse necrosis is commonly observable, with or without local regions of adenocarcinoma differentiation. The prognosis of LCNEC is obviously poorer than that of common malignant hepatobiliary tumors [40]. Okuyama et al. (2013) reported one case of a 2.5 cm-in-diameter LCNEC of the gallbladder, with multiple lymphatic, hepatic, and osseous metastasis [41].

Mixed Adenoneuroendocrine Carcinoma (MANEC)

The tumors consist of adenocarcinoma/squamous cell carcinoma and neuroendocrine tumor/carcinoma components. Adenocarcinoma components show varying degrees of differentiation, and the cells include columnar cells, goblet cells, and Paneth cells, forming tubular and papillary structures. PAS and Alcian blue staining show positive results. The squamous cell carcinoma components are nested masses, with or without keratin pearls. The neuroendocrine tumor/carcinoma is positive for NSE, CgA and CD56. Both of the

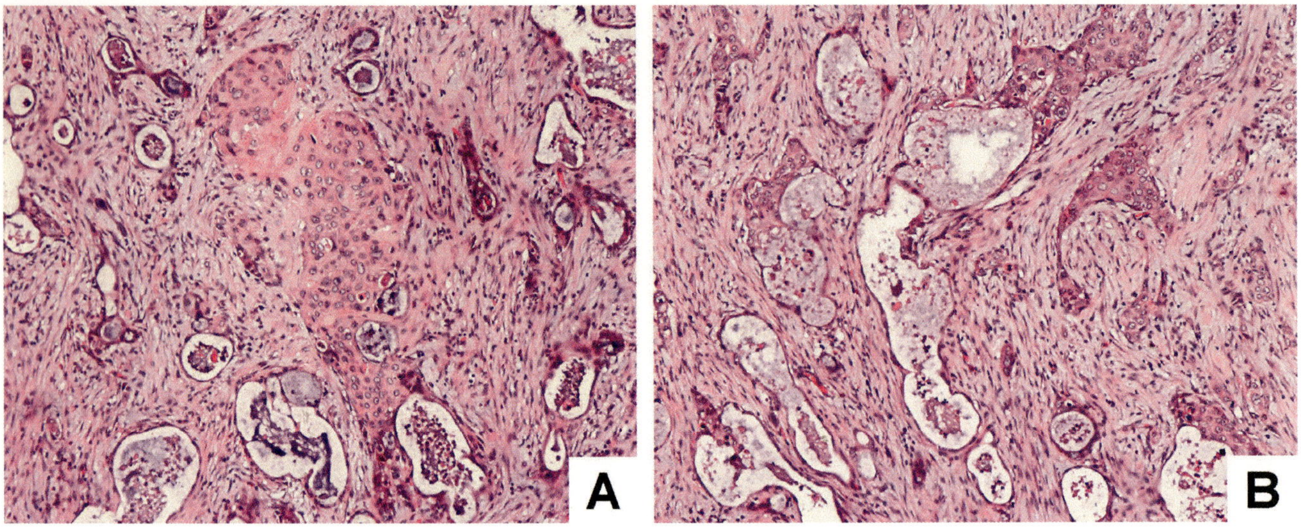

Fig. 9.25 Adenosquamous carcinoma of the gallbladder: (**a**) the tumor consists of two components, well-differentiated glands containing mucus and squamous differentiation regions with keratin pearls and intercellular bridges, and (**b**) there are transitional parts between these two components

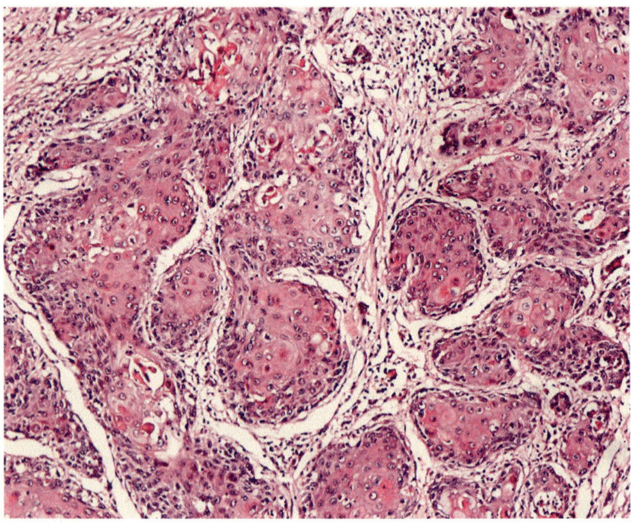

Fig. 9.26 The keratinized squamous carcinoma cells are arranged in nests, in an invasive growth pattern

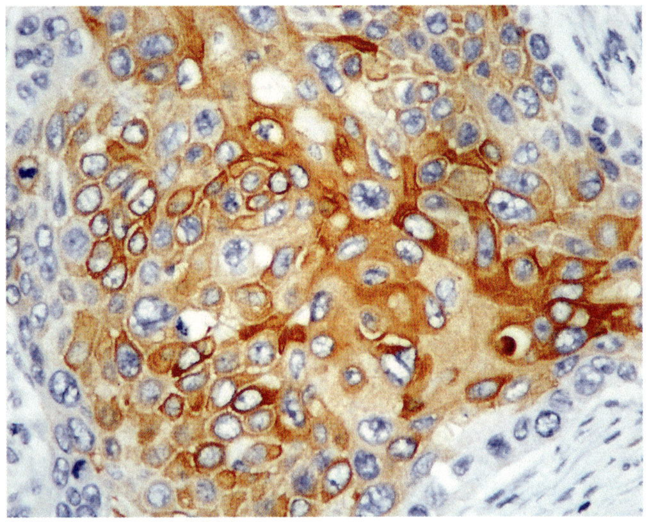

Fig. 9.27 The carcinoma cells are positive for CK19, with intercellular bridges

components can be CEA positive and account for 30% or more in proportion. MANECs may show no symptoms related to hormone hypersecretion. The biological behaviors of MANEC are highly malignant, often with hepatic invasion and lymphatic metastasis. Abe et al. (2013) reported one case of a malignant tumor of the gallbladder containing endocrine cells, adenocarcinoma, squamous cell carcinoma, and sarcoma components [42], speculating that these malignant components in different differentiated directions may derive from a common progenitor cell. In addition, Sośnik et al. (2006) reported a case of dual primary gallbladder carcinoma containing papillary adenocarcinoma and small cell neuroendocrine carcinoma [43].

Undifferentiated Carcinoma

Undifferentiated carcinoma, also known as sarcomatoid carcinoma, pleomorphic carcinoma, giant cell carcinoma, or spindle cell carcinoma, accounts for 5–20% of gallbladder carcinoma. Park et al. (2014) published a group of clinical pathological data, showing that the volume of undifferentiated carcinoma is often larger than that of common adenocarcinoma (5 cm versus 3 cm in average diameter), and the prognosis of the former is poorer than that of the latter (1-, 3-, and 5-year survival rates are 37.5%, 37.5%, and 18.8% versus 84.4%, 65.6%, and52.1%, respectively) [44]. The carcinoma cells are polygonal, spindle, or small cell-like (different from small cell carcinoma, it does not contain neuroendocrine particles) or sometimes contain multinucleated tumor giant cells (including osteoclast-like multinucleated giant cells) (Fig. 9.30), and they are inconsistent in size, with obvious atypia. The tumor cells sometimes form clear bounded nodules and lobules, containing large and vesicular nuclei, obvious nucleoli, similar to malignant lymphoma. About 10% of the cases contain intra- or extracellular PAS-positive translucent bodies, while the latter is positive for alpha fetoprotein. Lesions with osteoclast-like giant cells can also be observed, which is similar to osteoclastoma. Regions with differentiation of squamous cell carcinoma or adenocarcinoma are observed in a few cases. Albores et al. (2006) reported one case of benign giant cell tumor of the gallbladder, which can be differentiated from undifferentiated carcinoma with osteoclast-like giant cells using markers such as

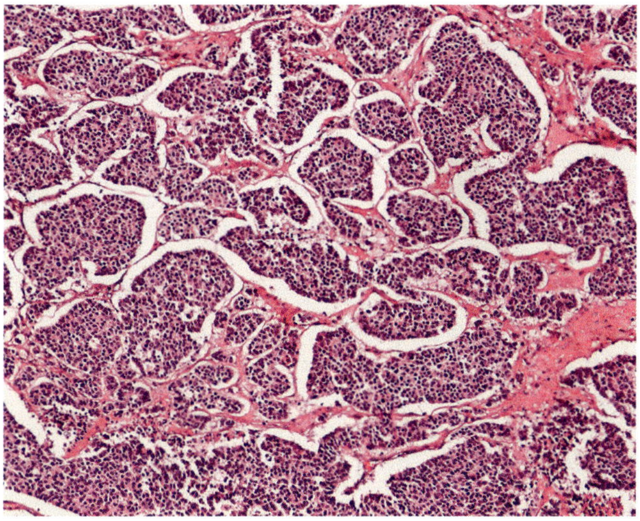

Fig. 9.28 Carcinoid of the gallbladder: the tumor cells are round or polygonal, arranged in nests, and they are consistent in size, with fine granular chromatin, pink cytoplasm, and fibrous stroma

CD163, CD68, HAM56, CK, etc. [45]. Generally, spindle cells or carcinoma cells in pleomorphic carcinoma regions are keratin positive, and lesions with only focal spindle cell and no sarcoma component can be diagnosed as sarcomatoid carcinoma.

Hepatoid Adenocarcinoma

Hepatoid adenocarcinoma is rare, and nine cases have been reported in the literature [46], morphologically identical to hepatoid adenocarcinoma in other organs, such as the stomach. It is highly malignant and tends to undergo hepatic and lymphatic metastasis. Microscopic observation mainly shows that the carcinoma tissues are displayed in trabecular or solid nest arrangement, and carcinoma cells are polygonal or cubic, rich in eosinophilic cytoplasm, similar to hepatocellular carcinoma cells, with or without production of bile and hepatocellular immunophenotypes (Fig. 9.31a–c). Immunohistochemistry shows it is positive for AFP, α1-antitrypsin, HCG, and NSE, and increased serum AFP can also be observed.

Cribriform Carcinoma

Cribriform carcinoma refers to invasive carcinoma with obvious cribriform structure, similar to invasive cribriform carcinoma of the breast in morphology, accounting for less than 1% of gallbladder carcinomas. The onset age for these patients is under that for adenocarcinoma of the gallbladder. And its occurrence is often associated with cholecystitis. The microscopic images show that the tumor cells are arranged in nests with the classic cribriform structure, small and consistent in morphology, containing less cytoplasm, small and round nuclei, and low to moderate degree of polymorphism and atypia. High-grade tumors contain vesicular nuclei, obvious nucleoli, and comedo necrosis. Different from breast

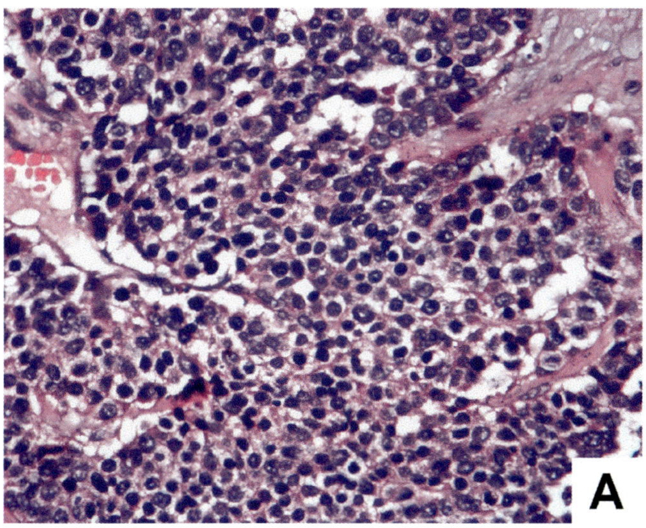

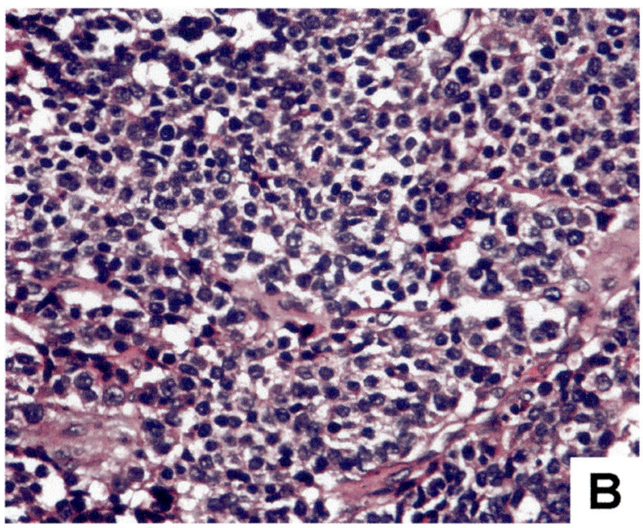

Fig. 9.29 Small cell neuroendocrine carcinoma of the gallbladder: (**a**) the small cells are distributed diffusely, and (**b**) with common mitotic figures

cancer, cribriform carcinoma of the gallbladder does not express estrogen and progesterone receptor [47].

9.2.1.6 Treatment and Prognosis

Researches show that it is insufficient to conduct simple cholecystectomy in patients with T1 (T1a and T1b) gallbladder carcinoma [48], and for gallbladder carcinoma in situ confined in the lamina propria and T1a cases, complete resection is the best choice, receiving a 5-year survival rate of 100%. And for patients with T_{1b} and T_2 tumors confined in the outer perimuscular layer, implementation of radical resection can achieve a 5-year survival rate of 55–90% [49]. However, approximately 80% of gallbladder carcinomas involve metastasis in the liver or other organs at diagnosis. Since the serosa of the gallbladder is weak, and there is no peritoneal covering on the contacting surface with the liver, gallbladder carcinoma tends to invade the adjacent liver tissue, or metastasize to the liver and lung by vascular invasion (cystic vein and portal vein). Lymphatic metastasis is the main migration pathway for the metastasis of gallbladder carcinoma, and 50–80% of gallbladder carcinomas are found to have lymphatic metastasis at surgery. The seventh edition (2010) TNM staging of gallbladder carcinoma (AJCC) grouped the lymph nodes related to metastasis into two groups. The first group includes lymph nodes around the neck of the gallbladder and upper-middle bile ducts, known as portal lymph nodes (N_1), and the second group includes those around the head of pancreas, superior mesenteric artery, and abdominal aortic, known as other drainage lymph nodes (N_2)(Table 9.1). And the prognosis of gallbladder carcinoma is generally poor, for it often has an insidious onset, late discovery, and low resection rate, and the 5-year survival rate is only about 5% [27].

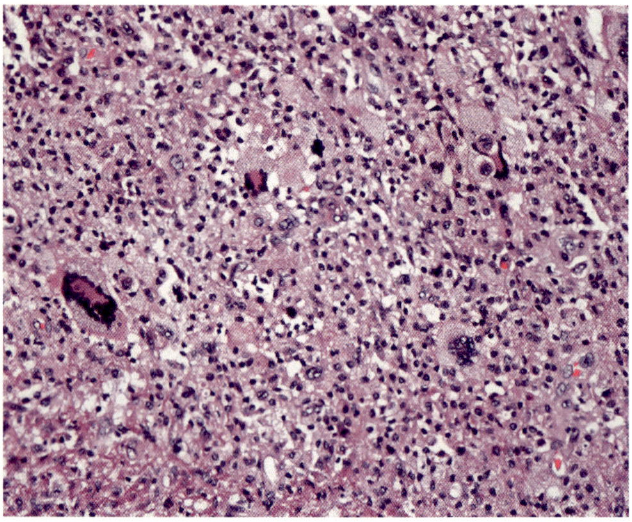

Fig. 9.30 Undifferentiated carcinoma of the gallbladder: the carcinoma cells are polygonal or spindle, with obvious atypia, and including osteoclast-like multinucleated giant cells

There are many factors affecting the prognosis of gallbladder carcinoma, including clinical stage and histological type of the tumor. For example, tumors confined to the gallbladder wall with papillary structures have a better prognosis, while poor prognosis is observed in cases of cystic wall penetrating or invading of the adjacent organs, with distal or lymphatic metastasis and vascular or perineuronal involvement. Also most undifferentiated carcinomas have a poor prognosis, and the median survival period for these patients is only around 6 months. In the aspect of growth pattern, if tumors cells grow by infiltrating among the muscular tissues without destruction of the structure of the gallbladder, the prognosis is significantly better than those that grow in an invasive and destructive pattern [30, 50]; molecular biomarkers such as mutation of 12th codon in oncogene *K-ras*, *APC* mutation, and expression of *PUMA*, *c-Myb*, *p53*, *N-cadherin*, and *P-cadherin* are closely associated with a poor prognosis of gallbladder carcinoma [51, 52]. In addition to surgery, neoadjuvant radiochemotherapy can be used to treat patients with advanced tumors. And reverse intensity-modulated radiation therapy (IMRT) can be adopted to improve the survival time [53]. It has been shown that single or combined chemotherapy of drugs, including *K-ras* downstream mole-

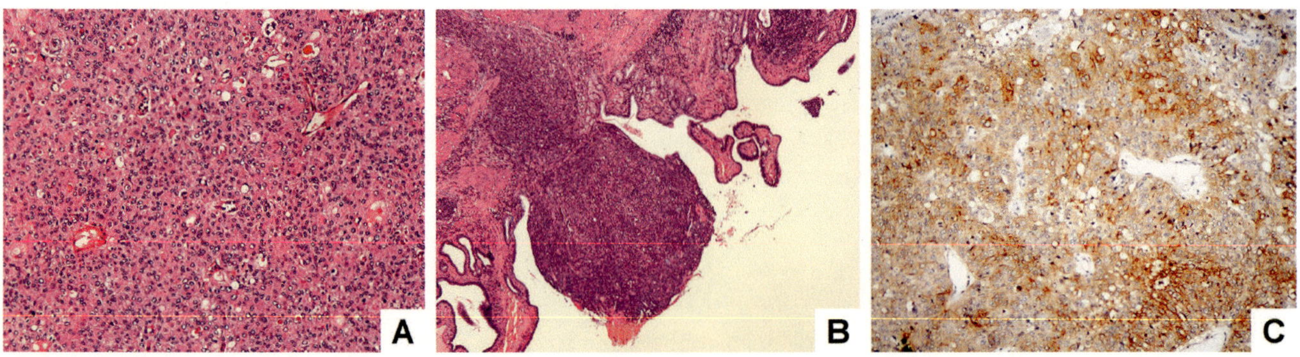

Fig. 9.31 Hepatoid adenocarcinoma of the gallbladder: (**a**) the carcinoma cells are polygonal or cubic, rich in eosinophilic cytoplasm, similar to hepatocellular carcinoma cells; (**b**) the tumor cells grow infiltratively under the mucosa; (**c**) the tumor cells are positive for GPC-3

Table 9.1 AJCC TMN staging of gallbladder carcinoma (2010)

Stage	TNM	Depth	Regional lymph node status	Distant metastases
0	Tis	In situ	None	None
Ia	$T_{1a}N_0M_0$	<Lamina propria	None	None
Ib	$T_{1b}N_0M_0$	<Muscular layer	None	None
II	$T_2N_0M_0$	<Perimuscular tissue; no extension beyond serosa or into the liver	None	None
IIIa	$T_3N_0M_0$	>Serosa and/or directly invades the liver and/or other adjacent organ or structure	None	None
IIIb	$T_{1\text{-}3}N_1M_0$	Any	Positive nodes along cystic duct bile, common bile duct, hepatic artery, and/or portal vein	None
IVa	$T_4N_0M_0$	Invades main portal vein, hepatic artery, or ≥ two extrahepatic organs/structures	None	None
	$T_2N_1M_0$	≤perimuscular tissue; no extension beyond serosa or into the liver	Positive nodes along cystic duct bile, common bile duct, hepatic artery, and/or portal vein	No
IVb	$T_{1\text{-}3}N_2M_0$	Any	Positive nodes: periaortic, pericaval, superior mesenteric artery and/or coeliac artery lymph nodes	None
	$T_{1\text{-}3}$ $N_{1\text{-}2}$ M_1	Any	Any	Yes

Reprint with permission from Compton, Gallbladder, Springer, 2012
TNM tumor-node-metastasis, *Tis* tumor in situ

cules in raf/MAPK signaling pathway targeted drugs, e.g., sorafenib, EGFR/HER2 targeted small molecular tyrosine kinase inhibitor gefitinib and monoclonal antibodies cetuximab and panitumumab, IGF-IR/PI3K signaling pathway targeted inhibitors, and antitumor angiogenesis targeted drugs, which aim at thymidine phosphorylase, may be the future direction of development in the individualized multimolecular targeted therapies for gallbladder carcinoma [54–60].

9.2.2 Malignant Mesenchymal Tumors of the Gallbladder

Over 100 cases of malignant mesenchymal tumors of the gallbladder have been reported in the current literature, accounting for about 1.5% of malignant tumors of the gallbladder [61]. And over 40 cases of gallbladder sarcoma have been reported, with a median diameter of 4.5 (2–14) cm. The median age of adult patients is 68.5(24–88) years old, while pediatric patients are aged 1.5–3 years old [62].

9.2.2.1 Leiomyosarcoma (LMS)

Griffon et al. (1897) reported the first case of LMS of the gallbladder, the incidence of which accounts for 0.14% in malignant lesions of the gallbladder. More than 20 cases of LMS of the gallbladder have been reported in the literature by 2012 [63], and it is the most common type of gallbladder sarcoma. The male to female ratio in the patients is 1:5, and the onset age is often 50–60 years old. Its pathogenesis may be related to infection of EBV. Clinical manifestations include right upper abdominal pain which is the main symptom, right upper abdominal masses, jaundice, or weight loss which are found in a few cases. On gross appearance, the tumors can be as large as 15 cm in diameter, and the sections are fishlike, grayish white or grayish red, with common hemorrhage and necrosis, or occasional cystic degeneration, often with invasion of the liver or common bile duct or metastasis to the adjacent lymph nodes and other organs. Under the microscope, the tumor cells are densely distributed with regions mainly consisting of spindle cells or polygonal cells, containing eosinophilic cytoplasm. Multinucleated giant tumor cells can be observed in rare cases. Mitotic figures are common. Perez-Montiel et al. (2004) reported one case of leiomyosarcoma which was malignant transformed from smooth muscle cells with adenomyomatous hyperplasia of the gallbladder [64]. Most of the leiomyosarcoma lesions are positive for desmin, H-caldesmon, and SMA; however, they should be differentiated from other spindle cell tumors, including fibrosarcoma, undifferentiated carcinoma (EMA, keratins, CEA positive), carcinosarcoma (AE1/AE3, CK, vimentin positive), gastrointestinal stromal tumors of the gallbladder (CD117, CD34, Dog-1 positive), etc. Al-Daraji et al. (2009) reported that LMS of the gallbladder may also be associated with infection of EBV [62]. LMS is highly malignant, and the incidence of LMS involving the liver reaches 75%. The 5-year survival rate of these patients is <5% [63].

9.2.2.2 Rhabdomyosarcoma (RMS)

Biliary RMS is relatively common, while RMS of the gallbladder is rare with only less than ten cases having been diagnosed. The reported cases are often elder females who are older than 60 years old and complicated by gallstones, while a few cases concern children, with tumors invading the liver or metastasis to lymph nodes or other organs at the time of diagnosis. These reported cases of RMA of the gallbladder include acinar type, embryonic type, mixed acinar/embryonic type, and botryoid RMS, and the latter is the same with biliary RMS showing protrusion into the cystic cavity [65] (Fig. 9.32a, b). Myo D1 (myoregulatory protein) and Myf4 (skeletal muscle-specific myogenin) are highly specific and sensitive for the diagnosis, and positive staining for both markers is located in the nuclei. RMS is highly malignant with a poor prognosis.

9.2.2.3 Angiosarcoma

Angiosarcoma of the gallbladder is rare, and 12 cases have been reported in the English literature by 2009 [62, 66–68]. It is a highly invasive vascular endothelial malignant tumor. The gallbladder wall can be as thick as 1.5 cm due to involvement of the tumor, with diffuse ulcer and necrosis of the mucosa, and hemorrhage and fibrous effusion on the serosa. The microscopic images show that the tumor cells are arranged in solid structures containing irregular cavities. The tumor cells can be epithelioid, with large, round or oval and vesicle nuclei and single and marked eosinophilic nucleolus; the mitotic figures are commonly observed.

9.2.2.4 Kaposi Sarcoma (KS)

KS is a malignant spindle cell tumor deriving from vascular endothelial cells, and infection of human herpesvirus 8 (HHV-8) is the main cause. Currently, less than five cases of primary KS of the gallbladder have been reported, and the patients were often around the age of 30 years old with AIDS [69].

9.2.2.5 Malignant Hemangiopericytoma

Gupta et al. reported one case of malignant hemangiopericytoma of the gallbladder in 1983 [70]. In 2001, Li-guo Sun et al. reported one case of a 29-year-old male patient with a 15 cm × 8 cm malignant hemangiopericytoma of the gallbladder, which was surgically excised. The tumor grew outward of the cavity and was fishlike. The microscopic observation showed that it contained abundant perithelial cells with atypia and staghorn-like interstitial blood vessels. In addition, Nestler G et al. (2007) reported one case of myogenic sarcoma with the morphology of hemangiopericytoma, and the immunohistochemistry showed that it was positive for vimentin and SMA, finally confirming it as a tumor with myogenic or myofibroblastic differentiation [71].

9.2.2.6 Liposarcoma

Jie Ma et al. (1996) reported one case of a 62-year-old female patient with a 16 cm × 14 cm × 9 cm myxoid liposarcoma of the gallbladder, which was surgically excised and weighted

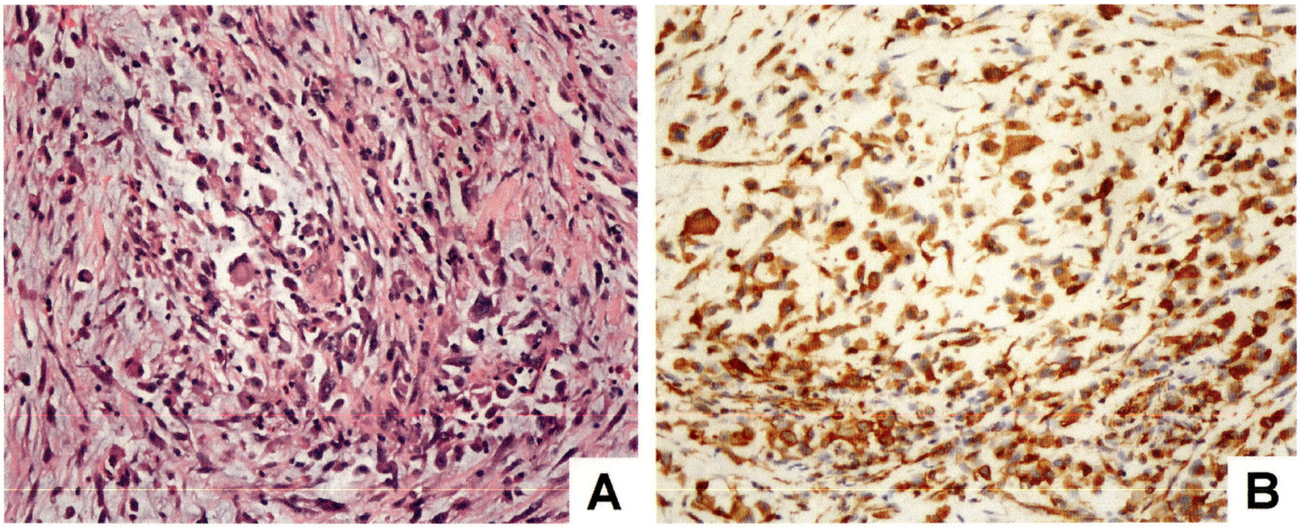

Fig. 9.32 Rhabdomyosarcoma of the gallbladder: (**a**) rhabdomyoblasts are elongated or round cells, exhibiting an embryonic morphology and containing eosinophilic granular cytoplasm rich in thick and thin filaments. (**b**) RMS cells are positive for myoglobin

1050 g. The microscopic images showed that the tumor consisted of spindle or round tumor cells scattered in the myxoid background, containing immature and claw-shaped blood vessels, with visible lipoblasts and multinucleated giant cells. Takashi et al. (2006) also reported one case of a huge liposarcoma of the gallbladder, which was 25 cm × 23 cm in size, and microscopic examination confirmed it was pleomorphic liposarcoma, with no mucus. The cells are spindle with obvious atypia, while some of them had the features of lipoblasts. Hamada et al. (2006) reported another case of 25 cm × 23 cm liposarcoma of the gallbladder which was surgically resected, and it was found to invade the muscular layer of the gallbladder wall [72]. Due to postsurgical recurrence in the liver and metastasis to the lung, the patient received a hepatectomy 10 months after the first surgery and a partial resection of the liver and the lung 29 months later, and the patient recovered well and was in healthy condition during the 3 years and 6 months' postsurgical follow-up.

9.2.2.7 Carcinosarcoma

Carcinosarcoma accounts for less than 1% of malignant gallbladder tumors, and less than 100 cases have been reported in both the foreign and domestic literatures [73, 74]. The tumor consists of sarcoma (vimentin positive) and adenocarcinoma (CK positive) components. The carcinoma component can be adenocarcinoma with or without squamous differentiation or squamous cell carcinoma, while the sarcoma component can be diverse, including leiomyosarcoma, fibrosarcoma, rhabdomyosarcoma, angiosarcoma, osteosarcoma, chondrosarcoma, and neurosarcoma. The proportions of the two components can be referred to adenosquamous carcinoma of the gallbladder (Fig. 9.33). Immunohistochemistry shows that different components express corresponding markers. Mesenchymal components are CK and CEA negative, which helps to make differential diagnosis from sarcomatoid carcinoma with spindle cells or giant cells. And if the mesenchymal part is sarcoma component and epithelial part is benign, the tumor is called as adenosarcoma. As to the histogenesis and pathogenesis, it is generally suggested that it is generated via dual differentiation of pluripotent stem cells to carcinoma and sarcoma, while it is also suggested that it derives from the malignant transformation of epithelial component or is the result of malignant transformation of both epithelial and mesenchymal components [75]. Carcinosarcoma is highly malignant, and invasion and metastasis can be found in early stages; thus, complete surgical resection should be implemented. For patients with carcinosarcoma of the gallbladder confined in the muscularis propria of the mucosa, the postsurgical 5-year survival rate can reach as high as 88.9% [73].

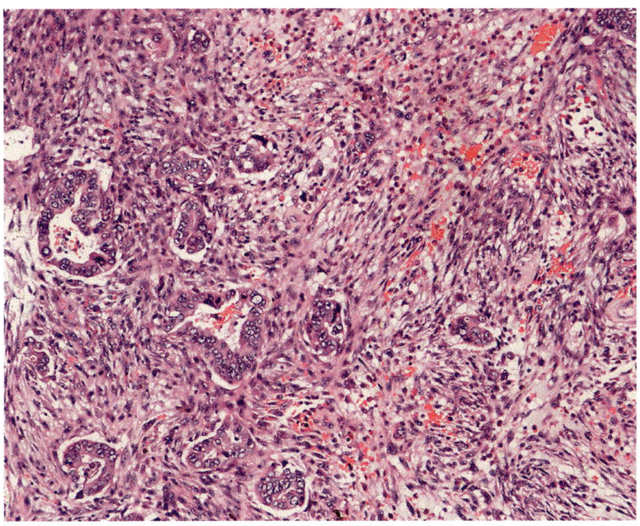

Fig. 9.33 Carcinosarcoma of the gallbladder: the carcinoma component is adenocarcinoma and the sarcoma component is fibrosarcoma

9.2.2.8 Adenosarcoma

Several cases of adenosarcoma of the gallbladder have been reported in domestic literature, and the basic characteristic of this tumor is a mixture of benign glands and spindle sarcomatoid stroma around the glands, showing a sleeve-like growth pattern, similar to the adenosarcoma in the uterus (Fig. 9.34a, b).

9.2.2.9 Malignant Melanoma

Hambi and Wieting reported the first case of primary malignant melanoma of the gallbladder in 1907, and only over 20 cases of this tumor have been reported in current English literature, and three cases have been found in domestic literature. Primary malignant melanoma of the gallbladder should be solitary and single tumor, deriving from mucosa, and generally papillary or polypoid, protruding into the cavity. It can metastasize to the common bile duct. And the most important diagnostic criterion is the existence of a junctional nevus-like region in the lesions (in the junctional region of epithelium and lamina propria, the melanoma cells are distributed in nests or sheets). Immunohistochemistry shows that the tumor is positive for HMB45, S-100, and vimentin, and Masson-Fontana-specific staining shows the intra- and extracellular melanin granules of the tumor cells. Primary malignant melanoma of the gallbladder has a poor prognosis, identical to that of the skin or mucosal cases, which is associated with the extension of infiltration, dissemination, and metastasis. Surgical resection is the main treatment method, and the 5-year survival rate of malignant melanoma is about 5% [76].

9.2.2.10 Lymphoma

Gallbladder lymphoma is rare, accounting for 0.1–0.2% of malignant biliary tumors. Over 50 cases of gallbladder lymphoma have been reported in foreign literature. The median

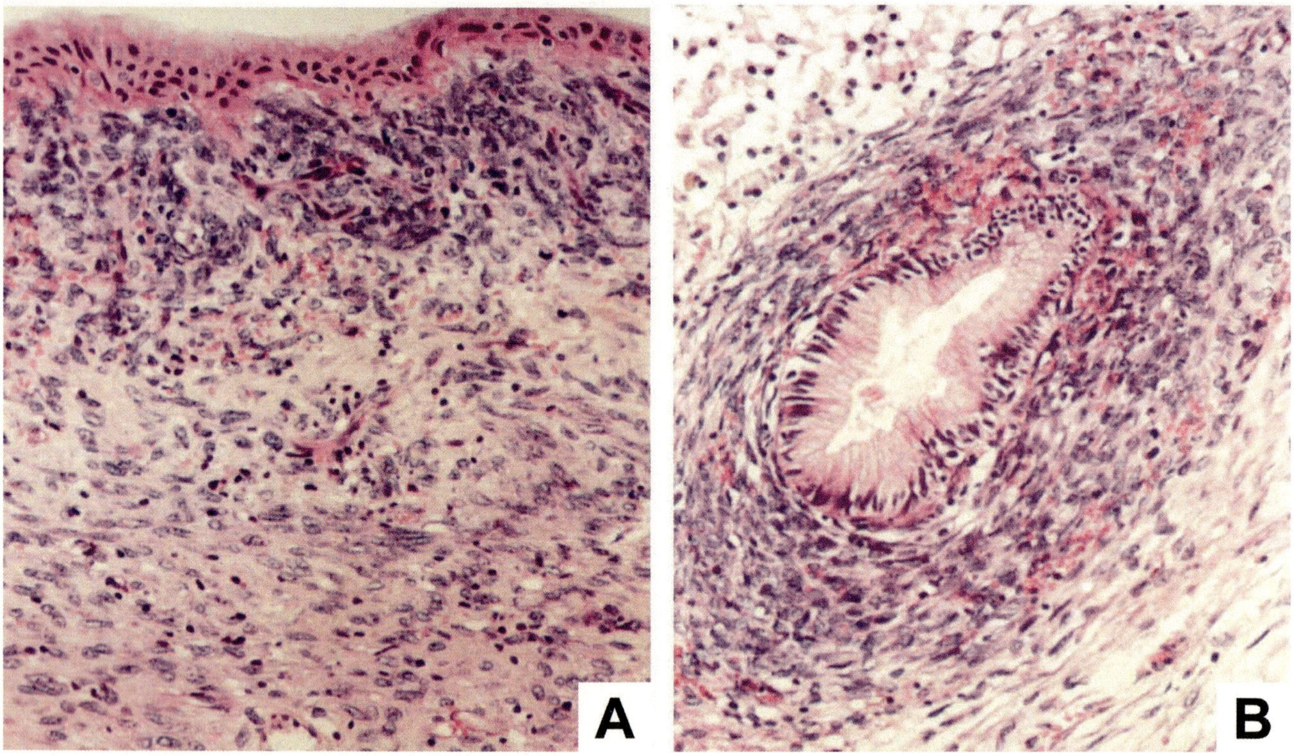

Fig. 9.34 A the sarcoma cells are spindle; B the spindle sarcomatoid cells are around the benign glands, showing a sleeve-like growth pattern

onset age is 63 (4–91) years old, and 54% of the patients have gallstones. The gross appearance of the tumor is mainly the thickened wall of the gallbladder, and the common histological types include diffuse large B-cell lymphoma, mucosa-associated lymphoid tissue lymphoma, extranodal marginal zone B-cell lymphoma, B lymphoblastic lymphoma, follicular lymphoma, etc. [77]. The pathogenesis may involve chronic bacterial inflammation of gallbladder mucosa, leading to formation of lymphoid follicles, and continuous antigenic stimulation results in mutation in lymphocytes.

9.2.2.11 Malignant Fibrous Histiocytoma (MFH)

Kristofferson (1983) reported the first case of MFH of the gallbladder, and Al-Daraji et al. reported that a total of 16 cases of MFH of the gallbladder have been found in the literature by 2009 [62], with pleomorphic MFH and myxoid MFH as the most common types, a male to female ratio of 5:11, and an average age of 66.8 (4–82) years old. The lesions are 2–14 cm in diameter and often single nodular. The histological morphology and immunohistochemistry phenotypes are the same with those in other organs, presenting a poor prognosis. However, Gruttadauria et al. (2001) reported one case which received surgical resection and chemotherapy with 46 weeks' disease-free survival period during the follow up.

9.2.2.12 Gastrointestinal Stromal Tumors (GIST)

Primary GIST of the gallbladder is extremely rare, and about ten cases of GIST of the gallbladder have been reported in the foreign literature [78]. GIST is a group of tumors with spontaneous differentiation and deriving from Cajal interstitial cells. Microscopic observation shows various kinds of spindle cells in interwoven bundles, mingled with sheet or focal epithelioid cells. Furihata et al. (2005) reported one case of malignant stromal tumors of the gallbladder with rhabdoid differentiation characteristics [79]. In the diagnosis of the disease, despite the diagnostic criteria of general GIST in morphology and immunohistochemistry, exclusion of gastrointestinal metastasis should be made. Currently, the volume of GIST (2 cm) and mitotic figures (5/50HPF) are the core indexes to make the risk evaluation. Most of the malignant GIST of the gallbladder are positive for Kit, and immunohistochemistry staining of CD117 (c-kit), Dog-1, and CD34 and testings of c-kit or PDGFRA gene mutations contribute to the diagnosis, evaluation of prognosis, prediction of the effects of targeted drugs, and treatments. Most of the Kit-positive GIST are sensitive for imatinib, and 80% of the GIST cases containing PDGFRA mutations are resistant to imatinib [80].

9.2.2.13 Ewing Sarcoma/Primitive Neuroectodermal Tumor (ES/PNET)

Song et al. reported a case of ES/PNET of the gallbladder in 2004 [81], concerning a 53 year old female patient, with a polypoid tumor of 7 cm × 4 cm × 3.5 cm in size and located on the bottom of the gallbladder. The section was grayish white, crisp in texture, with obvious necrosis. Under the microscope, the tumor consisted of diffuse sheets of monomorphic small round cells, mixed with fibrous and vascular stroma, as well as focal necrosis, common mitotic figures (20/10 HPF), and large amounts of characteristic Homer Wright rosette structures (Fig. 9.35). Immunohistochemistry showed that tumor cells were positive for MIC2/CD99, NSE, and Syn. The electron microscopic observation showed no neuroendocrine particles, without chromosome translocation of t(11; 22)(q24;q12) and t(21;22)(q22;q12). The patients presented no postsurgical recurrence during the 3 months of follow up.

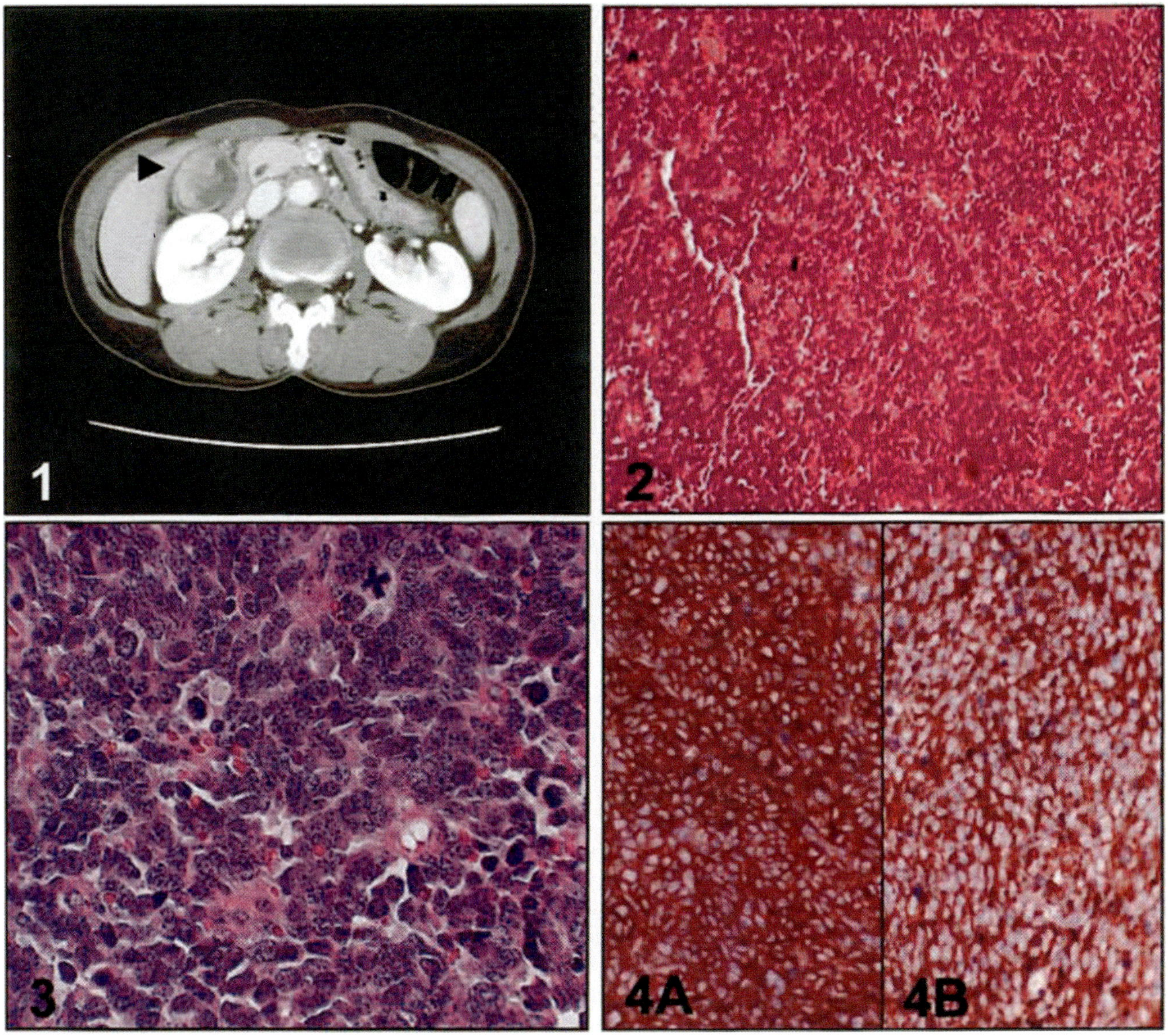

Fig. 9.35 (*1*) An abdominal and pelvic computed tomographic scan shows an intraluminal polypoid mass of the gallbladder with heterogenous enhancement (*arrowhead*). (*2*) The tumor shows diffuse sheets of monotonous small round cells with Homer Wright rosettes (hematoxylin-eosin, original magnification ×100). (*3*) The tumor cells have coarse or fine powdery chromatin, scanty cytoplasm, and inconspicuous nucleoli (hematoxylin-eosin, original magnification ×400). (*4*) The tumor cells demonstrate a diffuse, positive membranous immunoreactivity for MIC2 gene product (A) and positive cytoplasmic immunoreactivity for synaptophysin (B) (original magnifications ×200) (Cited from Song et al. [81])

9.3 Tumor-Like Lesions of the Gallbladder

9.3.1 Gallbladder Polyps

9.3.1.1 Pathogenesis and Mechanism

The pathogenesis of gallbladder polyps (GP) is complex, closely related to inflammation, gallstones, and cholesterol metabolism. With the advanced technology of medical examination, GP is easier to be discovered. GP accounts for 1–10% of surgically excised specimens in cholecystectomy, and the so-called pseudopolyps of the gallbladder belong to tumor-like lesions [2]. According to histological feature, GP can be divided into cholesterol polyps (50–90%), hyperplastic/metaplastic polyps (25%), granulation tissue polyps (12–15%), fibrous polyps (15%), and lymphoid polyps (<5%).

9.3.1.2 Clinical Features

Lymphoid polyps are common in female patients aged 65 (50–80) years old on average, and clinical manifestations mainly include symptoms due to chronic cholecystitis and cholelithiasis. Granulation tissue and fibrous polyps are mainly found in females older than 50 years old, while cholesterol polyps are commonly found in females aged 40–50 years old.

9.3.1.3 Gross Features

Cholesterol Polyp

Cholesterol polyps are small mulberry like, yellow in color, with thin pedicle connecting to the gallbladder, solitary or multiple, often <1 cm in diameter. Despite the small size, the polyps can be discovered via B-ultrasound and CT examination. Most of the cholesterol polyps are complicated by diffuse cholesterol deposition, while focal cholesterol deposition or gallstones can be found in a few cases.

Adenomatous Polyp

Generally, the diameter of adenomatous polyp is often <0.5 cm, multiple, with a pedicle or sessile and focal, granular, or villous projections.

Inflammatory Polyp

Also known as granulation tissue polyp, inflammatory polyps are often with wide pedicles connecting to the gallbladder. And few lesions are bigger than 1 cm in diameter, complicated by acute or chronic cholecystitis or xanthogranulomatous cholecystitis and gallstones.

Fibrous Polyp

Generally, fibrous polyp is often larger than inflammatory polyps, complicated by gallstones and chronic cholecystitis. Kim et al. (2003) reported a case of fibrous polyp of the gallbladder, with 1.2 cm × 0.8 cm in size which was excised via surgical resection [82].

Lymphoid Polyp

Lymphoid polyp can be solitary or multiple, showing small nodules prominent from the mucosa, 2–5 mm in diameter, with pedicles on the base, usually accompanied by chronic cholecystitis.

Mixed Polyp

It is a mixture of different types of polyps with the maximum diameter of 15 mm.

9.3.1.4 Microscopic Features

Cholesterol Polyps

The pedicle consists of vascular connective tissues, and the polyps contain varying numbers of villous projections, and lipid-phagocytized foamlike macrophages, lined with normal gallbladder epithelium (Fig. 9.36a, b).

Hyperplastic/Metaplastic Polyps

Hyperplastic/metaplastic polyps are often the nodular hyperplasia of pyloric gland, or papillary hyperplasia of gallbladder epithelium, or both, with or without intestinal metaplasia and/or metaplasia. Different from gallbladder adenomas, adenomatous polyps consist mainly of proliferated tall columnar epithelial structure (Fig. 9.37), with no obvious boundaries or fibrous capsule, and the papillary structure is less marked than adenoma, which is small with pedicles.

Granulation Tissue Polyps

Granulation tissue polyps often have a wide pedicle connected to the gallbladder, which contain abundant small blood vessels and inflammatory cells, such as neutrophils, lymphocytes, eosinophilic granulocytes, and plasma cells (Fig. 9.38).

Fibrous Polyps

Fibrous polyps are often lobulated, consisting of scattered glands or ductal structures and fibrous stromal components (Fig. 9.39), lined with gallbladder epithelium. In the fibrous stroma, varying degrees of edema can be observed, scattered with inflammatory cells, such as lymphocytes, similar to phyllodes tumors or fibrous adenomas of the breast.

Lymphoid Polyps

The proliferated lymphatic tissues form lymphoid follicles, with large germinal centers, lined with a layer of normal gallbladder epithelium, also known as lymphatic pseudotumor. Lymphoid polyps are often complicated by lymphatic hyperplasia of gallbladder mucosa, and the proliferated lym-

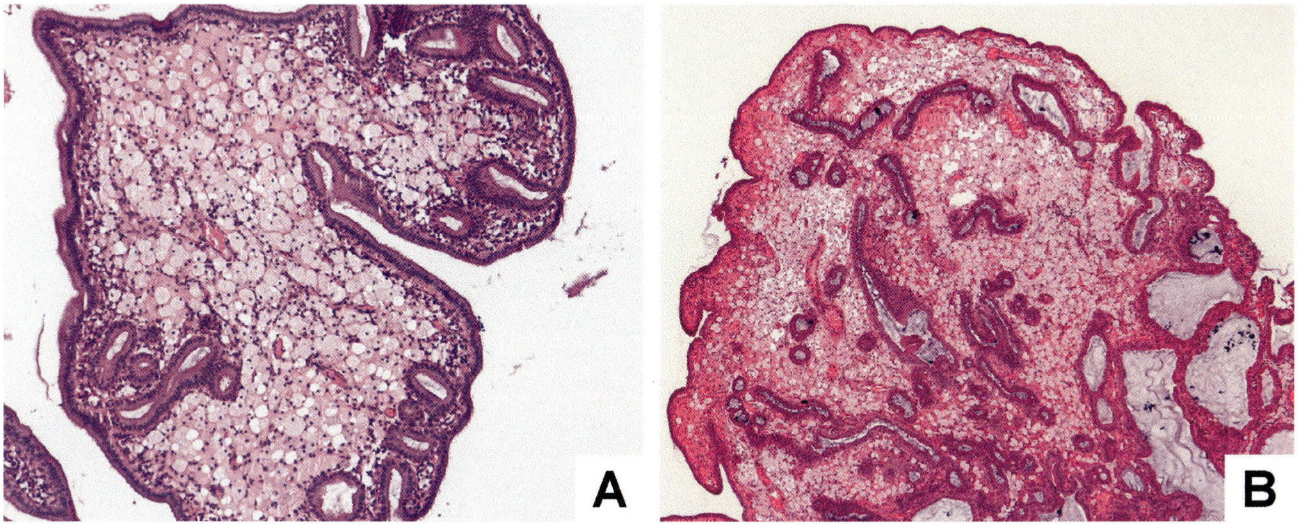

Fig. 9.36 Cholesterol polyps: (**a**) the polyps contain lipid-phagocytized foamlike macrophages; (**b**) the glands of the polyps are dilated, with mucus inside the glandular lumens

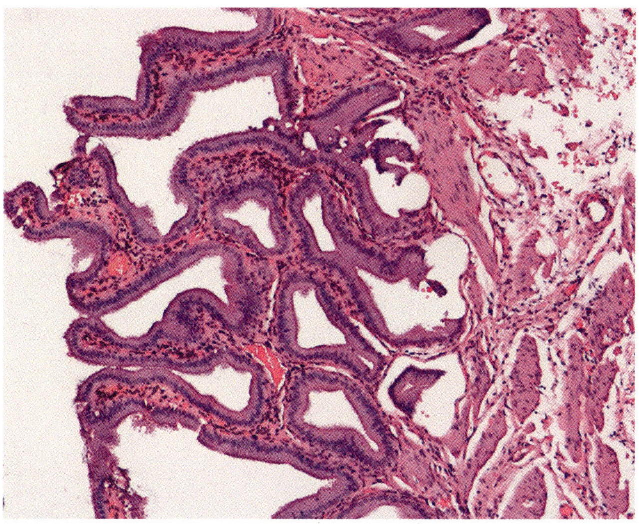

Fig. 9.37 Adenomatous polyps: adenomatous polyps consist mainly of proliferated tall columnar epithelium, forming pseudopapillary structures

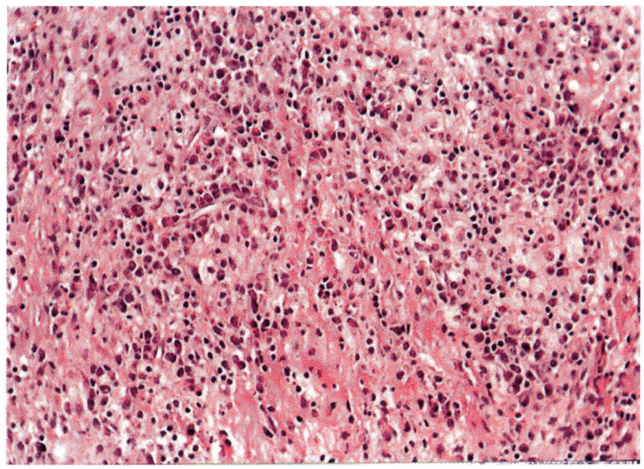

Fig. 9.38 Granulation tissue polyps: granulation tissue polyps contain abundant fiber connective tissues and inflammatory cells

phatic tissues can be confined to the lamina propria or even deep into the muscular layer of serosa.

Mixed Polyps

For instance, tubular adenoma component is complicated with cholesterol polyps (Fig. 9.40).

9.3.1.5 Differential Diagnosis

The pathological diagnosis is not difficult; however, the existence of dysplasia of the mucosal epithelium of the gallbladder should be carefully identified.

9.3.1.6 Treatment and Prognosis

In general, the canceration rate of the hyperplastic polyps/adenoma is about 0.2%, while malignant transformation of other kinds of polyps is rare. However, one case of cholesterol polyp of the gallbladder was reported to undergo malignant transformation in China (1999), which is worth to pay attention to.

9.3.2 Adenomyomatous Hyperplasia

9.3.2.1 Pathogenesis and Mechanism

Adenomyomatous hyperplasia (AMH), also known as adenomyomatosis or diverticulosis, refers to invagination or extraversion of the gallbladder mucosa, transversing through

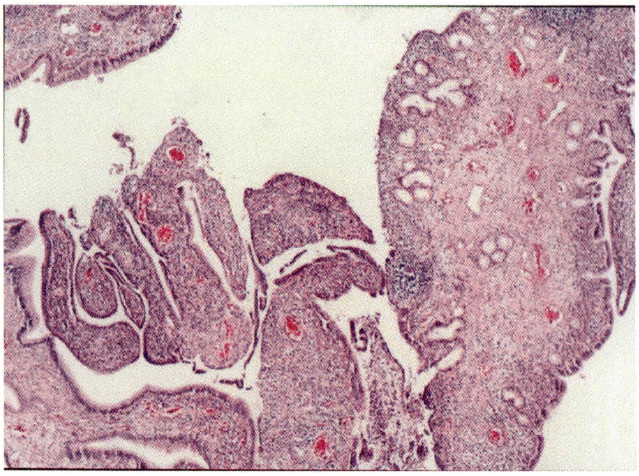

Fig. 9.39 Fibrous polyps: fibrous polyps consist of scattered glands or ductal structures and fibrous stromal components

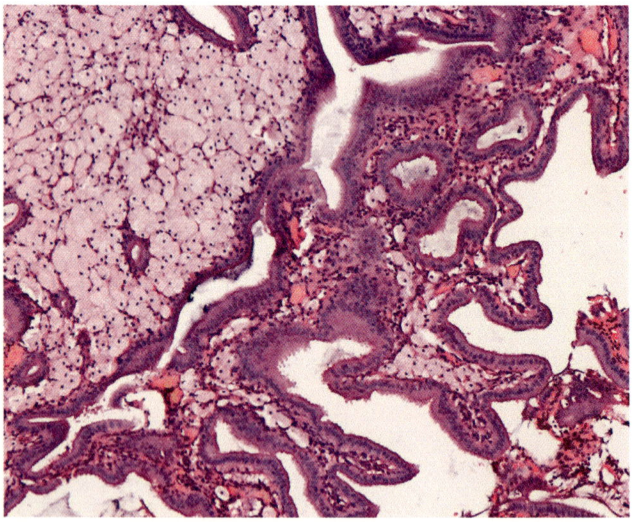

Fig. 9.40 The polyps consist of abundant foamlike macrophages and proliferative glands, forming pseudopapillary structures

intramuscular connective tissues complicated by smooth muscle hyperplasia, while focal nodular AMH was also known as adenomyoma [15]. More than 80% of the cases show varying degrees of chronic cholecystitis, suggesting that the disease is associated with hyperplasia of mucous glands and muscular layer, induced by long-term stimulation of chronic inflammation of the gallbladder, and gallstones are also a key pathogenic factor of AMH. The pathogenesis is related to abnormal contraction of gallbladder muscle or increased intracystic pressure caused by other factors.

9.3.2.2 Clinical Features

The vast majority of the patients have no obvious clinical symptoms, and some patients may come for diagnosis and treatment because of cholelithiasis-related symptoms. Some cases are discovered due to chronic cholecystitis or suspected gallbladder tumor, especially in cholecystectomy for gallbladder carcinoma.

9.3.2.3 Gross Features

Adenomyomatous hyperplasia of the gallbladder can be divided into diffuse, segmental, and focal type. Diffuse type: the lesions may involve the whole gallbladder, with the gallbladder wall as thick as five times the normal thickness and significant hyperplasia of Rokitansky-Aschoff sinus. Segmental type: lesions often involve a certain part of the gallbladder, with marked thickened wall of the involved regions. Focal type: also known as adenomyoma which is characteristically located on the bottom of the gallbladder, forming nodules with a diameter of 0.5–2.5 cm, and the section is grayish white, with multiple visible cystic cavities. The whole lesion can be hidden in the subserosa without capsules. Nishimura A et al. (2004) studied 156 cases of adenomyoma of the gallbladder and found the close relationship between segmental hyperplasia and chronic cholecystitis, suggesting the possible association of the structure and the result of gallstones [83].

9.3.2.4 Microscopic Features

It consists of Rokitansky-Aschoff sinus (columnar or cubic epithelium lined glands) and hyperplastic smooth muscle bundles in hybrid arrangement. The superficial epithelium often shows papillary hyperplasis, discontinuous with the inferior Rokitansky-Aschoff sinus, and the epithelium shows no atypia (Fig. 9.41). In chronic cholecystitis, invagination of the mucosa epithelium into the muscular layer often forms a few small Rokitansky-Aschoff sinuses (tubular structure without expanded cystic cavities), confined in the superficial part of the muscular layer, and no proliferated smooth mus-

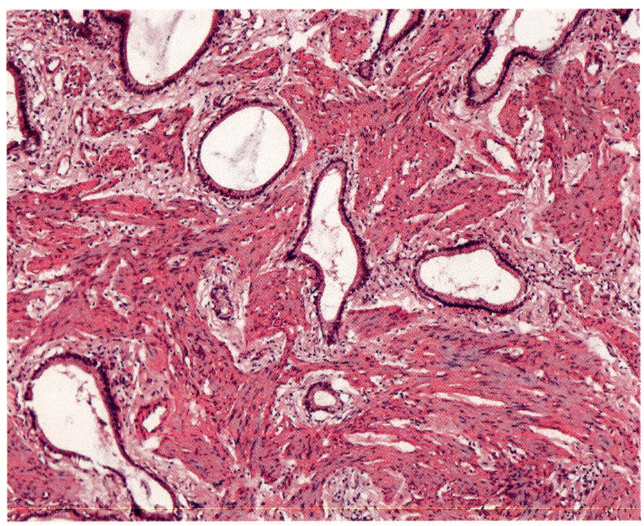

Fig. 9.41 Adenomyomatous hyperplasia of the gallbladder: the glands and smooth muscle bundles highly proliferated in hybrid arrangement, and the epithelium shows no atypia

cle tissue can be found around the Rokitansky-Aschoff sinus. The muscle tissue is intact in structure and arrangement, while adenocarcinoma of the gallbladder shows obvious atypia of the cells and tissues, without circular hyperplasia of smooth muscle, and the carcinoma tissues invade or destruct the gallbladder wall. Adenomyoma of the gallbladder or adenomyomatous hyperplasia is often complicated by severe dysplasia or carcinogenesis, characterized by normal superficial epithelium without atypia, but the underlying Rokitansky-Aschoff sinuses are dilated into cysts containing mucus or condensed bile, which are covered by tumorous biliary epithelium or columnar mucous epithelium.

9.3.2.5 Differential Diagnosis

The pathological diagnosis is not difficult; however, it should be carefully distinguished from well-differentiated adenocarcinoma with muscular infiltration. And when adenomyomatous hyperplasia shows focal epithelial atypia and pyloric gland metaplasia, or the glands are adjacent to or around nerve tissues, it should be noted that the lesions are not true neural invasion, and misdiagnosis of adenocarcinoma should be avoided. The lesions are generally without atypia, and it is helpful in the differential diagnosis to find Rokitansky-Aschoff sinuses which do not destruct the smooth muscle bundles and mild morphology of the large majority of the epithelial cells [84].

9.3.2.6 Treatment and Prognosis

Though adenomyoma of the gallbladder/adenomyomatous hyperplasia with severe atypical hyperplasia or adenocarcinoma is rare, a few cases have been reported occasionally [15, 85]. In principle, huge adenomyomatous hyperplasia of the gallbladder should be treated by cholecystectomy.

9.3.3 Xanthogranulomatous Cholecystitis

Xanthogranulomatous cholecystitis was first reported by Christensen and Ishak in1970, the histogenesis of which is diffuse or focal inflammatory lesions caused by effusion of bile from damaged Rokitansky-Aschoff sinuses into the gallbladder wall. The single nodular lesion can be up to2.5 cm in diameter, protruding from the surface of the gallbladder mucosa, connected to the wall via a wide pedicle on the bottom, or high thickening of the gallbladder wall (Fig. 9.42), often complicated by cholelithiasis. This disease can not be easily differentiated from malignant tumors based on clinical or imaging data, even on gross appearance. Inflammation can involve tissues out of the gallbladder wall, forming diffuse adhesion. Some cases show elevated tumor marker of CA19–9; thus, it may be easily misdiagnosed as gallbladder carcinoma. The microscopic observation shows formation of histiocytic granuloma in the deep muscular layer, consisting

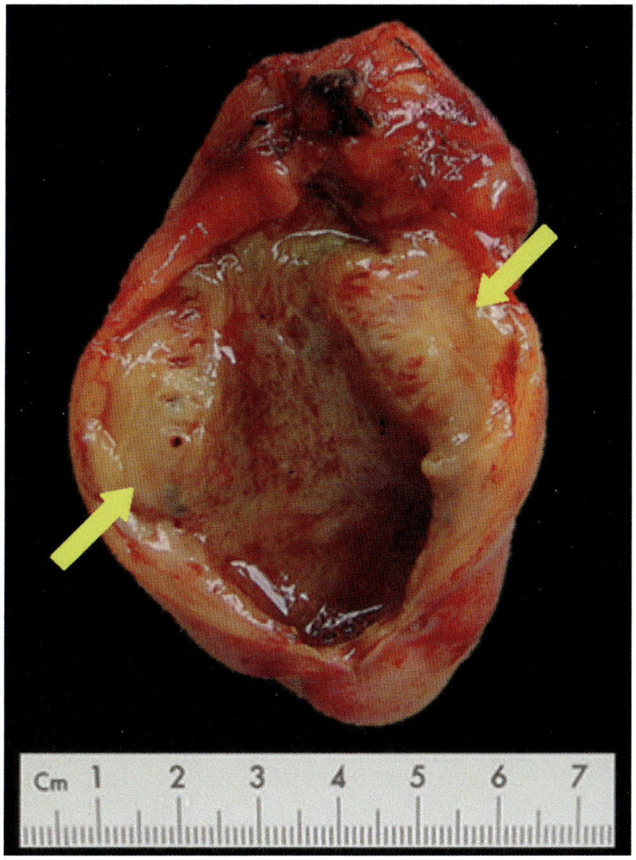

Fig. 9.42 Xanthogranulomatous cholecystitis: the gallbladder wall is highly thickened, and the lesion is grossly a *grayish yellow*, nodular mass

of lipoids and hemosiderin phagocytosed foamlike histocytes, Touton multinucleated giant cells, varying numbers of inflammatory cells, and fibrous tissues (Fig. 9.43a, b). The pathological diagnosis is not difficult, which should exclude the differential diagnosis of adenomyoma of the gallbladder, fibrosarcoma, malignant fibrous histiocytoma, and inflammatory myofibroblastic tumor. When it is difficult to make the diagnosis, immunohistochemistry labeling of histocyte marker, such as CD68, can facilitate the differential diagnosis of benign or malignant tumor, and differentiation should also be made from granulomatous lesions caused by tuberculosis, fungi, and parasites. Currently, multiple reports of the disease complicated with adenocarcinoma of the gallbladder have been reported [86, 87]; thus, particular attention should be paid in intraoperative frozen-section examination. Immunohistochemistry shows low expression of p53 and PCNA and membrane positive staining for β-catenin, which is different from the expression pattern of the gallbladder carcinoma. Generally xanthogranulomatous cholecystitis is not considered as a precancerous lesion of gallbladder carcinoma [88].

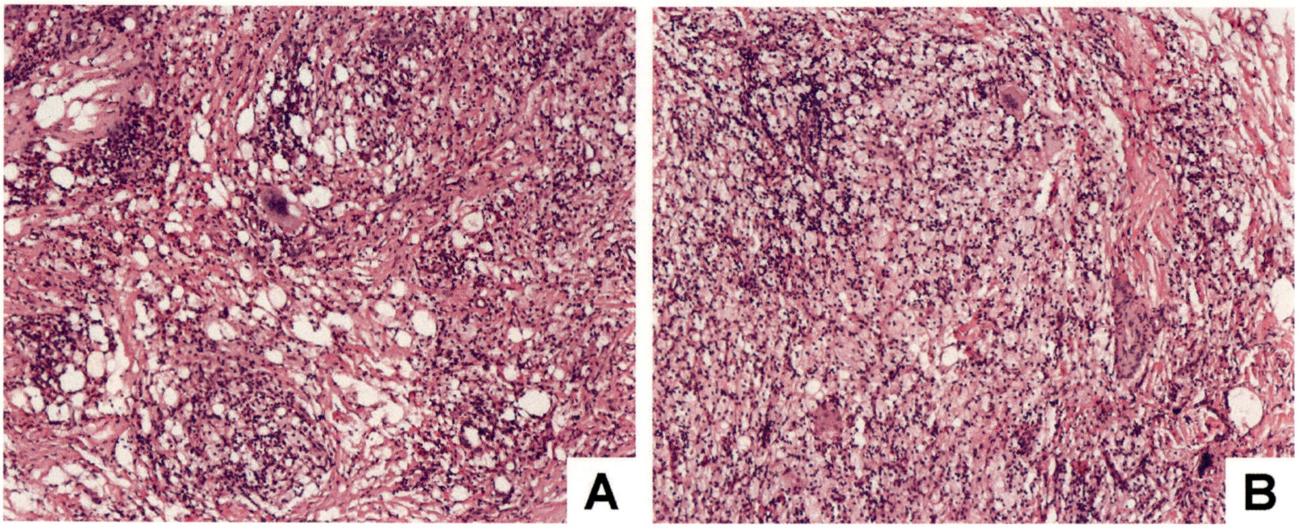

Fig. 9.43 Xanthogranulomatous cholecystitis: the lesion consists of foamlike histocytes, Touton multinucleated giant cells, varying numbers of inflammatory cells, and fibrous tissues (**a** & **b**)

In addition, rare cases of endometriosis of the gallbladder have been reported, and the microscopic lesions show endometrial glands and stroma, with deposition of hemosiderin, macrophage reaction, and fibrous hyperplasia [89].

References

1. Kwon W, Jang JY, Lee SE, et al. Clinicopathologic features of polypoid lesions of the gallbladder and risk factors of gallbladder cancer. J Korean Med Sci. 2009;24(3):481–7.
2. Sarkut P, Kilicturgay S, Ozer A, et al. Gallbladder polyps: factors affecting surgical decision. World J Gastroenterol. 2013;19(28):4526–30.
3. Acharya V, Ngai J, Whitelaw D, et al. Primary gallbladder lymphoma presenting as a polyp. BMJ Case Rep. 2014;2014:bcr2013202715.
4. Cheng Y, Jia Q, Xiong X, et al. Gallbladder tubulovillous adenoma in a patient with liver fluke infection. J Gastrointestin Liver Dis. 2013;22(4):374.
5. Adsay V, Jang KT, Roa JC, et al. Intracholecystic papillary-tubular neoplasms (ICPN) of the gallbladder (neoplastic polyps, adenomas, and papillary neoplasms that are >/=1.0 cm): clinicopathologic and immunohistochemical analysis of 123 cases. Am J Surg Pathol. 2012;36(9):1279–301.
6. Gokalp G, Dusak A, Topal NB, et al. Cystadenoma originating from the gallbladder. J Ultrasound Med. 2010;29(4):663–6.
7. Donthireddy KR, Ailawadhi S, Nasser E, et al. Malignant gastroparesis: pathogenesis and management of an underrecognized disorder. J Support Oncol. 2007;5(8):355–63.
8. Roa I, De Aretxabala X, Araya JC, et al. Preneoplastic lesions in gallbladder cancer. J Surg Oncol. 2006;93(8):615–23.
9. Hirata K, Ajiki T, Okazaki T, et al. Frequent occurrence of abnormal E-cadherin/beta-catenin protein expression in advanced gallbladder cancers and its association with decreased apoptosis. Oncology. 2006;71(1–2):102–10.
10. Kim K, Kim DH, Chae SW, et al. Expression of cell cycle-related proteins, p16, p53 and p63 as important prognostic markers in gallbladder adenocarcinoma. Pathol Oncol Res. 2013;20:409.
11. Pai RK, Mojtahed K. Mutations in the RAS/RAF/MAP kinase pathway commonly occur in gallbladder adenomas but are uncommon in gallbladder adenocarcinomas. Appl Immunohistochem Mol Morphol. 2011;19(2):133–40.
12. Albores-Saavedra J, Kloppel G, Adsay NV, et al. Carcinoma of the gallbladder and extrahepatic bile ducts. In: Bosman FT, Carneiro F, Hruban RH, et al., editors. WHO classification of tumours of the digestive system. Lyon: International Agency for Research on Cancer (IARC); 2010. p. 266–78.
13. Nakanishi Y, Zen Y, Kawakami H, et al. Extrahepatic bile duct carcinoma with extensive intraepithelial spread: a clinicopathological study of 21 cases. Mod Pathol. 2008;21(7):807–16.
14. Zhao H, Davydova L, Mandich D, et al. S100A4 protein and mesothelin expression in dysplasia and carcinoma of the extrahepatic bile duct. Am J Clin Pathol. 2007;127(3):374–9.
15. Albores-Saavedra J, Shukla D, Carrick K, et al. In situ and invasive adenocarcinomas of the gallbladder extending into or arising from Rokitansky-Aschoff sinuses: a clinicopathologic study of 49 cases. Am J Surg Pathol. 2004;28(5):621–8.
16. Segovia Lohse HA, Cuenca Torres OM. Prevalence and sequence of metaplasia-dysplasia-carcinoma of the gallbladder. A single centre retrospective study. Cir Esp. 2013;91(10):672–5.
17. Furukawa H. Leiomyoma, lipoma, myxoma, and fibroma of the gallbladder. Ryoikibetsu Shokogun Shirizu. 1996;1996(9):333–4.
18. Wachter DL, Buttner MJ, Grimm K, et al. Leiomyoma of the gallbladder: a case report with review of the literature and discussion of the differential diagnosis. J Clin Pathol. 2010;63(2):177–9.
19. Crucitti A, La Greca A, Antinori A, et al. Cavernous hemangioma of the gallbladder. Case report and review of the literature. Tumori. 2005;91(5):432–5.
20. Xia N-x, Qiu B-a, Liu P, et al. One case analysis of gallbladder lipoma. World Chin J Digestol 2008, 16(7): 796-797.
21. Sucandy I, Sharma D, Dalencourt G, et al. Gallbladder neurofibroma presenting as chronic epigastric pain - Case report and review of the literature. N Am J Med Sci. 2010;2(10):496–8.
22. Baker C, Bhagwat P, Wan A. Mesenteric paraganglioma with gallbladder paraganglion nest. J Surg Case Rep. 2012;2012(3):8.
23. Murakata LA, Ishak KG. Expression of inhibin-alpha by granular cell tumors of the gallbladder and extrahepatic bile ducts. Am J Surg Pathol. 2001;25(9):1200–3.
24. Boskovski MT, Saad A, Israel GM, et al. Lymphangioma of the gallbladder in adults: review of the literature and a case report. J Gastrointest Surg. 2012;16(3):663–8.

25. Stinton LM, Shaffer EA. Epidemiology of gallbladder disease: cholelithiasis and cancer. Gut Liver. 2012;6(2):172–87.
26. Maurya SK, Tewari M, Mishra RR, et al. Genetic aberrations in gallbladder cancer. Surg Oncol. 2012;21(1):37–43.
27. Hundal R, Shaffer EA. Gallbladder cancer: epidemiology and outcome. Clin Epidemiol. 2014;6:99–109.
28. Gabbi C, Kim HJ, Barros R, et al. Estrogen-dependent gallbladder carcinogenesis in LXRbeta−/− female mice. Proc Natl Acad Sci U S A. 2010;107(33):14763–8.
29. Park SK, Andreotti G, Rashid A, et al. Polymorphisms of estrogen receptors and risk of biliary tract cancers and gallstones: a population-based study in Shanghai. China Carcinog. 2010;31(5):842–6.
30. Okada K, Kijima H, Imaizumi T, et al. Clinical significance of wall invasion pattern of subserosa-invasive gallbladder carcinoma. Oncol Rep. 2012;28(5):1531–6.
31. Waldmann J, Zielke A, Moll R, et al. Cystadenocarcinoma of the gallbladder. J Hepato-Biliary-Pancreat Surg. 2006;13(6):594–9.
32. You Y, Bui K, Bui MM, et al. Histopathological and immunophenotypical features of intestinal-type adenocarcinoma of the gallbladder and its precursors. Cancer Control. 2014;21(3):247–50.
33. Dursun N, Escalona OT, Roa JC, et al. Mucinous carcinomas of the gallbladder: clinicopathologic analysis of 15 cases identified in 606 carcinomas. Arch Pathol Lab Med. 2012;136(11):1347–58.
34. Miyazawa M, Torii T, Toshimitsu Y, et al. Alpha-fetoprotein-producing clear cell carcinoma of the extrahepatic bile ducts. J Clin Gastroenterol. 2006;40(6):555–7.
35. Ohno Y, Kumagi T, Kuroda T, et al. Signet-ring cell carcinoma of the gallbladder complicated by pulmonary tumor thrombotic microangiopathy. Intern Med. 2014;53(11):1125–9.
36. Roa JC, Tapia O, Cakir A, et al. Squamous cell and adenosquamous carcinomas of the gallbladder: clinicopathological analysis of 34 cases identified in 606 carcinomas. Mod Pathol. 2011;24(8):1069–78.
37. Ishida M, Shiomi H, Naka S, et al. Clear cell neuroendocrine tumor G1 of the gallbladder without von Hippel-Lindau disease. Oncol Lett. 2012;4(6):1174–6.
38. Mahipal A, Gupta S. Small-cell carcinoma of the gallbladder: report of a case and literature review. Gastrointest Cancer Res. 2011;4(4):135–6.
39. Eltawil KM, Gustafsson BI, Kidd M, et al. Neuroendocrine tumors of the gallbladder: an evaluation and reassessment of management strategy. J Clin Gastroenterol. 2010;44(10):687–95.
40. Nakagawa T, Sakashita N, Ohnishi K, et al. Imprint cytological feature of large cell neuroendocrine carcinoma of the gallbladder: a case report. J Med Investig. 2013;60(1–2):149–53.
41. Okuyama Y, Fukui A, Enoki Y, et al. A large cell neuroendocrine carcinoma of the gall bladder: diagnosis with 18FDG-PET/CT-guided biliary cytology and treatment with combined chemotherapy achieved a long-term stable condition. Jpn J Clin Oncol. 2013;43(5):571–4.
42. Abe T, Kajiyama K, Harimoto N, et al. Composite adeno-endocrine carcinoma of the gallbladder with long-term survival. Int J Surg Case Rep. 2013;4(5):504–7.
43. Sosnik H, Sosnik K. Double cancer of the gallbladder – a case report. Pol J Pathol. 2006;57(4):213–5.
44. Park HJ, Jang KT, Choi DW, et al. Clinicopathologic analysis of undifferentiated carcinoma of the gallbladder. J Hepatobiliary Pancreat Sci. 2014;21(1):58–63.
45. Albores-Saavedra J, Grider DJ, Wu J, et al. Giant cell tumor of the extrahepatic biliary tree: a clinicopathologic study of 4 cases and comparison with anaplastic spindle and giant cell carcinoma with osteoclast-like giant cells. Am J Surg Pathol. 2006;30(4):495–500.
46. Lee JH, Lee KG, Paik SS, et al. Hepatoid adenocarcinoma of the gallbladder with production of alpha-fetoprotein. J Korean Surg Soc. 2011;80(6):440–4.
47. Albores-Saavedra J, Henson DE, Moran-Portela D, et al. Cribriform carcinoma of the gallbladder: a clinicopathologic study of 7 cases. Am J Surg Pathol. 2008;32(11):1694–8.
48. Hari DM, Howard JH, Leung AM, et al. A 21-year analysis of stage I gallbladder carcinoma: is cholecystectomy alone adequate? HPB (Oxford). 2013;15(1):40–8.
49. Andren-Sandberg A, Deng Y. Aspects on gallbladder cancer in 2014. Curr Opin Gastroenterol. 2014;30(3):326–31.
50. Okada K, Kijima H, Imaizumi T, et al. Wall-invasion pattern correlates with survival of patients with gallbladder adenocarcinoma. Anticancer Res. 2009;29(2):685–91.
51. Shu GS, Lv F, Yang ZL, et al. Immunohistochemical study of PUMA, c-Myb and p53 expression in the benign and malignant lesions of gallbladder and their clinicopathological significances. Int J Clin Oncol. 2013;18(4):641–50.
52. Yi S, Yang ZL, Miao X, et al. N-cadherin and P-cadherin are biomarkers for invasion, metastasis, and poor prognosis of gallbladder carcinomas. Pathol Res Pract. 2014;210(6):363–8.
53. Zhu AX, Hong TS, Hezel AF, et al. Current management of gallbladder carcinoma. Oncologist. 2010;15(2):168–81.
54. Bengala C, Bertolini F, Malavasi N, et al. Sorafenib in patients with advanced biliary tract carcinoma: a phase II trial. Br J Cancer. 2010;102(1):68–72.
55. Pignochino Y, Sarotto I, Peraldo-Neia C, et al. Targeting EGFR/HER2 pathways enhances the antiproliferative effect of gemcitabine in biliary tract and gallbladder carcinomas. BMC Cancer. 2010;10:631.
56. Malka D, Cervera P, Foulon S, et al. Gemcitabine and oxaliplatin with or without cetuximab in advanced biliary-tract cancer (BINGO): a randomised, open-label, non-comparative phase 2 trial. Lancet Oncol. 2014;15(8):819–28.
57. Hezel AF, Noel MS, Allen JN, et al. Phase II study of gemcitabine, oxaliplatin in combination with panitumumab in KRAS wild-type unresectable or metastatic biliary tract and gallbladder cancer. Br J Cancer. 2014;111(3):430–6.
58. Wolf S, Lorenz J, Mossner J, et al. Treatment of biliary tract cancer with NVP-AEW541: mechanisms of action and resistance. World J Gastroenterol. 2010;16(2):156–66.
59. Grierson JR, Brockenbrough JS, Rasey JS, et al. Synthesis and in vitro evaluation of 5-fluoro-6-[(2-iminopyrrolidin-1-YL)methyl] uracil, TPI(F): an inhibitor of human thymidine phosphorylase (TP). Nucleosides Nucleotides Nucleic Acids. 2010;29(1):49–54.
60. Jain HV, Rasheed R, Kalman TI. The role of phosphate in the action of thymidine phosphorylase inhibitors: Implications for the catalytic mechanism. Bioorg Med Chem Lett. 2010;20(5):1648–51.
61. Park EY, Seo HI, Yun SP, et al. Primary leiomyosarcoma of gallbladder. J Korean Surg Soc. 2012;83(6):403–7.
62. Al-Daraji WI, Makhlouf HR, Miettinen M, et al. Primary gallbladder sarcoma: a clinicopathologic study of 15 cases, heterogeneous sarcomas with poor outcome, except pediatric botryoid rhabdomyosarcoma. Am J Surg Pathol. 2009;33(6):826–34.
63. Savlania A, Behera A, Vaiphei K, et al. Primary leiomyosarcoma of gallbladder: a rare diagnosis. Case Rep Gastrointest Med. 2012;2012:287012.
64. Perez-Montiel D, Mucientes F, Spencer L, et al. Polypoid leiomyosarcoma of the gallbladder: study of a case associated with adenomyomatous hyperplasia. Ann Diagn Pathol. 2004;8(6):358–63.
65. Al-Jaberi TM, Al-Masri N, Tbukhi A. Adult rhabdomyosarcoma of the gall bladder: case report and review of published works. Gut. 1994;35(6):854–6.
66. Odashiro AN, Pereira PR, Odashiro Miiji LN, et al. Angiosarcoma of the gallbladder: case report and review of the literature. Can J Gastroenterol. 2005;19(4):257–9.
67. Costantini R, Di Bartolomeo N, Francomano F, et al. Epithelioid angiosarcoma of the gallbladder: case report. J Gastrointest Surg. 2005;9(6):822–5.

68. Husain EA, Prescott RJ, Haider SA, et al. Gallbladder sarcoma: a clinicopathological study of seven cases from the UK and Austria with emphasis on morphological subtypes. Dig Dis Sci. 2009;54(2):395–400.
69. Segarra P, Abril V, Gil M, et al. Kaposi's sarcoma of the bile ducts with cutaneous involvement in a patient with AIDS. Rev Esp Enferm Dig. 1996;88(9):637–9.
70. Gupta S, Padmanabhan A, Khanna S. Malignant hemangiopericytoma of the gallbladder. J Surg Oncol. 1983;22(3):171–4.
71. Nestler G, Halloul Z, Evert M, et al. Myogenous sarcoma of the gallbladder with a hemangiopericytomatous pattern. J Hepato-Biliary-Pancreat Surg. 2007;14(2):197–9.
72. Hamada T, Yamagiwa K, Okanami Y, et al. Primary liposarcoma of gallbladder diagnosed by preoperative imagings: a case report and review of literature. World J Gastroenterol. 2006;12(9):1472–5.
73. Khanna M, Khanna A, Manjari M. Carcinosarcoma of the gallbladder: a case report and review of the literature. J Clin Diagn Res. 2013;7(3):560–2.
74. Wang Y, Gu X, Li Z, et al. Gallbladder carcinosarcoma accompanied with bile duct tumor thrombi: a case report. Oncol Lett. 2013;5(6):1809–12.
75. Okabayashi T, Sun ZL, Montgomey RA, et al. Surgical outcome of carcinosarcoma of the gall bladder: a review. World J Gastroenterol. 2009;15(39):4877–82.
76. Haskaraca MF, Ozsoy M, Ozsan I, et al. Primary malignant melanoma of the gallbladder: a case report and review of the literature. Case Rep Surg. 2012;2012:693547.
77. Mani H, Climent F, Colomo L, et al. Gall bladder and extrahepatic bile duct lymphomas: clinicopathological observations and biological implications. Am J Surg Pathol. 2010;34(9):1277–86.
78. Kostov DV, Kobakov GL. Gastrointestinal stromal tumour of the gallbladder. HPB (Oxford). 2012;14(2):150.
79. Furihata M, Fujimori T, Imura J, et al. Malignant stromal tumor, so called "gastrointestinal stromal tumor", with rhabdomyomatous differentiation occurring in the gallbladder. Pathol Res Pract. 2005;201(8–9):609–13.
80. Corless CL, Schroeder A, Griffith D, et al. PDGFRA mutations in gastrointestinal stromal tumors: frequency, spectrum and in vitro sensitivity to imatinib. J Clin Oncol. 2005;23(23):5357–64.
81. Song DE, Choi G, Jun SY, et al. Primitive neuroectodermal tumor of the gallbladder. Arch Pathol Lab Med. 2004;128(5):571–3.
82. Kim DH, Kim SR, Song SY, et al. A large fibrous polyp of the gallbladder mimicking a polypoid carcinoma. J Gastroenterol. 2003;38(10):1009–12.
83. Nishimura A, Shirai Y, Hatakeyama K. Segmental adenomyomatosis of the gallbladder predisposes to cholecystolithiasis. J Hepato-Biliary-Pancreat Surg. 2004;11(5):342–7.
84. Albores-Saavedra J, Keenportz B, Bejarano PA, et al. Adenomyomatous hyperplasia of the gallbladder with perineural invasion: revisited. Am J Surg Pathol. 2007;31(10):1598–604.
85. Imai H, Osada S, Sasaki Y, et al. Gallbladder adenocarcinoma with extended intramural spread in adenomyomatosis of the gallbladder with the pearl necklace sign. Am Surg. 2011;77(3):E57–8.
86. Limaiem F, Chelly B, Hassan F, et al. Coexistence of xanthogranulomatous cholecystitis and gallbladder adenocarcinoma: a fortuitous association? Pathologica. 2013;105(4):137–9.
87. Al-Abed Y, Elsherif M, Firth J, et al. Simultaneous xanthogranulomatous cholecystitis and gallbladder cancer in a patient with a large abdominal aortic aneurysm. Korean J Intern Med. 2012;27(3):338–41.
88. Ghosh M, Sakhuja P, Agarwal AK. Xanthogranulomatous cholecystitis: a premalignant condition? Hepatobiliary Pancreat Dis Int. 2011;10(2):179–84.
89. Iafrate F, Ciolina M, Iannitti M, et al. Gallbladder and muscular endometriosis: a case report. Abdom Imaging. 2013;38(1):120–4.

10 Tumors of Extrahepatic Bile Duct

Wen-Ming Cong and You-Wen Qian

10.1 Benign Tumors of Extrahepatic Bile Duct

The rate of extrahepatic biliary benign tumors is very low, accounting for less than one tenth the rate of malignant biliary tumors, and the diameter of the tumor varies from several milimeters to centimeters; thus, intrabiliary growth often leads to stenosis of the bile ducts resulting in obstructive jaundice, of which adenoma is the most common type which accounts for about 75% of all benign tumors of extrahepatic bile duct.

10.1.1 Adenoma

The discovery rate of extrahepatic biliary adenoma (bile duct adenoma, BDA) in biliary surgeries is 0.1%, much lower than that of adenoma of the gallbladder. And two thirds of the extrahepatic BDA are solitary, and the most common site is the distal one third of the bile duct near the ampulla. BDA grows into the lumen of the bile duct which is often less than 1 cm in diameter, causing varying degrees of biliary stenosis and clinical symptoms due to biliary obstruction. Pathologically, it can be divided into three types:

① Tubular BDA is composed of small tubular glands which are densely arranged, and the gland epithelium is cubic or columnar, often with mucus secreting.

② Papillary BDA is the most common type with multigrade slender papillary branches on the surface [1], and the papilla consists of cubic or columnar epithelial cells containing mucus. The tumor size can reach 3 cm in diameter. It is also known as villous adenoma for the long and slender papilla-like villi (Fig. 10.1).

③ Tubular-papillary BDA consists of tubular glands and papillary structures, with each component accounting for more than 20%. Surgical resection is effective for the treatment of BDA. Dowdy et al. reviewed foreign literature and found 27 cases of BDA with complete pathological data from 1929 to 1960 [2], while Ming-yin Lan et al. (2012) analyzed the 17 cases of BDA reported at home and abroad from 1961 to 2011, including eight cases in upper part, one case in the middle part, and eight cases in the lower extrahepatic biliary system, showing that the male to female ratio was 5:12, the average age was 58.4 (21–73) years, and the clinical manifestations are nonspecific digestive and biliary symptoms.

Oshikiri et al. (2002) reported that glandular epithelium of papillary adenoma may contain atypical hyperplasia or focal carceration [3], and p53and Ki-67 staining can be carried out to evaluate the lesions. Tretiakova et al. (2012) reported that almost all of the extrahepatic biliary benign tumors, including BDA and low-grade dysplasia, were positive for CD10, with the number of positive stained cells ranging from 20 to 80%, and malignant tumors, including adenocarcinoma and high-grade dysplasia, were all CD10 negative, which can be considered as a key point in the differential diagnosis [4].

10.1.2 Granular Cell Tumor

10.1.2.1 Pathogenesis and Mechanism

Abrikossoff first reported granular cell tumor (GCT) in 1926, and in 1952, Coggins reported the first case of biliary GCT [5], also known as granular cell myoblastoma, which is a type of neurogenic tumor derived from Schwann cells based on the evidence in histology, immunohistochemistry, and electron microscopic observations. GCT is often found in the skin, subcutaneous tissues, tongue, breast, and gastrointestinal tract, while cases in the hepatobiliary system are rare with an incidence rate of less than 1% in all GCT. More than

W.-M. Cong (✉) • Y.-W. Qian
Department of Pathology, Eastern Hepatobiliary Surgery Hospital, Second Military Medical University, Shanghai, China
e-mail: wmcong@smmu.edu.cn

W.-M. Cong (ed.), *Surgical Pathology of Hepatobiliary Tumors*, DOI 10.1007/978-981-10-3536-4_10

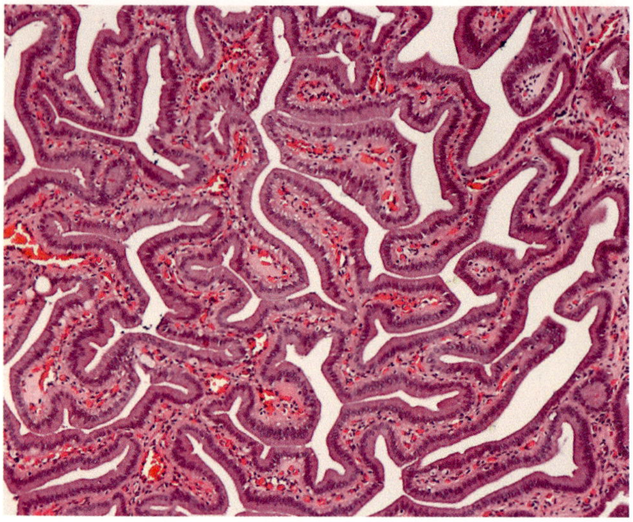

Fig. 10.1 Extrahepatic biliary adenoma: the adenoma cosists of multi-grade slender papillary branches on the surface, with fibrovascular cores, and the papilla consists of cubic or columnar epithelial cells containing mucus

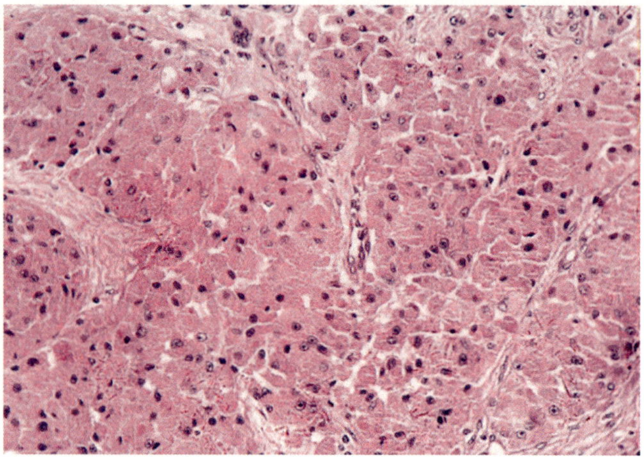

Fig. 10.2 Granular cell tumor of extrahepatic biliary: the tumor cells are arranged in acini, with abundant eosinophilic granular cytoplasm

70 cases of GCT in the extrahepatic biliary tree had been reported in the literature by 2012, accounting for less than 10% of biliary benign tumors [6, 7]. The tumor can show multicentric growth pattern, accompanied by GCT lesions in the gallbladder or skin.

10.1.2.2 Clinical Features

Foreign reports of granular cell tumor involve mainly the Negro population (60.5%) and young females (81%), with an average age of 33.9 (11–63) years. The clinical manifestations are similar to those of sclerosing cholangitis and cholangiocarcinoma, including abdominal pain (88%) and jaundice (53%). The lesions are often found in the junction of the cystic duct, common hepatic duct, and common bile duct [8], including common bile duct (58.1%), common hepatic duct (23.3%), cystic duct (14%), gallbladder, and duodenal ampulla (2.3%) [7]. Portal granular cell tumor can be similar to portal cholangiocarcinoma.

10.1.2.3 Gross Features

The lesions are often solitary without capsule, brownish yellow or yellowish white, and the average diameter is 1.6 (0.5–4) cm.

10.1.2.4 Microscopic Features

Tumor cells are arranged in sheets, acini, or clusters, with connective tissue separation. The tumor cells are polygonal or round in a larger size, rich in eosinophilic granular cytoplasm, with indistinct cell borders, and small and darkly stained nuclei (Fig. 10.2). These tumor cells can invade the whole layers of the bile duct wall, as well as nerve and small blood vessels in the biliary wall [7].

10.1.2.5 Immunohistochemistry

The tumor is positive for S-100, GFAP, and NSE staining.

10.1.2.6 Electron Microscopic Observation

Large quantities of lysozyme granules in the cytoplasm can be observed.

10.1.2.7 Differential Diagnosis

Although there is no report of malignant GCT of the bile duct, we should also pay attention to this kind of tumor. Generally, malignant GCT should show corresponding pathological biological behaviors, including invasion of surrounding tissues and cellular atypia, mitotic figures, rapid growth, tumor diameter >4 cm, metastasis and recurrence, etc.

10.1.2.8 Treatment and Prognosis

GCT of the gallbladder or cystic duct can be treated with simple cholecystectomy, and GCT of pancreatic segment of extrahepatic bile ducts often needs to be treated with Whipple surgery, while postsurgical radiotherapy and chemotherapy are not necessary for benign GCT lesions.

10.1.3 Cystadenoma

Ninety percent of cystadenoma are found in intrahepatic biliary system, and extrahepatic biliary adenoma is rare with about 100 cases in the current literature. Ninety-five percent of cystadenoma are mucinous, and the rest are serous. The average onset age of the patients is 48–58 years, and 80% of the patients manifest as obstructive jaundice. The serum CA19-9 can be elevated. Thickened cystic wall displayed on imaging, with calcification and papilla in the septa of the cystic cavity, suggests malignancy of the tumor [9]. Grossly, the tumor is often a solitary, spherical, or round mass, cyst-solid in texture, and the section shows multilocular structures, containing mucus or serous fluid. The tumor grows and extends along the biliary lumen of 2.5 28 cm in size. Histologically, 80% of cystadenomas are characterized by a monolayer of cubic or columnar epithelium and underlying ovary stroma (Fig. 10.3). The patients are predominantly females. Ovary stroma can be positive for ER and PR. However, cystadenoma without ovary stroma is often found in the elderly with no significant gender difference. The stromal component is hyalinized collagen connective tissue [10]. The postsurgical recurrence rate of biliary cyatadenoma is 10%, which may develop into cystadenocarcinoma. Studies have shown that the prognosis of hepatobiliary cystadenoma with ovary-like stroma is better than that of cases without ovary-like stroma [11]. This kind of tumor should be differentiated from simple cyst, cystic hamartoma, intraductal papillary tumor of bile duct, etc.

10.1.4 Papillomatosis

Caroli first described multiple papillomatosis of bile duct in 1958, and there have been nearly 140 biliary cases up to now, the pathogenesis of which may be related to bile stimulation and chronic inflammation of the bile duct, including bile duct stones, *Clonorchis sinensis*, Caroli's disease, ectopic pancreas, abnormal biliary tree, and primary sclerosing cholangitis [12]. Male patients are slightly more common with a male to female ratio of 2:1, and the common age range is 60–70 years. One case of the disease was found in the Department of Pathology, Eastern Hepatobiliary Surgery Hospital, Second Military Medical University, concerning a 54-year-old female, with multiple submucosal papillary lesions on the upper segment of common bile duct via choledochoscope, which was diagnosed as papillomatosis of the common bile duct based on the microscopic features (Fig. 10.4). Extrahepatic biliary papillomatosis may involve both the intrahepatic and extrahepatic biliary systems, and clinical manifestations are characterized as recurrent obstructive jaundice and cholangitis. ERCP examination is useful in establishing the diagnosis. Histologically, the tumor grows inward the biliary cavities with papillary structures and should be differentiated from canceration of papillomatosis or papillary adenocarcinoma based on the careful identification of the atypia of the tumor cells and the existence of biliary wall invasion. It has also been considered as a low malignant tumor according to its clinical and biological behaviors. Lee et al. (2004) suggested in a study that the canceration rate of biliary papillomatosis was as high as 83% [13]. Surgical resection is the preferred therapy; however, recurrence rate is high due to unresectable margin of the lesions or multi-lesion. Thus, for cases involving multigrade branches of bile ducts with high malignant potential, liver transplantation may be the best choice to improve the prognosis [14].

10.1.5 Adenofibromyomatous Hyperplasia

Adenofibromyomatous hyperplasia has a low incidence in extrahepatic bile duct, and most of the cases are found in the Vater ampulla at the end of the common bile duct. Imaging shows irregularly thickened wall of the common bile duct, and the formation of tumor-like nodules can be diagnosed as adenomyoma. Histologically, it presents hyperplasia of

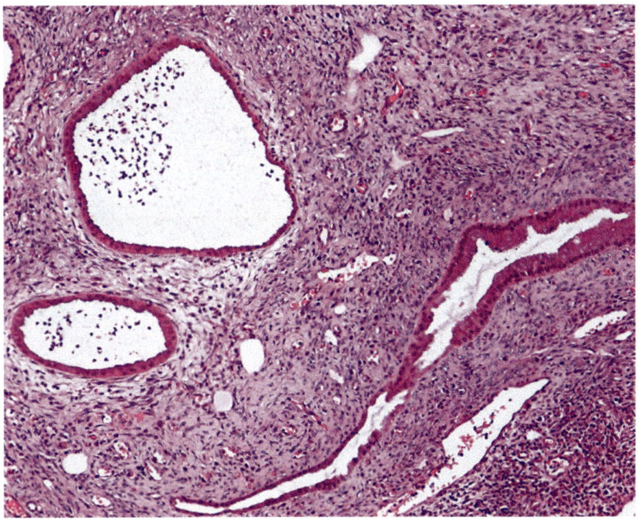

Fig. 10.3 Cystadenoma of extrahepatic biliary: the cystadenoma is characterized by a monolayer of cubic or columnar epithelium and underlying ovary stroma

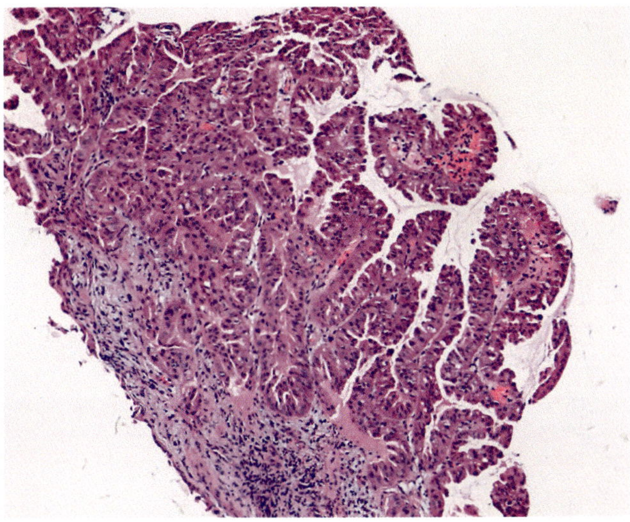

Fig. 10.4 Papillomatosis of extrahepatic biliary: the tumor grows inward the biliary cavities with papillary structures

submucosal glands and smooth muscles (Fig. 10.5). Muriel et al. (2009) reported one case of diffuse adenomyomatosis in the lower part of the common bile duct, extending a length of 4 cm, with microcysts of 1–3 mm in diameter on the cystic wall. The microscopic observation shows benign hyperplasia of glands with focal low-grade intraepithelial neoplasia [15]. Cases with atypia in the hyperplastic mucosal glands and obstructive jaundice should be differentiated from cholangiocarcinoma.

10.1.6 Angioleiomyoma

Pönkä et al. (1983) reported one case of an 80-year-old female with a space-occupying lesion in the common bile duct via ERCP, which was pathologically confirmed as angioleiomyoma [16].

10.1.7 Leiomyoma

So far, five cases of leiomyoma have been reported in the literature [17], including three cases of common bile duct leiomyoma which were all located in the pancreatic segment of the common bile duct, possibly related to the existence of the circular smooth muscle or sphincter. The tumor is only a few millimeters in diameter, and no other special symptoms or signs are found apart from obstruction jaundice. Serum CA19-9, CEA, and AFP were negative.

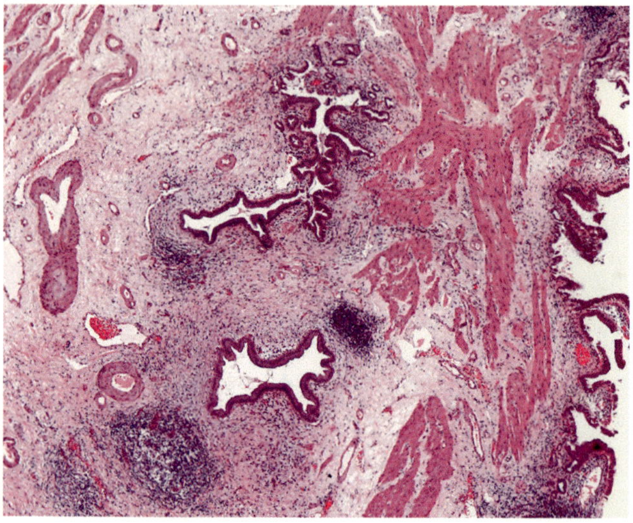

Fig. 10.5 Adenofibromyomatous hyperplasia of extrahepatic biliary: the lesion presents hyperplasia of submucosal glands and smooth muscles

10.1.8 Traumatic Neuroma

Traumatic neuroma is caused by tumor-like hyperplasia of the nerve and fibrous tissues in the injured bile duct wall, with varying components of the nervous tissues. It is often found in the residues of cystic duct after cholecystectomy. Herrera et al. (2009) reported 15 cases of traumatic neuroma in postsurgical extrahepatic biliary system after liver transplantation. The incidence rate of traumatic neuroma is 3.5% (15/428), and the lesions may originate in the common bile duct wall (type I) or the peripheral nerve tissue (type II) [18]. In addition, a few cases of neurofibromatous hyperplasia are found secondary to chronic cholecystitis.

10.1.9 Paraganglioma

Less than five cases of biliary paraganglioma have been reported in the literature, with the first case reported by Sarma et al. in 1980 [19]. Hitanant et al. (1984) reported a case of a 5 cm × 2 cm × 1.8 cm paraganglioma in the common hepatic duct which was surgically excised [20]. Caceres et al. (2001) reported one case of a 28-year-old female with surgically excised paraganglioma in the common bile duct, who manifested as right upper abdominal pain for more than 3 months, with normal serum catecholamine and no symptoms caused by biliary obstruction, and she showed good condition during the 6-year follow-up after the resection. Its microscopic features are similar to common paraganglioma, and the tumor consists of chief cells and supporting cells, forming cellular nests (cellular sphere), containing rich granular cytoplasm. Fibrous septa with abundant capillaries are found between these nests. Immunohistochemistry staining shows that the nest margin contains S-100-positive supporting cells containing neuroendocrine particles which can be found in electron microscopic images [21]. Malignant biliary paraganglioma has been reported in rare cases and should be carefully distinguished.

10.1.10 Neurofibroma

Neurofibroma is rare, and less than 20 of cases have been found in foreign literature so far [22]. Most of the tumors are associated with neurofibromatosis type 1 gene (NF1), but there are also reports of primary neurofibroma in the common bile duct [23]. Sukanta (2011) et al. reported one case of a 47-year-old female with neurofibroma in the common bile duct which was surgically excised. A lesion of 2 cm×2.5 cm of the common bile duct was found, causing stenosis and resulting in progressive obstructive jaundice. Two cases of extrahepatic biliary neurofibroma have been diagnosed in the Department of Pathology, Eastern Hepatobiliary Surgery Hospital, Second Military Medical University, concerning a 57-year-old male with a 2 cm × 1.8 cm lesion and a 68-year-old female with a 0.4 cm × 0.5 cm lesion, respectively. The tumors are grossly solid, grayish white, and nodular, while the microscopic observation shows that they are similar to common neurofibroma, with spindle tumor cells in wavy, spiral, or fence-like arrangement, and no atypia is observed. Immunohistochemistry shows that the tumors are positive for neural markers such as S-100 (Fig. 10.6).

10.1.11 Inflammatory Myofibroblastic Tumor

Extrahepatic biliary inflammatory myofibroblastic tumor (IMT) is a special type of inflammatory pseudotumor, which is more prone to present invasive behaviors, or is an independent type of lesions containing myofibroblasts. Its histological features are the same with those of intrahepatic IMT [24], and cases with positive expression of anaplastic lymphoma kinase (ALK) concern more young patients with a good prognosis. On the contrary, ALK negative cases are more common in elder patients with higher rate of metastasis. Biliary IMT lesions are often benign in nature; however, Kim et al. (2011) reported one case of portal IMT with high invasiveness, consisting of atypic tumor spindle cells, with common mitotic figures, and the myofibroblasts were positive for SMA and vimentin. Metastasis in the right chest wall was found 4 months after surgery, and malignant spindle cells were found in biopsy [25]. Thus, invasive IMT should be identified in the diagnosis of IMT.

10.1.12 Inflammatory Pseudotumor

Extrahepatic biliary inflammatory pseudotumor (IPT) has been reported in more than ten cases, and its histological features are the same with intrahepatic IPT. It consists of chronic inflammatory cells and hyperplastic fibrous connective tissues, causing biliary obstruction which leads to jaundice clinically, similar to the manifestation of portal cholangiocarcinoma or extrahepatic cholangiocarcinoma (ECC). Blanton et al. (2011) reported one case of a 20-year-old female with persistent jaundice. Abdominal CT showed dilatation of intrahepatic bile ducts, with obscure soft tissue densities in the portal area. ERCP demonstrated that an irregular stenosis was shown in the middle of the common hepatic duct, and choledochoscopic observation showed ulcerative changes. Cytological and choledochoscopic biopsy showed no definite malignant lesions. Postsurgical pathological examination confirmed the composition of spindle myofibroblasts, plasma cells, lymphocytes, eosinophilic granulocytes, and neutrophils, leading to obstruction and thickened wall of the common bile duct (incorrect, reference resource was not found), suggesting the possible existence of IPT in suspected cases of extrahepatic biliary malignant tumor. Some patients have IgG4-related sclerosing cholangitis in the background of autoimmune pancreatitis, with marked elevation of serum IgG4, and immunohistochemistry shows the presence of large quantities of IgG4-positive plasma cells. And these patients are sensitive for hormone therapy.

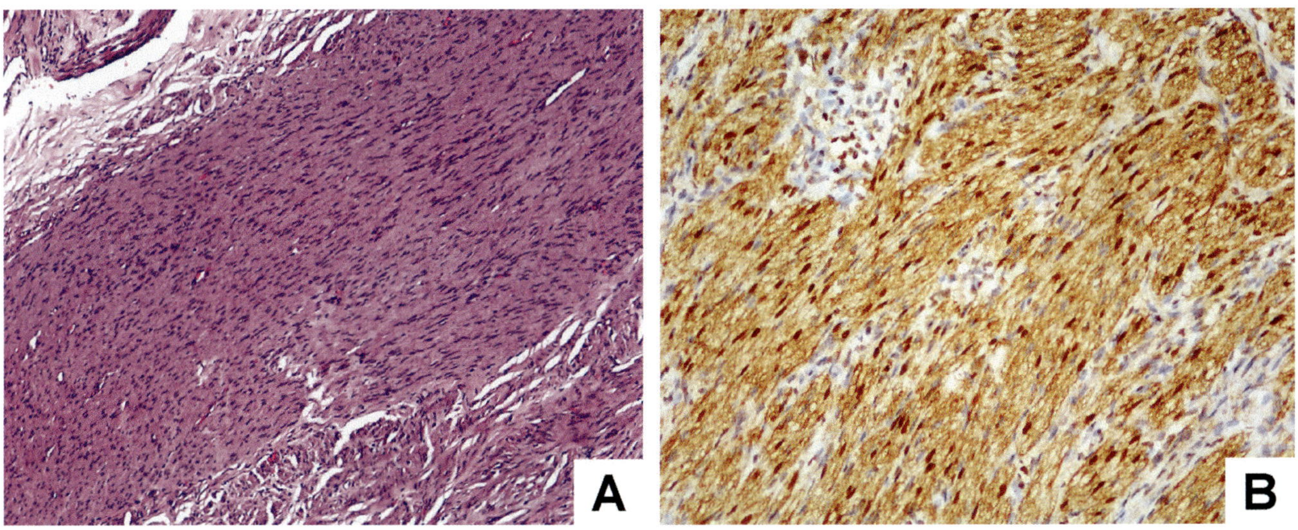

Fig. 10.6 Neurofibroma of extrahepatic biliary: (**a**) spindle tumor cells are in wavy, spiral, or fence-like arrangement and no atypia is observed; (**b**) immunohistochemistry shows that the tumor is positive for neural marker S-100

10.1.13 Gastrinoma

Gastrinoma is common in the pancreas and duodenum, while cases involving the extrahepatic biliary (including the common bile duct and common hepatic duct) are rare with only about ten cases reported in the literature, suggesting the possible origination in the stem cells of the ventral pancreatic bud. It manifests clinically as typical Zollinger-Ellison syndrome, but biliary obstruction or jaundice is rare. The tumor can form a mass larger than 1 cm in diameter on the biliary wall. Immunohistochemistry shows that it is positive for CgA and Syn and positive or negative for gastrin. Hepatic MRI and CT or single photon emission computed tomography of somatostatin receptor are helpful to exclude metastatic tumors originating from the liver or the "gastrinoma triangle." Early detection and surgical resection receive a good prognosis, with disappearance of clinical symptoms and return to normal serum gastrin [26].

10.1.14 Eosinophilic Cholangitis

According to statistics, about 10% of tumors causing portal stenosis are confirmed as benign tumors after surgical resection, which are also known as malignant masquerade. For instance, eosinophilic cholangitis in the common bile duct shows similar clinical and imaging features to cholangiocarcinoma. Dubay et al. (2010) reported one case of a 29-year-old female with upper abdominal pain and other digestive symptoms, and magnetic resonance cholangiopancreatography showed a 2 cm long stenosis in the middle of the common bile duct. Endoscopic ultrasound images showed an 8 mm focal wall thickening of the common bile duct, which was reactive bile duct epithelium shown in puncture examination, without tumor cells. The pathological examination showed that the thickened common bile duct wall contains infiltration of a large number of mature eosinophilic inflammatory cells and formation of eosinophilic abscess, with proliferated fibroblasts, and the pathological diagnosis was eosinophilic cholangitis. The disease often can be accompanied by increased eosinophilic granulocytes in the blood, and the differential diagnosis needs to be made to exclude the use of steroid hormone, parasite infection, and allergic reaction [27].

10.1.15 Neurilemmoma

Neurilemmoma derives from Schwann cells, also known as Schwannoma, and the predilection site is the digestive tract including the stomach, colon, and esophagus, while cases involving extrahepatic biliary system are rare with 15 cases reported in the foreign literature by 2012 [28]. Domestic cases of extrahepatic biliary neurilemmoma including those reported by our hospital can also be found [29]. The patients present a male to female ratio of 1:4, and an age range of 15–64 years (44 years old on average), and most of them (11/15) have symptoms of obstructive jaundice. The tumor originates in the Schwann cells of peripheral nerve of the biliary wall, with a capsule, and intratumorous hemorrhage, hyaline degeneration, and cystic degeneration can be found in some cases. The tumor consists of two main structures. Antoni A type contains densely distributed spindle or oval cells in the palisade and plexiform form. Antoni B type consists of loose and disordered tumor tissues in the myxoid matrix with edema. It is currently believed that neurilemmoma deriving in the digestive tract is mainly Antoni A type without mutations of neurofibromatosis type 2 gene (NF2) [30]. And it should be differentiated from neurofibroma, gastrointestinal stromal tumor, and leiomyoma. Immunohistochemistry shows that it is positive for S-100 and vimentin and negative for CD117 and CD34. Surgical resection prompts a good prognosis.

10.1.16 Heterotopias

Heterotopias of gastric mucosa into the extrahepatic biliary system are the most common type, and nine cases have been reported in the foreign literature with a male to female ratio of 2:1 and an average age of 37 (3–83) years. Of which six cases are found in the location near the junction of common bile duct and cystic duct, while the rest are located in the left hepatic duct, portal bile duct, and ampulla. The lesions are 3–25 mm in size, and the patients may present jaundice, abdominal pain, etc [31]. In addition, other ectopic tissues include pancrea, duodenum, accessory liver, adrenal gland, and thyroid gland, and imaging shows biliary occupying lesions. In histology, these ectopic tissues consist of normal parenchymal cells of the primary organs. However, malignancy has also been discovered in them and should be carefully observed when necessary.

Moreover, other benign non-epithelial tumors of the extrahepatic bile duct include lipomyoma, lymphangioma, angioma, melanoma, etc. The histomorphology is similar to those in soft tissues, which need not be repeated here.

10.2 Malignant Tumors of Extrahepatic Bile Duct

10.2.1 Extrahepatic Cholangiocarcinoma

10.2.1.1 Pathogenesis and Mechanism

Cholangiocarcinoma is usually abbreviated for extrahepatic cholangiocarcinoma (ECC). Extrahepatic bile ducts include the left and right hepatic duct, common hepatic duct, cystic duct, and common bile duct, and according to the orientation of the common bile duct and the relationship with the surrounding organs, it can be divided into superior duodenum, posterior-duodenum, and pancreatic and duodenal wall segments. The incidence of ECC is low and knowledge on ECC is far more less than that on intrahepatic cholangiocarcinoma. And 50–75% of the tumors are found in the upper one third of extrahepatic bile ducts including the portal area, and the lesions are more common in the confluence of thecommon bile duct, hepatic duct, and cystic duct. Cases in the middle one third (segment of the common bile duct between the cystic duct and the inferior margin of duodenum) account for 10–25%, while cases involving the lower one third segment (segment of the common bile duct between the inferior of duodenum and Vater ampulla) account for 10–20%. The predilection age is 60–70 years, and no gender difference is found related to the incidence. According to the domestic joint analysis on the 1979 autopsy cases of malignant tumors conducted by 38 departments of pathology of medical university, ECC accounted for only 0.07%. And according to the statistics provided by Shanghai Cancer Research Institute, male and female standardized incidences of gallbladder carcinoma and cholangiocarcinoma from 1978 to 2000 had been raised from 1.6/100000 and 2.3/100000 to 3.8/100000 and 5.4/100000, which were 2.46/100000 and 3.77/100000 in 2005, respectively, suggesting a drop in the incidence. Furthermore, it has been reported that new cases of gallbladder carcinoma and extrahepatic cholangiocarcinoma reached about 9810 in the USA in 2012, with 3200 death cases. And statistics of related data from 1985 to 2005 showed that the incidence of ECC in males and females were 1.1/100000 and 0.7/100000, respectively [32, 33].

The pathogenesis of ECC remains unclear, and the etiology may include ulcerative colitis (the incidence of which may be 9–21 times higher than that in normal population), primary biliary cirrhosis (PBC), primary sclerosing cholangitis (PSC), and several congenital biliary malformations such as congenital choledochocyst, congenital cyst of common bile duct (CCC), congenital malformation of the biliary tract, Carroli's disease, congenital hepatic fibrosis, polycystic liver and anomalous pancreatico-choledocho-ductal junction, biliary stones, parasitic infections (such as *Clonorchis sinensis*), exposure to chemical carcinogens, etc. (such as thorium anhydride), and patients with these lesions should be followed up closely. Other risk-increasing factors include diabetes, smoking, drinking, and infection of HBV/HCV [34–36]. Wang et al. (2011) made a meta-analysis on ECC, showing that 28–50% of the patients were (40% on average) p53 positive, the higher expression levels of which were associated with poorer staging of the tumor and histological type, vascular invasion, and lymphatic metastasis [37]. Chung et al. (2009) examined the tissue microarray of 221 cases of ECC and found elevation of phosphorylation AKT and mTOR levels [38], as well as reduction of PTEN expression in ECC, suggesting the possible application of PTEN, PTEN/p-AKT, and PTEN/p-mTOR as indicators for evaluation of the prognosis of ECC. Kawamoto et al. (2007) discovered that ECCs contain amplification of HER-2 gene (21.4%) and positive expression of the protein (31.3%); the practical significance needs further confirmation [39].

Nitta et al. (2014) found that the high expression rate of Ambra1, an autophagy protein, in cholangiocarcinoma was 71%, and the remaining 29% showed low expression. Ambra1 expression and lymphatic metastasis ($P = 0.0391$) or poor postsurgical 2-year overall survival rate ($P = 0.0209$) were significantly correlated, suggesting that autophagy played an important role in the invasive growth process of cholangiocarcinoma [40]. Nitta et al. (2014) found that epithelial-mesenchymal transition (EMT) is an important phenotype feature for cholangiocarcinoma and EMT associated markers showed significant correlation with the poor prognosis of cholangiocarcinoma, including E-cadherin ($P = 0.0208$), N-cadherin ($P = 0.0038$), and S-100A4 ($P = 0.0157$) [41].

10.2.1.2 Clinical Features

Wen-bing Wang et al. (2008) published a group of data showing that ECC patients were predominantly male, accounting for about 69% in all cases, while females accounted for only 31%, and the age range was 30–82 years with an average age of 58.6 years. Jaundice was the most common clinical symptom, which appeared earlier than that in gallbladder carcinoma with progression or volatility, found in 81.4% of all the cases. Other clinical manifestations included upper abdominal pain (29.2%), upper abdominal distension and discomfort (13.7%), itch (9.3%), fever (8.1%), and lack of appetite (5%) [42]. Laboratory tests showed elevation of tatal bilirubin and marked elevation of serum CEA and CA19-9. A total of 563 cases of surgically excised ECC were diagnosed in the Department of Pathology, Eastern Hepatobiliary Surgery Hospital, the Second Military Medical University from 2007 to 2014, and the average age of the patients was 59.1 (13–82) years, including 359 males and 204 females, with a male to female ratio of 1.76:1.

There are two basic points of the imaging features of ECC: ① biliarty obstruction caused by tumor lesions and ② direct signs of the tumor and the biliary invasion in imaging. The X-ray examination shows soft Rattan-like expansion of the bile ducts proximal to the obstruction, with irregular concentric or eccentric stenosis in the obstructive bile duct. And endoscopic retrograde cholangiopancreatography (ERCP) is very useful for the location of the ECC lesions, while endoscopic ultrasound has a diagnostic accuracy of 86% for detection of the infiltration depth of the ECC. Combined application of ERCP and percutaneous transhepatic cholangiography (PTC) can show the complete superior and inferior margins of the tumor, which is of crucial significance in determining the size, region, and treatment regime of the tumor; however, it may cause hemorrhage, bile leakage, biliary tract infection, pneumothorax, and other complications, due to its invasiveness. Magnetic resonance cholangiopancreatography (MRCP) is noninvasive, nonradioactive with arbitrary tomography and high resolution for soft tissues, etc., and the tumor is mainly the signal of soft tissue masses or thickened biliary wall, with irregular biliary stenosis. It is of important value in detection of the infiltration into the surrounding tissues and lymphatic metastasis, due to its good capacity in angiography, especially the advantage in the simultaneous imaging of both the superior and inferior segments of the obstructive bile duct after 3D reconstruction with high sensitivity and specificity. With the application of new technology of high-resolution ultrasound, detection rate of extrahepatic biliary cholangiocarcinoma can be up to 90.16% via color Doppler ultrasound [43].

10.2.1.3 Gross Features

In China, the incidence of ECC is higher than that of ICC, especially in portal ECC, accounting for 40–60% of malignant tumors of bile duct [44]. And the incidence for cholangiocarcinoma in foreign countries is 50% in portal area and 40% in extra-portal areas, while less than 10% of intrahepatic cholangiocarcinoma are found [45]. Since Klatskin first described the clinical and pathologcial features of hilar cholangiocarcinoma in 1965, it was also named as Klatskin tumor in former literatures and was preciously divided into four types: type I, tumor confined in the common hepatic duct; type II, tumor located in the confluence of the left and right hepatic ducts; type IIIa, tumor with invasion of the confluence of common hepatic duct and common bile duct and the right hepatic duct; type IIIb, tumor with invasion of the confluence of common hepatic duct and common bile duct and the left hepatic duct; and type IV, tumor with invasion of both the left and right hepatic duct.

On gross appearance, ECC can be divided into four types. ① Polypoid-papillary type: tumor is papillary, cauliflower, or polypoid, growing inward the biliary lumen, also known as intraductal type (Fig. 10.7). This type rarely invades the surrounding tissues and can be developed from multiple adenomas or papillomatosis, and papillary adenocarcinoma can grow in polypoid pattern occluding the lumen. Necrosis and detachment of the tumor may cause fluctuant jaundice. ② Nodular type: the tumor is nodular, with a diameter of 1–5 cm, surrounded by fibrous tissues. ③ Sclerosing type: the tumor grows invasively in the biliary wall, resulting in thickness and stiffness of the biliary wall and circular stenosis of the lumen, while the definite tumorous margin cannot be determined grossly, also known as interductal type. ④

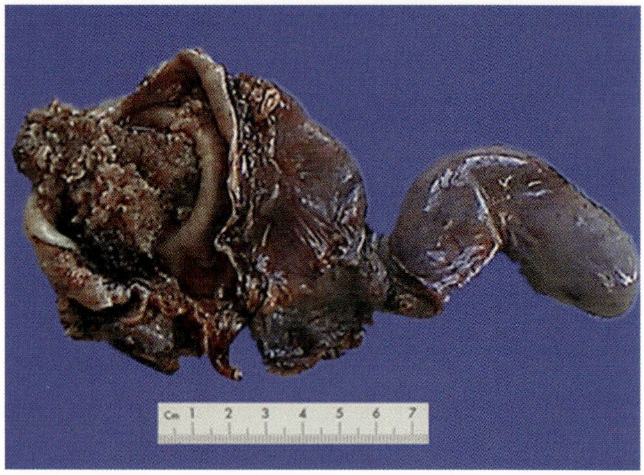

Fig. 10.7 Extrahepatic cholangiocarcinoma: polypoid-papillary type, the tumor is papillary, cauliflower, or polypoid, growing inward the biliary lumen

Diffusely infiltrating type: this type often grows and disseminates along the biliary lumen.

10.2.1.4 Microscopic Features

The vast majority of tumors are adenocarcinomas of varying degrees of differentiation, and well-differentiated cases are similar to biliary adenoma. The diagnosis of malignant cases is difficult to make, in which increased atypia, karyoplasmic ratio, and obvious nucleoli of the same glands, or stromal and perinervous infiltration, concentric interstitial reaction around the same glands, are the key features of malignancy in the diagnosis. According to the cellular morphology, the tumors can be divided into biliary type, intestinal type, and foveolar type, similar to the classification of adenocarcinoma of the gallbladder. However, biliary type of the tumor shows more mature appearance of extrahepatic biliary differentiation and contains more fibrous connective stroma. In addition, cholangiocarcinoma cells often produce mucus and express CEA, with metaplasia and dysplasia in the surrounding epithelium, such as squamous metaplasia and clear cell degeneration or neuroendocrine differentiation, or even with changes of small cell neuroendocrine carcinoma. Well-differentiated adenocarcinoma is rare, which is similar to adenoma consisting of gastric foveolar epithelium. On the basis of cellular arrangement, it can be divided into the following four categories.

10.2.2 Papillary Adenocarcinoma

The carcinoma cells are tall – columnar or cubic – forming papillary structures (Fig. 10.8a–c). About 72% of the papillary adenocarcinomas are located in bile ducts outside the portal area [35].

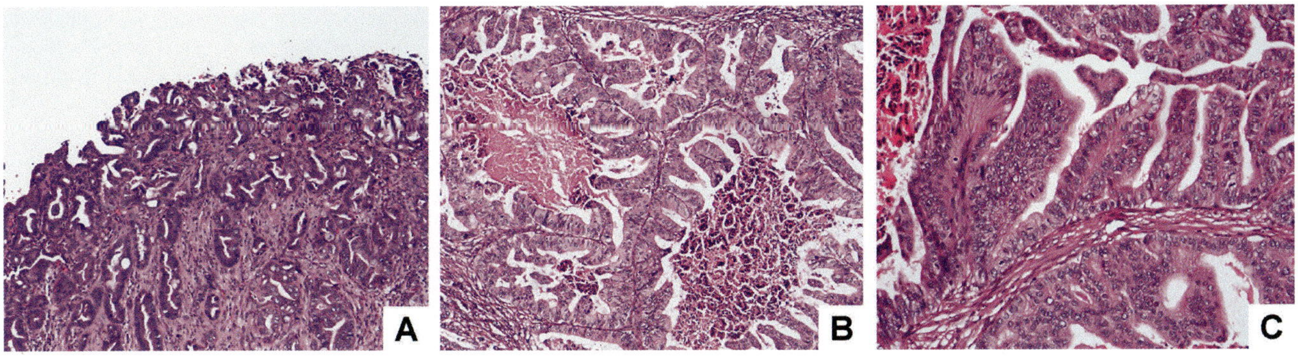

Fig. 10.8 Extrahepatic cholangiocarcinoma: (**a**) the carcinoma cells are tall, columnar or cubic, forming papillary structures, infiltrating from mucosal surface to submucosa; (**b**) tumor necrosis; (**c**) obvious mitotic figures

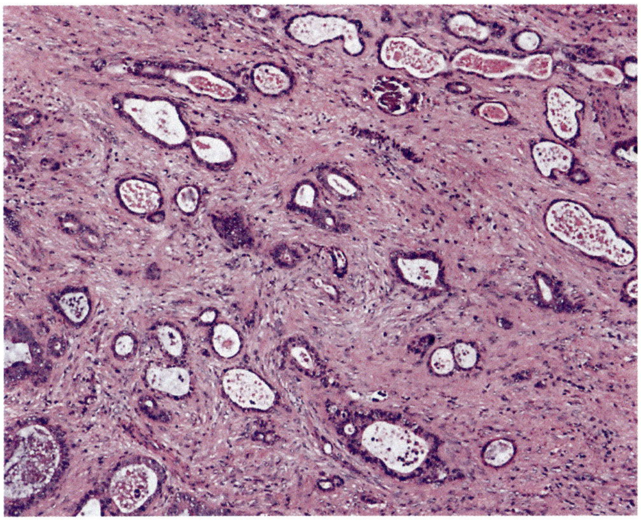

Fig. 10.9 Tubular adenocarcinoma of extrahepatic biliary: the carcinoma cells are arranged in irregular tubular structures and show an infiltrative growth pattern

10.2.3 Tubular Adenocarcinoma

The carcinoma cells are cubic and arranged in irregular tubular structures (Fig. 10.9).

10.2.4 Poorly Differentiated Adenocarcinoma

The tumor is solid in cord or sheet structures (Fig. 10.10a–b).

10.2.5 Undifferentiated Adenocarcinoma

The carcinoma cells are polymorphic, giant cell-like, or sarcomatoid and grow in diffuse distribution.

10.2.6 Other Types

Similar to the gallbladder, squamous cell carcinoma (Fig. 10.11), adenosquamous carcinoma (mucoepidermoid carcinoma), mucinous adenocarcinoma (Fig. 10.12a–b), signet ring cell carcinoma, clear cell adenocarcinoma, spindle cell carcinoma, etc. can also be found in extrahepatic biliary system.

10.2.6.1 Immunohistochemistry

The positive rate for CK7, EMA, and CEA can be higher than 85%, and the positive rate for CK19 and CA19-9 can also be high. And foveolar pattern is positive for MUC5AC. Specific staining shows normal bile duct epithelium and contains acid mucin, while sulfuric acid mucin is found in cells of ECC.

10.2.6.2 Pathological Staging

In 2010, WHO proposed the TNM staging system for distal cholangiocarcinoma (Table 10.1).

10.2.6.3 Treatment and Prognosis

The prognosis of ECC is significantly better than that of gallbladder carcinoma, possibly due to the early discovery and treatment of ECC because of jaundice, and the 5-year survival rate is 18–54% [46], while 5-year survival rates in cases with focal infiltration and metastasis are 24 and 2%, respectively. ECC shows focal invasiveness in growth pattern, and the resection rate is 10–90%, with focal postsurgical recurrence, which is a common and poor prognosis. The pathways for its metastasis include the following: from the cystic duct to gallbladder, direct invasion throughout the biliary wall to the liver, along the biliary nerve or nerve sheath (Fig. 10.13a–b), and vascular and lymphatic metastasis. Murakami et al. (2011) proposed the independent factors influencing the long-term prognosis for cholangiocarcinoma, including UICC TNM staging (P = 0.007), adjuvant chemotherapy

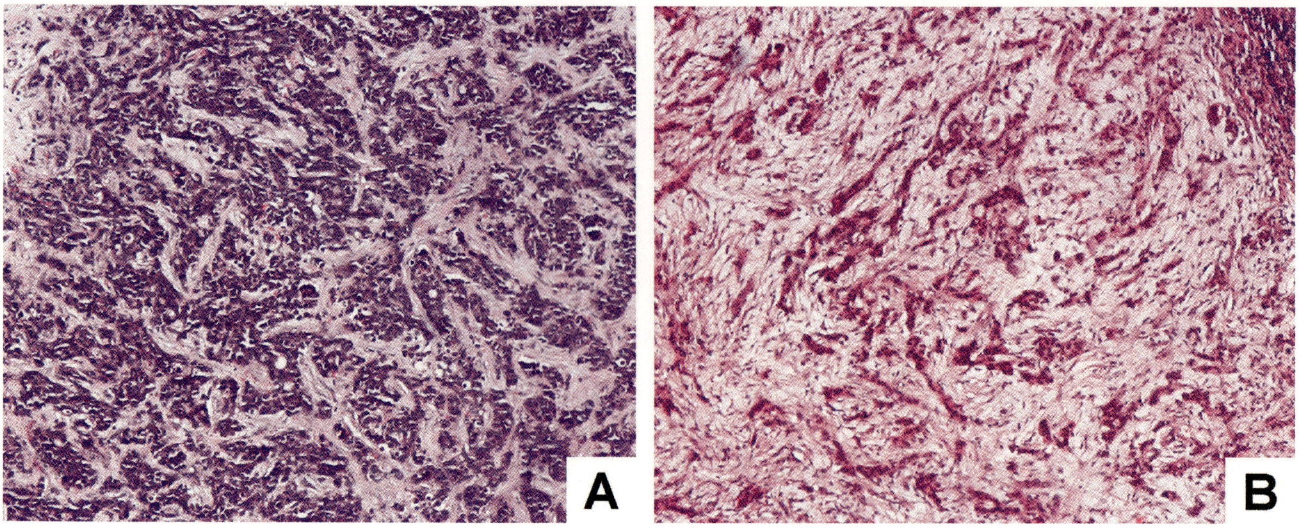

Fig. 10.10 Poorly differentiated adenocarcinoma of extrahepatic biliary: (**a**) sheet and nest structures; (**b**) cord structure

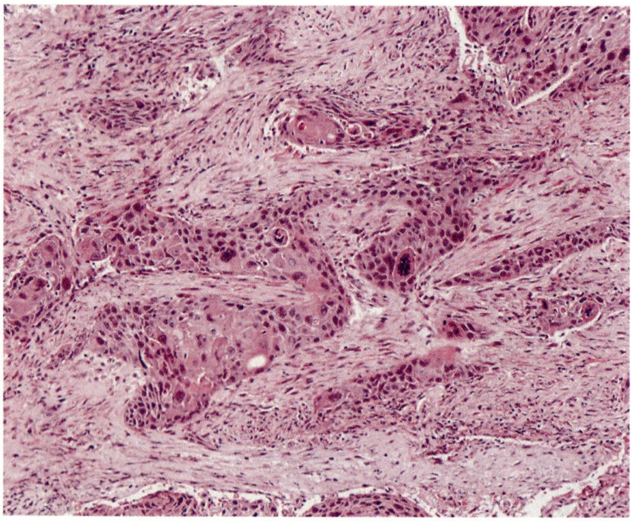

Fig. 10.11 Squamous cell carcinoma of extrahepatic biliary: squamous carcinoma is irregular cord-like, with keratin pearls, intercellular bridges and visible mitotic figures

(P = 0.009), surgical margin (P = 0.012), and lymphatic metastasis (P = 0.014). Yoshiaki et al. (2013) reported a group of 133 cases of ECC, with a neural invasion rate of 74% (98/133), and 5-year survival rates for cases with or without neural invasion of 28 and 74%, respectively, suggesting neural invasion is a crucial factor affecting the prognosis. The Chinese Chapter of the International Hepato-Pancreato-Biliary Association and Hepatosurgical group, Surgery Branch of Chinese Medical Association (2014), developed Diagnosis and Treatment for Cholangiocarcinoma (consensus of surgery experts), proposing that TNM staging should be the basis for the determination of indication and basic principles for surgeries of distal cholangiocarcinoma.

Stage 0–I: for tumors located in the upper and middle segments of the common bile duct, simple resection of related bile ducts is suitable. And for tumors in the distal end of the common bile duct, pancreaticoduodenectomy should be implemented.

StageIIA: combined resection of cholangiocarcinoma and adjacent involving tissues or pancreaticoduodenectomy.

StageIIB: tumors in the upper and middle segment of the common bile duct should be treated by resection of cholangiocarcinoma plus lymphadenectomy, and tumors of distal common bile duct should be treated with pancreaticoduodenectomy plus lymphadenectomy.

Stage III–IV: nonsurgical treatments.

For cases with clinical staging as 0, I, or IIA and suspected lymphatic metastasis, lymphadenectomy should also be implemented [47].

10.2.7 Hilar Cholangiocarcinoma

Hilar cholangiocarcinoma, also known as Klatskin tumor in the past, is a special subtype of cholangiocarcinoma, which originates in the confluence of the hepatic ducts and may extend a long segment of bile duct. Based on a domestic meta-analysis on 2280 cases of Klatskin tumor, Feng Li et al. (2013) found that the male to female ratio of Chinese patients with hilar cholangiocarcinoma was about 1.87:1 and the average age was 56.2(17–84) years. The clinical manifestations include jaundice (35%), abdominal distention and abdominal pain (26%), emaciation (13%), clay-colored stools (8%), itch (8%), hepatomegly (6%), fever (3%), and ascites (1%). The pathological classification on the 1380 lesions in the 2280 patients showed that well-differentiated

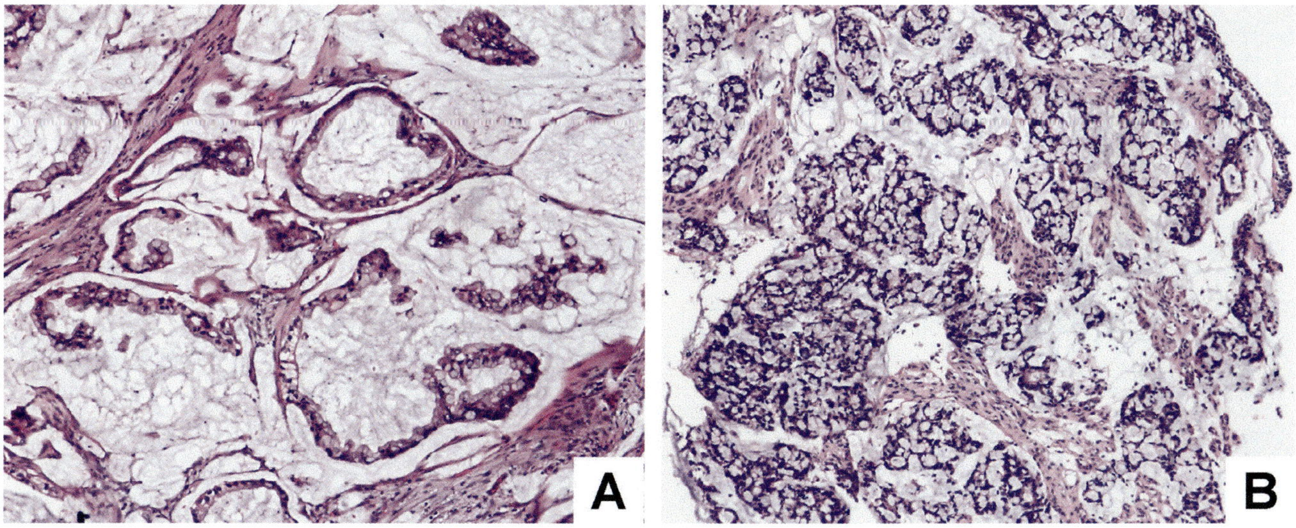

Fig. 10.12 Mucinous adenocarcinoma of extrahepatic biliary: (**a**) abundant mucus in the tumorous glands; (**b**) abundant mucus in the cytoplasm

Table 10.1 TNM staging for distal cholangiocarcinoma (AJCC 2010)

Primary tumor (T)			
T_x Primary tumor cannot be assessed			
T_0 No evidence of primary tumor			
Tis Carcinoma in situ			
T_1 Tumor confined to the bile duct histologically			
T_2 Tumor invades beyond the wall of the bile duct			
T_3 Tumor invades the gallbladder, pancreas, duodenum, or other adjacent organs without the involvement of the celiac axis or the superior mesenteric artery			
T_4 Tumor involves the celiac axis or the superior mesenteric artery			
Regional lymph nodes (N)			
N_x regional lymph nodes cannot be assessed			
N_0 No regional lymph node metastasis			
N_1 Regional lymph node metastasis			
Distant metastasis(M)			
M_0 No distant metastasis(no pathologic M_0; use clinical M to complete stage group)			
M_1 Distant metastasis			
Stage	**T**	**N**	**M**
0	Tis	N_0	M_0
IA	T_1	N_0	M_0
IB	T_2	N_0	M_0
IIA	T_3	N_0	M_0
IIB	T_1	N_1	M_0
	T_2	N_1	M_0
	T_3	N_1	M_0
III	T_4	Any N	M_0
IV	Any T	Any N	M_1

Reprint with permission from Compton, Perihilar Bile Ducts, Springer, 2012

adenocarcinoma or tubular papillary adenocarcinoma accounted only for 39.9% (550/1380), while moderately and poorly differentiated adenocarcinoma accounted for 38.6% (533/1380) [48]. The results were consistent with the recent reports in foreign literature [49], and it is also one of the main causes of the poor prognosis of hilar holangiocarcinoma. The pathological features are not identical to the previously described poorly differentiated adenocarcinoma by Klatskin, and current studies show that hilar holangiocarcinoma is mainly well-differentiated adenocarcinoma with focal infiltration, slow growth, and obvious fibrosis, while the rate of lymphatic and distal metastasis is low. The clinical course is long; however, the recurrence rate in cases with R0 (negative resectional margin) is as high as 50–70% [50]. Wen-long Yu et al. (2009) conducted a multifactorial analysis on a group of 205 cases of hilar cholangiocarcinoma, showing that lymphatic metastasis and depth of biliary infiltration are two independent risk factors impacting on the postsurgical long-term survival, and they advocated that intraoperative frozen sections should be inspected to evaluate the condition of lymph node regions with high incidence of metastasis such as portal area and base of common hepatic artery and the depth of the tumorous invasion into the biliary wall and the surrounding tissues, which can be relied on as a histological evidence for determing the region of surgical resection to improve the rate of R0 surgical resection and long-term therapeutic effects for the patients [51]. It should be differentiated from sclerosing cholangitis (TP53 negative) in diagnosis. In 2010, WHO proposed the TNM staging for hilar cholangiocarcinoma (Table 10.2).

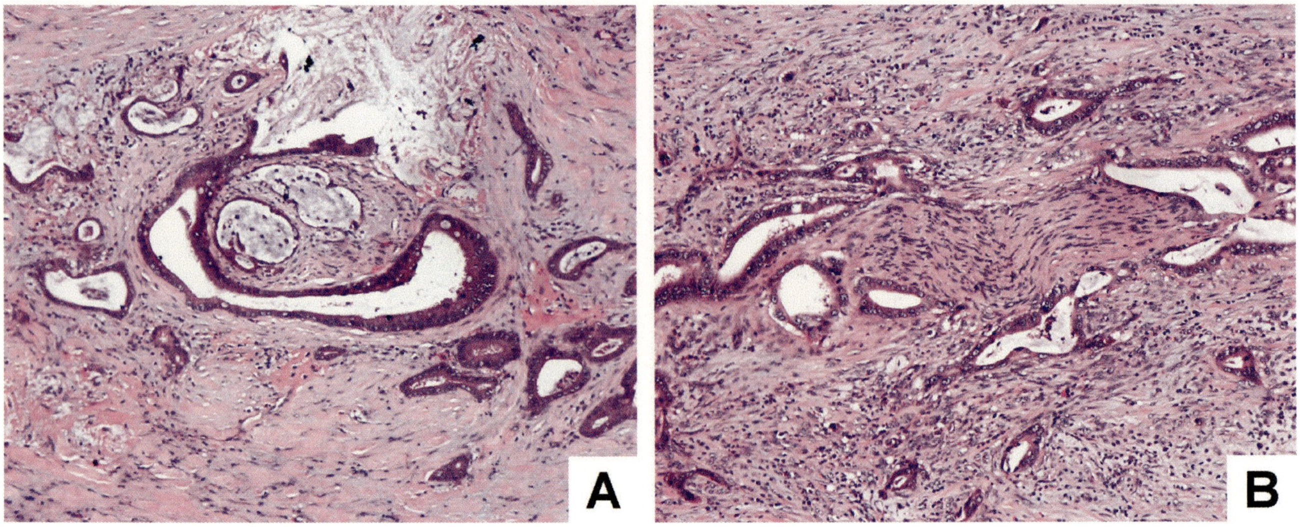

Fig. 10.13 Extrahepatic cholangiocarcinoma: tumorous glands are along or inside the biliary nerve or nerve sheath (**a** & **b**)

Table 10.2 TNM staging for hilar cholangiocarcinoma (AJCC 2010)

Primary tumor (T)			
T_x primary tumor cannot be assessed			
T_0 No evidence of primary tumor			
Tis Carcinoma in situ			
T_1 Tumor confined to the bile duct, with extension up to the muscle layer or fibrous tissue			
T_{2a} Tumor invades beyond the wall of the bile duct to surrounding adipose tissue			
T_{2b} Tumor invades adjacent hepatic parenchyma			
T_3 Tumor invades unilateral branches of the portal vein or hepatic artery			
T_4 Tumor invades main portal vein or its branches bilaterally, the common hepatic artery, the second-order biliary radicals bilaterally, and unilateral second-order biliary radicals with contralateral portal vein or hepatic artery involvement			
Regional lymph nodes (N)			
N_x Regional lymph nodes cannot be assessed			
N_0 No regional lymph node metastasis			
N_1 Regional lymph node metastasis (including nodes along the cystic duct, common bile duct, hepatic artery, and portal vein)			
N_2 Metastasis to periaortic, pericaval, superior mesenteric artery, and/or celiac artery lymph nodes			
Distal metastasis(M)			
M_0 No distant metastasis			
M_1 Distant metastasis			
Stage	**T**	**N**	**M**
0	Tis	N_0	M_0
I	T_1	N_0	M_0
II	$T_{2a\text{-}b}$	N_0	M_0
III A	T_3	N_0	M_0
III B	T_{1-3}	N_1	M_0
IV A	T_4	N_{0-1}	M_0
IV B	Any T	N_2	M_0
	Any T	Any N	M_1

Reprint with permission from Compton, Perihilar Bile Ducts, Springer, 2012

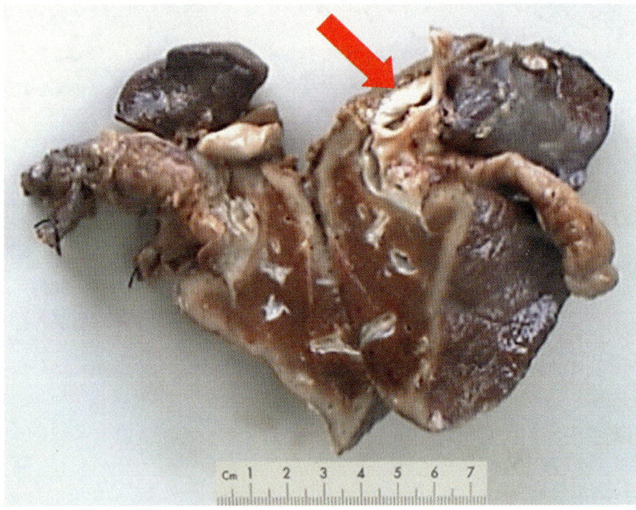

Fig. 10.14 Cystadenocarcinoma of extrahepatic biliary: the tumor is grossly cystic and solid and located in the portal area (*arrow* shows the tumor)

10.2.8 Cystadenocarcinoma

The extrahepatic biliary cystadenocarcinoma often manifests as jaundice in the corresponding patients. And when weight loss and ascites occur, exacerbation of the disease is indicated. Portal cystadenocarcinoma is often misdiagnosed as Klatskin tumor, and the tumor can be found in the bifurcation between the left and right hepatic ducts in the portal area. The tumor is grossly cystic and solid, with hemorrhage and necrosis, and grows invasively along the hepatic ducts (Fig. 10.14). Microscopic images show the tumor is tubular adenocarcinoma containing mucus in the lumen, and the cells are arranged in multilayers with focal dysplasia and moderate mitotic figures (Fig. 10.15). Radical resection of

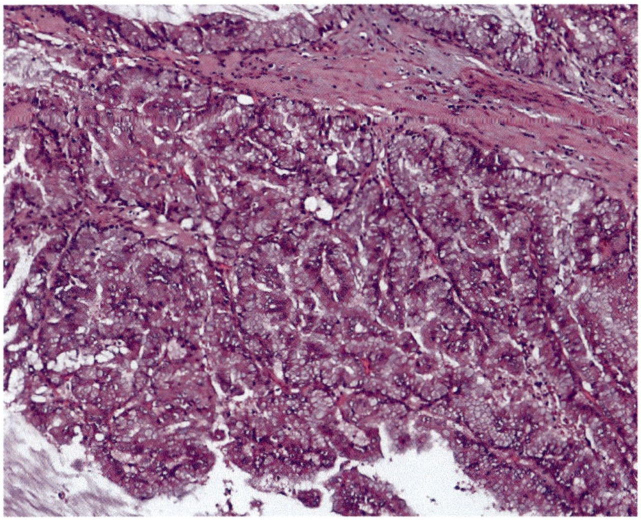

Fig. 10.15 Cystadenocarcinoma of extrahepatic biliary: the tumor is tubular adenocarcinoma, and the cells are tall-columnar and arranged in multilayers with focal invasion into the duct wall

the tumor plus partial resection of the liver tissue can lead to a good prognosis [52].

10.2.9 Fibrosarcoma

Fibrosarcoma (FS) found in extrahepatic biliary system is rare, and one related case was diagnosed in the Department of Pathology, Eastern Hepatobiliary Surgery Hospital, Second Military Medical University. The patient was a 37-year-old female who complained progressive dark urine with itchy skin. Ultrasound type B showed regular shape of the liver with smooth capsule, and a 3.4 cm × 2.4 cm flocculent echo was found in the median segment of the common bile duct. CT images showed a long and column mass in the right upper abdomen corresponding to the region posterior the duodenum, which was 6.5 cm × 3 cm in size with a clear boundary and homogeneous density. The lesion invaded upward to the portal area, compressing the common hepatic duct and portal vein with relatively smooth walls and marked tumorous surface adjacent to the liver. Significant homogeneous enhancement of the lesion was shown in arterial phase and decreased density in portal vein and delayed phases, which was still hyperdense compared to the liver on the same section. The liver is normal in size and morphology, and no abnormal densities were found in the liver parenchyma. Intrahepatic bile ducts were expanded in a rattern type, while no expansion was found in the inferior to the portal bile duct and the gallbladder underwent atrophy and collapse. MRI demonstrated that the liver had a smooth and even rim with soft and ratten-shaped intrahepatic bile ducts, which was dilated and broken at the middle of the portal bile duct. Density of soft tissue in the portal areas which was about 4 cm × 3 cm in size was enhanced significantly, and compression, narrowing, and translocation of the upper common bile duct were found. Serology showed AFP, 8.8 μg/L; CA19-9, 334.4 U/ml; and HBsAg negative. The preoperative diagnosis was portal cholangiocarcinoma. During the operation, it was observed that the liver was enlarged with cholestasis, reaching subcostal 2 cm, tawny, median textured, and no tumor nodules. A 5 cm × 6 cm sized and hard mass was palpated in extrahepatic biliary system. Complete resection of portal tumor was carried out.

On gross appearance, the extrahepatic biliary (including common bile duct) mass was 5.5 cm × 5.5 cm × 3 cm in size, and the section was grayish white or grayish yellow, without obvious hemorrhage or necrosis (Fig. 10.16). The microscopic observations showed that tumor cells were spindle or oval, arranged in herringbone, and the nuclei vary in size, with obvious atypia and common mitotic figures (Fig. 10.17). Immunohistochemistry investigations showed the tumor cells were vimentin and PCNA positive and SMA, S-100, and Hep Par-1 negative. The pathological diagnosis was fibrosarcoma (of the portal bile duct).

10.2.10 Rhabdomyosarcoma

Biliary rhabdomyosarcoma (RMS) mainly involves infants and children at an age of 0–14 years, with the average age of 3.5 years, and embryonal and botroyoid RMS account for 60% and 6% of the disease, respectively. By 2014, there have been 90 cases of hepatic and biliary RMS reported in the literature [53]. Tireli et al. (2005) reported one case of a 3-year-old patient with a surgically resected 8 cm × 4 cm × 3 cm embryonal RMS in the common bile duct [54], who was treated with postsurgical combined chemotherapy and radiotherapy, showing good condition during 1-year follow-up. One case of a 4-year-old patient with

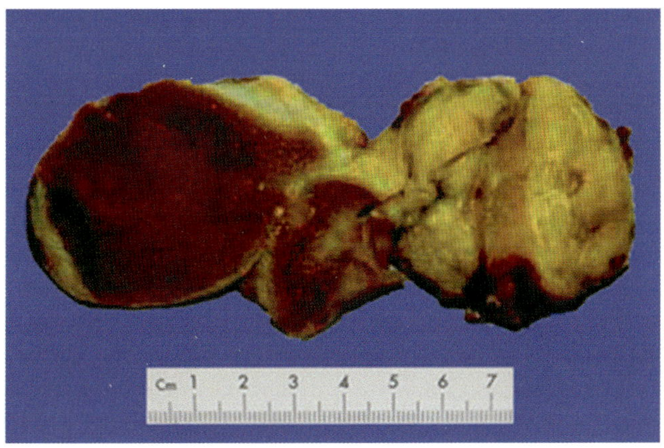

Fig. 10.16 Fibrosarcoma of extrahepatic biliary: the tumor on the *left* is *grayish yellow* and nodular; the gallbladder is on the *right*

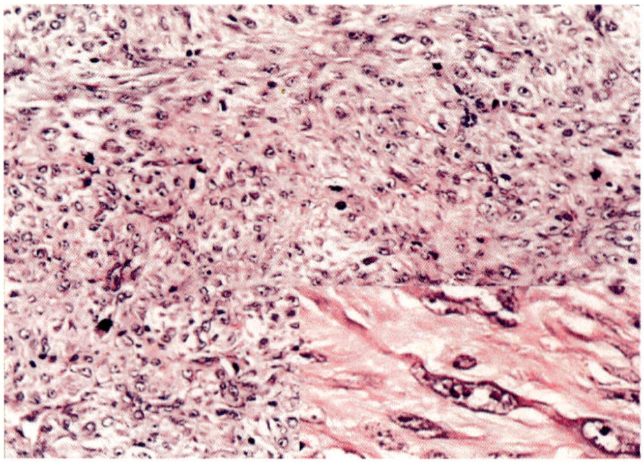

Fig. 10.17 Fibrosarcoma of extrahepatic biliary: the tumor cells were spindle or oval, arranged in herringbone, with collagenous fiber on both sides of the tumor giant cells (*lower right* shows the high magnification)

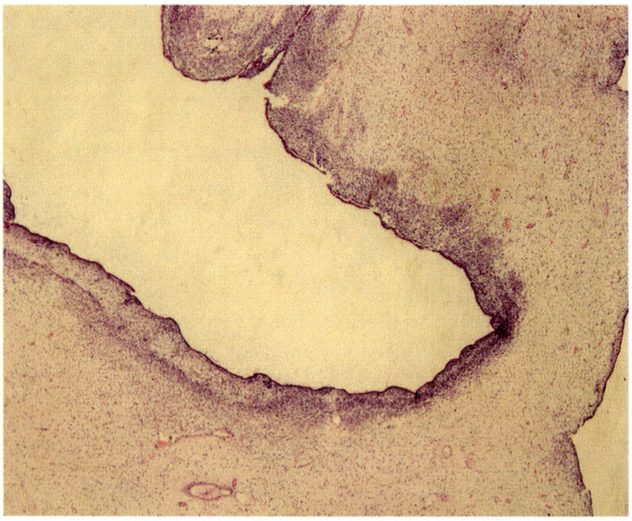

Fig. 10.18 Biliary botroyoid RMS: the tumor cells were densely distributed close to the inferior surface of biliary mucosal epithelium, forming characteristic "forming layer"

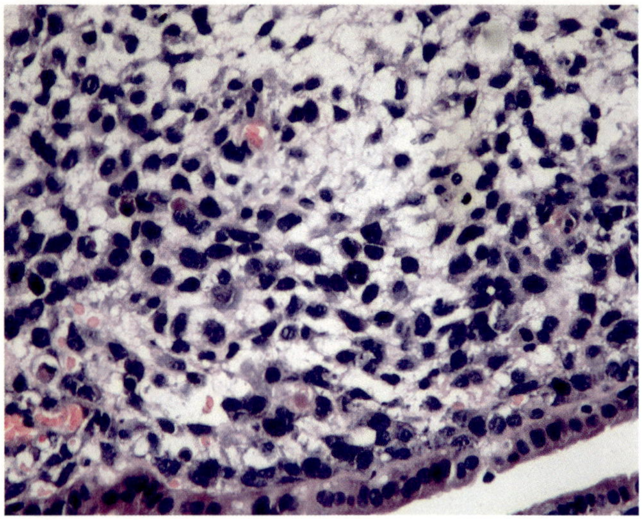

Fig. 10.19 Biliary botroyoid RMS: the nuclei were large and darkly stained, with active mitosis

RMS was diagnosed in the Department of Pathology, Eastern Hepatobiliary Surgery Hospital, Second Military Medical University, who received a surgical resection of botroyid RMS lesions involving the common bile duct and the left hepatic duct. The tumor showed a polypoid growth pattern to the luminal surface, and microscopic examination showed interstitial edema with mucus in the submucosal tissue of bile duct, and the tumor cells were densely distributed close to the inferior surface of biliary mucosal epithelium and around the proliferated mucous glands, forming characteristic "forming layer" (Fig. 10.18), while the bile duct walls below it contained much less tumor cells, and invasion could be found in individual neural tissues. The tumor cells were stellate, polygonal, or spindle, with little cytoplasm on both sides of the nuclei and no marked striations, and the nuclei were large and darkly stained, while bizarre cells and active mitosis (Fig. 10.19) could also be observed. Pathological factors which suggest good prognosis of RMS include no distal metastasis, complete resection of the lesions, botryooid type [55], diameter <5 cm, and onset age <10 years.

Other rare malignant tumors in extrahepatic biliary system include carcinoid, small cell carcinoma, large cell carcinoma [56–58], lymphoma, leiomyosarcoma, Kaposi sarcoma, carcinosarcoma, malignant melanoma, etc., the histomorphology of which is similar to that of correspondent tumors of the liver or soft tissues.

References

1. Lang M-y, Zhou M, Zhang M, et al. Report of three extrahepatic biliary adenomas and review of the literature. Fu Bu Wai Ke. 2012;25(5):297–9.
2. Dowdy Jr GS, Olin Jr WG, Shelton Jr EL, et al. Benign tumors of the extrahepatic bile ducts. Report of three cases and review of the literature. Arch Surg. 1962;85:503–13.
3. Oshikiri T, Kashimura N, Katanuma A, et al. Mucin-secreting bile duct adenoma--clinicopathological resemblance to intraductal papillary mucinous tumor of the pancreas. Dig Surg. 2002;19(4):324–7.
4. Tretiakova M, Antic T, Westerhoff M, et al. Diagnostic utility of CD10 in benign and malignant extrahepatic bile duct lesions. Am J Surg Pathol. 2012;36(1):101–8.
5. Coggins RP. Granular-cell myoblastoma of common bile duct; report of a case with autopsy findings. AMA Arch Pathol. 1952;54(4):398–402.
6. Bilanovic D, Boricic I, Zdravkovic D, et al. Granular cell tumor of the common hepatic duct presenting as cholangiocarcinoma and acute acalculous cholecystitis. Acta Chir Iugosl. 2008;55(4):99–101.

7. Saito J, Kitagawa M, Kusanagi H, et al. Granular cell tumor of the common bile duct: a Japanese case. World J Gastroenterol. 2012;18(43):6324–7.
8. Karakozis S, Gongora E, Zapas JL, et al. Granular cell tumors of the biliary tree. Surgery. 2000;128(1):113 5.
9. Chandrasinghe PC, Liyanage C, Deen KI, et al. Obstructive jaundice caused by a biliary mucinous cystadenoma in a woman: a case report. J Med Case Rep. 2013;7:278.
10. Hennessey DB, Traynor O. Extrahepatic biliary cystadenoma with mesenchymal stroma: a true biliary cystadenoma? A case report. J Gastrointestin Liver Dis. 2011;20(2):209–11.
11. Buetow PC, Buck JL, Pantongrag-Brown L, et al. Biliary cystadenoma and cystadenocarcinoma: clinical-imaging-pathologic correlations with emphasis on the importance of ovarian stroma. Radiology. 1995;196(3):805–10.
12. Adioui T, Seddik H, Baba H, et al. Successful surgical treatment of extrahepatic biliary papillomatosis diagnosed with endoscopic retrograde cholangiopancreatography: a case report. J Med Case Rep. 2014;8:148.
13. Lee SS, Kim MH, Lee SK, et al. Clinicopathologic review of 58 patients with biliary papillomatosis. Cancer. 2004;100(4):783–93.
14. Vibert E, Dokmak S, Belghiti J. Surgical strategy of biliary papillomatosis in Western countries. J Hepatobiliary Pancreat Sci. 2010;17(3):241–5.
15. Genevay M, Frossard JL, Huber O, et al. High-grade common bile duct stricture caused by diffuse adenomyomatosis. Gastrointest Endosc. 2009;69(6):1167–8.
16. Ponka A, Laasonen L, Strengell-Usanov L. Angioleiomyoma of the common bile duct. Acta Med Scand. 1983;213(5):407–10.
17. Goo JC, Yi MY, Jeon WJ, et al. A case of leiomyoma in the common bile duct. Korean J Gastroenterol. 2006;47(1):77–81.
18. Herrera L, Martino E, Rodriguez-Sanjuan JC, et al. Traumatic neuroma of extrahepatic bile ducts after orthotopic liver transplantation. Transplant Proc. 2009;41(3):1054–6.
19. Sarma DP. Paraganglioma of the hepatic duct: A personal commentary. South Med J. 2006;99(7):785–6.
20. Hitanant S, Sriumpai S, Na-Songkla S, et al. Paraganglioma of the common hepatic duct. Am J Gastroenterol. 1984;79(6):485–8.
21. Caceres M, Mosquera LF, Shih JA, et al. Paraganglioma of the bile duct. South Med J. 2001;94(5):515–8.
22. Ray S, Das K, Mridha AR, et al. Neurofibroma of the common bile duct: a rare cause of obstructive jaundice. Am J Surg. 2011;202(1):e1–3.
23. Bechade D, Boulanger T, Palazzo L, et al. Primary neurofibroma of the common bile duct. Gastrointest Endosc. 2010;72(4):895–7.
24. Kim BS, Joo SH, Kim GY, et al. Aggressive hilar inflammatory myofibroblastic tumor with hilar bile duct carcinoma in situ. J Korean Surg Soc. 2011;81(Suppl 1):S59–63.
25. Blanton C, Kalarickal J, Joshi V. Biliary obstruction from a bile duct mass. Gastroenterology. 2011;141(3):812–3.. 1129
26. Price TN, Thompson GB, Lewis JT, et al. Zollinger-Ellison syndrome due to primary gastrinoma of the extrahepatic biliary tree: three case reports and review of literature. Endocr Pract. 2009;15(7):737–49.
27. Dubay D, Jhala N, Eloubeidi M. Eosinophilic cholangitis. Clin Gastroenterol Hepatol. 2010;8(8):A22.
28. Fonseca GM, Montagnini AL, Rocha Mde S, et al. Biliary tract schwannoma: a rare cause of obstructive jaundice in a young patient. World J Gastroenterol. 2012;18(37):5305–8.
29. Yu W-l, Shi S, Yang J, et al. One case of extrahepatic biliary neurilemmoma. Journal of Hepatopancreatobiliary Surgery. 2007;19(5):331–2.
30. Lasota J, Wasag B, Dansonka-Mieszkowska A, et al. Evaluation of NF2 and NF1 tumor suppressor genes in distinctive gastrointestinal nerve sheath tumors traditionally diagnosed as benign schwannomas: s study of 20 cases. Lab Investig. 2003;83(9):1361–71.
31. Fukuda S, Mukai S, Shimizu S, et al. Heterotopic gastric mucosa in the hilar bile duct mimicking hilar cholangiocarcinoma: report of a case. Surg Today. 2013;43(1):91–5.
32. Shen M-c, Chu Q, Zhan R-z, et al. Preliminary observation of pathologic characteristics of biliary tract cancers in Shanghai: Analysis of 487 cases. Tumori. 2005;25(6):596–9.
33. Siegel R, Naishadham D, Jemal A. Cancer statistics, 2012. CA Cancer J Clin. 2012;62(1):10–29.
34. Matsumoto K, Onoyama T, Kawata S, et al. Hepatitis B and C virus infection is a risk factor for the development of cholangiocarcinoma. Intern Med. 2014;53(7):651–4.
35. Ye XH, Huai JP, Ding J, et al. Smoking, alcohol consumption, and the risk of extrahepatic cholangiocarcinoma: a meta-analysis. World J Gastroenterol. 2013;19(46):8780–8.
36. Zhang LF, Zhao HX. Diabetes mellitus and increased risk of extrahepatic cholangiocarcinoma: a meta-analysis. Hepato-Gastroenterology. 2013;60(124):684–7.
37. Wang J, Wang X, Xie S, et al. p 53 status and its prognostic role in extrahepatic bile duct cancer: a meta-analysis of published studies. Dig Dis Sci. 2011;56(3):655–62.
38. Chung JY, Hong SM, Choi BY, et al. The expression of phospho-AKT, phospho-mTOR, and PTEN in extrahepatic cholangiocarcinoma. Clin Cancer Res. 2009;15(2):660–7.
39. Kawamoto T, Krishnamurthy S, Tarco E, et al. HER Receptor Family: Novel Candidate for Targeted Therapy for Gallbladder and Extrahepatic Bile Duct Cancer. Gastrointest Cancer Res. 2007;1(6):221–7.
40. Nitta T, Sato Y, Ren XS, et al. Autophagy may promote carcinoma cell invasion and correlate with poor prognosis in cholangiocarcinoma. Int J Clin Exp Pathol. 2014;7(8):4913–21.
41. Nitta T, Mitsuhashi T, Hatanaka Y, et al. Prognostic significance of epithelial-mesenchymal transition-related markers in extrahepatic cholangiocarcinoma: comprehensive immunohistochemical study using a tissue microarray. Br J Cancer. 2014;111(7):1363–72.
42. Wang W-b, Zhang X-h, Shi Y-m, et al. Surgical procedure and prognotic analysis of extrahepatic cholangiocarcinoma: a report of 161 cases. Tumori. 2008;28(3):251–5.
43. Hou X-y, Zhou S-y. The use of color doppler ultrasound in the diagnosis of extrahepatic cholangiocarcinoma. Chin J Clin Rational Drug Use. 2012;5(19):160.
44. Zheng S-g, Xiang C-h, Feng X-b, et al. The diagnosis and treatment guidelines of hilar cholangiocarcinoma. Chin J Surg. 2013;51(10):865–71.
45. Deoliveira ML, Cunningham SC, Cameron JL, et al. Cholangiocarcinoma: thirty-one-year experience with 564 patients at a single institution. Ann Surg. 2007;245(5):755–62.
46. Murakami Y, Uemura K, Sudo T, et al. Prognostic factors after surgical resection for intrahepatic, hilar, and distal cholangiocarcinoma. Ann Surg Oncol. 2011;18(3):651–8.
47. Chinese Chapter of International Hepato-Pancreato-Biliary Association, Hepatic Surgery Group, Chinese Society of Surgery, Chinese Medical Association. Diagnosis and treatment of cholangiocarcinoma: surgical expert consensus. J Huazhong Univ Sci Technolog Med Sci. 2014;34(4):469–75.
48. Li F, Zhou G-w. Hilar cholangiocarcinoma: a meta-analysis of 2280 cases. Chin J Hepatobiliary Surg. 2013;19(3):171–6.
49. Clary B, Jarnigan W, Pitt H, et al. Hilar cholangiocarcinoma. J Gastrointest Surg. 2004;8(3):298–302.
50. Soares KC, Kamel I, Cosgrove DP, et al. Hilar cholangiocarcinoma: diagnosis, treatment options, and management. Hepatobiliary Surg Nutr. 2014;3(1):18–34.
51. Yu W-l, Zhang Y-j, Dong H, et al. Biopathological characteristics of hilar cholangiocarcinoma and the clinical significance. Chin J Surg. 2009;47(15):1162–6.

52. Pais-Costa SR, Martins SJ, Araujo SL, et al. Extrahepatic biliary cystadenocarcinoma mimicking Klatskin tumor. Arq Bras Cir Dig. 2013;26(1):66–8.
53. Nakib G, Calcaterra V, Goruppi I, et al. Robotic-assisted surgery approach in a biliary rhabdomyosarcoma misdiagnosed as choledochal cyst. Rare Tumors. 2014;6(1):5173.
54. Tireli GA, Sander S, Dervisoglu S, et al. Embryonal rhabdomyosarcoma of the common bile duct mimicking choledochal cyst. J Hepato-Biliary-Pancreat Surg. 2005;12(3):263–5.
55. Margain-Deslandes L, Gelas T, Bergeron C, et al. A botryoid rhabdomyosarcoma diagnosed as a choledochal cyst. Pediatr Blood Cancer. 2013;60(12):2089–90.
56. Jethava A, Muralidharan V, Mesologites T, et al. An unusual presentation of a carcinoid tumor of the common bile duct. JOP. 2013;14(1):85–7.
57. Kim BC, Song TJ, Lee H, et al. A case of small cell neuroendocrine tumor occurring at hilar bile duct. Korean J Gastroenterol. 2013;62(5):301–5.
58. Sasatomi E, Nalesnik MA, Marsh JW. Neuroendocrine carcinoma of the extrahepatic bile duct: case report and literature review. World J Gastroenterol. 2013;19(28):4616–23.

Liver Biopsy for the Diagnosis of Liver Neoplasms

11

Stephen C. Ward and Swan N. Thung

11.1 Biopsy Diagnosis of Hepatocellular Carcinoma and Other Hepatocellular Lesions

Hepatocellular carcinoma (HCC) is the most common primary malignant neoplasm of the liver. Approximately 90% of these tumors arise in the background of cirrhosis secondary to an underlying liver disease, such as infection with hepatitis B or C virus, alcoholic liver disease, nonalcoholic steatohepatitis, or autoimmune hepatitis. In most cases, larger tumors can be reliably diagnosed on imaging studies when they show arterial enhancement and portal venous washout on dynamic contrast-enhanced CT or MRI studies. This characteristic imaging pattern is due to the increased arterial supply of the tumor compared to the surrounding liver. Smaller tumors may be more difficult to characterize by imaging studies. Tumors smaller than 2 cm may be classified as a very early or "vaguely nodular" HCC which have a poorly defined border or progressed HCC which have a more distinct border [1, 2]. These very early HCCs do not generally have the complete alterations in the blood supply characteristic of progressed tumors and thus lack the features required for diagnosis on imaging. According to the American Association for the Study of Liver Diseases practice guidelines, tumors arising in a cirrhotic liver that are larger than 1 cm and show the characteristic findings of arterial enhancement and portal venous washout on dynamic imaging can be diagnosed as HCC without the need for a biopsy, while liver biopsy may be required when the imaging features are not characteristic [3]. As the understanding of the molecular pathogenesis of HCC advances, tissue samples may soon be required even in radiologically diagnosed HCC for the purposes of assessing prognosis and tailoring therapy.

S. C. Ward • S.N. Thung (✉)
Division of Hepatopathology, Department of Pathology, Icahn School of Medicine at Mount Sinai, New York, NY, USA
e-mail: swan.thung@mountsinai.org

Classically HCC consists of large tumor cells with relatively abundant eosinophilic cytoplasm and centralized nuclei that contain prominent nucleoli. Tumors often recapitulate the trabecular architecture of the normal liver, though the trabeculae are thickened to more than three cells wide (Fig. 11.1). Bile production may also be seen and when present is definitive evidence of hepatocellular differentiation (Fig. 11.2). Other morphologic patterns include pseudoglandular, solid, scirrhous, clear cell, and steatohepatitic (Fig. 11.3). On resection specimens, HCCs may show various morphologic patterns, but classic areas of HCC are often still apparent elsewhere. Diagnosing well-differentiated HCC on biopsy, however, can be difficult. For this reason it is recommended that liver from non-lesional area is also sampled for comparison. Diagnosing HCC on biopsy becomes even more challenging in several settings, including distinguishing well-differentiated HCC from high-grade dysplastic nodules in cirrhotic livers, distinguishing well-differentiated HCC from hepatocellular adenoma, identifying malignant transformation of a hepatocellular adenoma, and distinguishing poorly differentiated HCC (Fig. 11.4) from poorly differentiated cholangiocarcinoma and metastatic lesions. This section will focus on differentiating HCC from benign hepatocellular lesions, while later sections will focus on distinguishing HCC from other primary and metastatic tumors of the liver.

11.1.1 Benign Hepatocellular Lesions

High-grade dysplastic nodules are considered premalignant lesions that arise in the cirrhotic liver. They are characterized by architectural atypia, i.e., nodule within nodule, and/or cellular atypia, the most frequent being an increase in cell density with increased nuclear to cytoplasmic ratio, so-called small cell change. These lesions may have thickened trabeculae, but not greater than three hepatocytes thick. The hepatocyte nuclei are round and isochromatic. Occasional unpaired arteries can be seen. It is important to remember

W.-M. Cong (ed.), *Surgical Pathology of Hepatobiliary Tumors*, DOI 10.1007/978-981-10-3536-4_11

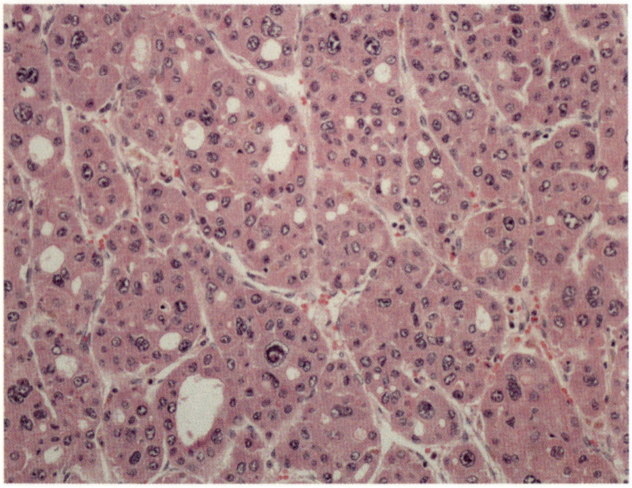

Fig. 11.1 Hepatocellular carcinoma with eosinophilic cytoplasm and thick trabeculae outlined by endothelial cells

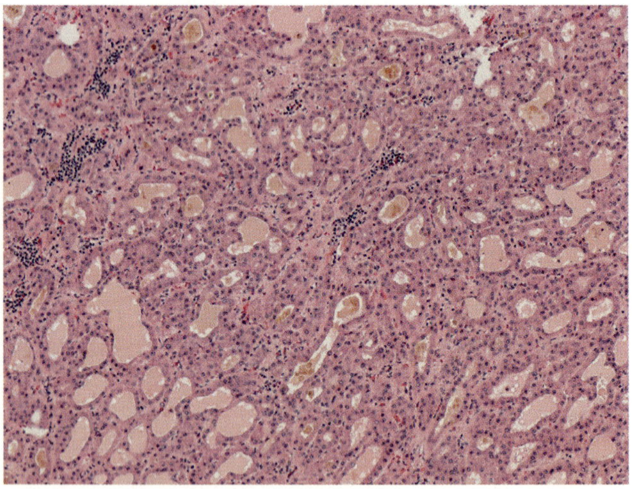

Fig. 11.2 Hepatocellular carcinoma with bile in the pseudoglands

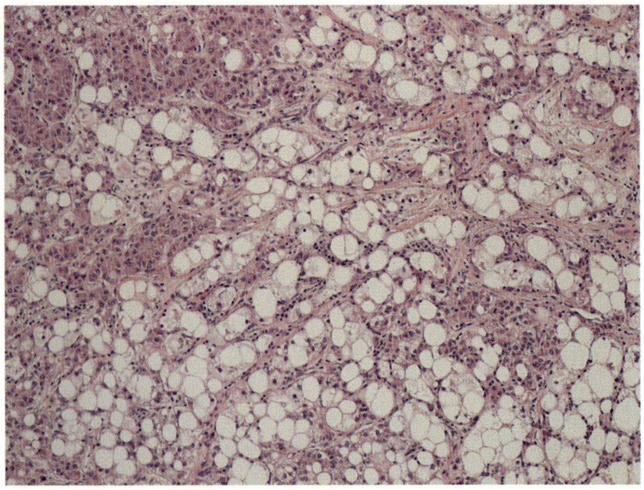

Fig. 11.3 Hepatocellular carcinoma with steatotic and ballooned tumor cells

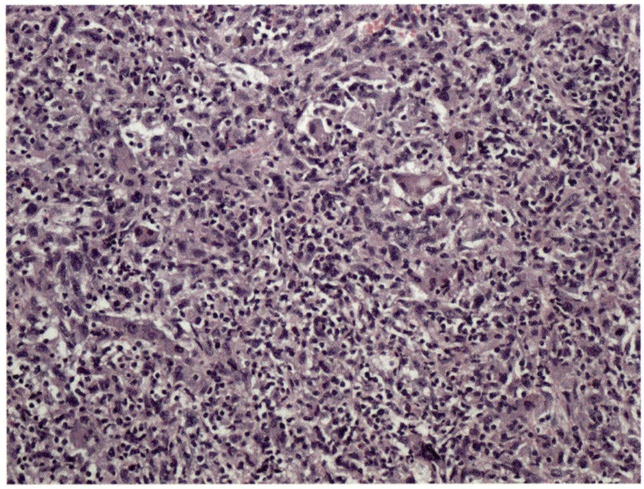

Fig. 11.4 Hepatocellular carcinoma, poorly differentiated without the characteristic eosinophilic cytoplasm or trabecular formation

that malignant transformation usually arise from the center of a high-grade dysplastic nodule and may not be represented when biopsy specimen is taken from the periphery of a lesion (Fig. 11.5). In the setting of genetic hemochromatosis, identification of nodules with decreased iron content compared to the surrounding liver (iron-free foci) indicates a proliferative, likely preneoplastic lesion [4].

Hepatocellular adenomas (HCAs) are benign clonal proliferations of hepatocytes that are encountered in noncirrhotic livers. Certain subtypes of HCAs have the potential to undergo malignant transformation, which will be described in more detail below. Focal nodular hyperplasia is a benign non-clonal proliferation of hepatocytes secondary to vascular changes and these lesions are not associated with significant malignant potential.

Currently, HCAs are classified into four distinct subtypes with differing clinical, morphological, immunohistochemical, and molecular features. These subtypes are designated as hepatocyte nuclear factor 1 alpha-mutated (H-HCA), inflammatory (I-HCA), and beta-catenin-mutated (b-HCA and b-IHCA) [5]. Hepatocellular adenomas that do not fit within these three groups are designated unclassified (U-HCA). H-HCAs usually arise sporadically or in the setting of maturity-onset diabetes of the young and are characterized histologically by steatosis and show no significant cytologic atypia. These tumors have no significant potential for malignant transformation. By immunohistochemistry, these tumors demonstrate loss of staining with liver fatty acid-binding protein (Fig. 11.6a, b), which helps in separating H-HCA from steatotic vaguely nodular HCC. b-HCAs are hepatocellular adenomas with malignant potential that show nuclear staining for beta-catenin and/or diffuse cytoplasmic staining with glutamine synthetase. These adenomas occur more frequently in men and often show cytologic atypia (Fig. 11.7a, b). I-HCA tumors may be associated with systemic inflammatory disorders and may act as a source of systemic inflammation. These tumors are characterized by a chronic inflammatory infiltrate, dilated and/or telangiectatic sinusoids, and portal tract-like structures which demonstrate ductular reaction but do not contain native bile ducts (Fig. 11.8a). These tumors show positive staining for the inflammatory markers, serum amyloid A protein and/or C-reactive protein (Fig. 11.8b). A subset of I-HCAs that harbor a beta-catenin mutation (b-IHCA) have a potential for malignant transformation. As the understanding of the malignant potential for subgroups of HCAs has grown, biopsy is becoming more important in the decision-making process of managing these patients. An immunohistochemical panel consisting of beta-catenin, glutamine synthetase, liver fatty acid-binding protein, serum amyloid A, and C-reactive protein is recommended to appropriately classify the tumor. If limited tissue is available, staining with glutamine synthetase is the most useful in determining malignant potential and has the added benefit of ruling out focal nodular hyperplasia, which has a characteristic "maplike" staining pattern (see below). In addition, glutamine synthetase immunoreaction of centrilobular hepatocytes is also useful in identifying non-lesional areas.

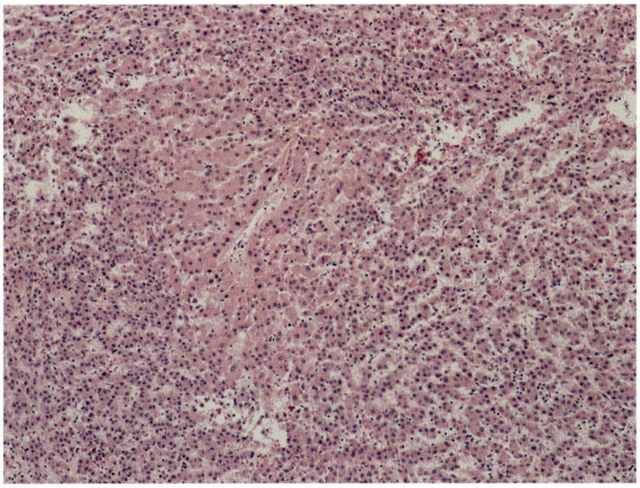

Fig. 11.5 Hepatocellular carcinoma arising in high-grade dysplastic nodule. A non-tumorous area still remains in the center

Focal nodular hyperplasia (FNH) is a benign non-clonal hepatocellular proliferation that develops in response to vascular changes within the liver. These tumors usually arise in young women without underlying liver disease. FNH has a classic pattern on imaging, demonstrating central scar, and most cases do not require biopsy for diagnosis. Fibrolamellar carcinoma is a malignant hepatocellular neoplasm that also often arises in young women in the absence of known liver disease and also often shows a central scar on imaging studies. Liver biopsy may be indicated in differentiating these tumors and will be discussed below. The inflammatory subtype of HCA can also mimic FNH on imaging and histology. Because HCAs have the potential for malignant transformation, especially when they contain a beta-catenin mutation, and carry a high risk for bleeding, their differentiation from FNHs on needle biopsy is essential. On histology, FNH consists of a nodular proliferation of cytologically bland hepatocytes with arteries which demonstrate irregular and eccentric wall thickening. The larger vessels are embedded in fibrous septa, which do not contain bile ducts, though ductular reaction can be seen along their periphery (Fig. 11.9a). It is important to have the appropriate clinical information (age, sex, and presence or absence of underlying liver disease)

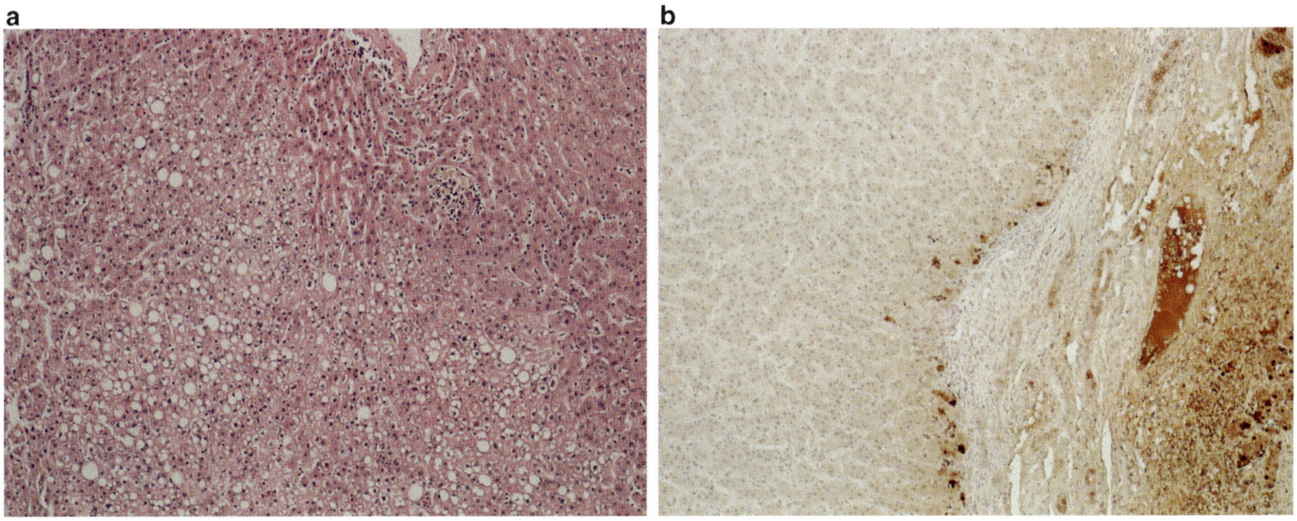

Fig. 11.6 Hepatocellular adenoma with steatosis, typically seen in HNF1α mutation (**a**); liver fatty acid-binding protein immunostain is absent in the adenoma (*left*) but is positive in the surrounding liver parenchyma (**b**)

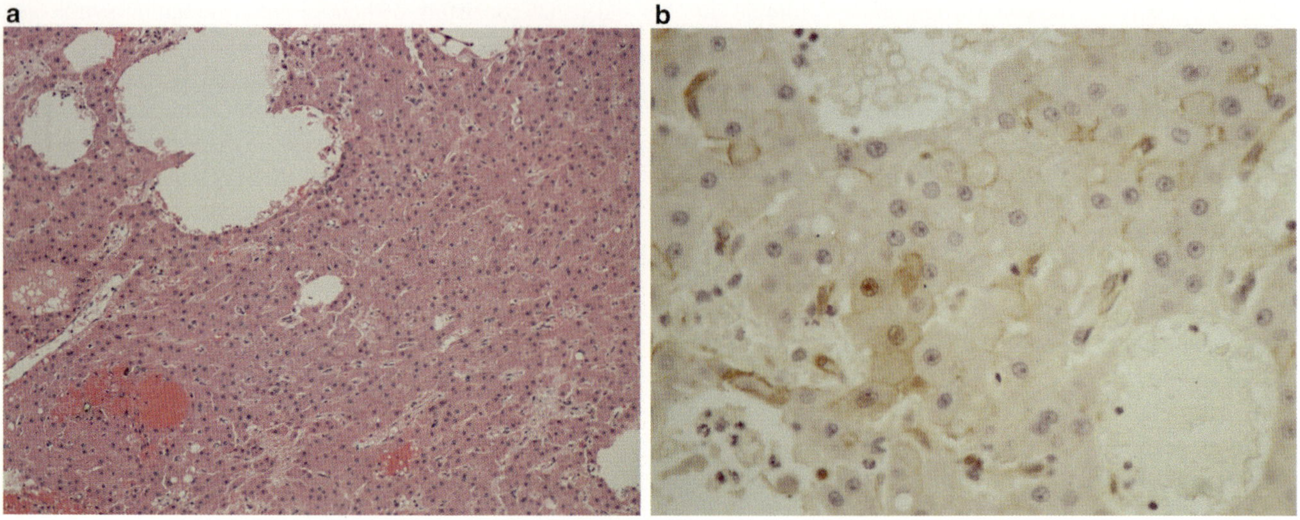

Fig. 11.7 β-catenin-mutated hepatocellular adenoma with atypia (**a**) and nuclear immunostaining for β-catenin (**b**)

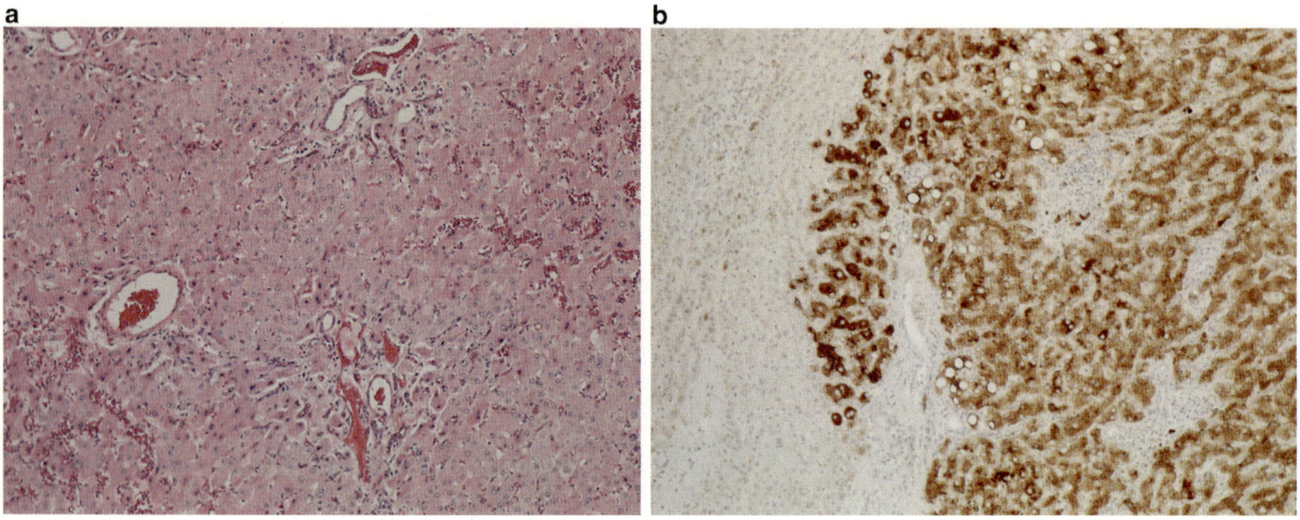

Fig. 11.8 Inflammatory hepatocellular adenoma with telangiectatic vessels and mild inflammation (**a**) and diffuse serum amyloid A immunostain of the adenoma (*right*) (**b**)

when considering the diagnosis of FNH on needle biopsy. Depending on the portion of the lesion that is biopsied, the lesion can mimic cirrhotic liver or an HCA. Recognition of eccentrically thickened arteries is key to making the diagnosis; however, these are not always sampled. Immunohistochemical stain for glutamine synthetase can be very helpful, especially if these eccentrically thickened vessels are not seen on the biopsy. Glutamine synthetase demonstrates a "maplike" staining pattern of hepatocytes away from the vascularized fibrous septa with absence of staining of periseptal regions [6] (Fig. 11.9b). This can be used to distinguish these lesions from HCAs which will either be diffusely positive in b-HCAs, or spotty, or negative in other subtypes of HCAs. The I-HCA subtype will demonstrate diffuse staining for serum amyloid A protein and/or C-reactive protein, which is not seen in FNH.

11.1.2 Well-Differentiated Hepatocellular Carcinoma

Well-differentiated HCC is characterized by tumor cells with relatively abundant eosinophilic cytoplasm with central round nuclei and containing nucleoli. Well-differentiated HCC generally demonstrates trabecular or pseudoglandular growth patterns. The pseudoglandular patterns of HCC can be readily distinguished from the nonneoplastic liver by pattern alone, while the trabecular pattern can present more difficulty, especially on a small biopsy (Fig. 11.10a, b) [7]. In

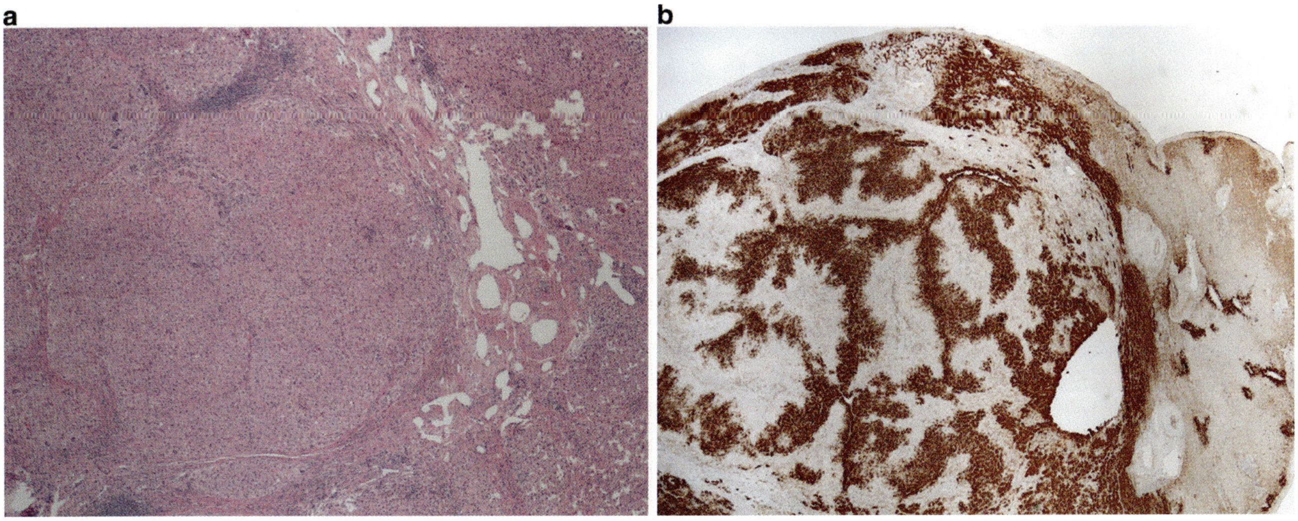

Fig. 11.9 Focal nodular hyperplasia with dystrophic blood vessels and fibrous septa (**a**) and characteristic maplike pattern of glutamine synthetase immunostain (*left*) (**b**)

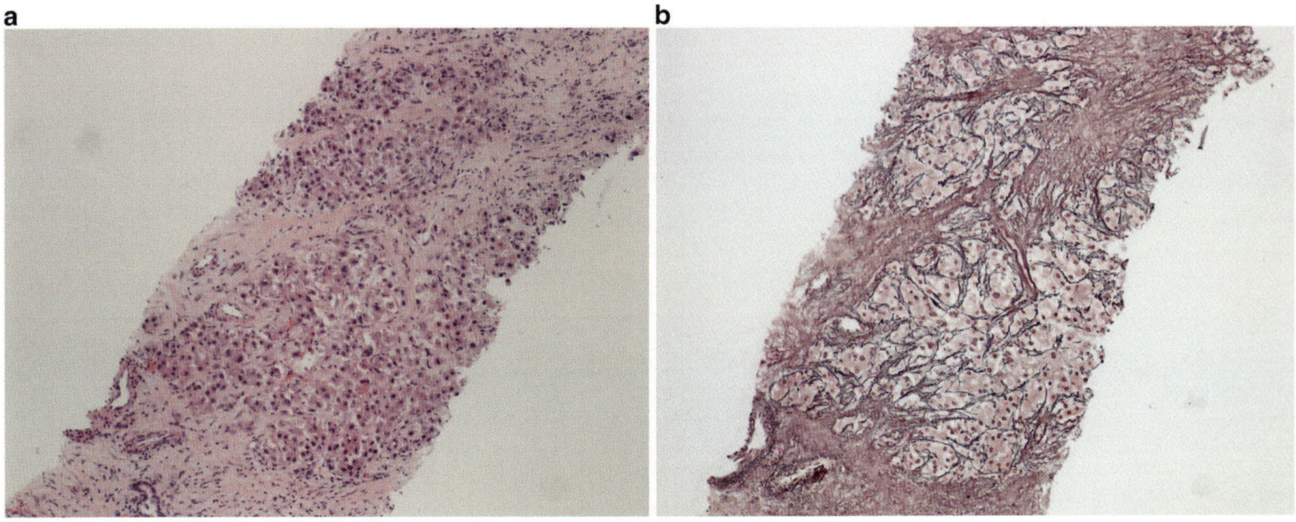

Fig. 11.10 Well-differentiated hepatocellular carcinoma (**a**) with altered but not decreased reticulin fibers (**b**)

general, a lesion with trabeculae more than three hepatocytes thick indicates a malignant lesion. Additionally, identifying unpaired arteries (i.e., arteries without an accompanying bile duct) also suggests a neoplastic process [8], though this feature does not help in distinguishing HCA or high-grade dysplastic nodule from HCC. Stromal invasion is a histologic feature that, when present is indicative of malignancy in a vaguely nodular lesion. Stromal invasion is characterized by neoplastic hepatocytes invading a portal tract or fibrous septum (Fig. 11.11) [9]. Crystal blue or trichrome stains may be useful in identifying areas of stromal invasion [10]. Steatosis may be present in well-differentiated HCC and is observed in 40% of vaguely nodular HCC (Fig. 11.12). The International Consensus Group for Hepatocellular Neoplasia lists the following features that may be present in various combinations in HCC: increased cell density to two times the surrounding liver tissue with increased nuclear to cytoplasmic ratio and irregular thin trabeculae pattern, varying number of portal tracts within the tumor, pseudoglandular pattern, diffuse fatty change, and varying numbers of unpaired arteries. While these features can be helpful, many can also be seen in high-grade dysplastic nodules and individually are thus not specific for HCC. If present on the biopsy specimen, stromal invasion remains the most useful histologic feature of malignancy [11]. Several ancillary studies can be useful in supporting the diagnosis of HCC. Reticulin stain outlines the trabeculae of normal hepatocytes, while this staining pattern can be lost or altered in malignant processes (Fig. 11.10b) [12]. Reticulin stain can also be useful in assessing the thickness of the trabeculae. The hepatic sinusoids in the nonneo-

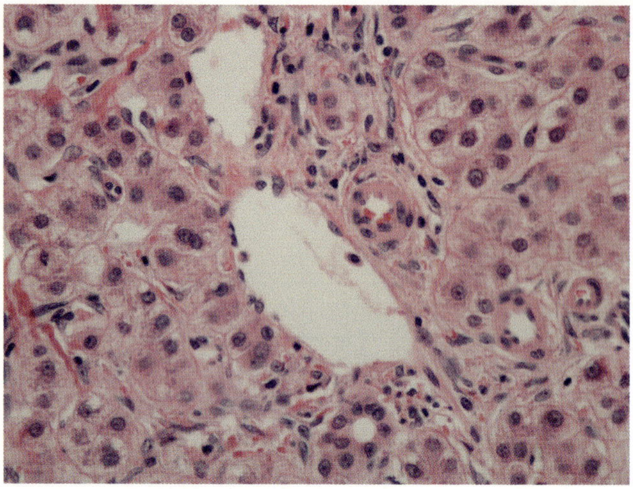

Fig. 11.11 Well-differentiated hepatocellular carcinoma with stromal invasion of tumor cells in the portal tract

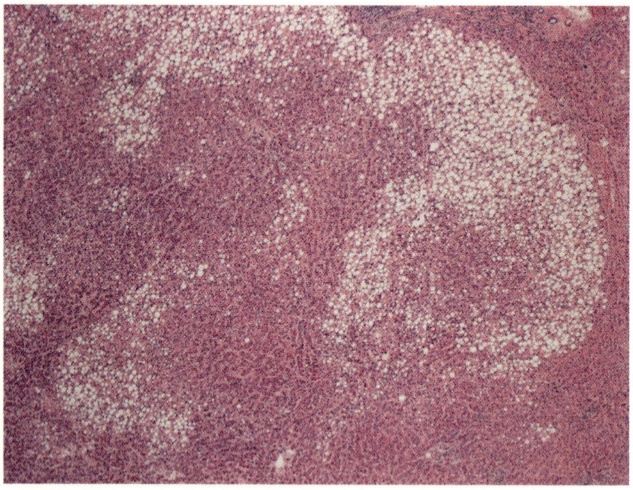

Fig. 11.12 Vaguely nodular hepatocellular carcinoma with steatosis and ill-defined borders

plastic liver are lined by a modified endothelium that does not stain for CD34, while the endothelial lining cells are often altered resulting in immunoreactivity for CD34 in HCC [8, 13]. A panel of three immunostains consisting of glypican-3, heat shock protein 70, and glutamine synthetase has been devised which demonstrates a 49% sensitivity and a 100% specificity in differentiating early HCC from high-grade dysplastic nodule on needle biopsy when any two markers are positive [14]. A panel of two immunostains of glypican-3 and heat shock protein 70 also showed a 67% sensitivity and 100% specificity in distinguishing HCC from HCA when either marker was positive. Glutamine synthase is not useful in this setting [15]. Of note, cholangiocarcinoma can also demonstrate trabecular architecture, especially at its periphery, though usually these tumors demonstrate fibrosis in the center of the tumor, and the tumor cells usually lack nucleoli (Fig. 11.13).

Fibrolamellar carcinoma is a rare malignant liver tumor with characteristic clinical and morphologic features. These tumors usually arise in young patients with no known underlying liver disease. Recently, a DNAJB1-PRKACA chimeric transcript has been identified in fibrolamellar carcinoma which may play a role in the pathogenesis [16]. On imaging, these tumors often show a central scar, similar to FNH. On histology, these tumors are very distinctive. They are characterized by large oncocytic tumor cells with prominent nuclei within a dense lamellated collagenous background (Fig. 11.14). Some tumor cells may contain large amphophilic cytoplasmic inclusions termed "pale bodies." [17] These tumors demonstrate hepatocellular differentiation, staining positively for HepPar-1. Unlike HCC, these tumors are almost universally positive for CK7 [18], EMA [19], and CD68 [20] (Fig. 11.15), and many also show positivity for other biliary markers such as B72.3, CK19, EpCAM, or monoclonal CEA by immunohistochemistry [19].

Hepatoblastoma is the most common primary malignant liver tumor in infancy and young children. They rarely occur in older children or adults. Hepatoblastoma can be classified as epithelial type or mixed epithelial and mesenchymal type. The epithelial type can be further subdivided into pure fetal, mixed fetal and embryonal, mixed fetal and macrotrabecular, and mixed fetal and small cell undifferentiated, while the mixed epithelial and mesenchymal type can be further divided into those with and without teratoid features [21]. The fetal morphology consists of an alternating pattern of pale and darker staining epithelial cells resembling hepatocytes (Fig. 11.16). The embryonal type consists of angulated darker cells with high nucleus to cytoplasm ratio arranged in sheets or clusters or singly. The macrotrabecular subtype consists of thickened trabeculae (more than ten cells thick), and the small cell undifferentiated subtype consists of discohesive small round blue cells with minimal cytoplasm. The mixed epithelial and mesenchymal type consists of an epithelial component plus a mesenchymal component, such as mature or immature fibrous tissue, cartilage, or osteoid-like tissue. Mixed tumors with other mesenchymal and epithelial components such as skeletal muscle, bone, cartilage, and stratified squamous epithelium are considered teratoid. Differentiating fetal subtype of hepatoblastoma, especially when macrotrabecular component is present, from a well-differentiated HCC, can be difficult on a biopsy specimen, especially in older children or adolescents in which either type of tumor may be seen [22]. Identification of the pattern of alternating pale and darker staining cells is a key feature in diagnosing the fetal subtype of hepatoblastoma in these cases.

a b

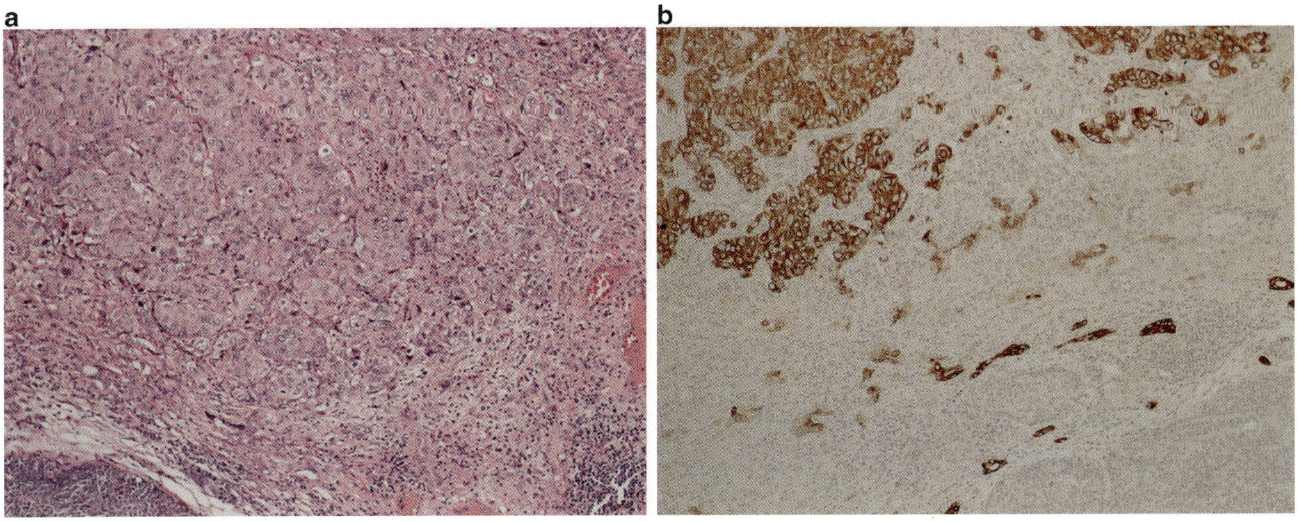

Fig. 11.13 Trabecular-like arrangement of tumor cells at the periphery of intrahepatic cholangiocarcinoma (**a**). Tumor cells are positive for CK7 (**b**)

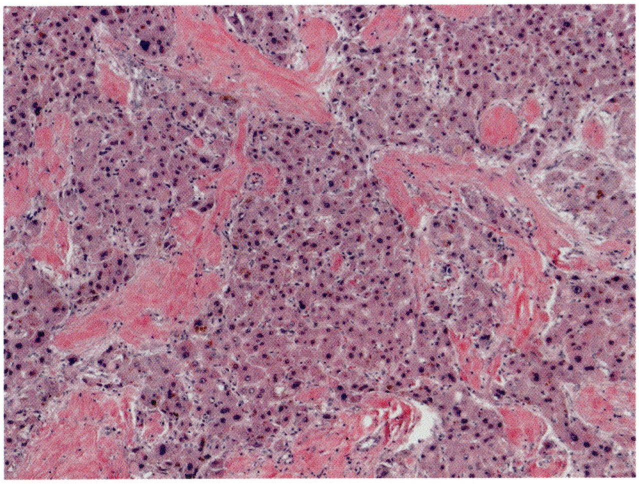

Fig. 11.14 Fibrolamellar carcinoma with large eosinophilic cells separated by hyaline fibrous septa

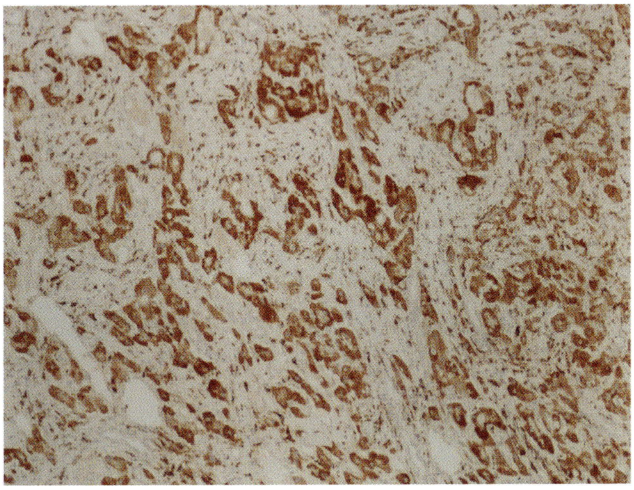

Fig. 11.15 Fibrolamellar carcinoma with CD68 positive tumor cells

11.2 Biopsy Diagnosis of Cholangiocarcinoma, Combined Hepatocellular-Cholangiocarcinoma, Mixed Primary Liver Carcinoma, and Benign Biliary Proliferations

Intrahepatic cholangiocarcinoma (ICCA) usually arises in a non-cirrhotic liver and less commonly in hepatitis B, hepatitis C, and alcoholic-related cirrhosis. It can be subdivided into mass-forming, periductal infiltrating, and intraductal types. The periductal infiltrating type is characterized by tumor growth along the biliary tree, without a clear mass lesion, while the intraductal type is characterized by a papillary growth of biliary epithelium within the duct lumen which may cause cystic dilatation (Figs. 11.17 and 11.18). These types are much less common than the mass-forming types and may require resection in order to appreciate the architecture and establish the diagnosis. Mass-forming ICCA is often indistinguishable from metastatic carcinoma and less frequently from hepatocellular carcinoma on imaging, and a biopsy may be required for diagnosis.

The diagnosis of ICCA is essentially a diagnosis of exclusion as metastatic lesions must be ruled out clinically and/or histologically. Several morphologic patterns can be seen in cholangiocarcinoma as these tumors can range from well to moderately to poorly differentiated carcinoma. The well-differentiated tumors are characterized by proliferation of regular glands with cuboidal or columnar lining and round regular nuclei. Moderately differentiated tumors may show more tortuous or less defined glands and are often lined by cells with more atypical nuclei (Fig. 11.19). Poorly differen-

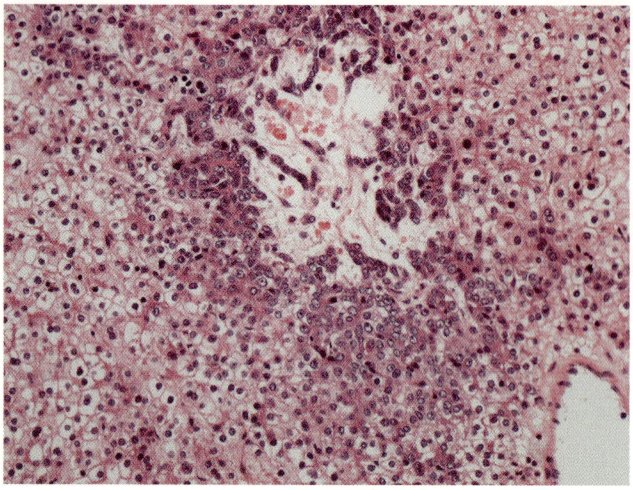

Fig. 11.16 Hepatoblastoma with characteristic darker and lighter-stained tumor cells

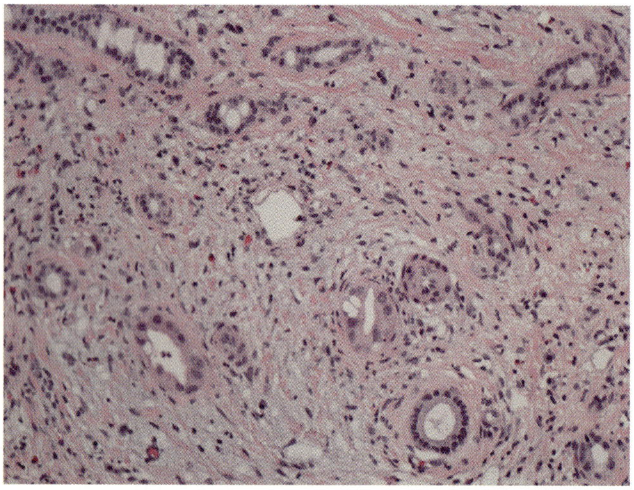

Fig. 11.17 Cholangiocarcinoma with periductal invasion

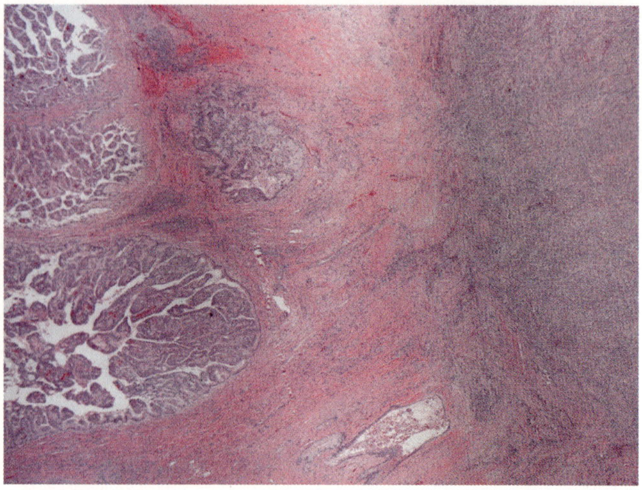

Fig. 11.18 Intraductal papillary cholangiocarcinoma

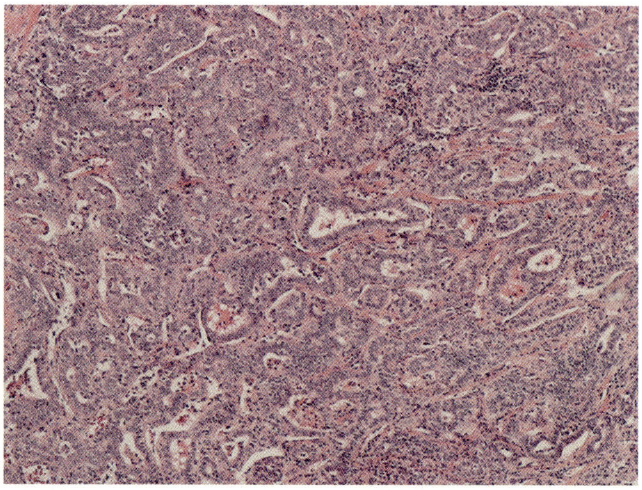

Fig. 11.19 Intrahepatic cholangiocarcinoma, moderately differentiated

tiated tumors may show cells with scanty cytoplasm arranged in sheets, nests, trabeculae, or occasionally cribriform structures sometimes with comedonecrosis (Fig. 11.20). There is no obvious glandular formation. Undifferentiated cholangiocarcinomas consisting of markedly atypical cells with no discernable architectural structure are only rarely seen. Some tumors may show features more frequently seen in hilar and extrahepatic cholangiocarcinomas, including more pronounced mucin production, large glands with tall columnar cells, infiltration of the portal structures, and papillary growth pattern. These may represent tumors that originated as intraductal papillary neoplasms and progressed to form a mass lesion. ICCAs almost always initiate desmoplastic reaction. Interestingly, some ICCAs are comprised of polygonal eosinophilic tumor cells arranged in a prominent trabecular growth pattern, and these tumors may be difficult to distinguish from HCC. Trabecular growth may also be seen at the periphery of typical cholangiocarcinoma (Fig. 11.13). Helpful features in distinguishing these tumors from HCC include a more prominent fibrous stroma, especially in the center of the tumor, and lack of nucleoli. Bile production by the tumor is definitive evidence of hepatocellular, rather than biliary differentiation, although bile trapping sometimes is seen in ICCA. Immunohistochemical stains can usually resolve any difficult cases. Immunohistochemical evidence of hepatocellular carcinoma include positive staining for HepPar-1, cytoplasmic staining for TTF-1 (certain clone of antibody such as 8G7G3/1), and canalicular staining pattern with CD10 and pCEA. Cholangiocarcinomas are positive for CK7 and negative for the above markers of hepatocytic differentiation [7]. Of note, HCC can occasionally show focal positive staining for CK7, particularly the scirrhous type, a rare variant which is characterized by a dense fibrous stroma which may also demonstrate less staining with HepPar-1 [23].

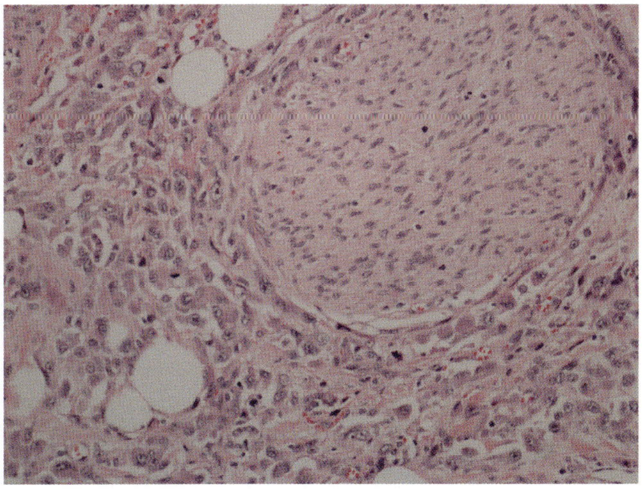

Fig. 11.20 Poorly differentiated cholangiocarcinoma without glandular formation in perineural spaces

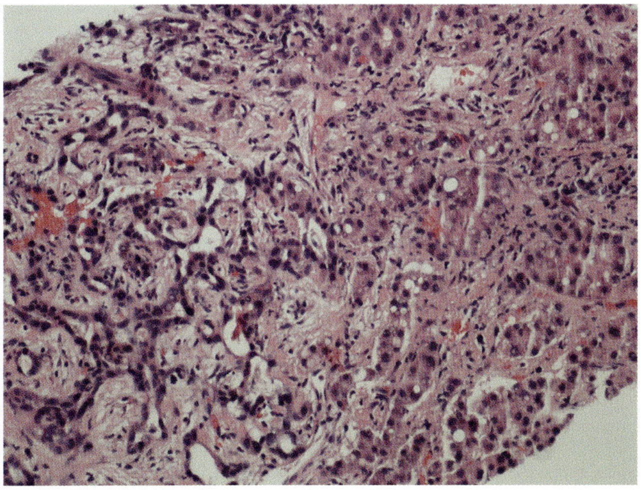

Fig. 11.21 Both hepatocellular carcinoma (*right*) and cholangiocarcinoma (*left*) components are present in combined cholangio-hepatocellular carcinoma

Evaluation of adenocarcinoma in the liver requires clinical and pathological correlation. If a primary site is known, comparison with the prior specimen or a focused immunohistochemical panel (e.g., TTF-1 if a history of primary lung is known) can confirm or rule out metastasis from this site. While there are no specific immunohistochemical stains that can be used to definitively diagnose cholangiocarcinoma, immunohistochemistry is helpful in ruling out metastatic lesions from other sites. If a primary tumor site is not clinically apparent, a panel of immunohistochemical stains including CK7, CK20, CDX-2, TTF-1, PAX8, GATA3, p63, plus WT1, ER, PR, BRST-2, and mammaglobin in women, or PSA and prostatic acid phosphatase in men, may be useful in guiding the search for primary site by ruling in or out lower gastrointestinal, lung, thyroid, kidney, urinary bladder, breast, mullerian, or prostate tumors. ICCAs are generally positive for CK7 and CK19, variably positive for CK20, and negative for the remaining markers listed above, though weak nuclear staining with CDX-2 can be seen. Pancreas, gallbladder, and upper gastrointestinal (stomach and small intestine) primaries also share this immune profile and thus cannot be distinguished by immunohistochemistry and morphology; and therefore clinical correlation is essential.

A tumor may contain areas or show features of both hepatocellular carcinoma and cholangiocarcinoma, and these are designated combined hepatocellular-cholangiocarcinomas (see Chap. 10 for more in-depth discussion). Diagnosis of a combined hepatocellular-cholangiocarcinoma cannot usually be made on biopsy since it is unlikely that there would be sufficient tissue from both components in a small biopsy specimen to document the dual nature of this tumor. This diagnosis should be considered especially if a tumor is showing features of both HCC and cholangiocarcinoma (Fig. 11.21).

Cholangiolocellular carcinoma is a rare liver tumor that morphologically is characterized by cords of bland-looking cells within a fibrous stroma that closely resembles ductular reaction or bile duct adenoma (Fig. 11.22). This tumor is often in association with classic cholangiocarcinoma or hepatocellular carcinoma. Cholangiolocellular carcinoma is thought to arise from the canals of Herring and is positive for biliary markers such as CK7 and CK19 as well as N-CAM. Some tumors may be positive for p53. This tumor can be distinguished from classical cholangiocarcinoma by positivity for N-CAM; however, distinguishing this tumor from benign ductular reaction is more difficult, especially on biopsy. This is an important distinction since ductular reaction may be present at the interface of a tumor and the uninvolved liver parenchyma. Immunostain for p53 can be useful, if positive, to favor a cholangiocellular carcinoma; however, a negative result does not rule out this tumor [7].

11.2.1 Mixed Primary Liver Carcinoma (See Chap. 5)

11.2.1.1 Benign Biliary Proliferations

Bile duct adenoma consists of a benign proliferation of duct-like structures with variable stroma (Fig. 11.23). Grossly, these lesions are usually small firm subcapsular nodules, and they are often identified when surveying the abdomen at the time of surgery for resection of a non-liver tumor. A frozen section is often requested to rule out metastatic carcinoma. On histology, these lesions are characterized by closely packed tubular structures with small lumen and minimal intervening stroma. Cytologically, the cells are bland, with abundant cytoplasm and regular nuclei. Eosinophilic round to oval inclusions, containing alpha1-antitrypsin, are some-

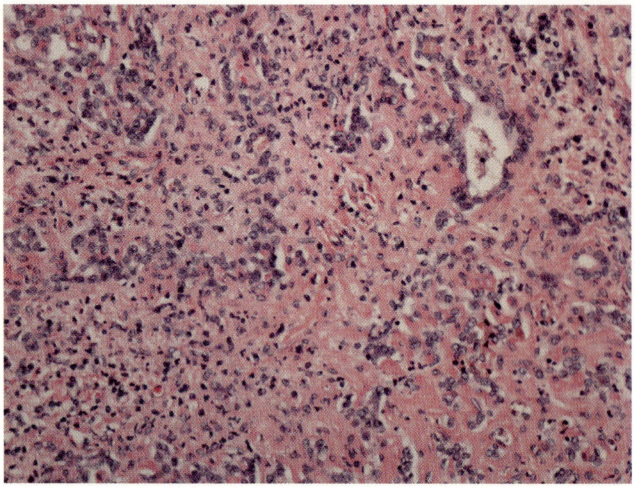

Fig. 11.22 Cholangiolocellular carcinoma with cords of bland-looking ductular-like cells within fibrotic stroma

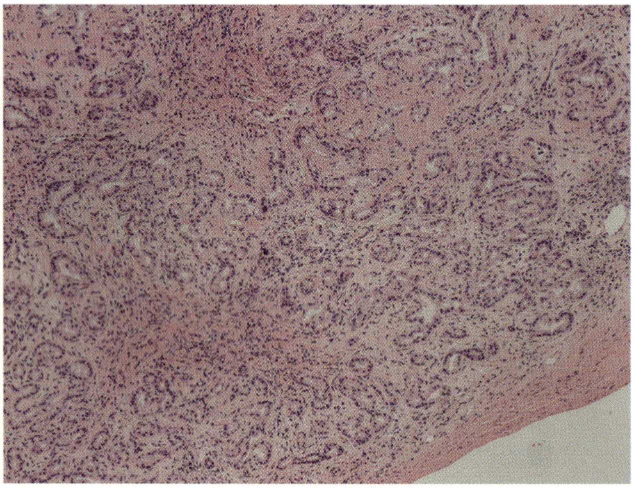

Fig. 11.23 Subcapsular bile duct adenoma

times observed. Occasional cases may show some atypia, and case reports have described cholangiocarcinomas arising from these lesions, but the vast majority of bile duct adenomas are benign.

Bile duct hamartoma, or von Meyenburg complex, is another small firm lesion which may be multiple and present anywhere in the liver (Fig. 11.24). Subcapsular bile duct hamartoma may be identified at the time of surgery and sent for frozen section to rule out metastatic carcinoma. These lesions are always associated with portal tracts and are generally characterized by more abundant stroma than bile duct adenoma. The lumens of the duct-like structures are usually patent, tortuous, and often contain bile. Cytologically, these lesions are bland, though, like bile duct adenoma, rare cases have been reported in association with cholangiocarcinoma. In situ carcinoma, however, has not been documented.

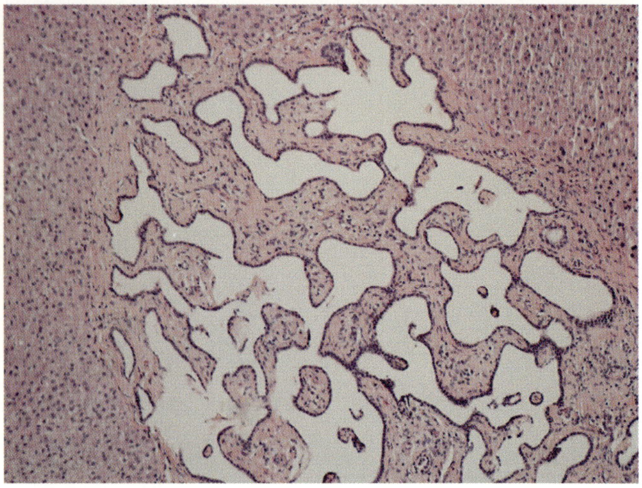

Fig. 11.24 von Meyenburg complex within a portal tract

Biliary adenofibroma is a larger benign biliary lesion that morphologically resembles a von Meyenburg complex with characteristic complex tubulocystic proliferation of biliary epithelium within a fibroblastic stroma (Fig. 11.25). Additionally, intraluminal bile concretions, apocrine-like epithelial change, acute inflammation, and granulomas may also be seen [24].

11.2.1.2 Biopsy Diagnosis of Other Liver Tumors

Neuroendocrine tumors, especially of gastrointestinal tract origin, often metastasize to the liver. Many will be low-grade tumors which would show relative uniformity of the tumor cells which have a "salt and pepper" chromatin pattern. More poorly differentiated tumors may resemble large and small cell carcinomas analogous to those seen in the lung. Neuroendocrine tumors may also arise as primary tumors in the liver. This diagnosis requires careful exclusion of other primary sites of origin [25]. Primary and metastatic neuroendocrine tumors will demonstrate immunohistochemical evidence of neuroendocrine differentiation with positive staining for synaptophysin, chromogranin, neuron specific enolase, and/or CD56. Immunohistochemical stain for Ki-67 is useful in determining the proliferation index and grade of these tumors. Primary hepatic signet ring cell neuroendocrine tumor is a rare primary liver tumor that morphologically resembles a signet ring cell carcinoma with a clear vacuole-like space. Ancillary tests show that this space is not a mucin-containing vacuole but rather is composed of cytokeratin filaments (Fig. 11.30). The tumor cells are also positive for neuroendocrine markers such as synaptophysin and chromogranin. This tumor should be considered when a tumor with signet ring morphology is encountered in the absence of a known primary tumor such as gastric primary [26].

Several vascular tumors can arise as primary hepatic neoplasms in the pediatric and adult patient population. Hemangiomas are the most common primary tumor of the liver and consist of a benign vascular proliferation. These tumors are usually readily diagnosed by imaging studies and biopsy is avoided due to bleeding risk. Histologically, they consist of dilated vascular spaces lined by benign endothelium within a fibrotic stroma. These tumors may become hyalinized or sclerotic. Occasionally a sclerotic hemangioma may be noted during surgery for another reason and a frozen section may be requested to rule out metastatic carcinoma. In these cases, the outline of the prior vascular spaces can usually be appreciated, leading to the correct diagnosis.

Epithelioid hemangioendothelioma is a rare vascular tumor that can mimic intrahepatic cholangiocarcinoma. The tumor is characterized by eosinophilic epithelioid tumor cells which invade the liver sinusoids. The epithelioid cells may contain intracellular lumens that can mimic signet ring cells. Identification of red blood cells within these intracytoplasmic lumens is very helpful in correctly identifying this tumor. The tumor may also contain spindle or stellate dendritic cells and cells with an intermediate morphology between epithelioid cells and dendritic cells (Fig. 11.26a). When the diagnosis of epithelioid hemangioendothelioma is suspected, confirmation can be made by demonstrating positive staining with vascular markers such as CD31, CD34, and factor VIII-associated antigen (Fig. 11.26b). Most epithelioid hemangioendotheliomas harbor a WWTR1-CAMTA1 gene fusion [27, 28], while a distinct subset harbors a YAP1-TFE3 gene fusion [29] both of which can be detected with molecular techniques. These tumors may also demonstrate staining for cytokeratin which may lead to the misdiagnosis of this tumor as a carcinoma.

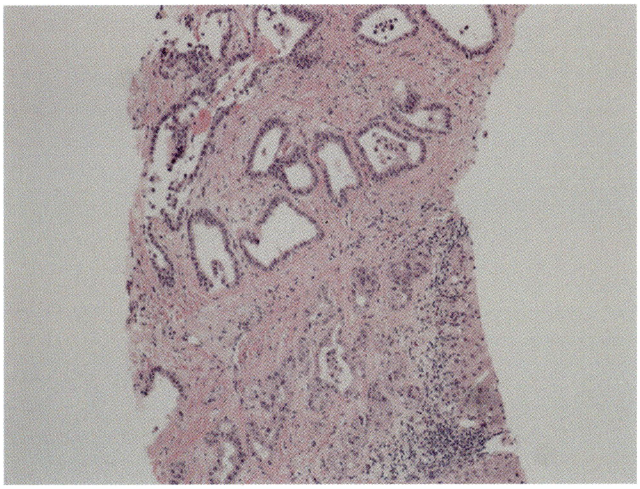

Fig. 11.25 Biliary adenofibroma containing tubulocystic proliferation of biliary epithelium in its stroma

Primary angiosarcoma of the liver can also rarely be encountered. These tumors demonstrate features similar to angiosarcoma in other locations, containing irregular vascular spaces lined by atypical endothelial cells with prominent nuclei which protrude into the lumen of the vascular spaces giving them a hobnail appearance (Fig. 11.27). These tumors will also be positive for vascular markers such as CD31 and CD34.

Infantile hemangioma is a benign vascular proliferation that occurs in infancy. These tumors tend to follow a course of proliferation, maturation, and involution and can cause serious complications including heart failure and rupture. Histologically, these tumors are characterized by a proliferation of vascular channels lined by bland endothelial cells at the periphery and more fibrous tissue in the center of the

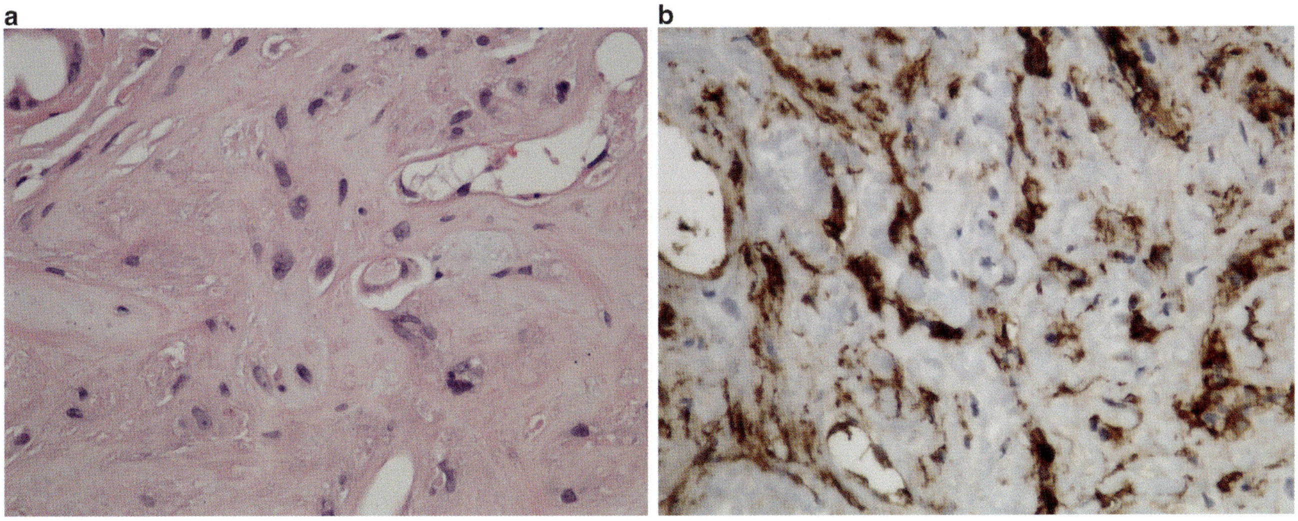

Fig. 11.26 Epithelioid hemangioendothelioma with plump, spindle, and stellate endothelial tumor cells and fibrotic background (**a**) and immunostaining of tumor cells for CD34 (**b**)

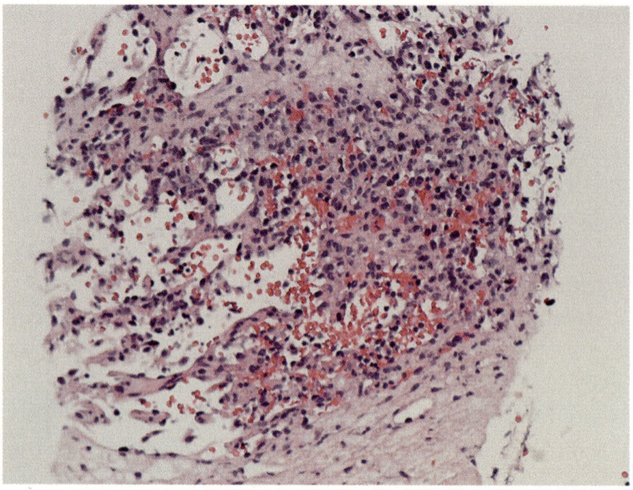

Fig. 11.27 Angiosarcoma with pleomorphic tumor cells in vascular channels and forming solid area of tumor cells

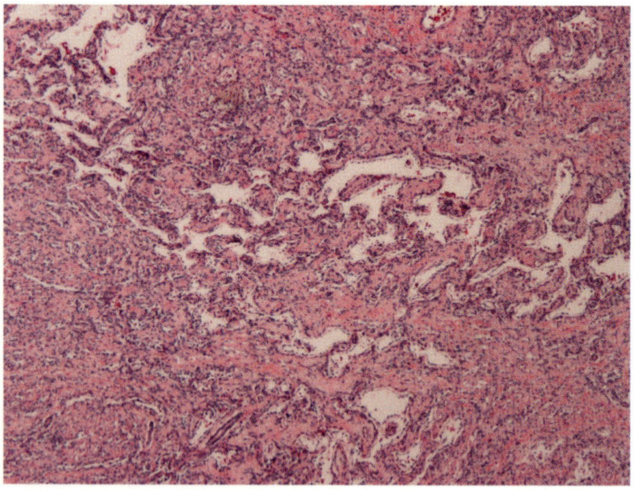

Fig. 11.28 Infantile hemangioendothelioma with proliferative vascular channels lined by endothelial cells

lesion (Fig. 11.28). Hepatocytes and bile ducts are often entrapped at the edges of the tumor. Infantile angiosarcoma is the very rare malignant correlate which is characterized by vascular channels lined by pleomorphic and hyperchromatic endothelial cells that demonstrate budding and branching and often an accompanying spindle cell component.

Angiomyolipoma is a tumor with malignant potential that can arise in the liver. These tumors are characterized by adipose tissue, blood vessels, and spindle or epithelioid cells in various proportions (Fig. 11.29a). Depending on the composition and sampling of the tumor, this entity can mimic a lipoma, a mesenchymal tumor, or an epithelial tumor. The epithelioid component of angiomyolipoma has sometimes been mistaken as well-differentiated HCC. Rare cases of malignant angiomyolipoma have been reported. Immunohistochemical stains for melanoma markers HMB-45 and melan-A are positive in these tumors, distinguishing these tumors from carcinomas and other mesenchymal tumors (Fig. 11.29b).

The liver can give rise to a variety of cystic neoplasms. The majority are cysts that contain clear serous fluid and are lined by benign biliary or mesothelial cells, though in many cases the lining cells may become denuded. Mucinous cystic neoplasms can also be seen in the liver. These cysts are similar to the mucinous cystic neoplasms encountered in the pancreas. They contain mucus and are lined by mucinous epithelium with surrounding ovarian-like stroma which is positive for estrogen receptor (ER), progesterone receptor (PR), inhibin, and CD10 by immunohistochemistry. Unlike the simple biliary cysts, mucinous cystic neoplasms can develop dysplasia and invasive carcinoma; thus, it is important that these tumors are removed entirely. Occasionally, a cystic lesion will be biopsied, or a frozen section will be performed to rule out a mucinous cystic neoplasm to guide the surgical management. Finding the mucinous lining with the ovarian-like stroma is necessary in establishing the diagnosis of mucinous neoplasm (Fig. 11.30). Immunohistochemical stains for ER, PR, and inhibin and CD10 may be useful in identifying or confirming the presence of ovarian-like stroma. It is also important to distinguish these lesions from echinococcal cysts which would have a fibrotic lining with a laminated membrane and germinal membrane. Protoscolices may also be seen.

Inflammatory pseudotumor is a mass-forming proliferation of myofibroblasts and fibrous tissue with prominent plasma cell infiltration. Most lesions are thought to be reactive, though some may show overexpression of ALK-1 and may be neoplastic. Some cases may fall under the expanding group of IgG4-related diseases that are seen in other organ systems, such as the pancreas. These lesions may be biopsied to rule out a malignant process. The finding of a prominent plasma cell proliferation in the background of a myofibroblastic proliferation without significant atypia is important in distinguishing this lesion from a malignant lymphoma or other tumors. Immunohistochemical stains may show a prominence of IgG4-positive cells in inflammatory pseudotumors.

Lymphoma may involve the liver as a primary process or metastatic disease. The tumor may present as a mass-forming lesion or an infiltrative process. Hepatitis C, primary biliary cirrhosis, and autoimmune hepatitis have also been associated with primary hepatic diffuse large B-cell lymphoma and mucosa-associated lymphoid tissue (MALT) lymphoma (Fig. 11.31) [30]. A liver mass may be biopsied to reveal a malignant lymphocytic proliferation. Clinical correlation would be necessary to distinguish primary or secondary involvement of the liver. Some lymphomas, such as hepatosplenic T-cell lymphoma, may present as an infiltrative process, and a biopsy may be performed due to altered liver

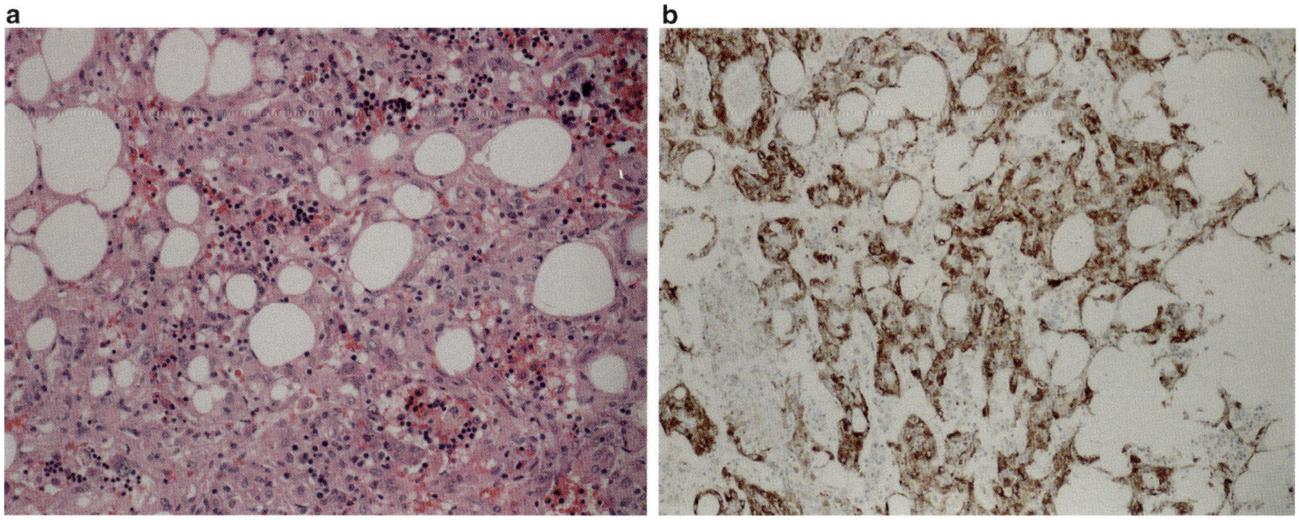

Fig. 11.29 Angiomyolipoma with epithelioid muscle cells and adipose tissue (**a**) and HMB-45 immunostain (**b**)

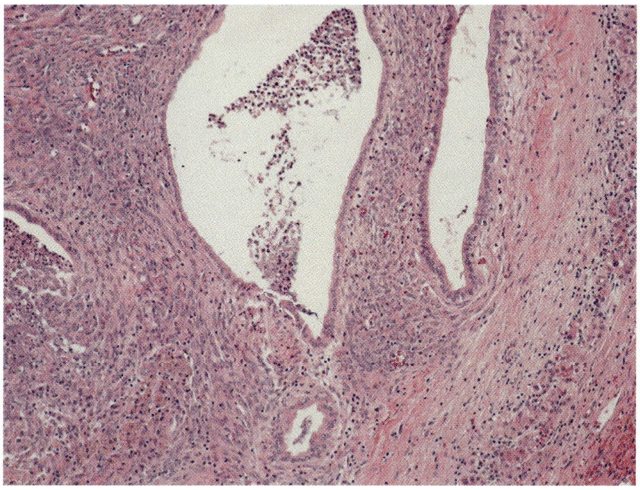

Fig. 11.30 Mucinous cystic neoplasm with mucinous epithelium and underlying "ovarian-like" stroma

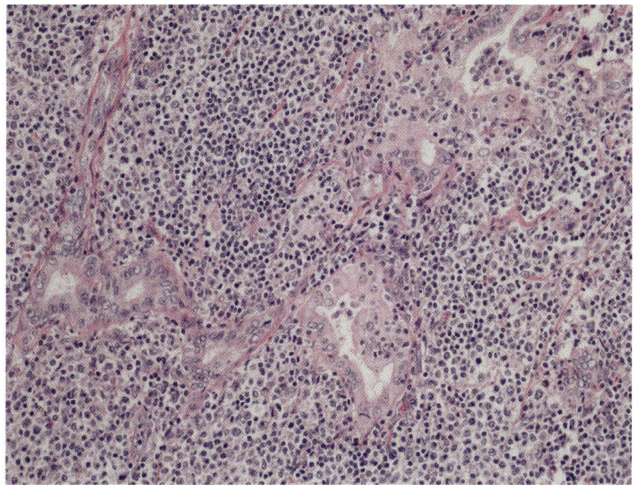

Fig. 11.31 Mucosa-associated lymphoid tissue (MALT) lymphoma with tumor cells surrounding distorted bile duct

enzyme levels without an identifiable mass (Fig. 11.32). In these cases, the malignant lymphoid cells diffusely infiltrate the sinusoidal spaces. Special care should be taken in evaluating the cells within the sinusoids to avoid missing this diagnosis. A panel of immunohistochemical stains and possibly molecular studies may be required to evaluate an atypical lymphoid proliferation encountered on liver biopsy.

Two additional mesenchymal tumors that may also be encountered in the pediatric population are mesenchymal hamartoma and embryonal sarcoma. Mesenchymal hamartoma is a multicystic tumorlike lesion of the liver that develops before birth and is usually diagnosed before the age of 3. On histology, the lesion consists of a loose myxoid or collagenous connective tissue arranged around duct or duct-like structures. Embryonal sarcoma is a malignant mesenchymal tumor that most often affects children aged 6–15 years of age. The tumor is composed of loose or myxoid stroma with spindle cells, polymorphous cells, giant cells, and stellate cells with marked pleomorphism. Intracytoplasmic hyaline globules are commonly seen in the large polymorphous cells. Some tumors may show a storiform pattern and others may show anaplastic components or osteoid formation. Entrapped islands of hepatocytes and bile duct-like structures may be seen. Immunohistochemically, embryonal sarcomas are strongly positive for vimentin and may show positivity for desmin, cytokeratin, alpha smooth muscle actin, alpha-1-anti-trypsin, CD10, CD68, and calponin. Importantly, embryonal sarcoma is negative for MyoD1, which is helpful in differentiating this tumor from rhabdomyosarcoma, and does not show nuclear staining with beta-catenin, which is helpful in differentiating this tumor from hepatoblastoma.

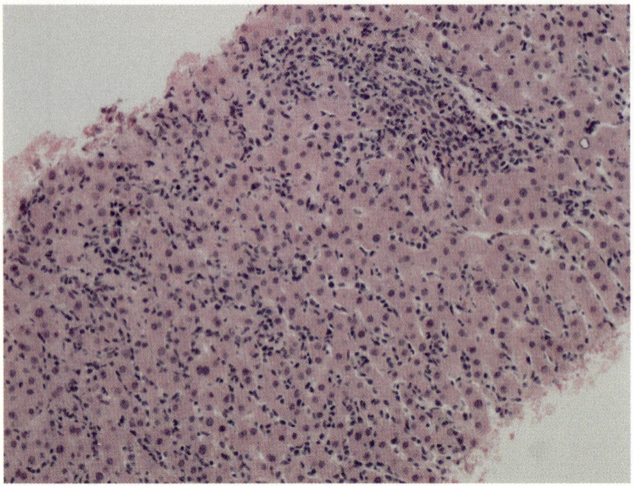

Fig. 11.32 Hepatosplenic T-cell lymphoma with tumor cells in sinusoids

Many other tumors may be seen as primary lesions in the liver, including lymphangioma, solitary fibrous tumor, Kaposi sarcoma, leiomyosarcoma, rhabdomyosarcoma, synovial sarcoma, teratoma, and yolk sac tumors. These tumor show similar morphologic and immunohistochemical features to these tumors located in soft tissue and other sites and will not be further discussed here.

11.3 Biopsy in Differential Diagnosis of Liver Tumors

Liver biopsy is a very useful procedure in diagnosing liver tumors. The clinical information, especially age and sex of the patient, presence of underlying liver disease, and history of prior malignancy, are crucial for the accurate diagnosis. It is often helpful if the biopsy specimen contains tissue from the tumor as well as the non-tumor liver, especially in distinguishing well-differentiated HCC from a regenerative nodule in the setting of cirrhosis or differentiating hepatic adenoma from surrounding nonneoplastic liver. Examination of the non-tumor liver may also provide important information, such as identifying previously undiagnosed liver disease such as steatohepatitis, hemochromatosis, alpha-1 antitrypsin deficiency, and autoimmune hepatitis or staging and grading of known liver disease such as viral hepatitis. The approach to the biopsy of a liver mass should be guided by the clinical scenario of the biopsy.

In an adult patient with established cirrhosis and a liver mass with equivocal imaging findings, the primary differential diagnosis will be between HCC and a regenerative or dysplastic nodule. Significant cytologic atypia or pseudoglandular architecture would indicate malignancy, as well as identification of stromal invasion or vascular invasion. Helpful, but less specific, histologic features that would favor malignancy include presence of unpaired arteries and trabecular architecture with trabeculae more than three hepatocytes thick. If the histologic features remain equivocal, additional studies may be required. Demonstration of the loss or increased (in well-differentiated HCC) of the reticulin staining pattern supports the diagnosis of HCC. A panel of immunohistochemical stains for glypican-3, HSP-70, and glutamine synthetase may also be useful. If the tumor is positive for two or more of these stains, this is strong evidence of malignancy, though approximately half of HCCs will not show this staining pattern. If these additional studies are inconclusive, then the diagnosis rests on the balance of histologic features that would favor either a well-differentiated HCC or a dysplastic or regenerative nodule.

In an adult patient with a liver mass without known liver disease, a metastatic tumor must first be ruled out. Imaging characteristics may be able to differentiate a glandular lesion from a hepatocytic lesion. If an adenocarcinoma is identified on biopsy, a careful review of the clinical history is crucial in identifying a possible source of a metastatic lesion. This could then be confirmed on biopsy by morphology and immunohistochemical stains. If no primary site is identified, a panel consisting of CK7, CK20, CDX-2, TTF-1, PAX8, GATA3, p63 plus WT1, ER, PR, BRST-2, and mammaglobin in women, or PSA and prostatic acid phosphatase in men, may be helpful in directing the search for a primary lesion. If the lesion is only positive for CK7, the differential would include a primary intrahepatic cholangiocarcinoma in addition to a metastatic lesion from the pancreas or upper gastrointestinal tract. If signet ringlike cells are seen, epithelioid hemangioendothelioma should be considered. Some of these tumors may show red blood cells within the intracellular spaces, strongly suggestive of epithelioid hemangioendothelioma. These tumors may be positive for cytokeratins but importantly are also positive for vascular markers such as CD31, CD34, FLI-1, and factor VIII-associated antigen. If a lesion is biopsied that shows the morphology of ductular reaction, this would most likely represent ductular reaction adjacent to a tumor; however, a cholangiocellular carcinoma should also be considered. Immunopositivity for p53 would favor cholangiocellular carcinoma, though a negative result would not rule out this tumor and re-biopsy may be indicated.

If a hepatocytic lesion is identified at biopsy in a noncirrhotic liver, the primary differential diagnosis would be FNH, HCA, HCC, and fibrolamellar carcinoma. FNH has characteristic imaging features with a central scar and demonstrates eccentrically thickened vessels on biopsy. Immunohistochemical stain for glutamine synthetase shows a maplike staining pattern in these benign lesions. HCAs are a benign neoplastic proliferation of hepatocytes, some of which have the potential for malignant transformation. Many of the same features described above (pseudoglandular architecture, thickened trabeculae, stromal invasion, and loss of reticulin staining) are useful in distinguishing a well-differentiated HCC from a HCA. Positivity for glypican-3 and HSP-70 is highly suggestive of HCC in this setting, though approximately one third of HCCs will not show this staining pattern. Glutamine synthetase will either be diffusely positive or negative in HCAs, distinguishing these lesions from FNH which demonstrate the" maplike" pattern. An immunohistochemical panel consisting of beta-catenin, glutamine synthetase, liver fatty acid-binding protein, serum amyloid A, and C-reactive protein is recommended to appropriately classify the tumor into H-HCA, I-HCA, b-HCA, b-IHCA, and U-HCA (see above). Importantly, demonstration of a beta-catenin mutation by diffuse staining with glutamine synthetase or nuclear staining with beta-catenin indicates a lesion with increased malignant potential.

Identification of a spindle cell neoplasm on a biopsy of a liver mass in an adult may indicate a primary tumor or, much more likely, a metastatic lesion. If a primary site is known or suspected, the tumor can be compared to prior specimen if available, or a few directed immunostains can be used to confirm this as the site of origin. If a primary site is not known, angiomyolipoma, solitary fibrous tumor, gastrointestinal stromal tumor, and melanoma should be considered as well as tumors of muscle, vascular, or glial origin. Immunohistochemical stains can guide the search for a primary tumor. A panel including vimentin, smooth muscle actin, desmin, CD31, CD34, factor VIII-related antigen, CD117, DOG-1, HMB-45, melan-A, S100, and BCL-2 should be considered to use for differential diagnosis should also be considered to rule out a sarcomatoid carcinoma. If a poorly differentiated neoplasm is encountered, an initial round of immunohistochemical stains should be aimed at determining epithelial (AE1/AE3, CAM5.2), mesenchymal (vimentin), or lymphoid (CD45, CD3, CD20) origin. Immunostainings for various cytokeratins should be attempted to definitively rule out a carcinoma. Once the lineage has been established, additional site-specific immunostains can be used to further classify the tumor, as described above.

In infants and young children without known liver disease, the most likely hepatocytic tumor is hepatoblastoma. In older children, especially those with underlying liver disease such as perinatally acquired hepatitis B infection, differentiating hepatoblastoma from HCC may become an issue. Most subtypes of hepatoblastoma can be easily recognized and distinguished from HCC by their morphologic pattern, though the fetal subtype can cause difficulty, especially when it contains macrotrabecular component or in recurrent hepatoblastoma. The key feature distinguishing the fetal subtype of hepatoblastoma from HCC is the identification of the alternating "light and dark" pattern on low magnification representing differential glycogen and lipid content in the tumor cells and high serum level of alpha-fetoprotein in hepatoblastoma. Embryonal sarcoma and mesenchymal hamartoma would also be in the differential diagnosis of a tumor in this age group.

References

1. Nakashima O, Sugihara S, Kage M, Kojiro M. Pathomorphologic characteristics of small hepatocellular carcinoma: a special reference to small hepatocellular carcinoma with indistinct margins. Hepatology. 1995;22:101–5.
2. Forner A, Reig ME, de Lope CR, Bruix J. Current strategy for staging and treatment: the BCLC update and future prospects. Semin Liver Dis. 2010;30:61–74.
3. Bruix J, Sherman M, American Association for the Study of Liver Diseases. Management of hepatocellular carcinoma: an update. Hepatology. 2011;53:1020–2.
4. Deugnier YM, Charalambous P, Le Quilleuc D, Turlin B, Searle J, Brissot P, Powell LW, Halliday JW. Preneoplastic significance of hepatic iron-free foci in genetic hemochromatosis: a study of 185 patients. Hepatology. 1993;18:1363–9.
5. Sempoux C, Chang C, Gouw A, Chiche L, Zucman-Rossi J, Balabaud C, Bioulac-Sage P. Benign hepatocellular nodules: what have we learned using the patho-molecular classification. Clin Res Hepatol Gastroenterol. 2013;37:322–7.
6. Bioulac-Sage P, Laumonier H, Rullier A, Cubel G, Laurent C, Zucman-Rossi J, Balabaud C. Over-expression of glutamine synthetase in focal nodular hyperplasia: a novel easy diagnostic tool in surgical pathology. Liver Int. 2009;29:459–65.
7. Sempoux C, Jibara G, Ward SC, Fan C, Qin L, Roayaie S, Fiel MI, Schwartz M, Thung SN. Intrahepatic cholangiocarcinoma: new insights in pathology. Semin Liver Dis. 2011;31(1):49–60.
8. Park YN, Yang CP, Fernandez GJ, Cubukcu O, Thung SN, Theise ND. Neoangiogenesis and sinusoidal "capillarization" in dysplastic nodules of the liver. Am J Surg Pathol. 1998;22:656–62.
9. Kondo F, Kondo Y, Nagato Y, Tomizawa M, Wada K. Interstitial tumour cell invasion in small hepatocellular carcinoma. Evaluation in microscopic and low magnification views. J Gastroenterol Hepatol. 1994;9:604–12.
10. Nakano M, Saito A, Yamamoto M, Doi M, Takasaki K. Stromal and blood vessel wall invasion in well-differentiated hepatocellular carcinoma. Liver. 1997;17:41–6.
11. International Consensus Group for Hepatocellular Neoplasia. Pathologic diagnosis of early hepatocellular carcinoma: a report of the international consensus group for hepatocellular neoplasia. Hepatology. 2009;49:658–64.
12. Roncalli M. Hepatocellular nodules in cirrhosis: focus on diagnostic criteria on liver biopsy. A Western experience. Liver Transpl. 2004;10(2 Suppl 1):S9–15.
13. Ruck P, Xiao JC, Kaiserling E. Immunoreactivity of sinusoids in hepatocellular carcinoma. An immunohistochemical study using lectin UEA-1 and antibodies against endothelial markers, including CD34. Arch Pathol Lab Med. 1995 Feb;119(2):173–8.
14. Di Tommaso L, Destro A, Seok JY, Balladore E, Terracciano L, Sangiovanni A, Iavarone M, Colombo M, Jang JJ, Yu E, Jin SY, Morenghi E, Park YN, Roncalli M. The application of markers (HSP70 GPC3 and GS) in liver biopsies is useful for detection of hepatocellular carcinoma. J Hepatol. 2009;50:746–54.
15. Lagana SM, Salomao M, Bao F, Moreira RK, Lefkowitch JH, Remotti HE. Utility of an immunohistochemical panel consisting of glypican-3, heat-shock protein-70, and glutamine synthetase in the distinction of low-grade hepatocellular carcinoma from hepatocel-

lular adenoma. Appl Immunohistochem Mol Morphol. 2013;21(2):170–6.
16. Honeyman JN, Simon EP, Robine N, Chiaroni-Clarke R, Darcy DG, Lim II, Gleason CE, Murphy JM, Rosenberg BR, Teegan L, Takacs CN, Botero S, Belote R, Germer S, Emde AK, Vacic V, Bhanot U, LaQuaglia MP, Simon SM. Detection of a recurrent DNAJB1-PRKACA chimeric transcript in fibrolamellar hepatocellular carcinoma. Science. 2014;343(6174):1010–4.
17. Craig JR, Peters RL, Edmondson HA, Omata M. Fibrolamellar carcinoma of the liver: a tumor of adolescents and young adults with distinctive clinico-pathologic features. Cancer. 1980;46:372–9.
18. Van Eyken P, Sciot R, Brock P, Casteels-Van Daele M, Ramaekers FC, Desmet VJ. Abundant expression of cytokeratin 7 in fibrolamellar carcinoma of the liver. Histopathology. 1990;17:101–7.
19. Ward SC, Huang J, Tickoo SK, Thung SN, Ladanyi M, Klimstra DS. Fibrolamellar carcinoma of the liver exhibits immunohistochemical evidence of both hepatocyte and bile duct differentiation. Mod Pathol. 2010;23:1180–90.
20. Ross HM, Daniel HD, Vivekanandan P, Kannangai R, Yeh MM, Wu TT, Makhlouf HR, Torbenson M. Fibrolamellar carcinomas are positive for CD68. Mod Pathol. 2011;24:390–5.
21. Ishak G, Goodman ZD, Stocker JT. Hepatoblastoma and hepatocellular carcinoma. In: Tumors of the liver and intrahepatic bile ducts. Washington, DC: Armed Forces Institute of Pathology; 2001. p. 159–183 and 199–230.
22. Ward SC, Thung SN, Lim KH, Tran TT, Hong TK, Hoang PL, Jang JJ, Park YN, Abe K. Hepatic progenitor cells in liver cancers from Asian children. Liver Int. 2010;30:102–11.
23. Matsuura S, Aishima S, Taguchi K, Asayama Y, Terashi T, Honda H, Tsuneyoshi M. 'Scirrhous' type hepatocellular carcinomas: a special reference to expression of cytokeratin 7 and hepatocyte paraffin 1. Histopathology. 2005;47(4):382–90.
24. Tsui WM, Loo KT, Chow LT, Tse CC. Biliary adenofibroma. A heretofore unrecognized benign biliary tumor of the liver. Am J Surg Pathol. 1993;17:186–92.
25. Fenoglio LM, Severini S, Ferrigno D, Gollè G, Serraino C, Bracco C, Castagna E, Brignone C, Pomero F, Migliore E, David E, Salizzoni M. Primary hepatic carcinoid: a case report and literature review. World J Gastroenterol. 2009;15:2418–22.
26. Zhu H, Sun K, Ward SC, Schwartz M, Thung SN, Qin L. Primary hepatic signet ring cell neuroendocrine tumor: a case report with literature review. Semin Liver Dis. 2010;30:422–8.
27. Tanas MR, Sboner A, Oliveira AM, Erickson-Johnson MR, Hespelt J, Hanwright PJ, Flanagan J, Luo Y, Fenwick K, Natrajan R, Mitsopoulos C, Zvelebil M, Hoch BL, Weiss SW, Debiec-Rychter M, Sciot R, West RB, Lazar AJ, Ashworth A, Reis-Filho JS, Lord CJ, Gerstein MB, Rubin MA, Rubin BP. Identification of a disease-defining gene fusion in epithelioid hemangioendothelioma. Sci Transl Med. 2011;3:98ra82.
28. Errani C, Zhang L, Sung YS, Hajdu M, Singer S, Maki RG, Healey JH, Antonescu CR. A novel WWTR1-CAMTA1 gene fusion is a consistent abnormality in epithelioid hemangioendothelioma of different anatomic sites. Genes Chromosom Cancer. 2011;50:644–53.
29. Antonescu CR, Le Loarer F, Mosquera JM, Sboner A, Zhang L, Chen CL, Chen HW, Pathan N, Krausz T, Dickson BC, Weinreb I, Rubin MA, Hameed M, Fletcher CD. Novel YAP1-TFE3 fusion defines a distinct subset of epithelioid hemangioendothelioma. Genes Chromosom Cancer. 2013;52:775–84.
30. Kikuma K, Watanabe J, Oshiro Y, Shimogama T, Honda Y, Okamura S, Higaki K, Uike N, Soda T, Momosaki S, Yokota T, Toyoshima S, Takeshita M. Etiological factors in primary hepatic B-cell lymphoma. Virchows Arch. 2012;460:379–87.

Appendix

Abbreviations

AE	Alveolar echinococcosis
AML	Angiomyolipoma
APC	Adenomatous polyposis coli
ARMS	Acinar rhabdomyosarcoma
AS	Angiosarcoma
BAF	Biliary adenofibroma
BCA	Biliary cystadenoma
BCLC	Barcelona Clinic Liver Cancer
BDA	Bile duct adenoma
BDH	Bile duct hamartoma
BH	Biliary hamartoma
BilIN	Biliary intraepithelial neoplasia
BMH	Biliary microhamartoma
CCA	Cholangiocarcinoma
CCC	Congenital choledochal cyst
CE	Cystic echinococcosis
CEA	Carcinoembryonic antigen
CgA	Chromogranin A
CHB	Chronic hepatitis B
CHC	Combined hepatocellular-cholangiocarcinoma
CHF	Congenital hepatic fibrosis
CHFC	Ciliated hepatic foregut cyst
CLC	Cholangiocellular carcinoma
CLH	Compensatory lobar or segmental hyperplasia
CL-HCC	Cirrhosis-like HCC
CLM	Cutaneous larva migrans
CNSET	Calcifying nested stromal-epithelial tumors
DC	Dendritic cells
DF	Dysplastic foci
DLBCL	Diffuse large B-cell lymphoma
DN	Dysplastic nodules
DNSCT	Desmoplastic nested spindle cell tumor
DPHCC	Dual-phenotype HCC
DSRCT	Desmoplastic small round cell tumor
ECC	Extrahepatic cholangiocarcinoma
EHE	Epithelioid hemangioendothelioma
EMP	Extramedullary plasmacytoma
ERCP	Endoscopic retrograde cholangiopancreatography
ERMS	Embryonal rhabdomyosarcoma
ES/PNET	Ewing sarcoma/primitive neuroectodermal tumor
FDCT	Follicular dendritic cell tumor
FFC	Focal fatty change
FL-HCC	Fibrolamellar hepatocellular carcinoma
FNH	Focal nodular hyperplasia
FS	Fibrosarcoma
GCT	Granular cell tumor
GFAP	Glial fibrillary acidic protein
GIST	Gastrointestinal stromal tumor
GPC-3	Glypican-3
AML	Angiomyolipoma
HB	Hepatoblastoma
HBV	*Hepatitis B virus*
HCC	Hepatocellular carcinoma
HCL	Hairy cell lymphoma
HCV	*Hepatitis C virus*
HFD	Hepatobiliary fibrocystic disease
HGDN	High-grade dysplastic nodule
HHT	Hereditary hemorrhagic telangiectasia
HHV-8	*Human herpesvirus* type 8
HPCs	Hepatic progenitor cells
HSTCL	Hepatosplenic T-cell lymphoma
ICC	Intrahepatic cholangiocarcinoma
IDC	Interdigitating dendritic cell
IH	Infantile hemangioma
IHC	Immunohistochemistry
I-HCA	Inflammatory hepatocellular adenoma
IHE	Infantile hemangioendothelioma
IMT	Inflammatory myofibroblastic tumor
IPNB	Intraductal papillary neoplasms of the bile ducts
IPMN	Intraductal papillary mucinous biliary neoplasm
IPN	Intraductal papillary neoplasms
IPT	Inflammatory pseudotumor
KS	Kaposi's sarcoma
LCD	Liver cell dysplasia
LELC	Lymphoepithelioma-like carcinoma
LEL-CCC	Lymphoepithelioma-like cholangiocarcinoma
LEL-HCC	Lymphoepithelioma-like hepatocellular carcinoma

W.-M. Cong (ed.), *Surgical Pathology of Hepatobiliary Tumors*, DOI 10.1007/978-981-10-3536-4

LGDN Low-grade dysplastic nodule
LMS Leiomyosarcoma
LS Liposarcoma
MALT-L Mucosa-associated lymphoid tissue lymphoma
MCBH Multicystic biliary hamartoma
MCN Mucinous cystic neoplasms of the liver
MH Mesenchymal hamartoma
MO Multicentric occurrence
MPBTs Mucin-producing bile duct tumors
MPNST Malignant peripheral nerve sheath tumor
MRCP Magnetic resonance cholangiopancreatography
MRN Macroregenerative nodule
MRT Malignant rhabdoid tumor
MVI Microvascular invasion
NEC Neuroendocrine carcinoma
NEMH Nodular extramedullary hematopoiesis
NEN Neuroendocrine neoplasms
NET Neuroendocrine tumor
NF2 Neurofibromatosis type 2
NRH Nodular regenerative hyperplasia
NSET Nested stromal-epithelial tumor
OCGTs Osteoclast-like giant cell tumors
OPN Osteoponin
OS Osteosarcoma
PAS Periodic acid-Schiff reaction
PBC Primary biliary cirrhosis
PEComa Perivascular epithelioid cell neoplasms
PHL Primary hepatic lymphoma
PLD Polycystic liver disease
PLG Polypoid lesions of the gallbladder
PNT Partial nodular transformation
pPNET Peripheral primitive neuroectodermal tumor
PSC Primary sclerosing cholangitis
PTC Percutaneous transhepatic cholangiography
RHCC Recurrent hepatocellular carcinoma
RMS Rhabdomyosarcoma
SFT Solitary fibrous tumor
SHC Simple hepatic cysts
SHCC Small hepatocellular carcinoma
SNN Solitary necrotic nodules
Syn Synaptophysin
TACE Transcatheter arterial chemoembolization
UES Undifferentiated embryonal sarcoma
VHL Von Hippel-Lindau disease
VIP Vipoma
VLM Visceral larva migrans

Index

W.-M. Cong (ed.), *Surgical Pathology of Hepatobiliary Tumors*, DOI 10.1007/978-981-10-3536-4